# ANESTHESIOLOGY
# MANUAL

## Best Practices and Case Management

### 2025 EDITION

Authors
**Admir Hadzic, MD, PhD**
**Catherine Vandepitte, MD, PhD**

Contributors:

Jirka Cops, PhD | Darren Jacobs, MSc | Jill Vanhaeren, MSc
Stien Beyens, MSc | William Aerts, MD | Angela Lucia Balocco, MD
Emil Bosinci, MD | Robbert Buck, MD | Jasper Gevaert, MD | Jef Grieten, MD
Ivan Keser, MD | Isabelle Lenders, MD | Ana Lopez Gutiérrez, MD, PhD
Edward R. Mariano, PD, PhD | Leander Mancel, MD | Dieter Mesotten, MD, PhD
Laurens Peene, MD | Sarah Shiba, MD | Walter Staelens, MD
Hendrik Stragier, MD | Sam Van Boxstael, MD, PhD | Imré Van Herreweghe, MD
Jan Van Zundert, MD, PhD | Rony Atiyeh, MD | Andy De Baerdemaeker, MD
Max Feinstein, MD | Victor Coll Sijercic, BS | Richard Southgate, MD
Dusica Stamenkovic, MD, PhD

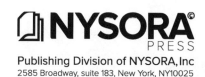

**NYSORA**
PRESS

**Publishing Division of NYSORA, Inc**
2585 Broadway, suite 183, New York, NY10025
info@nysora.com. www.nysora.com

# REVIEWERS

- Sonalika Tudimilla, MD | Department of Anaesthesiology, Dr. D. Y. Patil Medical College, Hospital and Research Centre, Dr. D. Y. Patil Vidyapeeth, Pimpri, Pune, India
- Marie-Camille Vanderheeren, MD | Department of Anesthesiology and Resuscitation, UZ Leuven, Leuven, Belgium
- Prof. André Van Zundert, MD, PhD, MSc., FHEA FRCA FASRA EDRA FANZCA | Department of Anaesthesia & Perioperative Medicine, Royal Brisbane and Women's Hospital, Herston-Brisbane, Australia | Faculty of Medicine, The University of Queensland, Brisbane, Australia
- Drisya V L, DNB | Department of Anesthesiology, KB Bhabha Hospital, Mumbai, India
- Hrvoje Vučemilović, MD | Department of Anaesthesiology, University hospital of Split, Split, Croatia
- Dennis Warfield Jr., MD | Department of Anesthesiology & Perioperative Medicine, Penn State Health Milton S. Hershey Medical Center, Hershey, USA
- Baber Zaheer, MBBS, FCAI, DESA, FRCA, FCPS | Anesthesia and Critical Care Directorate, Dartford and Gravesham NHS Trust, UK

# INTRODUCTION

Welcome to the world of anesthesiology, where science, precision, and compassion converge to ensure the safety and comfort of patients. This book is designed to be your comprehensive guide to the best clinical practices and case management protocols in the field, brought to you by the dedicated team at NYSORA.

Anesthesiology is a dynamic and ever-evolving specialty, requiring practitioners to stay abreast of the latest advancements and techniques. Our goal with this book is to provide you with a reliable, up-to-date resource that will enhance your knowledge, skills, and confidence in delivering exceptional patient care. Whether you are a student, a seasoned practitioner, or anywhere in between, you will find valuable insights and practical guidance tailored to meet the demands of modern anesthesiology.

We have meticulously compiled the expertise of our NYSORA's team, fellows, and NYSORA's Educational Board members from within key opinion leaders across various subfields, including acute and chronic pain medicine, musculoskeletal medicine, and point-of-care ultrasound. Our collective knowledge and wisdom, combined with our team's educational excellence and innovative illustrations, ensures that this book stands as a definitive reference in the field.

We encourage you enjoy reading these pages filled with deep knowledge curiosity and enthusiasm. Let this book be your trusted companion as you navigate the complexities and challenges of practical, clinical anesthesiology. Together, we can continue to advance the field, improve patient outcomes, and foster a community of lifelong learners dedicated to excellence in patient care. Welcome to your journey in anesthesiology; we are thrilled that you have chosen to start your Journey with NYSORA.

# DEDICATION

This book is dedicated to all students and practitioners of anesthesiology whose relentless pursuit of excellence ensures the safety and comfort of patients worldwide. Your dedication, skill, and compassion are the pillars of our profession, and this work is a testament to your unwavering commitment to advancing the field.

# FOREWORD

The field of anesthesiology is both a science and an art, demanding a unique blend of technical skill, comprehensive knowledge, and compassionate patient care. It is with great pride and enthusiasm that we present this book, a culmination of the collective expertise of NYSORA's team of education specialists, illustrators, and an educational board composed of over 150 key opinion leaders across anesthesiology, acute and chronic pain medicine, musculoskeletal (MSK) medicine, and point-of-care ultrasound (POCUS).

This comprehensive volume offers the most up-to-date review of best clinical practices and practical case management protocols ever published in our field. It is NYSORA's continuous contribution and dedication to improving clinical practice and the safety of patients requiring anesthesia and pain medicine. Through meticulously curated content, detailed infographics, and evidence-based guidelines, this book serves as a valuable resource for both seasoned practitioners and those new to the field.

Our aim is to equip readers with the knowledge and tools necessary to excel in their practice, enhance patient outcomes, and navigate the complexities of anesthesiology with confidence. Each chapter is designed to provide practical insights and actionable protocols, ensuring that this book becomes an indispensable reference for daily clinical use.

At NYSORA, we are convinced that this book will become the bible for generations of anesthesiologists and pain medicine specialists dedicated to patient care. The collaboration and expertise poured into this work reflect our commitment to advancing the field and supporting the continuous education of its practitioners.

We hope this book not only enhances your clinical practice but also inspires you to strive for excellence in every aspect of patient care. It is through your dedication and passion that the field of anesthesiology continues to evolve, ensuring the highest standards of safety and efficacy for patients worldwide.

Sincerely,

Authors, on behalf of the NYSORA Team

# ACKNOWLEDGMENTS

The creation of this book has been a monumental endeavor, made possible by the collective efforts of many dedicated individuals. We extend our deepest gratitude to everyone who contributed to this comprehensive resource on anesthesiology best practices and clinical case management protocols.

First and foremost, we would like to thank the exceptional team of education specialists, illustrators, and members of our educational board. Your unwavering commitment to excellence, attention to detail, and innovative approach to education have been instrumental in bringing this book to life. Your expertise has ensured that the content is both accurate and accessible, making it an invaluable resource for practitioners at all levels.

We are profoundly grateful NYSORA collaborators and Educational Board members who are opinion leaders across the fields of anesthesiology, acute and chronic pain medicine, musculoskeletal (MSK) medicine, and point-of-care ultrasound (POCUS) who generously shared their knowledge and insights. Your contributions have enriched this book with a wealth of practical wisdom and cutting-edge practices, reflecting the latest advancements in our field.

A special thanks to the NYSORA team, fellows, nurses, and our colleagues at ZOL, Genk, Belgium for their tireless dedication to this project. Your passion for advancing the field of anesthesiology and improving patient care is evident in every page of this book. Your collaborative spirit and relentless pursuit of excellence have set a new standard for educational resources in our profession.

We would also like to acknowledge the patients and families whose experiences have shaped our understanding and practices. Your trust and collaboration have been invaluable in refining the protocols and approaches presented in this book.

Finally, to all the students, practitioners, and educators who use this book, we thank you for your commitment to continuous learning and improvement. It is your dedication to the highest standards of patient care that inspires us to strive for excellence in everything we do.

With sincere appreciation,

Authors, on behalf of the entire NYSORA Team

# NOTICE / DISCLAIMER

# LIBRARY OF CONGRESS IDENTIFICATION

**Authors**:

- Admir Hadzic, MD, PhD
- Catherine Vandepitte, MD, PhD

**Contributors**:

- Jirka Cops, PhD
- Darren Jacobs, MSc
- Jill Vanhaeren, MSc
- Stien Beyens, MSc
- William Aerts, MD
- Angela Lucia Balocco, MD
- Emil Bosinci, MD
- Robbert Buck, MD
- Jasper Gevaert, MD
- Jef Grieten, MD
- Ivan Keser, MD
- Isabelle Lenders, MD
- Ana Lopez Gutiérrez, MD, PhD
- Edward R. Mariano, PD, PhD
- Leander Mancel, MD
- Dieter Mesotten, MD, PhD
- Laurens Peene, MD
- Sarah Shiba, MD
- Walter Staelens, MD
- Hendrik Stragier, MD
- Sam Van Boxstael, MD, PhD
- Imré Van Herreweghe, MD
- Jan Van Zundert, MD, PhD
- Rony Atiyeh, MD
- Andy De Baerdemaeker, MD
- Max Feinstein, MD
- Victor Coll Sijercic, BS
- Richard Southgate, MD
- Dusica Stamenkovic, MD, PhD

Title: **Anesthesiology Manual**
Subtitle: **Best Practices and Case Management**

**2025 Edition**
Identifiers:
**Library of Congress Control Number: 2024913720**
**ISBN 979-8-9899218-3-6**

# Table of Contents

## AIRWAY ISSUES

Airway abscess & infection ........................................................................................................ 18
Airway trauma ........................................................................................................................... 20
Difficult airway management ..................................................................................................... 22
Expanding neck hematoma .........................................................................................................27
Lung protective ventilation .........................................................................................................29
Microlaryngoscopy and airway laser ......................................................................................... 30
Penetrating neck injuries ........................................................................................................... 32
Pulmonary aspiration ................................................................................................................. 34
Rigid bronchoscopy ....................................................................................................................36
Tracheostomy ............................................................................................................................. 38

## CARDIAC DISEASES

Adult congenital heart disease (ACHD) ...................................................................................... 41
Aortic dissection ........................................................................................................................ 43
Aortic regurgitation (AR) ............................................................................................................ 46
Aortic stenosis ........................................................................................................................... 48
Atrial fibrillation (AF) ................................................................................................................. 50
Atrial septal defect (ASD) .......................................................................................................... 52
Brugada syndrome (BRS) ........................................................................................................... 54
Cardiac contusion .......................................................................................................................56
Cardiac implantable electronic devices (CIEDS) ....................................................................... 58
Cardiac tamponade .................................................................................................................... 62
Cardiomyopathies ...................................................................................................................... 64
Coronary artery disease ............................................................................................................. 68
Infective endocarditis: Prophylaxis ........................................................................................... 70
Intraoperative arrhythmias .........................................................................................................73
Mitral regurgitation .....................................................................................................................77
Mitral stenosis ............................................................................................................................79
Pulmonary hypertension (PH) .................................................................................................... 81
QT prolongation .......................................................................................................................... 83
Right heart failure ...................................................................................................................... 85
Transplanted heart ..................................................................................................................... 90
Tricuspid regurgitation (TR) ....................................................................................................... 91
Wolff-Parkinson-White syndrome ...............................................................................................93

## CRITICAL CARE

Abdominal compartment syndrome (ACS) .................................................................................. 96
Acute Respiratory Distress Syndrome (ARDS) ...........................................................................99
Transfusion of blood products ..................................................................................................102
Burns .........................................................................................................................................104
Crush injuries ............................................................................................................................109
Drowning ................................................................................................................................... 111
Inhalation injury ........................................................................................................................113
Organ donation ..........................................................................................................................115
Pregnant trauma patients .........................................................................................................117
Sepsis ........................................................................................................................................122
Trauma .......................................................................................................................................126

# EMERGENCIES

Advanced life support ..................................................................................129
Airway fire..............................................................................................132
Anaphylaxis............................................................................................134
Bronchospasm.........................................................................................137
Compartment syndrome ............................................................................139
Delayed emergence ..................................................................................143
Dental luxation, fracture, or avulsion...........................................................147
Extravasation injuries ..............................................................................149
Fat embolism syndrome ............................................................................151
Full stomach ..........................................................................................153
High or total spinal anesthesia ...................................................................155
Hypertension...........................................................................................157
Hypoglycemia..........................................................................................161
Hypotension ...........................................................................................163
Hypovolemia ...........................................................................................165
Hypoxemia .............................................................................................169
Increased airway pressure .........................................................................171
Increased intracranial pressure ..................................................................173
Laryngospasm.........................................................................................175
Local anesthetic systemic toxicity (LAST).....................................................178
Malignant hyperthermia ...........................................................................180
Perioperative bleeding ..............................................................................182
Perioperative myocardial infarction/injury (PMI) ...........................................190
Postoperative visual loss (POVL)..................................................................192
Seizures ................................................................................................194
Status epilepticus....................................................................................196
Tension pneumothorax..............................................................................199
Transfusion reactions...............................................................................201
Venous air embolism (VAE) ........................................................................203
Venous thromboembolism (VTE) .................................................................205

# ENDOCRINOLOGY

Acromegaly .............................................................................................208
Adrenocortical insufficiency.......................................................................210
Alcohol withdrawal syndrome.....................................................................214
Anorexia nervosa.....................................................................................218
Carcinoid ...............................................................................................220
Cushing's syndrome..................................................................................223
Diabetes insipidus....................................................................................226
Diabetic ketoacidosis................................................................................229
Diabetes mellitus type 2 ...........................................................................231
Euglycemic diabetic ketoacidosis................................................................236
Hyperaldosteronism..................................................................................238
Hypercapnia............................................................................................240
Hyperglycemia.........................................................................................242
Hyperkalemia..........................................................................................244
Hypernatremia.........................................................................................246
Hyperparathyroidism.................................................................................248
Hyperthyroidism/thyroid storm...................................................................250

Hypokalemia ........................................................................................................................ 252
Hyponatremia ...................................................................................................................... 254
Hypoparathyroidism ............................................................................................................ 256
Hypothyroidism ................................................................................................................... 259
Malnutrition ........................................................................................................................ 262
Metabolic acidosis .............................................................................................................. 266
Metabolic alkalosis ............................................................................................................. 269
Multiple endocrine neoplasia syndromes ............................................................................ 271
Obesity ............................................................................................................................... 275
Panhypopituitarism ............................................................................................................. 280
Parathyroidectomy .............................................................................................................. 284
Pheochromocytoma ............................................................................................................. 286
Perioperative steroids ......................................................................................................... 288
Porphyria ............................................................................................................................ 290
SIADH ................................................................................................................................. 295
Thyroidectomy .................................................................................................................... 297

## HEMATOLOGY

Acute leukemia ................................................................................................................... 301
Antiphospholipid antibody syndrome .................................................................................. 303
Coagulopathy ...................................................................................................................... 307
Disseminated Intravascular Coagulation (DIC) .................................................................... 309
Factor V Leiden ................................................................................................................... 311
G6PD deficiency .................................................................................................................. 313
Hemophilia .......................................................................................................................... 315
Heparin-induced thrombocytopenia (HIT) ........................................................................... 318
Idiopathic thrombocytopenic purpura (ITP) ........................................................................ 321
Jehovah's witness patients .................................................................................................. 323
Perioperative anemia .......................................................................................................... 326
Polycythemia (erythrocytosis) ............................................................................................ 328
Sickle cell disease .............................................................................................................. 331
Thalassemia ........................................................................................................................ 333
Tumor lysis syndrome .......................................................................................................... 335
Von Willebrand's Disease (VWD) ......................................................................................... 337

## HEPATIC DISEASES

End Stage Liver Disease (ESLD) ........................................................................................... 342
Jaundiced patient ............................................................................................................... 345
Liver resection .................................................................................................................... 348
Patient with a liver transplant ............................................................................................. 351

## MISCELLANEOUS

Awareness during anesthesia ............................................................................................. 354
Bariatric surgery ................................................................................................................. 356
Beach chair position ........................................................................................................... 358
Bleomycin exposure ............................................................................................................ 359
Cannabis use ...................................................................................................................... 361
Corneal abrasion ................................................................................................................ 364
Extravasation of NMBDs ...................................................................................................... 366
Fluid and electrolyte balance ............................................................................................. 367

Gastroesophageal reflux disease .................................................................................................... 370
Geriatric patients ........................................................................................................................... 372
Inflammatory bowel disease ........................................................................................................... 374
Laparoscopic surgery ..................................................................................................................... 377
Methemoglobinemia ....................................................................................................................... 379
Non-operating room anesthesia (NORA) ......................................................................................... 381
Perioperative hypothermia ............................................................................................................. 382
Perioperative malnutrition .............................................................................................................. 384
Perioperative stroke ....................................................................................................................... 387
Postoperative delirium (POD) .......................................................................................................... 390
Postoperative nausea and vomiting (PONV) ..................................................................................... 392
Postoperative nerve injuries ........................................................................................................... 394
Postoperative neurocognitive disorder ............................................................................................ 398
Postoperative pain management ..................................................................................................... 400
Prone position ................................................................................................................................ 402
Succinylcholine myalgias ................................................................................................................ 404

## NEUROANESTHESIA

Acute spinal cord injury .................................................................................................................. 406
Aneurysm coiling ............................................................................................................................ 408
Autonomic dysreflexia ..................................................................................................................... 410
Chiari malformation ........................................................................................................................ 412
Craniotomy ..................................................................................................................................... 414
Epilepsy .......................................................................................................................................... 416
Hydrocephalus ................................................................................................................................ 419
Ménière's disease ........................................................................................................................... 421
Pituitary surgery ............................................................................................................................. 424
Posterior fossa surgery ................................................................................................................... 426
Spina bifida .................................................................................................................................... 429
Spine surgery ................................................................................................................................. 432
Subarachnoid hemorrhage .............................................................................................................. 436
Traumatic brain injury ..................................................................................................................... 440

## NEUROMUSCULAR DISEASES

Amyotrophic lateral sclerosis (ALS) ................................................................................................. 443
Guillain-barré syndrome .................................................................................................................. 446
Lambert-Eaton myasthenic syndrome (LEMS) ................................................................................. 448
Multiple sclerosis ............................................................................................................................ 450
Myasthenia gravis ........................................................................................................................... 452
Myotonic dystrophy ......................................................................................................................... 456
Parkinson's disease ......................................................................................................................... 460
Polymyositis and dermatomyositis ................................................................................................... 465

## OBSTETRICS

Amniotic fluid embolism .................................................................................................................. 469
Antepartum bleeding ....................................................................................................................... 471
Breastfeeding patient ...................................................................................................................... 473
Breech presentation ........................................................................................................................ 476
Cesarean delivery ........................................................................................................................... 478
Cervical cerclage ............................................................................................................................ 485

Challenges in obstetric anesthesiology ..........................................................................................................487
Dyspnea during pregnancy ...........................................................................................................................490
External cephalic version ...............................................................................................................................492
Fetal distress...................................................................................................................................................494
Gestational diabetes.......................................................................................................................................496
Hysterectomy ..................................................................................................................................................498
Multiple gestation...........................................................................................................................................501
Non-obstetric surgery.....................................................................................................................................503
Peripartum cardiac arrest ..............................................................................................................................506
Peripartum cardiomyopathy...........................................................................................................................512
Physiological changes during pregnancy ......................................................................................................515
Placenta accreta..............................................................................................................................................517
Placenta praevia..............................................................................................................................................519
Placental abruption .........................................................................................................................................521
Post-dural puncture headache (PDPH).........................................................................................................524
Postpartum hemorrhage .................................................................................................................................526
Preeclampsia...................................................................................................................................................528
Prelabor rupture of membranes (PROM) ......................................................................................................532
Umbilical cord prolapse ..................................................................................................................................534
Uterine inversion .............................................................................................................................................536
Uterine rupture ................................................................................................................................................538

# PEDIATRICS

Bronchopulmonary dysplasia...........................................................................................................................541
Cerebral palsy..................................................................................................................................................545
CHARGE syndrome..........................................................................................................................................549
Cleft lip and palate..........................................................................................................................................552
Congenital diaphragmatic hernia....................................................................................................................557
Craniofacial dysostosis....................................................................................................................................560
Croup/Laryngotracheobronchitis ....................................................................................................................562
DiGeorge syndrome .........................................................................................................................................565
Down syndrome ...............................................................................................................................................568
Duchenne muscular dystrophy........................................................................................................................570
Epiglottitis .......................................................................................................................................................572
Fontan physiology............................................................................................................................................574
Foreign body aspiration ...................................................................................................................................576
Genetic syndromes: General considerations...................................................................................................578
Goldenhar syndrome........................................................................................................................................579
Mitochondrial disease .....................................................................................................................................581
Mucopolysaccharidoses..................................................................................................................................583
Necrotizing enterocolitis .................................................................................................................................586
Omphalocele and gastroschisis......................................................................................................................589
Patent ductus arteriosus..................................................................................................................................592
Pediatric anxiety..............................................................................................................................................594
Pediatric patient..............................................................................................................................................596
Pierre-Robin sequence ....................................................................................................................................600
Premature infant..............................................................................................................................................604
Pyloric stenosis ...............................................................................................................................................607
Scoliosis...........................................................................................................................................................609
Status epilepticus in pediatric patients ..........................................................................................................612

Strabismus surgery........................................................................................................614
Tetralogy of Fallot........................................................................................................616
Tonsillectomy................................................................................................................619
Tracheoesophageal fistula............................................................................................621
Treacher Collins syndrome...........................................................................................623
Upper respiratory tract infection..................................................................................625
VACTERL........................................................................................................................627

## PSYCHIATRIC DISORDERS

Electroconvulsive therapy (ECT)...................................................................................631
Monoamine oxidase inhibitors (MAOI).........................................................................633
Neuroleptic malignant syndrome.................................................................................635
Serotonin syndrome.....................................................................................................637

## RARE CO-EXISTING DISEASES

Amyloidosis...................................................................................................................640
Glycogen storage disorders.........................................................................................643
Hereditary angiedema (C1 Esterase Deficiency)..........................................................646
Hereditary hemorrhagic telangiectasias......................................................................648
HIV and AIDS.................................................................................................................650
Huntington's disease....................................................................................................653
Neurofibromatosis........................................................................................................655
Periodic paralysis.........................................................................................................657
Sarcoidosis...................................................................................................................659

## RENAL DISEASES

Acute kidney injury (AKI)..............................................................................................662
Chronic kidney disease (CKD).......................................................................................664
Hemolytic uremic syndrome........................................................................................666
Nephrectomy................................................................................................................668
Nephrotic syndrome.....................................................................................................670
Renal transplant...........................................................................................................673
TURP and TURP syndrome............................................................................................678

## RESPIRATORY & THORACICS

Anterior mediastinal mass............................................................................................682
Asthma..........................................................................................................................684
Bronchiectasis...............................................................................................................686
Bronchopleural fistula...................................................................................................687
Bullous lung disease.....................................................................................................689
Chronic obstructive pulmonary disease.......................................................................691
Cystic fibrosis................................................................................................................694
Esophagectomy............................................................................................................697
Lung cancer..................................................................................................................699
Massive hemoptysis......................................................................................................701
Mediastinoscopy..........................................................................................................704
Obstructive sleep apnea...............................................................................................706
Pneumonectomy..........................................................................................................710
Pneumonia....................................................................................................................712
Post-lung transplant patient........................................................................................715

Pulmonary embolism................................................................................................................................717
Restrictive lung disease .........................................................................................................................720
Smoking ....................................................................................................................................................722
Thymectomy..............................................................................................................................................723
Transfusion-related acute lung injury (TRALI)....................................................................................724

## SKIN & MUSCULOSKELETAL DISORDERS

Achondroplasia.........................................................................................................................................727
Ankylosing spondylitis............................................................................................................................729
Ehlers-Danlos syndrome .........................................................................................................................732
Marfan syndrome .....................................................................................................................................735
Osteogenesis imperfecta........................................................................................................................737
Psoriasis....................................................................................................................................................740
Rhabdomyolysis........................................................................................................................................743
Rheumatoid arthritis................................................................................................................................746
Scleroderma..............................................................................................................................................749
Sjogren's syndrome .................................................................................................................................751
Stevens-Johnson syndrome ...................................................................................................................753
Systemic lupus erythematosus..............................................................................................................755
Granulomatosis with polyangiitis ..........................................................................................................758

## ANESTHETIC TECHNIQUES

Blind nasal intubation .............................................................................................................................761
Closed circle anesthesia .........................................................................................................................763
Fiberoptic intubation................................................................................................................................765
One-lung anesthesia ...............................................................................................................................768
Preoperative fasting ................................................................................................................................770
Prolonged anesthesia..............................................................................................................................772
Total intravenous anesthesia (TIVA) ......................................................................................................774
Videolaryngoscopy...................................................................................................................................777

## TOXICITIES

Beta-blocker overdose.............................................................................................................................781
Calcium channel blocker toxicity...........................................................................................................783
Carbon monoxide poisoning....................................................................................................................785
Cocaine intoxication.................................................................................................................................787
Cyanide poisoning....................................................................................................................................789
Digoxin toxicity .........................................................................................................................................791
Heroin or opioid toxicity...........................................................................................................................793
Lithium toxicity..........................................................................................................................................795
MAOI toxicity .............................................................................................................................................797
MDMA (exctasy) toxicity ..........................................................................................................................799
Methamphetamine toxicity......................................................................................................................802
Methanol and ethylene glycol poisoning...............................................................................................804
Opioid tolerance or methadone-using patients....................................................................................807
Organophosphates toxicity .....................................................................................................................811
Paracetamol overdose.............................................................................................................................813
Salicylate toxicity .....................................................................................................................................816
TCA toxicity................................................................................................................................................818

# VASCULAR DISORDERS

Abdominal Aortic Aneurysm (AAA) Repair ..................................................................................................................................822
Carotid Endarterectomy ....................................................................................................................................................................827

# INTRODUCTION

Welcome to the "Anesthesiology Manual: Best Practices and Case management." This manual has been meticulously designed to serve as a comprehensive guide for both students and practitioners in the field of anesthesiology. To get the most out of this manual, here are some tips on how to effectively use it:

### Organization and Structure

This manual is organized into sections that cover the entire spectrum of the practice of anesthesiology, pain and perioperative medicine. Each section is divided into specific topics that provide detailed information on best practices, and clinical protocols.

### Navigating the Content

- **Table of Contents:** Start by reviewing the Table of Contents to familiarize yourself with the structure and flow of the manual. This will help you quickly locate the sections and topics relevant to your needs.

### Practical Application

- **Step-by-Step Protocols:** Follow the step-by-step protocols for various procedures to ensure adherence to the latest standards and best practices. These protocols are intended to guide you through each process with precision and clarity.

### Keeping Up-to-Date

- **Regular Updates:** Medical practices and standards are continuously evolving. Stay updated by cross the information in this manual with the latest guidelines and research. This will ensure that you are always practicing the most current and effective techniques.

### Safety and Compliance

- **Adherence to Protocols:** Always adhere to the protocols and guidelines established by your institution. While this manual provides a comprehensive overview, institutional protocols take precedence and are tailored to specific environments and patient populations.
- **Equipment Checks:** Regularly verify that the information regarding equipment and medications is up-to-date. This includes checking for any updates in product information and ensuring all equipment is functioning correctly before use.

### Collaborative Learning

- **Discussion and Consultation:** Use this manual as a basis for discussion and consultation with colleagues. Collaborative learning and peer review are essential components of professional development and ensuring high standards of patient care. Free-register to NYSORALMS.COM, engage in professional information exchange case discussions and provide or ask for feedback on specific topics of interest.

By following these steps, you can maximize the benefits of this manual and enhance your practice or teaching in anesthesiology. We hope this resource serves as a valuable tool in your ongoing education and professional growth.

# AIRWAY ISSUES

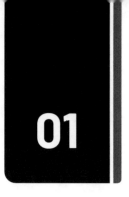

# AIRWAY ABSCESS & INFECTION

## LEARNING OBJECTIVES

- The consequences of airway infection and retropharyngeal abscess during intubation
- Management of airway infection and retropharyngeal abscess

---

## DEFINITION AND MECHANISM

- Upper respiratory or ear infections can lead to retropharyngeal abscess formation (collection of pus in the retropharyngeal space)
- Tracheal intubation will be difficult due to distorted airway anatomy, edema, decreased mouth opening, and immobile tissue
- Vocal cords can be difficult to visualize
- A retropharyngeal abscess can rupture and aspiration of the content can occur during intubation
- Induction of general anesthesia may precipitate complete airway closure
- It affects mostly children between 2 and 4, but adults too can develop abscesses. Usually, the infection involves multiple types of bacteria

## SIGNS AND SYMPTOMS

| Upper airway infection | Retropharyngeal abscess |
|---|---|
| Cough | Severe sore throat |
| Runny nose | Swollen lymph nodes |
| Sneezing | Difficulty breathing |
| Throat pain | Difficulty speaking |
| Fever | Noisy breathing |
| Trouble swallowing or difficulty swallowing | Severe headache |
| | Stiff neck |
| | Coughing |
| | Fever |

## COMPLICATIONS OF A RETROPHARYNGEAL ABSCESS

- Blocked airway/compresion of the airway
- Aspiration pneumonia
- Swelling and inflammation in the thorax
- Sepsis
- Epidural abscess and discitis osteomyelitis
- Carotid artery erosion (haemorrhage, thrombosis) and jugular vein thrombosis
- Mediastinitis

## RISK FACTORS & COMORBIDITIES

- Adults: HIV, IV drug use, diabetes, head & neck malignancies, alcohol
- Immunosuppression
- Pediatric: upper respiratory tract infections

## MANAGEMENT

- Investigate the airway using an X-ray or CT-scan, MRI and point of care ultrasound (high resolution linear transducer)
- Perform preoxygenation
- Intubate using awake fiberoptic intubation
- Consider a tracheostomy if endotracheal intubation is not possible
  - Challenge: distorted anatomy affects the location of landmarks
- Treat retropharyngeal abscess with broadspectrum IV antibiotics
- Consider draining the abscess

## KEEP IN MIND

- Full stomach & need for rapid sequence induction (RSI) vs difficult airway
- Full stomach & need for RSI plus need for deep level of anesthesia vs. risk of hemodynamic instability (sepsis)
- Awake fiberoptic intubation does not visualize ETT passing abscess & therefore potential for abscess rupture
- Consider the use of a videolaryngoscope
- Be prepared to use a tracheostomy as back-up strategy in case of respiratory distress.

### SUGGESTED READING

- Apfelbaum JL, Hagberg CA, Connis RT, et al. 2022 American Society of Anesthesiologists Practice Guidelines for Management of the Difficult Airway. Anesthesiology. 2022;136(1):31-81.
- Cho SY, Woo JH, Kim YJ, et al. Airway management in patients with deep neck infections: A retrospective analysis [published correction appears in Medicine (Baltimore). 2016 Oct 21;95(42):e36c2]. Medicine (Baltimore). 2016;95(27):e4125.
- Davies I, Jenkins I. Paediatric airway infections. BJA Educ. 2017;17(10):341-345.
- Straker, Tracey, Shobana Rajan, and Mazen A. Maktabi (eds), ' Anesthetic Management of the Patient with Retropharyngeal Abscess with Emphasis on Perioperative and Airway Management', in Tracey Straker, Shobana Rajan, and Magdalena Anitescu (eds), Anesthesiology: A Problem-Based Learning Approach, Anesthesiology A Problem Based Learning (New York, 2018; online edn, Oxford Academic, 1 Nov. 2018)

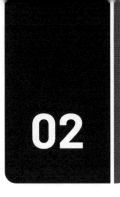

# AIRWAY TRAUMA

## LEARNING OBJECTIVES

- Recognize airway trauma
- Management of airway trauma

## DEFINITION AND MECHANISM

- A life-threatening condition resulting from blunt and penetrating injuries to the head, neck and chest, as well as from medical procedures that may injure the airway
- Maxillofacial, neck, laryngeal or tracheobronchial injuries
- Airway obstruction or obstruction by blood, secretions, tissue edema, debris, and vomitus
- Airway trauma can be associated with cervical spine injury which will worsen during intubation

## SIGNS AND SYMPTOMS

- Neck pain
- Hoarseness
- Dysphagia
- Cough
- Dysphonia
- Laryngeal dyspnea
- Loss of consciousness

- Stridor
- Cyanosis
- Hypoxemia
- Hamman's sign or a mediastinal crunch (a crunching, rasping sound, heard over the precordium in mediastinal emphysema)
- Subcutaneous emphysema

| Anatomical territory | Associated problems | Caution: red flag signs and symptoms |
|---|---|---|
| Maxillofacial | Traumatic brain injury and base of skull fracture<br>Cervical spine fracture<br>Ophthalmic injury<br>Vascular injury<br>Pulmonary aspiration of blood and debris | Signs of increased intracranial pressure<br>Neurological deficit<br>Neurogenic shock<br>Significant bleeding from fracture displacement<br>Bilateral anterior mandible fractures and airway obstruction<br>Ventilatory failure |
| Laryngotracheal | Cervical fracture<br>Vascular injury<br>Oesophageal injury<br>Rib fractures and flail segment<br>Pneumothorax<br>Hemothorax<br>Pneumomediastinum<br>Pulmonary contusion | Massive hemoptysis and stridor have previously been reported as cardinal features of severe laryngotracheal trauma<br>Massive surgical emphysema<br>Ventilatory failure<br>Cardiovascular collapse |
| Trachea and bronchi | Vascular injury<br>Oesophageal injury<br>Rib fractures and flail segment<br>Tension pneumothorax<br>Hemothorax<br>Pneumomediastinum<br>Pulmonary contusion | Massive hemoptysis<br>Massive surgical emphysema<br>Ventilatory failure<br>Cardiovascular collapse |

# MANAGEMENT

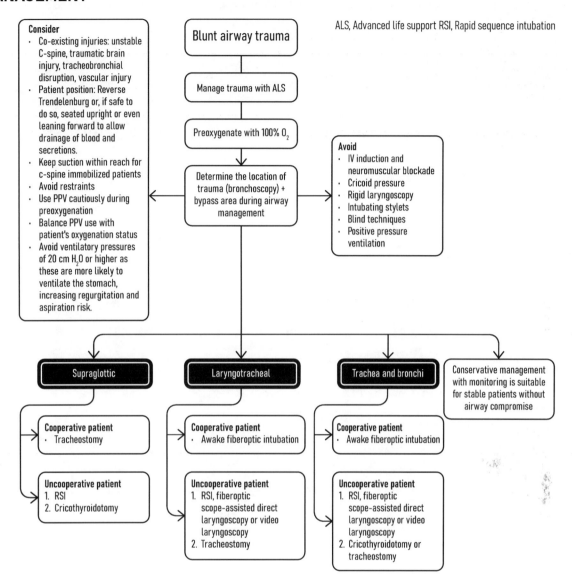

**Consider**
- Co-existing injuries: unstable C-spine, traumatic brain injury, tracheobronchial disruption, vascular injury
- Patient position: Reverse Trendelenburg or, if safe to do so, seated upright or even leaning forward to allow drainage of blood and secretions.
- Keep suction within reach for c-spine immobilized patients
- Avoid restraints
- Use PPV cautiously during preoxygenation
- Balance PPV use with patient's oxygenation status
- Avoid ventilatory pressures of 20 cm $H_2O$ or higher as these are more likely to ventilate the stomach, increasing regurgitation and aspiration risk.

**Blunt airway trauma**

ALS, Advanced life support RSI, Rapid sequence intubation

Manage trauma with ALS

Preoxygenate with 100% $O_2$

Determine the location of trauma (bronchoscopy) + bypass area during airway management

**Avoid**
- IV induction and neuromuscular blockade
- Cricoid pressure
- Rigid laryngoscopy
- Intubating stylets
- Blind techniques
- Positive pressure ventilation

**Supraglottic**

**Cooperative patient**
- Tracheostomy

**Uncooperative patient**
1. RSI
2. Cricothyroidotomy

**Laryngotracheal**

**Cooperative patient**
- Awake fiberoptic intubation

**Uncooperative patient**
1. RSI, fiberoptic scope-assisted direct laryngoscopy or video laryngoscopy
2. Tracheostomy

**Trachea and bronchi**

**Cooperative patient**
- Awake fiberoptic intubation

**Uncooperative patient**
1. RSI, fiberoptic scope-assisted direct laryngoscopy or video laryngoscopy
2. Cricothyroidotomy or tracheostomy

Conservative management with monitoring is suitable for stable patients without airway compromise

# KEEP IN MIND

- Full stomach vs difficult airway vs need for double-lumen tube
- Airway management may be difficult in the uncooperative or pediatric patient
- Keep the neck in a neutral position due to the potentially unstable cevical spine by C-collar or manual in-line stabilization (MILS)
- Airway management is potentialy complicated if facial fractures or airway burns are present
- Team work and additional experts might be helpful (oral and maxillofacial surgery and ENT)

## SUGGESTED READING

- Athanassoglou V, Rogers A, Hofmeyr R. In-hospital management of the airway in trauma. BJA Education 2024; 24(7): 238e244.
- Jain U, McCunn M, Smith CE, Pittet JF. Management of the Traumatized Airway. Anesthesiology. 2016;124(1):199-206.
- Mercer SJ, Jones CP, Bridge M, Clitheroe E, Morton B, Groom P. Systematic review of the anaesthetic management of non-iatrogenic acute adult airway trauma. Br J Anaesth. 2016;117 Suppl 1:i49-i59.
- Prokakis C, Koletsis EN, Dedeilias P, Fligou F, Filos K, Dougenis D. Airway trauma: a review on epidemiology, mechanisms of injury, diagnosis and treatment. J Cardiothorac Surg. 2014;9:117.
- Shilston J, Evans DL, Simons A, Evans DA. Initial management of blunt and penetrating neck trauma. BJA Educ. 2021;21(9):329-335.

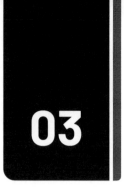

# 03

# DIFFICULT AIRWAY MANAGEMENT

## LEARNING OBJECTIVES

- Getting familiar with an evidence-based, structured approach to managing a difficult airway

## SIGNS AND SYMPTOMS

- Failure to ventilate or intubate a patient
- Airway edema and trauma from repeated intubation attempts
- Desaturation and subsequent hypoxia
- Absent or minimal end-tidal $CO_2$
- Insufficient tidal volumes
- Cyanosis
- Cardiac arrest

## RISK FACTORS

| Difficult intubation | Difficult laryngeal mask airway | Difficult front-neck access |
|---|---|---|
| History of difficult intubation<br>Distorted airway anatomy<br>Airway bleeding or hematoma<br>Tumor<br>Foreign body<br>Snoring<br>Obstructive sleep apnea<br>Diabetes mellitus<br>Increasing Mallampati and modified Mallampati scores<br>Thyromental distance < 6 cm<br>Sternomental distance < 12.5 cm<br>Interincisor distance < 4 cm<br>Large neck circumference<br>Reduced neck mobility<br>Acquired or congenital disease:<br>- Ankylosing spondylitis<br>- Degenerative osteoarthritis<br>- Treacher-collins<br>- Klippel-Feil syndrome<br>- Down syndrome | Anatomical variations<br>Obesity<br>Beard<br>Poor dentition<br>History of radiation to the neck<br>Airway abnormalities | Obesity<br>Anatomical abnormalities<br>Presence of goiter or thyroid enlargement<br>Limited neck extension<br>Prior surgery or radiation<br>Infection or inflammation |

# DIFFICULT INTUBATION GUIDELINES

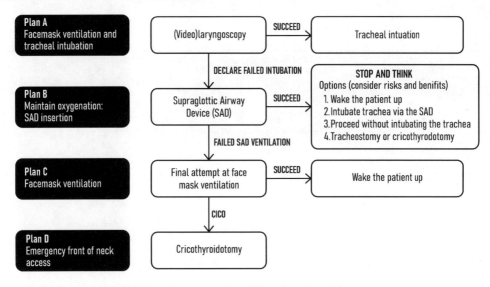

SAD, Supraglottic airway device; CICO, can't intubate, can't oxygenate

# MANAGEMENT OF UNANTICIPATED DIFFICULT TRACHEAL INTUBATION IN ADULTS

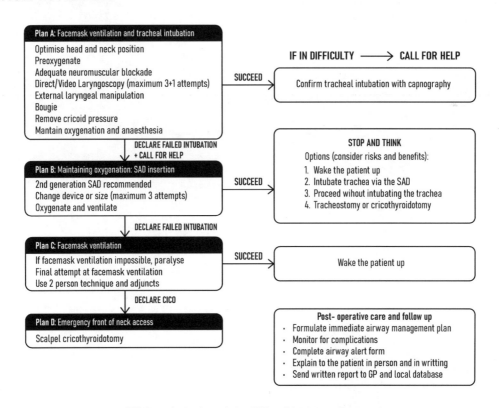

SAD, Supraglottic airway device; CICO, can't intubate, can't oxygenate

## FAILED INTUBATION, FAILED OXYGENATION IN THE PARALYZED, ANESTHETIZED PATIENT

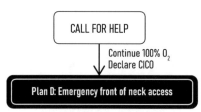

CALL FOR HELP

Continue 100% $O_2$
Declare CICO

**Plan D: Emergency front of neck access**

Continue to give oxygen via upper airway
Ensure neuromuscular blockade
Position patient to extend neck

---

**Scalpel cricothyroidotomy**

Equipment: 1. Scalpel (number 10 blade)
2. Bougie
3. Tube (cuffed 6.0 mm ID)

**Laryngeal handshake to identify cricothyroid membrane**

**Palpable cricothyroid membrane**

Transverse stab incision through cricothyroid membrane
Turn blade through 90° (sharp edge caudally)
Slide coude tip of bougie along blade into trachea
Railroad lubricated 6.0 mm cuffed tracheal tube into trachea
Ventilate, inflate cuff and confirm position with capnography
Secure tube

**Impalpable cricothyroid membrane**

Make an 8-10 cm vertical skin incision, caudad to cephalad
Use blunt dissection with fingers of both hands to separate tissues
Identify and stabilize the larynx
Proceed with technique for palpable cricothyroid membrane as above

---

**Post-operative care and follow up**

- Postpone surgery unless immediately life treatening
- Urgent surgical review of cricothyroidotomy site
- Document and follow up as in main flow chart

# MANAGEMENT

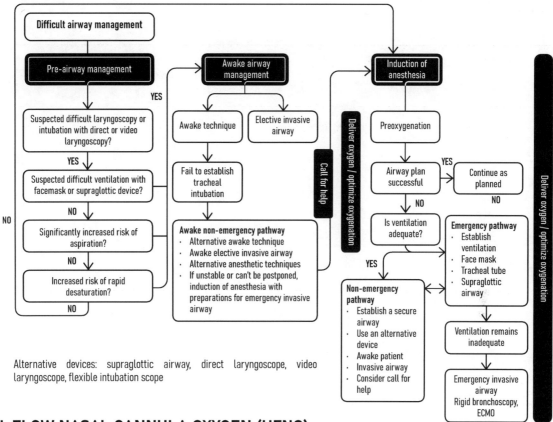

Alternative devices: supraglottic airway, direct laryngoscope, video laryngoscope, flexible intubation scope

## HIGH-FLOW NASAL CANNULA OXYGEN (HFNO) THERAPY

- High-flow nasal oxygen improves preoxygenation before intubation and maximizes apnoea time before desaturation
- Maintains adequate oxygenation even in apnea and allows time for intubation or alternative airway management
- The major advantage of high-flow nasal oxygen is its ability to be administered continuously during airway procedures, unlike oxygen delivered via a face mask, which must be discontinued after the induction of general anesthesia
- This method of preoxygenation may be especially advantageous for patients who have diminished functional residual capacity or an elevated oxygen demand due to conditions such as pregnancy, obesity, or sepsis

### HFNO Contraindications

- Consciousness disorder if aspiration concern
- Agitated or uncooperative patient
- Facial injury (risk of airway soiling)
- High secretion load
- Patients at high risk of aspiration
- Base of skull fractures (risk of pneumocephalus)
- Complete or impending airway obstruction

## VORTEX APPROACH

- The Vortex Approach is a high-acuity tool designed to streamline complex decision-making and actions in emergency airway management situations This approach rests on the foundation that there are three primary non-surgical 'lifelines' for establishing and verifying alveolar oxygen delivery:
  - Face mask
  - Supraglottic airway
  - Endotracheal tube
- Failure to restore alveolar oxygen delivery after a 'best effort' with any of the lifelines necessitates a transition to the next available lifeline, as visualized in the tool's circular layout, which allows for any lifeline to be accessed first and followed by others in any sequence deemed suitable for the situation
- Should a 'best effort' with each of these lifelines fail, it indicates a 'can't intubate, can't oxygenate' (CICO) scenario, necessitating the initiation of emergency front-of-neck access
- The tool includes a list of five optimization categories applicable to each lifeline, these categories are designed to enhance the chances of success during the 'best effort' phase, guiding the options available to maximize effective airway management

# THE VORTEX

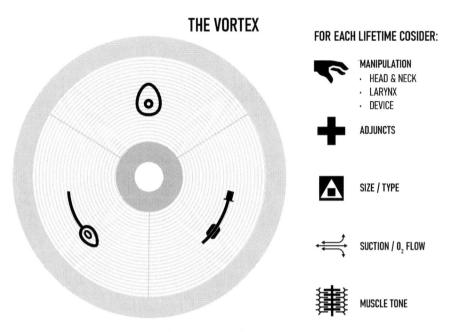

**FOR EACH LIFETIME COSIDER:**

- MANIPULATION
  - HEAD & NECK
  - LARYNX
  - DEVICE
- ADJUNCTS
- SIZE / TYPE
- SUCTION / $O_2$ FLOW
- MUSCLE TONE

**Maximum three attempts at each lifeline (unless gamechanger) at least one attempt should be by most experienced clinician priming status escalates with unsuccesful best effort at any lifetime**

Figure adapted from vortexapproach.org.

## KEEP IN MIND

- Always screen for a difficult airway
- When a difficult airway is suspected, consider an awake intubation
- Plan, anticipate, and communicate when a difficult airway is suspected
- Call for help early
- Know your team, your environment, and your tools and devices
- Allocate tasks to the team members
- Never neglect the basics: Positioning and pre-oxygenation
- Ensure adequate depth of anesthesia and muscle relaxation
- Keep track of time and oxygen saturation, oxygenation should be prioritized at all times
- Video laryngoscopy is an essential skill and should be promptly available
- A supraglottic airway and bag-mask ventilation are essential backup strategies, switch strategies when they prove unsuccessful
- When non-invasive strategies fail and a CICO (can't intubate, can't oxygenate) occurs, a scalpel cricothyroidotomy is the recommended rescue technique
- After a successful difficult intubation, reassess ABCD and make a plan for extubation
- Inform the patient about any airway difficulties encountered and ensure proper documentation for future anesthetic plans

## SUGGESTED READING

- Ang KS, Green A, Ramaswamy KK, Frerk C. Preoxygenation using the Optiflow™ system. Br J Anaesth. 2017;118(3):463-464.
- Apfelbaum JL, Hagberg CA, Connis RT, et al. 2022 American Society of Anesthesiologists Practice Guidelines for Management of the Difficult Airway. Anesthesiology. 2022;136(1):31-81.
- Frerk C, Mitchell VS, McNarry AF, et al. Difficult Airway Society 2015 guidelines for management of unanticipated difficult intubation in adults. Br J Anaesth. 2015;115(6):827848.
- Lee MH, Kim HJ. Application of high-flow nasal oxygenation as a rescue therapy in difficult videolaryngoscopic intubation. SAGE Open Med Case Rep. 2021;9:2050313X211010015.
- Shallik N, Karmakar A. Is it time for high flow nasal oxygen to be included in the difficult airway algorithm?. Br J Anaesth. 2018;121(2):511-512.
- https://vortexapproach.org/

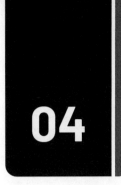

# EXPANDING NECK HEMATOMA

## LEARNING OBJECTIVES

- Recognize an expanding neck hematoma
- Management of an expanding neck hematoma

## DEFINITION AND MECHANISM

- Hematoma is caused by blunt neck trauma leading to the dissection of a major blood vessel or bleeding from a soft tissue injury
- May result from recent surgery or spontaneous as with a ruptured thyroidal cyst, thyroidal vessel, or parathyroid adenoma
- Affects the pharynx, larynx, esophagus, and trachea and results in airway compromise
- Theoretical potential for hemodynamic instability due to compression of the carotid sinus with resulting bradycardia/hypotension

## CAUSES

- Injuries to the internal and/or external carotid arteries, external carotid artery deep branches, or internal jugular veins
- Injuries to the cervical fascial layers (barriers of deep spaces) that facilitate the pooling of blood and hematoma

## MANAGEMENT

```
                     Expanding neck hematoma
                    /                          \
         Expanding hematoma          Minimal hematoma with
                                        no progression
                |                              |
    Rapidly assess the situation + keep   Conservative approach + monitoring
            patient calm
                |
    Provide supplemental oxygen + call for
            help
                |
    Intubate immediately with symptoms of
          airway compromise
                |
    Perform decompression of the wound →
          relief from hypoxia
                |
    Explore neck/wound surgically in OR  →
                |
    Anticoagulation therapy can be
    restarted after the hematoma resolves
        with monitoring of PT-INR
```

- Release of sutures
- Open the platysma
- Evacuate the blood clot below the deep fascia
- Identify the source of the hematoma
- Manage bleeding after hematoma evacuation with gentle pressure

**Signs and symptoms**
- Change in voice quality
- Neck tightness
- Neck pain/pressure
- Neck swelling
- Dysphagia
- Sweating
- Agitation
- Anxiety

Respiratory symptoms occur later:
- Stridor
- Hypoxia
- Dyspnea
- Tachypnea
- Tracheal deviation

## KEEP IN MIND

- Intubation may be difficult and should be performed by an experienced anesthesiologist
- In case of inability to intubate, a surgical airway should be performed early

**SUGGESTED READING**

- Alfraidy, D, Helmi, H, Alamodi Alghamdi, M, Bokhari, A, Alsaif, A. Rare cause of acute neck hematoma. Clin Case Rep. 2019; 7: 1378– 1381.
- Barash PG, Cahalan MK, Cullen BF, Stock C, Stoelting RK, Ortega R, Sharar SR, Holt H. Clinical anesthesia. 2017. Eight edition. Wolters Kluwer.
- Shuker ST. Expanding Hematoma's Life-Threatening Neck and Face Emergency Management of Ballistic Injuries. J Craniofac Surg. 2 016;27(5):1282-1285.
- Shakespeare WA, Lanier WL, Perkins WJ, Pasternak JJ. Airway management in patients who develop neck hematomas after carotid endarterectomy. Anesth Analg. 2010;110(2):588-593.

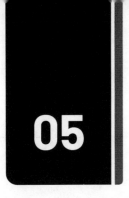

# LUNG PROTECTIVE VENTILATION

## LEARNING OBJECTIVES

- Understand the basic principles behind lung protective ventilation

**05**

- Lung protective ventilation (LPV) is a ventilation strategy aiming to reduce pulmonary complications after mechanical ventilation
- Perioperative lung injury is a spectrum of disease that includes inflammation, impaired gas exchange, radiographic abnormalities, and respiratory failure
- It is reasonable to use LPV as the default ventilation strategy in all mechanically ventilated patients

## VENTILATOR SETTINGS (MANAGEMENT)

- Tidal volume of 6-8 mL/kg predicted body weight
- Plateau pressures < 30 cm $H_2O$
- Start positive end-expiratory pressure (PEEP) at 5 cm $H_2O$
- When performing recruitment maneuvers use:
  - The lowest effective pressure
  - The shortest effective time
  - The least amount of breaths

## KEEP IN MIND

- Ventilator induced lung injury (VILI) occurs via:
  - Volutrauma: high tidal volumes
  - Barotrauma: high inspiratory pressures
  - Atelectotrauma: repetitive and rapid opening of the alveoli
- Biotrauma:
  - Inflammatory damage
  - Apoptotic/fibroproliferative processes
  - The translocation of bacteria and pro-inflammatory mediators
- VILI shares common pathophysiological features with acute respiratory distress syndrome (ARDS)
- ARDS is caused by:
  - Pneumonia, sepsis, or aspiration pneumonitis (in 85% of cases)
  - Blood transfusion, hemorrhagic shock, burns, inhalation injury
  - Surgical factors: trauma, retraction injury, cardiopulmonary bypass, and ischemia-reperfusion injury
- VILI occurs most often in patients with predisposing factors for ARDS
- In patients at risk for ARDS or with ARDS, LPV:
  - Improves oxygenation and pulmonary physiology
  - Reduces postoperative pulmonary complications
  - Reduces the relative risk of death at day 28

**SUGGESTED READING**

- Beitler JR, Malhotra A, Thompson BT. Ventilator-induced Lung Injury. Clin Chest Med. 2016;37(4):633-646.
- O'Gara B, Talmor D. Perioperative lung protective ventilation. BMJ. 2018;362:k3030. Published 2018 Sep 10. doi:10.1136/bmj.k3030
- Petrucci N, De Feo C. Lung protective ventilation strategy for the acute respiratory distress syndrome. Cochrane Database Syst Rev. 2013;2013(2):CD003844. Published 2013 Feb 28.
- Young CC, Harris EM, Vacchiano C, et al. Lung-protective ventilation for the surgical patient: international expert panel-based consensus recommendations. Br J Anaesth. 2019;123(6):898-913.

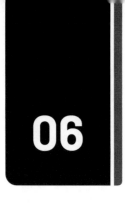

# MICROLARYNGOSCOPY AND AIRWAY LASER

**06**

## LEARNING OBJECTIVES

- Airway management during microlaryngoscopy and laser procedures

## DEFINITION AND MECHANISM

- Microlaryngoscopy allows visualizing the vocal cords with a microscope to remove lesions from the vocal cords or to reduce the narrowing of the larynx and trachea
- Potential for dynamic airway obstruction with induction, positive pressure ventilation & paralysis:
  □ Double setup with rigid bronchoscope available
- Shared airway with the need to optimize surgical conditions/safety
- Airway laser is a source of energy that can be focused on extreme high intensity and is capable of vaporizing tissues or photocoagulation
- The advantages of lasers are microscopic precision, a bloodless operative field, reduction of tissue reaction, preservation of normal tissue, and complete sterility
- Complications:
  □ Airway obstruction, laryngospasm
  □ Laser: airway fire, burns, venous air embolism with Yttrium Aluminum Garnett (YAG) laser (deeper), pneumothorax
  □ Jet ventilation: barotrauma, abnormal ventilation/oxygenation
  □ Unprotected airway & aspiration risk

| Microlaryngoscopy | Airway laser surgery |
|---|---|
| Benign growth nodules, polyps, cysts | Laryngeal cancers |
| Granulomas | Papilloma excision |
| Vocal cord dysfunction | Vocal cord dysfunction or nodule/cyst removal |
| Obstructing tumor | Obstructing tumor |
| Foreign body | Postcorrosive or traumatic tracheal stenosis |

## MANAGEMENT

- Patients who are not at risk of respiratory obstruction can have standard endotracheal intubation following preoxygenation
- If obstruction of the airway is anticipated, difficult airway equipment is mandatory
- Different sizes of laryngoscope blades, oral and nasal airways, fiberoptic bronchoscope or video endoscope, rigid bronchoscope, and tracheostomy trays should be available
- Laser-resistant/non-combustible endotracheal tubes are recommended by the American Society of Anesthesiologists as the default endotracheal airway during laser surgery of the respiratory tract to protect the operating field
- The cuff is the most vulnerable part of the endotracheal tube (ETT), as, the cuff is inflated with air (or saline) to occlude the trachea external to the tube and thus directs all the gas flows from the endotracheal tube (ETT) exclusively to the trachea, and vice versa
- A dye such as methylene blue is typically instilled into the cuff for such cases, so there is an obvious visual alert if the balloon is inadvertently popped
- Airway management classified in a closed or open system:
- Closed system (intubation)
  □ General anesthesia with ETT (microlaryngoscopic tube or laser tube)

- Open system (no intubation, tubeless technique):
  - Topical/local anesthesia with sedation
  - General anesthesia without intubation
  - Apnea & intermittent intubation/bag-mask ventilation
  - Tubeless spontaneous ventilation technique
  - Jet ventilation with Sanders technique: supraglottic vs subglottic, via catheter/rigid scope
  - High-frequency jet ventilation

Risks/complications:
- Difficulty maintaining oxygenation/ventilation in morbid obesity, stiff thorax, restrictive/obstructive pneumopathy, lung fibrosis, reduced alveolar-capillary diffusion capacity (pulmonary edema)
- Risk of dynamic hyperinflation if obstructed airway with barotrauma (subcutaneous emphysema, pneumothorax/pneumomediastinum, tracheobronchial injury), hypoxemia, hypercarbia/hypocarbia, gastric distension & regurgitation due to scope malalignment, possible vocal cord motion if supraglottic, drying of laryngeal mucosa, the distal spread of particulate matter with potential tracheobronchial viral or tumor seeding

## KEEP IN MIND

- Jet ventilation avoids the risk of ETT complications (kinked, obstructed, displaced, damaged, ignited)
- Contraindication to jet ventilation & need for airway laser
- Full stomach & laser surgery: laser ETT vs jet ventilation
- Maintain the $FiO_2$ below 30% as ventilation with 100% $FiO_2$ creates risk of fire during MLS

**■ SUGGESTED READING ■**

- Hemantkumar, Indrani. (2017). Anesthesia for Laser Surgery of the Airway. An International Journal Otorhinolaryngology Clinics. 9. 1-5. 10.5005/jp-journals-10003-1250.
- Novakovic D, Sheth M, Fellner A, Zoszak A, Liew S, Nguyen DD. Microlaryngeal Laser Surgery Using High-flow Nasal Ventilation at Two Oxygen Concentration Deliveries. Laryngoscope. 2023 Mar;133(3):634-639.
- Pearson, K., Mguire, B., 2017. Anaesthesia for laryngo-tracheal surgery, including tubeless field techniques. BJA Education 17, 242-248

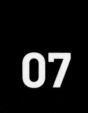

# PENETRATING NECK INJURIES

## LEARNING OBJECTIVES

- Recognize penetrating neck injuries
- Management of penetrating neck injuries

## DEFINITION AND MECHANISM

- Trauma to the neck by breaching the platysma muscle
- Caused by stab wounds, gunshot wounds, self-harm, road traffic accidents, and other high-velocity objects
- Partial or complete occlusion, dissection, pseudoaneurysm, extravasation of blood, or arteriovenous fistula formation

- Potential for serious & life-threatening injuries
  - Laryngeal/tracheobronchial tree disruption
  - Tension/open pneumothorax, massive hemothorax
  - Major vascular disruption
  - Esophageal tear
  - Spinal cord injury, nerve injury

## Anatomical zones of penetrating neck injury

| Zone | Anatomical boundaries | Anatomical structures at risk |
|------|----------------------|------------------------------|
| 1 | Superior boundary: skull base<br>Inferior boundary: angle of the mandible | Pharynx<br>Carotid arteries<br>Internal jugular veins<br>Cranial nerves<br>Sympathetic chain<br>Parotid gland |
| 2 | Superior boundary: angle of the mandible<br>Inferior boundary: cricoid cartilage | Laryngotracheal complex<br>Pharynx<br>Oesophagus<br>Carotid artery<br>Jugular veins<br>Vertebral arteries<br>Spinal cord<br>Vagus and phrenic nerves |
| 3 | Superior boundary: cricoid cartilage<br>Inferior boundary: clavicles | Trachea<br>Oesophagus<br>Carotid artery<br>Jugular veins<br>Thoracic duct<br>Spinal cord<br>Cranial nerves<br>Vertebral arteries |

## SIGNS AND SYMPTOMS

- Shock
- Active hemorrhage
- Pulsatile bleeding or expanding hematoma
- Audible bruit or palpable thrill
- Airway compromise
- Wound bubbling
- Subcutaneous emphysema
- Stridor
- Hoarseness
- Difficulty/pain when swallowing
- Hemiparesis
- Neurological deficits

## MANAGEMENT

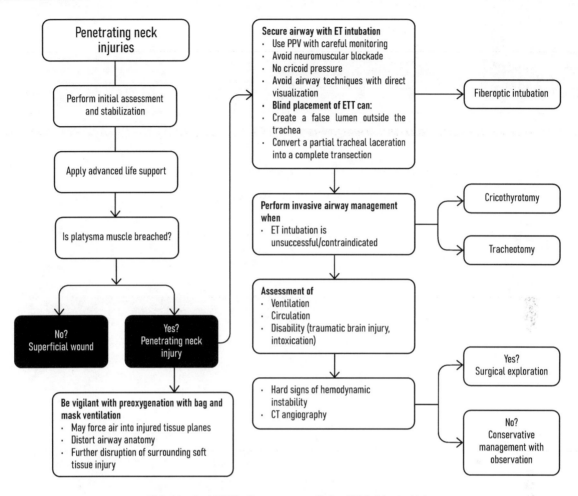

ET, Endotracheal; PPV, Positive pressure ventilation; ETT, Endotracheal tube

## KEEP IN MIND

- Full stomach/rapid sequence intubation (RSI) vs potentially challenging airway
- Uncooperative patient vs. awake fiberoptic bronchoscopic intubation
- Securing airway vs. consequences of PPV

## SUGGESTED READING

- Huh H, Han JH, Chung JY, et al. Anesthetic management of penetrating neck injury patient with embedded knife -A case report-. Korean J Anesthesiol. 2012;62(2):172-174.
- McCann C, Watson A, Barnes D. Major burns: Part 1. Epidemiology, pathophysiology and initial management. BJA Educ. 2022;22(3):94-103.
- Nowicki JL, Stew B, Ooi E. Penetrating neck injuries: a guide to evaluation and management. Ann R Coll Surg Engl. 2018;100(1):6-11.

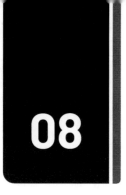

# PULMONARY ASPIRATION

## LEARNING OBJECTIVES

- Identification of patients at risk for pulmonary aspiration
- Reducing the risk of pulmonary aspiration
- Management of pulmonary aspiration

## DEFINITION AND MECHANISM

- The inhalation of oropharyngeal or gastric contents into the larynx and the respiratory tract
- Aspiration accounts for more deaths than failure to intubate or ventilate
- May lead to chemical pneumonitis, bacterial pneumonia, or acute respiratory distress syndrome

## SIGNS AND SYMPTOMS

- Symptoms can range from none to respiratory failure and subsequent cardiac arrest in a massive aspiration event

| Risk factors | |
| --- | --- |
| Patient factors | Full stomach<br>Emergency surgery<br>Inadequate fasting time<br>Gastrointestinal obstruction |
| Delayed gastric emptying | Systemic diseases, including diabetes mellitus and chronic kidney disease<br>Recent trauma<br>Opioids<br>Increased intracranial pressure<br>Previous gastrointestinal surgery<br>Pregnancy (including active labor) |
| Incompetent lower oesophageal sphincter | Hiatus hernia<br>Recurrent regurgitation<br>Dyspepsia<br>Previous upper gastrointestinal surgery<br>Pregnancy |
| Esophageal diseases | Previous gastrointestinal surgery<br>Morbid obesity |
| Surgical factors | Upper gastrointestinal surgery<br>Lithotomy or head down position<br>Laparoscopy<br>Cholecystectomy |
| Anesthetic factors | Light anesthesia<br>Supra-glottic airways<br>Positive pressure ventilation<br>Length of anaesthetic time > 2 h<br>Difficult airway |
| Device factors | First-generation supra-glottic airway devices |

| Prevention | |
|---|---|
| Reducing gastric volume | Preoperative fasting<br>Nasogastric aspiration<br>Prokinetic premedication |
| Avoidance of general anesthetics | Regional anesthesia |
| Reducing pH of gastric contents | Antacids<br>H2 histamine antagonists<br>Proton pump inhibitors |
| Airway protection | Tracheal intubation<br>Second-generation supraglottic airway devices |
| Prevent regurgitation | Cricoid pressure<br>Rapid sequence induction |
| Extubation | Awake after return of airway reflexes<br>Position (lateral, head down or upright) |

# MANAGEMENT

- Anesthesiologists should have a low index of suspicion for aspiration
- Emergency anesthesia on its own is an important risk factor for aspiration
- Management is supportive
- The trachea should be suctioned after securing a safe airway, ideally before positive pressure ventilation to prevent the distal displacement of aspirated material
- Antibiotics should only be used if pneumonia develops, early antibiotics may lead to the selection of virulent bacteria including pseudomonas
- There is no evidence that using steroids either reduces mortality or improves outcome

## SUGGESTED READING

- Asai T. Editorial II: Who is at increased risk of pulmonary aspiration?. Br J Anaesth. 2004;93(4):497-500.
- Michael Robinson, MB ChB FRCA, Andrew Davidson, MA MBBS FRCA FFICM, Aspiration under anaesthesia: risk assessment and decision-making, Continuing Education in Anaesthesia Critical Care & Pain, Volume 14, Issue 4, August 2014, Pages 171-175.

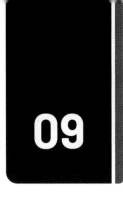

# RIGID BRONCHOSCOPY

## LEARNING OBJECTIVES

- Indications for rigid bronchoscopy
- Advantages and disadvantages of rigid bronchoscopy
- Anesthesia management for rigid bronchoscopy

## DEFINITION AND MECHANISM

- To gain better access to the patient's airway
- Allows insertion of instruments or airway devices
- Diagnosis of infections, cancers, inflammatory conditions, sarcoidosis, and lymphoma
- Treatment of airway obstruction, airway narrowing (stenosis), airway cancers, bleeding
- Removal of foreign or aspirated objects
- Considerations for surgical technique: stenting, laser, endobronchial electrosurgery, argon plasma coagulation, & balloon bronchoplasty

| Advantages | Disadvantages |
|---|---|
| Can be inserted past airway obstruction | Always requires general anesthesia |
| The airway is secure during the procedure | Oral and pharyngeal damage |
| Allows for:<br>Larger biopsies<br>Tamponade (stop) bleeding areas<br>Removal of airway tumors and foreign objects<br>Deploying airway devices (tracheobronchial stents) to keep a collapsing airway open | Limited visualization |
| | Nonflexible metal rod |

## FACTORS THAT COMPLICATE RIGID BRONCHOSCOPY

- Patients requiring high levels of supplemental $O_2$
- Patients with baseline hypercarbia and hemodynamic instability
- Unstable cervical spine or diminished range of motion of the cervical spine caused by spondylosis
- Maxillofacial trauma or oral disease preventing opening of the jaw (stenosis, obstructing neoplasms)
- Procedure-specific complications: hemorrhage, airway trauma, perforation, fire, systemic gas embolism, & dissemination of post-obstructive pneumonia

## KEEP IN MIND

- Full stomach vs. unsecured airway
- High oxygen requirements with risk of fire ignition
- Jet ventilation through obstructing stenoses with risk of air trapping & barotrauma

Rigid bronchoscopy

# MANAGEMENT

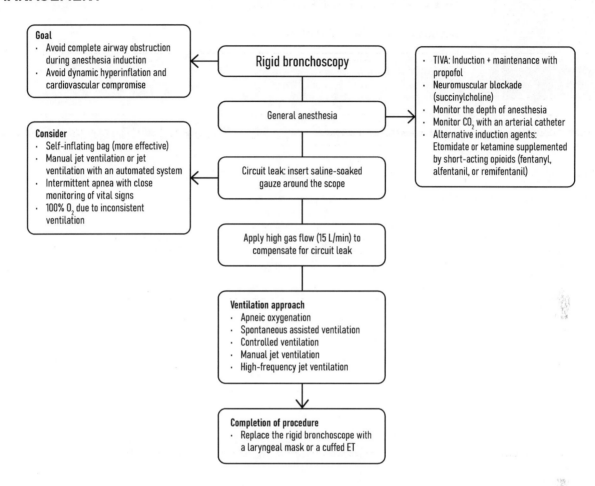

**Goal**
- Avoid complete airway obstruction during anesthesia induction
- Avoid dynamic hyperinflation and cardiovascular compromise

**Rigid bronchoscopy**

- TIVA: Induction + maintenance with propofol
- Neuromuscular blockade (succinylcholine)
- Monitor the depth of anesthesia
- Monitor $CO_2$ with an arterial catheter
- Alternative induction agents: Etomidate or ketamine supplemented by short-acting opioids (fentanyl, alfentanil, or remifentanil)

**General anesthesia**

**Consider**
- Self-inflating bag (more effective)
- Manual jet ventilation or jet ventilation with an automated system
- Intermittent apnea with close monitoring of vital signs
- 100% $O_2$ due to inconsistent ventilation

**Circuit leak: insert saline-soaked gauze around the scope**

**Apply high gas flow (15 L/min) to compensate for circuit leak**

**Ventilation approach**
- Apneic oxygenation
- Spontaneous assisted ventilation
- Controlled ventilation
- Manual jet ventilation
- High-frequency jet ventilation

**Completion of procedure**
- Replace the rigid bronchoscope with a laryngeal mask or a cuffed ET

## SUGGESTED READING

- Galway U, Zura A, Khanna S, Wang M, Turan A, Ruetzler K. Anesthetic considerations for bronchoscopic procedures: a narrative review based on the Cleveland Clinic experience. J Thorac Dis. 2019;11(7):3156-3170.
- Kabadayi, Selin & Bellamy, Mark. (2016). Bronchoscopy in critical care. BJA Education. 17. mkw040. 10.1093/bjaed/mkw040.
- Pathak V, Welsby I, Mahmood K, Wahidi M, MacIntyre N, Shofer S. Ventilation and anesthetic approaches for rigid bronchoscopy. Ann Am Thorac Soc. 2014;11(4):628-634.

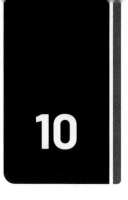

# TRACHEOSTOMY

## LEARNING OBJECTIVES

- Identify conditions requiring a tracheostomy
- Management of a tracheostomy

---

## DEFINITION AND MECHANISM

- Surgical incision into the trachea that forms a temporary or permanent opening, when intubation is expected to last > 1-2 weeks
- Very short and wide tube directly placed into trachea → decreased risk of pneumonia
- Commonly performed in the OR under general anesthesia
- Create access to remove secretions from the lungs
- Often needed when health problems require long-term use of a machine (ventilator) to help you breathe
- Emergency tracheostomy is performed when the airway is suddenly blocked due to a traumatic injury to the face or neck
- Patients with a tracheostomy can be weaned from a ventilator faster than patients with a ETT
- Consider: shared airway, difficult airway
  - Close communication with surgeon, backup plan discussed

## INDICATIONS

- Prolonged mechanical ventilation
- Pulmonary toilet
- Airway protection
- Part of a surgical procedure
- Upper airway obstruction
- Aspiration risk

## CONDITIONS REQUIRING A TRACHEOSTOMY

- Congenital abnormalities of the airway
- Airway burns from the inhalation of corrosive material
- Obstruction of the airway by a foreign object
- Obstructive sleep apnea
- Injury to the larynx
- Severe neck or mouth injuries
- Bilateral vocal cord paralysis
- Facial burns or surgery
- Chronic lung disease
- Anaphylaxis
- Coma
- Cancers that affect the head and neck
- Infection
- Neck tumors
- Paralysis of the muscles used in swallowing
- Injury to the chest wall
- Dysfunction affecting the diaphragm

| Early | Short-term | Long-term |
|---|---|---|
| Hemorrhage | Blockage | Tracheomalacia |
| Aspiration | Tube displacement | Tracheal stenosis |
| Pneumothorax | Pneumothorax | Tracheocutaneous fistula |
| Failure of procedure | Surgical emphysema | Decannulation problems |
| | Infection | |
| | Delayed hemorrhage | |
| | Tracheal necrosis | |
| | Tracheo-arterial fistula | |

## MANAGEMENT

- High-flow nasal oxygen therapy to slow the time to desaturation where intubation or face-mask ventilation is difficult/impossible
  - Risk of fire as $FiO_2$ is close to 1.0 if diathermy is used
- Check the position and size of the tracheostomy tube with a combination of capnography + endoscopy + cuff pressure
  - If the tube is too short: the cuff may herniate up into the superior larynx (within the vocal cords) thereby causing reduced pulmonary compliance, persistent cuff leaks, or tracheal damage
  - If the tube too long: risk of endobronchial tube placement

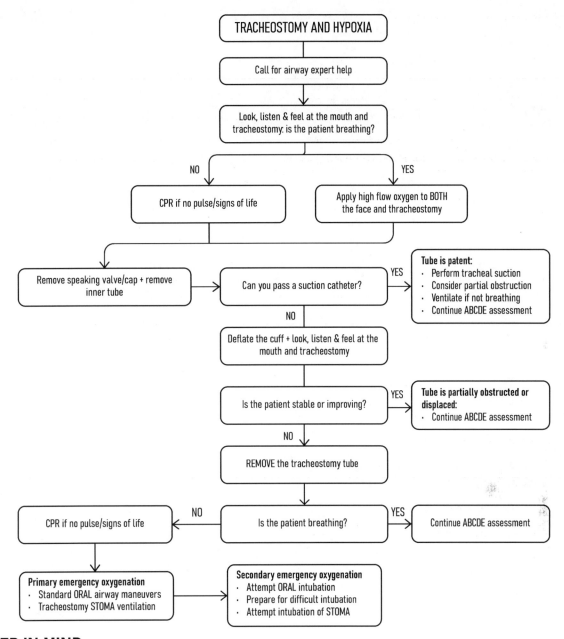

**TRACHEOSTOMY AND HYPOXIA**

Call for airway expert help

Look, listen & feel at the mouth and tracheostomy: is the patient breathing?

**NO** → CPR if no pulse/signs of life

**YES** → Apply high flow oxygen to BOTH the face and thracheostomy

Remove speaking valve/cap + remove inner tube

Can you pass a suction catheter?

**YES** → **Tube is patent:**
- Perform tracheal suction
- Consider partial obstruction
- Ventilate if not breathing
- Continue ABCDE assessment

**NO**

Deflate the cuff + look, listen & feel at the mouth and tracheostomy

Is the patient stable or improving?

**YES** → **Tube is partially obstructed or displaced:**
- Continue ABCDE assessment

**NO**

REMOVE the tracheostomy tube

Is the patient breathing?

**NO** → CPR if no pulse/signs of life

**YES** → Continue ABCDE assessment

**Primary emergency oxygenation**
- Standard ORAL airway maneuvers
- Tracheostomy STOMA ventilation

**Secondary emergency oxygenation**
- Attempt ORAL intubation
- Prepare for difficult intubation
- Attempt intubation of STOMA

## KEEP IN MIND

- A laryngectomy tube can be used instead of a tracheostomy tube for intraoperative ventilation of the lungs during surgery
- Difficult BMV & supraglottic device ventilation (air leak)
- Dangerous placement of ETT (direct vision preferred)
- Comorbid disease:
  - ICU patient with multi-organ failure, sepsis, lung injury, etc
  - Neuromuscular disorders, chronic high spinal cord injury
- Ensure emergency tracheostomy equipment is available: various sizes of cuffed/uncuffed tracheostomy tubes, suction catheters, graspers, Ambu bags & ties

## ■ SUGGESTED READING ■

- Lewith H, Athanassoglou V. Update on management of tracheostomy. BJA Educ. 2019;19(11):370-376.
- Rosero EB, Corbett J, Mau T, Joshi GP. Intraoperative Airway Management Considerations for Adult Patients Presenting With Tracheostomy: A Narrative Review. Anesth Analg. 2021;132(4):1003-1011.

# CARDIAC DISEASES

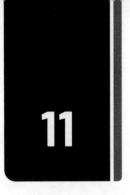

# ADULT CONGENITAL HEART DISEASE (ACHD)

## LEARNING OBJECTIVES

- Describe the implications and comorbidities of ACHD
- Classify the severity and assess the anesthetic risk factors of ACHD
- The anesthetic management of patients with ACHD

## DEFINITION AND MECHANISM

- Congenital heart disease (CHD) is the most common birth defect in humans, affecting nearly 1% of live births
- Defects range from mild to severe
- Just a few decades ago: Children with CHD faced high mortality rates
- Today, more than 80% of children with CHD survive adolescence and reach adulthood

| Classification | |
|---|---|
| Simple ACHD: Simple lesions conferring no functional limitations, or those who have undergone curative surgery | Unrepaired lesion:<br>- Isolated aortic valve disease (13/1000 live births)<br>- Isolated mitral valve disease (excluding mitral cleft or parachute valve)<br>- Isolated patent foramen ovale, small atrial septal defect, or ventricular septal defect<br>Mild pulmonary stenosis<br>Repaired lesion<br>- Ligated or occluded ductus arteriosus<br>- Repaired sinus venosus or secundum atrial septal defect<br>- Repaired ventricular septal defect |
| Moderate complexity ACHD: Moderately complex disease that may pose some day-to-day limitations, or patients who have undergone surgery likely to require reoperation | Aorta to left ventricular fistula<br>Partial or total anomalous pulmonary venous drainage<br>Atrioventricular canal defects (partial or complete)<br>Coarctation of the aorta<br>Ebstein's anomaly<br>Significant infundibular right ventricular outflow tract obstruction<br>Ostium primum or sinus venosus atrioseptal defect<br>Unrepaired ductus arteriosus<br>Moderate-to-severe pulmonary stenosis or regurgitation<br>Sinus of Valsalva fistula or aneurysm<br>Subvalvular or supravalvular aortic stenosis<br>Tetralogy of Fallot<br>Ventricular septal defect with associated anomaly, e.g., aortic regurgitation, absent valve, subaortic stenosis, mitral valve disease, right ventricular outflow tract obstruction, straddling atrioventricular valve |
| Severe complexity ACHD: Adults with severe complexity ACHD with significant functional limitation, they may have had palliative surgery or been deemed not amenable to intervention | Conduits: valved or non-valved<br>All types of cyanotic heart disease<br>Double-outlet ventricle<br>Eisenmenger syndrome<br>Fontan procedure or total cavopulmonary connection<br>Mitral, tricuspid, or pulmonary atresia<br>Pulmonary hypertension<br>Any single-ventricle circulation<br>Transposition of the great vessels<br>Truncus arteriosus<br>Very rare complex anomalies, e.g., criss-cross heart, isomerism, ventricular inversion, heterotaxy syndromes |

# COMMON COMORBIDITIES

- Heart failure
- Arrhythmias
- Sudden cardiac death
- Infectious endocarditis
- Additionally acquired heart diseases

- Pulmonary hypertension
- Neurological complications
- Hematological impairments
- Rheological impairments

| Risk factors | |
| --- | --- |
| Anatomic lesion | Single ventricle<br>Biventricular physiology with systemic RV |
| Physiologic status | Poor exercise tolerance and/or decreased ventricular function (EF < 25% or NYHA 3-4)<br>Cyanosis (SaO$_2$ < 80%)<br>Pulmonary hypertension (systemic or suprasystemic PAP)<br>Neurodevelopmental delay |
| Comorbidities | Obesity (BMI > 35)<br>COPD (FEV1 < 30% of predicted)<br>Diabetes mellitus type 1<br>Chronic renal insufficiency (GFR < 30%) |
| Intraprocedural complications | Inotropy or vasopressor need<br>Arrhythmia requiring treatment<br>Blood product transfusion |

EF, ejection fraction; NYHA, New York Heart Association; SaO2, Arterial oxygen saturation; PAP, pulmonary arterial pressure; COPD, chronic obstructive pulmonary disease; FEV1, forced expiratory volume; GFR, glomerular filtration rate

# MANAGEMENT

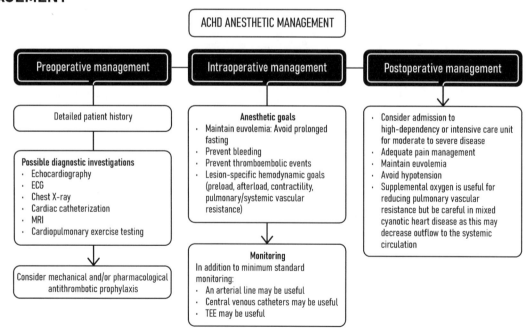

## SUGGESTED READING

- Baehner T, Ellerkmann RK. Anesthesia in adults with congenital heart disease. Current Opinion in Anesthesiology. 2017;30(3).
- Motta P, Manrique AM, Partington SL, Ullah S, Zabala LM. Congenital heart disease in adults (when kids grow up) pediatric geriatric anesthesia. Curr Opin Anaesthesiol. 2020;33(3):335-342.
- Weale J, Kelleher AA. Adult congenital heart disease. Anaesthesia & Intensive Care Medicine. 2021;22(5):290-6.

Adult congenital heart disease (ACHD)

# 12

# AORTIC DISSECTION

## LEARNING OBJECTIVES

- Define and classify aortic dissection
- Describe the risk factors for aortic dissection
- Diagnose aortic dissection
- Manage patients with aortic dissection

## DEFINITION AND MECHANISM

- Life-threatening emergency
- Most common type of acute aortic syndrome
- Occurs when a tear in the aortic intima allows blood to dissect into the wall of the aorta
- Can result from abnormalities in underlying tissue structure (Marfan syndrome, Loeys-Dietz syndrome)
- Can also occur in previously asymptomatic patients with no known genetic aortopathy
- Often associated with an increase in physical activity or stress, leading to acute hypertension

## CLASSIFICATION

- There are several classification systems for aortic dissection:

| DeBakey | |
|---------|---|
| Type I | Tear in the ascending portion; involves all portions of the thoracic aorta |
| Type II | Tear in the ascending aorta; involves the ascending aorta only, stopping before the innominate artery |
| Type III | Tear located in the descending segment; almost always involves the descending thoracic aorta only, starting distal to the left subclavian artery; can propagate proximally into the arch |
| **Stanford** | |
| Type A | All dissections involving the ascending aorta irrespective of the site of tear |
| Type B | All dissections that do not involve the ascending aorta |

## DIAGNOSIS

- Imaging
  - CT
    - The triple rule-out protocol is the one-stop CT examination for chest pain designed to differentiate acute coronary syndrome, pulmonary embolism, and acute aortic dissection
  - Transthoracic echocardiography (TTE)
  - Transesophageal echocardiography (TEE)
    - Provides more complete imaging of the aorta than TTE
  - MRI
    - Can combine anatomical and functional information in one examination and provide a comprehensive evaluation of aortic dissection
- Biomarkers
  - D-dimer and fibrin degradation products
  - Smooth muscle myosin heavy chain
  - Matrix metalloproteinase-9
- Elastin degradation products
  - Calponin
  - Transforming growth factor-beta (TGFβ)

Aortic dissection

# MANAGEMENT

| Risk factors | | |
|---|---|---|
| Lifestyle factors | Long-term arterial hypertension<br>Smoking<br>Dyslipidemia<br>Cocaine, crack cocaine, or amphetamine use | |
| Connective tissue disorders | Marfan's syndrome<br>Loeys-Dietz's syndrome<br>Ehlers-Danlos syndrome<br>Turner's syndrome | |
| Hereditary vascular disease | Bicuspid aortic valve<br>Coarctation of the aorta | |
| Vascular inflammation | Autoimmune disorders:<br>· Giant-cell arteritis<br>· Takayasu's arteritis<br>· Behçet's disease<br>· Ormond's disease | Infection:<br>· Syphilis<br>· Tuberculosis |
| Deceleration trauma | Motor vehicle accident | |
| Iatrogenic factors | Catheter or instrument intervention | Valvular or aortic surgery:<br>· Side-clamping, cross-clamping, or aortotomy<br>· Graft anastomosis<br>· Patch aortoplasty |

# MANAGEMENT

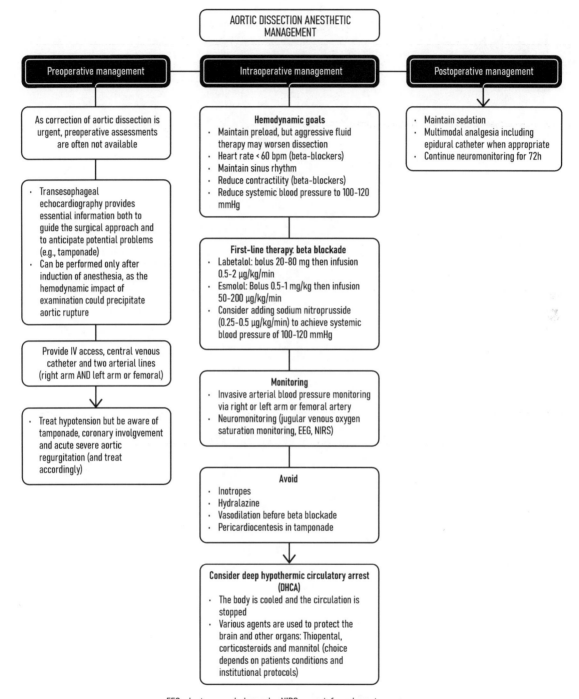

| AORTIC DISSECTION ANESTHETIC MANAGEMENT |

**Preoperative management**

As correction of aortic dissection is urgent, preoperative assessments are often not available

- Transesophageal echocardiography provides essential information both to guide the surgical approach and to anticipate potential problems (e.g., tamponade)
- Can be performed only after induction of anesthesia, as the hemodynamic impact of examination could precipitate aortic rupture

Provide IV access, central venous catheter and two arterial lines (right arm AND left arm or femoral)

- Treat hypotension but be aware of tamponade, coronary involgvement and acute severe aortic regurgitation (and treat accordingly)

**Intraoperative management**

**Hemodynamic goals**
- Maintain preload, but aggressive fluid therapy may worsen dissection
- Heart rate < 60 bpm (beta-blockers)
- Maintain sinus rhythm
- Reduce contractility (beta-blockers)
- Reduce systemic blood pressure to 100-120 mmHg

**First-line therapy: beta blockade**
- Labetalol: bolus 20-80 mg then infusion 0.5-2 µg/kg/min
- Esmolol: Bolus 0.5-1 mg/kg then infusion 50-200 µg/kg/min
- Consider adding sodium nitroprusside (0.25-0.5 µg/kg/min) to achieve systemic blood pressure of 100-120 mmHg

**Monitoring**
- Invasive arterial blood pressure monitoring via right or left arm or femoral artery
- Neuromonitoring (jugular venous oxygen saturation monitoring, EEG, NIRS)

**Avoid**
- Inotropes
- Hydralazine
- Vasodilation before beta blockade
- Pericardiocentesis in tamponade

**Consider deep hypothermic circulatory arrest (DHCA)**
- The body is cooled and the circulation is stopped
- Various agents are used to protect the brain and other organs: Thiopental, corticosteroids and mannitol (choice depends on patients conditions and institutional protocols)

**Postoperative management**

- Maintain sedation
- Multimodal analgesia including epidural catheter when appropriate
- Continue neuromonitoring for 72h

EEG, electroencephalography; NIRS, near-infrared spectroscopy

# SUGGESTED READING

- Agarwal S, Kendall J, Quarterman C. Perioperative management of thoracic and thoracoabdominal aneurysms. BJA Educ. 2019;19(4):119-125.
- Gregory SH, Yalamuri SM, Bishawi M, Swaminathan M. The Perioperative Management of Ascending Aortic Dissection. Anesth Analg. 2018;127(6):1302-1313.
- Nienaber CA, Clough RE. Management of acute aortic dissection. Lancet. 2015;385(9970):800-811. doi:10.1016/S0140-6736(14)61005-9

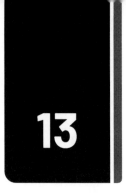

# AORTIC REGURGITATION (AR)

## LEARNING OBJECTIVES

- Describe the underlying mechanisms of AR
- Recognize the symptoms of AR
- Manage patients with AR

## DEFINITION AND MECHANISM

- Aortic regurgitation (AR) is defined as diastolic reversal of blood flow from the aorta into the left ventricle
- Most common etiology: Rheumatic heart disease, aortic root dilation, or congenital bicuspid aortic valve are common causes
- Acute AR:
  - May develop from:
    - Valvular abnormalities (most commonly infective endocarditis)
    - Marfan syndrome and other connective tissue disorders
    - Aortic abnormalities (mostly aortic dissection)
    - Iatrogenic causes such as traumatic injury (i.e., motor vehicle accident) or during transcutaneous aortic valve procedures
  - Characterized by an abrupt increase in left ventricular end-diastolic volume
  - In severe cases, patients often present with pulmonary edema and even cardiogenic shock
- Chronic AR:
  - Most commonly caused by atherosclerotic degeneration of the aortic valve and/or congenital bicuspid aortic valve
  - In the early phases, compensatory mechanisms keep the left ventricular ejection fraction in the normal range
  - Over time, the LV dilates and hypertrophies to normalize wall stress by maintaining the ratio of ventricular wall thickness to cavity radius
  - Compensatory mechanisms allow patients to remain stable and asymptomatic for many years, even in the presence of severe AR
  - If wall thickening fails to keep up with the volume overload, there is an increase in wall stress which then results in a reduction in LV systolic function and LVEF due to myocyte damage
  - As LV filling pressures rise, symptoms of fatigue and dyspnea may appear
  - Angina can develop even in the presence of normal coronary arteries
  - Pulmonary edema and heart failure can occur due to chronically elevated left-sided filling pressures

## SIGNS & SYMPTOMS

- Symptoms
  - Chronic AR
    - Patients with chronic AR remain asymptomatic for years. When symptoms appear, they are due to left heart failure:
      - Chest pain
      - Palpitations
      - Increasing exercise intolerance
      - Dyspnea
      - Paroxysmal nocturnal dyspnea
      - Orthopnea
  - Acute AR
    - Because of a lack of chronic compensation, patients usually present with pulmonary edema and heart failure refractory to optimal medical therapy
    - Patients are often hypotensive and clinically appear to be on the verge of cardiovascular collapse
- Diagnostic signs
  - Collapsing pulse and wide pulse pressure
  - Displaced apex inferolaterally
  - Early diastolic high-pitched murmur
  - An Austin-Flint murmur may be heard in mid-diastole at the apex
  - De Musset's sign – head nodding with each pulse
  - Corrigan's sign – visible carotid pulsation

## SEVERITY ASSESSMENT

- Echocardiography is the best diagnostic tool to evaluate the severity of AR. A rough guideline for approximating severity is the width of the AR jet compared to the width of the left ventricular outflow tract:
  - Mild < 25%
  - Moderate 25-65%
  - Severe > 65%
- Other ways to measure severity are vena contracta width, pressure half time, regurgitant volume/fraction and effective regurgitant orifice area

## ACUTE SEVERE AR MANAGEMENT

- Sudden aortic incompetence results in acute pulmonary congestion
- Immediate management:
  - Afterload reduction (nitroprusside)
  - Enhancement of contractility and heart rate (dobutamine)
  - Emergency surgical intervention is likely necessary
  - Intra-aortic balloon pump is contraindicated

## MANAGEMENT

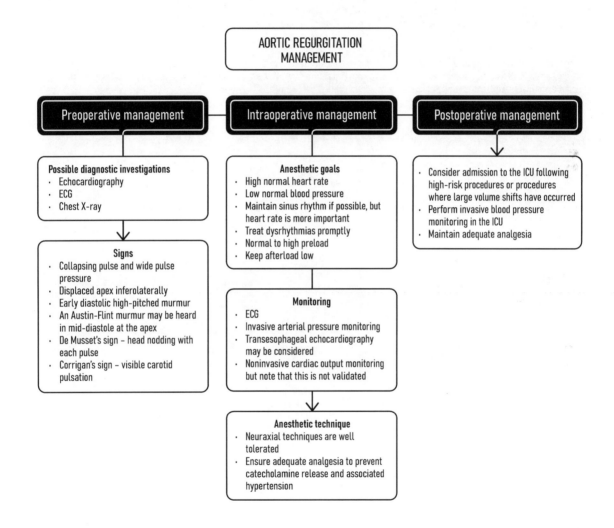

AORTIC REGURGITATION MANAGEMENT

**Preoperative management**

Possible diagnostic investigations
- Echocardiography
- ECG
- Chest X-ray

Signs
- Collapsing pulse and wide pulse pressure
- Displaced apex inferolaterally
- Early diastolic high-pitched murmur
- An Austin-Flint murmur may be heard in mid-diastole at the apex
- De Musset's sign – head nodding with each pulse
- Corrigan's sign – visible carotid pulsation

**Intraoperative management**

Anesthetic goals
- High normal heart rate
- Low normal blood pressure
- Maintain sinus rhythm if possible, but heart rate is more important
- Treat dysrhythmias promptly
- Normal to high preload
- Keep afterload low

Monitoring
- ECG
- Invasive arterial pressure monitoring
- Transesophageal echocardiography may be considered
- Noninvasive cardiac output monitoring but note that this is not validated

Anesthetic technique
- Neuraxial techniques are well tolerated
- Ensure adequate analgesia to prevent catecholamine release and associated hypertension

**Postoperative management**

- Consider admission to the ICU following high-risk procedures or procedures where large volume shifts have occurred
- Perform invasive blood pressure monitoring in the ICU
- Maintain adequate analgesia

### SUGGESTED READING

- Flint N, Wunderlich NC, Shmueli H, Ben-Zekry S, Siegel RJ, Beigel R. Aortic Regurgitation. Curr Cardiol Rep. 2019;21(7):65.
- Hines, R. L. (2017). Stoelting's anesthesia and co-existing disease (7th ed.). Elsevier - Health Sciences Division
- Nishimura RA, Otto CM, Bonow RO, et al. 2014 AHA/ACC Guideline for the Management of Patients With Valvular Heart Disease: executive summary: a report of the American College of Cardiology/American Heart Association Task Force on Practice Guidelines [published correction appears in Circulation. 2014 Jun 10;129(23):e650]. Circulation. 2014;129(23):2440-2492.
- Pollard BJ, Kitchen, G. Handbook of Clinical Anaesthesia. Fourth Edition. CRC Press. 2018. 978-1-4987-6289-2.

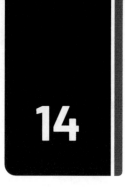

# AORTIC STENOSIS

## LEARNING OBJECTIVES

- Define and recognize aortic stenosis
- Describe the pathophysiology of aortic stenosis and its consequences
- Describe the general anesthetic management principles for aortic stenosis

## DEFINITION AND MECHANISM

- Aortic stenosis occurs when the aortic valve narrows and blood cannot flow normally
- Severe aortic stenosis is a risk factor for perioperative cardiac complications in non-cardiac surgery
- Age-related calcific degeneration is the most common cause of aortic stenosis in the elderly
- There are several causal mechanisms:
  - Degenerative calcific aortic stenosis: Progressive fibrosis and calcification due to mechanical stress over time
  - Congenital bicuspid aortic valve: Abnormal valve structure, with two rather than three leaflets, which can produce fibrosis and calcifications
  - Rheumatic aortic stenosis: Long-term consequence of acute rheumatic fever

### AORTIC STENOSIS (AS) PATHOPHYSIOLOGY

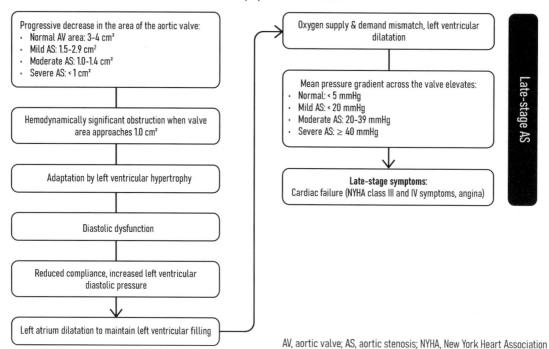

AV, aortic valve; AS, aortic stenosis; NYHA, New York Heart Association

## SEVERITY ASSESSMENT

|  | Aortic sclerosis | Mild | Moderate | Severe |
|---|---|---|---|---|
| Peak velocity (m/s) | ≤ 2.5 m/s | 2.6–2.9 | 3.0–4.0 | ≥ 4.0 |
| Mean gradient (mmHg) | < 20 | < 20 | 20–40 | ≥ 40 |
| AVA (cm²) | > 2.5 | > 1.5 | 1.0–1.5 | < 1.0 |
| Indexed AVA (cm²/m²) | > 1.2 | > 0.85 | 0.60–0.85 | < 0.6 |
| Velocity ratio | > 0.50 | > 0.50 | 0.25–0.50 | < 0.25 |

## MANAGEMENT

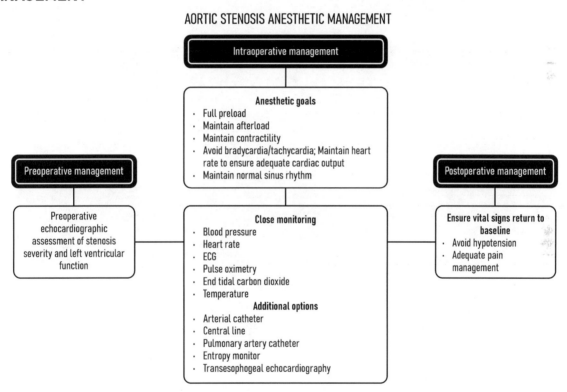

AORTIC STENOSIS ANESTHETIC MANAGEMENT

AV, aortic valve; AS, aortic stenosis; NYHA, New York Heart Association

## KEEP IN MIND

- All necessary medications and equipment to ensure stable vital signals and to treat irregularities must be available during the procedure

**SUGGESTED READING**

- Baumgartner H Chair, Hung J Co-Chair, Bermejo J, et al. Recommendations on the echocardiographic assessment of aortic valve stenosis: a focused update from the European Association of Cardiovascular Imaging and the American Society of Echocardiography. Eur Heart J Cardiovasc Imaging. 2017;18(3):254-275.
- Brown J, Morgan-Hughes NJ. Aortic stenosis and non-cardiac surgery. Continuing Education in Anaesthesia Critical Care & Pain. 2005;5(1):1-4.
- Schneider AC. A review of aortic stenosis: an anesthetic perspective. J Anesth Crit Care Open Access. 2018;10(6):262-264.

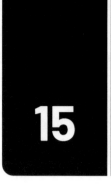

# ATRIAL FIBRILLATION (AF)

## LEARNING OBJECTIVES

- Describe the overall mechanisms of AF
- Recognize risk factors for perioperative AF
- Manage patients with AF or risk of AF

## DEFINITION AND MECHANISM

- Atrial fibrillation (AF) is the most common sustained arrhythmia
- Very rapid and uncoordinated atrial activity
- Twofold increase in premature mortality
- Important factor in major adverse cardiovascular events such as heart failure, severe stroke, and myocardial infarction
- Initiation and maintenance of AF can be linked to "trigger" (initiating event) and "substrate" (atrial remodeling that maintains AF)

## RISK FACTORS FOR PERIOPERATIVE AF

| Patient-related | Surgery-related |
| --- | --- |
| Age | Hypovolemia and hypervolemia |
| Race (lower risk in African population) | Hypoxia |
| History of atrial fibrillation | Intraoperative hypotension |
| Congestive heart failure | Catecholamine versus noncatecholamine vasopressor use |
| Ischemic heart disease | Trauma |
| Hypertension | Pain |
| Chronic renal failure | Type of surgery |
| Sepsis | Hypoglycemia |
| Asthma | Electrolyte abnormalities (primarily hypokalemia and hypomagnesemia) |
| Cardiac valvular disease | Anemia |
| Obstructive sleep apnea | |
| Obesity | |
| Alcohol use | |

## KEEP IN MIND

- Patients who develop perioperative AF have higher in-hospital mortality and longer length of hospital stay
- Those with preexisting AF who develop perioperative AF have similar outcomes compared with patients who develop perioperative AF de novo

# MANAGEMENT

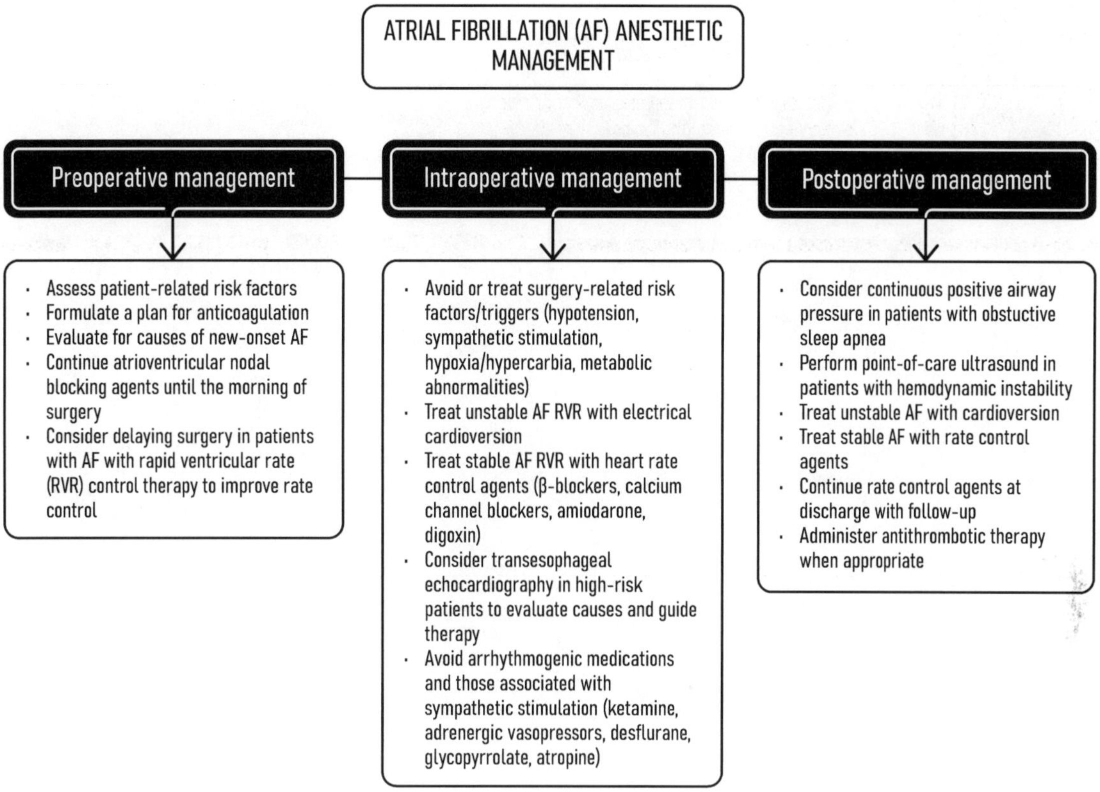

ATRIAL FIBRILLATION (AF) ANESTHETIC MANAGEMENT

**Preoperative management**

- Assess patient-related risk factors
- Formulate a plan for anticoagulation
- Evaluate for causes of new-onset AF
- Continue atrioventricular nodal blocking agents until the morning of surgery
- Consider delaying surgery in patients with AF with rapid ventricular rate (RVR) control therapy to improve rate control

**Intraoperative management**

- Avoid or treat surgery-related risk factors/triggers (hypotension, sympathetic stimulation, hypoxia/hypercarbia, metabolic abnormalities)
- Treat unstable AF RVR with electrical cardioversion
- Treat stable AF RVR with heart rate control agents (β-blockers, calcium channel blockers, amiodarone, digoxin)
- Consider transesophageal echocardiography in high-risk patients to evaluate causes and guide therapy
- Avoid arrhythmogenic medications and those associated with sympathetic stimulation (ketamine, adrenergic vasopressors, desflurane, glycopyrrolate, atropine)

**Postoperative management**

- Consider continuous positive airway pressure in patients with obstuctive sleep apnea
- Perform point-of-care ultrasound in patients with hemodynamic instability
- Treat unstable AF with cardioversion
- Treat stable AF with rate control agents
- Continue rate control agents at discharge with follow-up
- Administer antithrombotic therapy when appropriate

AF, atrial fibrillation; RVR, rapid ventricular rate; AF RVR, atrial fibrilation rapid ventricular rate rate

## SUGGESTED READING

- Karamchandani K, Khanna AK, Bose S, Fernando RJ, Walkey AJ. Atrial Fibrillation: Current Evidence and Management Strategies During the Perioperative Period. Anesthesia & Analgesia. 2020;130(1).
- Wijesurendra RS, Casadei B. Mechanisms of atrial fibrillation. Heart. 2019;105(24):1860-1867

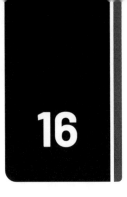

**16**

# ATRIAL SEPTAL DEFECT (ASD)

## LEARNING OBJECTIVES

- Describe the causes and consequences of ASD
- Recognize risk factors for ASD
- Diagnose ASD
- Anesthetic management of patients with ASD

## DEFINITION AND MECHANISM

- Atrial septal defect (ASD) is one of the most common types of congenital heart defects, occurring in about 25% of children
- Failure to close the septum between the right and left atria
- Small defects usually close spontaneously during childhood
- Large defects that do not close spontaneously may require percutaneous or surgical intervention
- Blood flows from the left atrium to the right atrium causing a left-to-right shunt
- Increase in pulmonary vascular resistance due to chronic volume overload, resulting in pulmonary hypertension
- Once pulmonary pressures equal systemic pressures, the shunt across the ASD reverses, and deoxygenated blood flows into the left atrium (Eisenmenger syndrome)
- Other complications:
  - Atrial dysrhythmias
  - Right-sided congestive heart failure
  - Transient ischemic attack/stroke

| Risk factors | |
|---|---|
| Secondary to inherited disorder | Down syndrome<br>Treacher-Collins syndrome<br>Thrombocytopenia-absent radii syndrome<br>Turner syndrome<br>Noonan syndrome |
| Maternal exposures | Rubella<br>Alcohol<br>Drugs, e.g., cocaine |

## ASD TYPES

- Ostium secundum defect: Increased reabsorption of the septum primum in the atrium's roof, or the septum secundum does not occlude the ostium secundum
- Ostium primum defect: Failure of the septum primum to fuse with the endocardial cushions
- Sinus venosus defect: Superior and inferior defects occur, and neither involves the true membranous septum:
  - Superior defect: The orifice of the superior vena cava overrides the atrial septum above the oval fossa and drains both the left and right atria
  - Inferior defect: The orifice of the inferior vena cava overrides both atria
- Coronary sinus defect: A defect or hole in the common wall between the left atrium and the coronary sinus creates a communication between the right and left atria

## DIAGNOSIS

- Transthoracic echocardiogram (gold standard diagnostic imaging modality)
- Cardiac CT and MRI
- Exercise testing can help determine the reversibility of shunt flow and the response of patients with pulmonary artery hypertension to activity
- Cardiac catheterization is contraindicated in young patients who present with small, uncomplicated ASDs.
- Differential diagnosis:
  - Atrioventricular septal defect
  - Ventricular septal defect
  - Cyanotic congenital heart disease (sinus venosus defects and coronary sinus defects)
    - Total anomalous pulmonary venous return
    - Pulmonary stenosis
    - Truncus arteriosus
    - Tricuspid atresia

# MANAGEMENT

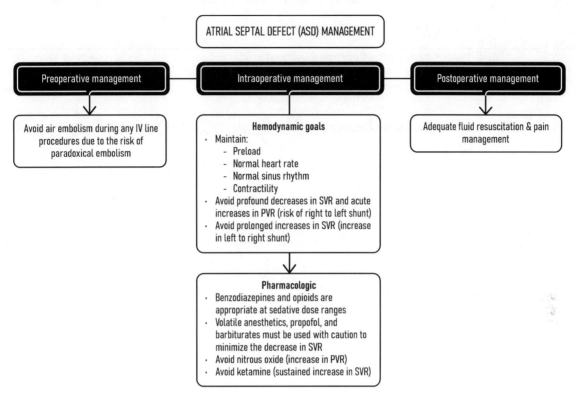

**ATRIAL SEPTAL DEFECT (ASD) MANAGEMENT**

**Preoperative management**

Avoid air embolism during any IV line procedures due to the risk of paradoxical embolism

**Intraoperative management**

**Hemodynamic goals**
- Maintain:
  - Preload
  - Normal heart rate
  - Normal sinus rhythm
  - Contractility
- Avoid profound decreases in SVR and acute increases in PVR (risk of right to left shunt)
- Avoid prolonged increases in SVR (increase in left to right shunt)

**Pharmacologic**
- Benzodiazepines and opioids are appropriate at sedative dose ranges
- Volatile anesthetics, propofol, and barbiturates must be used with caution to minimize the decrease in SVR
- Avoid nitrous oxide (increase in PVR)
- Avoid ketamine (sustained increase in SVR)

**Postoperative management**

Adequate fluid resuscitation & pain management

SVR, systemic vascular resistance; PVR, pulmonary vascular resistance

## SUGGESTED READING

- Calvert PA, Klein AA. Anaesthesia for percutaneous closure of atrial septal defects. Continuing Education in Anaesthesia Critical Care & Pain. 2008;8(1):16-20.
- Menillo AM, Lee LS, Pearson-Shaver AL. Atrial Septal Defect. [Updated 2022 Aug 8]. In: StatPearls [Internet]. Treasure Island (FL): StatPearls Publishing; 2022 Jan-. Available from: https://www.ncbi.nlm.nih.gov/books/NBK535440/
- Yen P. ASD and VSD Flow Dynamics and Anesthetic Management. Anesth Prog. 2015;62(3):125-130.

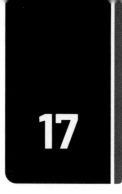

# BRUGADA SYNDROME (BrS)

## LEARNING OBJECTIVES

- Recognize sings & symptoms of Brugada syndrome
- Diagnose Brugada syndrome
- Manage patients with Brugada syndrome

## DEFINITION AND MECHANISM

- Brugada syndrome (BrS) is an abnormality of cardiac ion channels that increases the risk of ventricular fibrillation and sudden cardiac death
- Linked to 19 genetic mutations that encode for sodium, calcium, or potassium channels and result in either increase or decrease in their activity
- In up to 80% of patients, no causative genetic mutation can be found
- Thought to be responsible for up to 40% of sudden cardiac death cases in a structurally normal heart

## SIGNS & SYMPTOMS

- Palpitations
- Chest discomfort
- Syncope and nocturnal agonal respiration
- Monomorphic ventricular tachycardia is rare but is more often seen in infants and children
- Events typically occur during sleep with increased vagal tone, with fever, or can be precipitated by drugs, alcohol, and electrolyte disorders
- Between 20 and 30% of patients: supraventricular tachycardias (atrial flutter, atrioventricular nodal re-entry, Wolff-Parkinson-White syndrome), atrial fibrillation is seen most frequently
- In critical care, the most common presentation will be a patient with aborted sudden cardiac death
- Many patients remain asymptomatic

## DIAGNOSIS

Diagnosis is based on fulfilling the BrS ECG morphological criteria:
- Type 1: A cove shaped (with T-wave inversion) ST-segment elevation ≥ 2 mm in V1 and/or V2 when placed in a standard or superior position, either spontaneously or after Na-channel blocking agent administration (e.g., ajmaline/flecainide)
- Additional ECG morphologies:
  □ Type 2: Saddleback-shaped (with positive T-wave) ST-segment 1 mm in V1 and/or V2
  □ Type 3: Saddleback or cove-shaped ST-segment elevation < 1 mm in V1 and/or V2
  □ Neither are diagnostic

- The ECG morphology can change with time and an individual with true BrS can manifest all three different morphologies at different times
- Many conditions can reproduce a type 1 Brugada ECG, differential diagnosis:
  □ Early repolarisation
  □ Athlete's heart
  □ Acute coronary events
  □ Pulmonary embolism
  □ Electrolyte disturbance
  □ Pericarditis
  □ Myocarditis
  □ Dissecting aortic aneurysm
  □ Arrhythmogenic right ventricular cardiomyopathy

# MANAGEMENT

### RISK ASSESSMENT

Risk factors for arrhythmic events in Brugada syndrome:
- Spontaneous type 1 ECG pattern
- Male sex
- Syncopal episodes
- Nocturnal agonal respiration
- Previous ventricular tachycardia/ventricular fibrillation
- Fragmented QRS complex (i.e., increased number of deflections)
- Prolonged QRS
- T-wave alternans
- Ventricular refractory period
- Early repolarization pattern in inferolateral leads
- Family history of sudden cardiac death

### MEDICATIONS TO AVOID

- Class 1A and 1C antiarrhythmic drugs
- Lithium
- Tricyclic antidepressants should prefferably be avoided, although no substantial evidence on arrhythmia provoking
- Other antiarrhythmics (amiodarone, verapamil, alpha-adrenergic agonists, beta-adrenergic blockers, vagotonic agents, selective serotonin reuptake inhibitors, tetracyclic antidepressants)
- Certain antiepileptics (carbamazepine, phenytoin, lamotrigine)

### PERIOPERATIVE MANAGEMENT

- Take a thorough history
- 12-lead ECG may be valuable, but ECG patterns can vary greatly
- Check electrolytes and correct when needed
- Keep serum magnesium in normal range
- Disable ICD when present
- Continuous ECG monitoring
- Means for external defibrillation should be immediately available and, if possible, apply pads be pre-emptively
- Isoprenaline and, if possible, quinidine should be available
- Consider the risks and benefits when using propofol
- Thiopental has been used without issue
- Ketamine and etomidate are associated with ST-segment elevation
- Opioids can be used safely (with caution)
- When local anesthetics are used, minimize the dose and systemic absorption, use lidocaine with adrenaline in favor of bupivacaine
- Avoid alpha-2-agonists such as clonidine

### ELECTRICAL (ARRHYTHMIC) STORM MANAGEMENT

- Defined as more than two episodes of ventricular tachycardia (VT) or ventricular fibrillation (VF) in a 24-hour period
- Immediate management of VT/VT: defibrillation
- Acute pharmacological treatment: isoprenaline 0.003 µg/kg/min
- Avoid amiodarone
- Discontinue provocative agents
- Treat pyrexia with antipyretics and active cooling
- Optimize electrolytes
- When there is no return of consciousness or ongoing arrhythmia: Standard post-arrest management in ICU

QRS, QRS complex; ICD, implantable cardioverter defibrillator; VF, ventricular fibrillation; SSRI, selective serotonin reuptake inhibitors; TCA, tricyclic antidepressants; VT, ventricular tachycardia

## SUGGESTED READING

- Kloesel B, Ackerman MJ, Sprung J, Narr BJ, Weingarten TN. Anesthetic management of patients with Brugada syndrome: a case series and literature review. Can J Anaesth. 2011;58(9):824-836.
- Levy D, Bigham C, Tomlinson D. Anaesthesia for patients with hereditary arrhythmias part I: Brugada syndrome. BJA Educ. 2018;18(6):159-165.
- Li KHC, Lee S, Yin C, et al. Brugada syndrome: A comprehensive review of pathophysiological mechanisms and risk stratification strategies [published correction appears in Int J Cardiol Heart Vasc. 2020 Dec 19;32:100699]. Int J Cardiol Heart Vasc. 2020;26:100468. Published 2020 Jan 21.

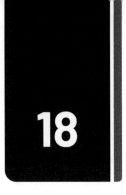

# CARDIAC CONTUSION

## LEARNING OBJECTIVES

- Identify patients at risk for cardiac contusion
- Diagnose cardiac contusion
- Manage patients with (suspected) cardiac contusion

## DEFINITION AND MECHANISM

- Bruising or (microscopically small) hemorrhaging of the heart muscle
- Generally caused by blunt thoracic trauma: A decelerating force on the anterior side of the thorax

## SIGNS & SYMPTOMS

- Mechanical injuries (e.g., rupture of atria or chordae)
- Arrhythmias (premature ventricular complexes, atrial fibrillation, ventricular fibrillation), most commonly within 24h after trauma
- In the emergency department, many patients do not show symptoms of cardiac contusion after trauma, but severe arrhythmia or even cardiac arrest can occur within 72h
- Patients with hemodynamic changes but without clear bleeding or cardiac tamponade are suspected of cardiac contusion

## DIAGNOSIS

Diagnosis for cardiac contusion remains controversial, diagnostic tools include:
- ECG
- Echocardiography
- Measurement of cardiac biomarkers (troponin T, troponin I, CK-MB) but note that troponin levels are sensitive but not specific for cardiac contusion

# MANAGEMENT

## CARDIAC CONTUSION

### Preoperative management

**Assessment**
- Thorough preoperative assessment including history, physical examination, and review of any imaging studies (e.g., echocardiogram, CT scan)
- Determine the extent of trauma (ECG, ultrasound, cardiac biomarkers)
- Assess cardiac function and intracardiac volume
- Check for signs of heart failure or arrhythmias

**Monitoring**
- Continuous ECG monitoring to detect arrhythmias
- Consider invasive monitoring (e.g., arterial line, central venous pressure monitoring) for hemodynamic instability

**Medication review**
- Review current medications and their impact on cardiac function
- Discontinue medications that may exacerbate myocardial depression or arrhythmias

### Intraoperative management

**Anesthetic agents**
- Use agents with minimal myocardial depressant effects
- Prefer short-acting agents to allow rapid adjustment
- Avoid agents that can exacerbate arrhythmias (e.g., halothane, high doses of volatile anesthetics)

**Induction and maintenance**
- Induction should be slow and controlled to avoid sudden changes in heart rate and blood pressure
- Consider using etomidate (0.2-0.3 mg/kg IV) or ketamine (1-2 mg/kg IV) for induction due to their relatively stable hemodynamic profiles (0.2-0.5 mg/kg for anesthesia)
- Maintenance with a combination of low-dose volatile anesthetics (e.g., sevoflurane, titrated to effect, typically 0.5-2% end-tidal concentration) and opioids (e.g., fentanyl, 1-2 mcg/kg IV bolus, with additional doses as needed; continuous infusion at 0.5-1 mcg/kg/hr) to minimize myocardial depression

**Hemodynamic management**
- Maintain normovolemia and avoid both hypovolemia and fluid overload
- Use vasopressors or inotropes, e.g., norepinephrine (0.01-0.1 mcg/kg/min IV infusion, titrated to desired blood pressure), dobutamine (2-20 mcg/kg/min IV infusion, titrated to desired cardiac output) if needed to support blood pressure and cardiac output
- Avoid sudden changes in heart rate; beta-blockers (e.g., esmolol, 0.5 mg/kg IV bolus over 1 minute, followed by infusion at 50-200 mcg/kg/min) or calcium channel blockers (e.g., diltiazem, 0.25 mg/kg IV bolus over 2 minutes, followed by infusion at 5-15 mg/hr) may be required for rate control

**Monitoring**
- Continuous ECG monitoring for arrhythmias
- Invasive blood pressure monitoring for real-time assessment of hemodynamic status
- Consider transesophageal echocardiography (TEE) if available, especially in unstable patients or during major surgeries

### Postoperative management

**Monitoring**
- Continued close monitoring in a high-dependency unit or ICU
- Monitor for late arrhythmias and signs of myocardial dysfunction
- Perform regular follow-up echocardiography to monitor recovery

**Pain control**
- Adequate pain management to avoid sympathetic stimulation, which can exacerbate myocardial strain
- Use multimodal analgesia to minimize opioid requirements and their potential for respiratory depression
  - Acetaminophen: 1 g IV or PO every 6 hours
  - NSAIDs: (e.g., Ibuprofen) 400-800 mg PO every 6-8 hours, if not contraindicated
  - Local anesthetics: (e.g., lidocaine with adrenaline) dose based on surgical site and volume required

**Hemodynamic support**
- Continue supportive care to maintain adequate cardiac output and tissue perfusion
- Adjust medications based on postoperative cardiac function and hemodynamic status

## SUGGESTED READING

- Thiele H, Ohman EM, Desch S, Eitel I, de Waha S. Management of cardiogenic shock. European Heart Journal. 2015;36(20):1223-30.
- Van Lieshout EMM, Verhofstad MHJ, Van Silfhout DJT, Dubois EA. Diagnostic approach for myocardial contusion: a retrospective evaluation of patient data and review of the literature. Eur J Trauma Emerg Surg. 2021;47(4):1259-1272.

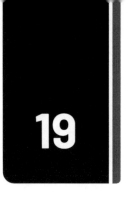

# CARDIAC IMPLANTABLE ELECTRONIC DEVICES (CIEDS)

## LEARNING OBJECTIVES

- Preoperative assessment and precautions for patients with a CIED
- Intraoperative and postoperative management of patients with a CIED

## DEFINITION AND MECHANISM

- Cardiac implantable electronic device (CIED) refers to any permanently implantable cardiac pacemaker or any implantable cardioverter–defibrillator (ICD), as well as any cardiac resynchronization therapy device

| Possible perioperative adverse events | |
|---|---|
| Device function | Oversensing: Resulting in asystole<br>Pacemaker mediated tachycardia<br>Failure of CRT function: Resulting in exacerbation of heart failure<br>Lead damage/migration: With insertion of Central Venous Catheters<br>Inability to place magnet or magnet displacement: Prone position<br>MRI-related risks: Magnet switch closure, myocardial injury, reprogramming, lead failure, inappropriate high pacing.<br>Inappropriate ICD firing (Cardioversion or defibrillation)<br>CRT causing Torsade de Pointes.<br>Inappropriate management of ICD with Pacemaker function by magnet placement: Will not turn Pacemaker into asynchronous mode.<br>Activation of rate modulation at upper limit: Ventilator is interpreted as "exercise"<br>Inappropriate reprogramming of asynchronous mode to a heart rate that is insufficient to meet patient's metabolic demands under surgery.<br>Inappropriate reprogramming of asynchronous mode to a lower heart rate not fast enough to override the patient's native rhythm and therefore competes with it (R on T phenomenon).<br>Direct damage to pulse generator. |
| Clinical | Hypotension<br>Tachyarrhythmia and bradyarrhythmia<br>Myocardial tissue damage<br>Myocardial ischemia and infarction |

## MAGNET USE

- Electromagnetic radiation properties and CIED distance from the magnet, as well as CIED design, materials, shielding, programming, sensitivity, and filtering properties, modulate the extent of the magnet interference and effect on function of the CIED
- Application of a magnet to pacemaker produces an asynchronous mode of pacing to protect a patient from the effects of electromagnetic interference
- A magnet can be secured over the pulse generator of an ICD to suspend the arrhythmia detection function and prevent discharge. Subsequent removal of the magnet promptly reactivates the ICD

## MANAGEMENT

- **Preoperative**
  - Determine whether the patient has a CIED
  - Determine the CIED type, manufacturer, and primary indication for placement
  - Determine whether the patient is pacing-dependent
  - Determine the CIED's current settings and that it is functioning properly by interrogating the cardiac implantable electronic device or obtaining the most recent interrogation report
  - Determine possible sources of electromagnetic interference:
    - Electrosurgery (monopolar > bipolar)
    - Evoked potential monitors
    - Nerve stimulators Twitch/Train of Four (TOF) monitors, peripheral nerve stimulators or spinal cord stimulators)
    - Fasciculations
    - Shivering
    - Large tidal volumes
    - External defibrillation
    - Magnetic resonance imaging
    - Radiofrequency ablation or lesioning
    - Extracorporeal shock wave lithotripsy
    - Electroconvulsive therapy
  - Determine precautions:
    - See infographic

Cardiac implantable electronic devices (CIEDs)

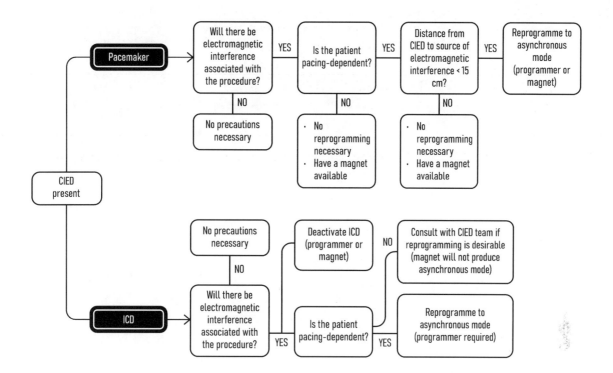

- **Intraoperative**
  - Continuously monitor and display the electrocardiogram and $SpO_2$
  - Perform continuous peripheral pulse monitoring for all patients
  - If unanticipated CIED interactions occur, temporarily suspend the procedure until the source of interference can be identified and eliminated or managed
  - Interference source management:

| Intraoperative | |
|---|---|
| Electrosurgery | Position the electrode so that the current does not pass through or near the CIED generator and leads Avoid proximity of the electrical current to the generator or leads When possible, use bipolar electrosurgery instead of monopolar When monopolar electrosurgery is necessary, use intermittent and irregular bursts at the lowest feasible energy levels Use an ultrasonic (harmonic) scalpel If monopolar electrosurgery is planned superior to the umbilicus, ensure that the pacing function is altered to an asynchronous pacing mode in pacing-dependent patients and suspend an ICD's antitachycardia function, if present. Ensure that the patient is in a monitored environment |
| Radiofrequency ablation | Keep the radiofrequency current path (electrode tip to current return pad) as far away from the generator and leads as possible If radiofrequency ablation is planned superior to the umbilicus, ensure that the pacing function is altered to an asynchronous pacing mode in pacing-dependent patients and suspend an ICD's antitachycardia function, if present. Ensure that the patient is in a monitored environment |
| Lithotripsy | Avoid focus of the lithotripsy beam near the generator |

Cardiac implantable electronic devices (CIEDs)

| Intraoperative | |
|---|---|
| Magnetic resonance imaging (MRI) | Move the patient outside of the immediate MRI area |
| | Interrogate the CIED before the MRI scan |
| | Suspend the antitachycardia function of an ICD before the MRI scan |
| | Alter the pacing function to an asynchronous pacing mode in pacing-dependent patients before the MRI scan |
| | Ensure that someone capable of programming the CIED remains in attendance for the duration of the MRI scan |
| | Ensure that someone capable of performing advanced life support remains in attendance for the duration of the MRI scan |
| | Reinterrogate the CIED and restore its permanent settings after the MRI is completed |
| Radiofrequency identification devices | Avoid the use of these devices in close proximity to the CIED |
| | Monitor for signs of electromagnetic interference and be prepared to stop using the radiofrequency identification device if interference occurs |
| Electroconvulsive therapy | Alter the pacing function to an asynchronous pacing mode in pacing-dependent patients |
| | Suspend an IDC's antitachycardia function, if present |
| | Monitor for and be prepared to manage postconvulsive sinus tachycardia |
| | Monitor for and treat ventricular arrhythmias that may occur secondary to the hemodynamic effects of electroconvulsive therapy |

## EMERGENCY CARDIOVERSION OR DEFIBRILLATION

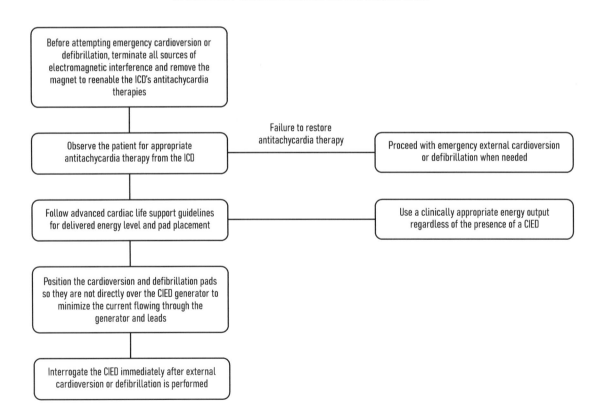

- **Postoperative**

# CARDIAC IMPLANTABLE ELECTRONIC DEVICES: POSTOPERATIVE MANAGEMENT

Continue to monitor and display cardiac rate and rhythm as indicated by the patient's medical condition

For a CIED that was reprogrammed pre- or intraoperatively:
- Ensure that back-up pacing and cardioversion-defibrillation equipment are immediately available until the CIED's permanent settings are restored (e.g., until the antitachycardia function of an ICD is reenabled)
- Ensure the cardiac rate and rhythm are continuously monitored and displayed until the CIED's permanent settings are restored
- Ensure the patient remains in a monitored environment until the CIED's permanent settings are restored

Perform a postoperative CIED interrogation whenever:
- Emergency surgery occurred without appropriate preoperative CIED evaluation
- There is suspicion that antitachycardia therapy might have been disabled rather than temporarily suspended with magnet placement
- The delivery of antitachycardia therapy was observed or suspected
- There is concern for CIED malfunction (i.e., significant electromagnetic interference occurred in close proximity to the CIED, an invasive procedure was performed in close proximity to a CIED generator or lead, or large fluid shifts occurred)

If interrogation determines that the CIED settings are inappropriate, reprogram to newly appropriate settings

---

**SUGGESTED READING**

- Practice advisory for the perioperative management of patients with cardiac implantable electronic devices: pacemakers and implantable cardioverter-defibrillators 2020. Apfelbaum JL, Schulman PM, Mahajan A, Connis RT, Agarkar M. Anesthesiology. 2020;132:225-252.
- Stone ME, Salter B, Fischer A. Perioperative management of patients with cardiac implantable electronic devices. British Journal of Anaesthesia. 2011;107:i16-i26.
- Thomas H, Plummer C, Wright IJ, Foley P, Turley AJ. Guidelines for the peri-operative management of people with cardiac implantable electronic devices: Guidelines from the British Heart Rhythm Society. Anaesthesia. 2022;77(7):808-817.

Cardiac implantable electronic devices (CIEDs)

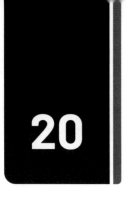

# CARDIAC TAMPONADE

## LEARNING OBJECTIVES

- Describe the overall mechanisms of cardiac tamponade
- Recognize sings and symptoms of cardiac tamponade
- Diagnose cardiac tamponade
- Anesthetic management of patients with cardiac tamponade

## DEFINITION AND MECHANISM

- Cardiac tamponade is characterized by compression of the heart chambers caused by an accumulation of fluid in the pericardial space
- Common causes:
  - Pericarditis
  - Tuberculosis
  - Trauma
  - Malignancy
  - Aortic dissection
  - Iatrogenic after cardiac surgery and invasive procedures
- Intrapericardial pressure increases, causing an increase in right (RV) and left ventricular (LV) filling pressures
- Increased intrapericardial pressure eventually compresses all the cardiac chambers causing a decrease in cardiac output
- Tamponade leads to an exaggerated shift of the interventricular septum to the left during inspiration resulting in impairment of LV filling
- Decrease in systemic arterial pressure by > 10 mmHg during inspiration (pulsus paradoxus)
- Crucial factors in the development of tamponade:
  - Rate of fluid accumulation relative to the pericardial stretch
  - Presence or absence of compensatory mechanisms
- Gradually developing effusions are largely asymptomatic, rapidly accumulating effusions can present with tamponade

## SIGNS & SYMPTOMS

- Symptoms:
  - Dyspnea (usually the first and most sensitive)
  - Orthopnea
  - Chest discomfort
- Clinical manifestations are consistent with low cardiac output and high central venous pressure:
  - Low mean arterial pressure
  - Cool peripheries
  - Signs of poor end-organ perfusion (e.g., low urine output)
- Palpating the pulse reveals an apparent variation in pulse volume due to pulsus paradoxus
- Jugular venous pressure is typically increased, with distended neck veins apparent
- Sympathetic tone is increased and manifests as tachycardia, diaphoresis, anxiety and poor distal perfusion
- A pericardial rub might be heard on auscultation in patients with inflammatory pericardial disease

## DIAGNOSIS

- Chest X-ray: Enlarged globular cardiac silhouette in chronic large pericardial effusions
- ECG:
  - QRS complexes may be lower in amplitude
  - Sinus tachycardia is common
  - Atrial dysrhythmias may be present
  - Beat-to-beat variation in both the amplitude and axis of the QRS complexes may be present in patients with large effusions
- Transthoracic (TTE) or transesophageal echocardiography (TEE): determine the size, location, and hemodynamic effects of the pericardial effusion:

  - Effusions up to 10 mm in thickness during diastole are considered small, between 10 and 20 mm are considered moderate, and greater than 20 mm are considered large
  - Collapse of the cardiac chambers
  - Inferior vena cava dilatation
  - Increased respiratory variation in the intracardiac blood flow measured with Doppler
  - Excessive leftward shift of the interventricular septum during spontaneous inspiration
- Differential diagnoses:
  - Epicardial fat
  - Pleural effusions

Cardiac tamponade

# ANESTHETIC MANAGEMENT

### HEMODYNAMIC GOALS (FULL, FAST, FORWARD, STRONG)

- Maintain or ideally augment preload, particularly in patients with hypovolemia
- Avoid bradycardia, treat promptly if it occurs
- Maintain sinus rhythm
- Maintain systemic vascular resistance (SVR)
- Maintaining compensatory cardiovascular mechanisms (tachycardia and raised SVR) during the induction of anesthesia is essential.
- Maintain contractility
- Avoid myocardial depressants

### PREOPERATIVE MANAGEMENT

- Emergency medications should be available before induction:
  - Vasopressors (metaraminol, ephedrine, norepinephrine)
  - Inotropes (epinephrine)
- Attach defibrillator pads before induction

### INTRAOPERATIVE MANAGEMENT

- Ideal induction choice: Minimal effect on heart rate, contractility and SVR (e.g., ketamine, etomidate, midazolam)
- Spontaneous breathing techniques may be advantageous for induction
- Invasive arterial pressure monitoring is essential
- Central venous access is desirable, but should not delay urgent pericardial drainage
- Provide large bore IV cannula with running intravenous fluids to restore preload and ensure vasopressors reach their targets
- Avoid high positive end-expiratory pressure and large tidal volumes
- Maintain anesthesia with a balanced technique using volatile inhalation agents, intravenous opioids, ketamine and short- or intermediate-acting neuromuscular blocking agents
- Intraoperative transesophageal echocardiography can be useful to monitor hemodynamic management
- Deepen anesthesia and reduce vasopressors when rebound hypertension occurs

### POSTOPERATIVE MANAGEMENT

- Analgesia: Long-acting opioids (morphine, oxycodone) or regional anesthesia (e.g., intercostal nerve block)

# KEEP IN MIND

- Cardiac tamponade is an emergency requiring immediate of the pressure effect of the pericardial fluid
- This is achieved by percutaenous or open surgical draining

## SUGGESTED READING

- Clinical Anesthesiology. 5th Edition, Morgan, GE, Mikhail, MS, Murray, MJ. Anesthesia for Cardiac Surgery. Cardiac Tamponade. 474-76.
- Essence of Anesthesia Practice: 4th Edition, Fleisher, LA, Roizen, Michael, F, Roizen. Cardiac Tamponade. 76.
- Madhivathanan PR, Corredor C, Smith A. Perioperative implications of pericardial effusions and cardiac tamponade. BJA Educ. 2020;20(7):226-234.

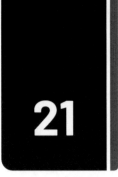

**21**

# CARDIOMYOPATHIES

## LEARNING OBJECTIVES

- Recognize the different classes of cardiomyopathies
- Anesthetic management of patients with cardiomyopathy

## DEFINITION AND MECHANISM

- Cardiomyopathy is a myocardial disorder in which the heart muscle is structurally and functionally abnormal
- Can be inherited or acquired
- Can affect all age groups
- Affects the shape, function, and electrical system of the heart
- Signs and symptoms can usually be managed successfully and patients can have a good life expectancy

## DILATED CARDIOMYOPATHY

- Dilatation of the left and right ventricles, impaired systolic function
- Major cause of heart failure and arrhythmia in young adults
- Two-thirds of cases are idiopathic
- Possible causes:
  - Familial association
  - Post-viral infection
  - Part of a disease process (ischemic heart disease, hypertension, diabetes, malformation syndrome, alcohol, neuromuscular disorder, inborn errors of metabolism, exposure to cardiotoxic agents)
- Asymptomatic in early stages
- Symptoms of heart failure (dyspnea, fatigue, ascites, peripheral edema, arrhythmias)
- Embolic events and sudden death may occur at a later stage
- Diagnosis: Echocardiography, chest radiograph, electrocardiography, blood tests, detailed medical and family history, physical examination

# MANAGEMENT

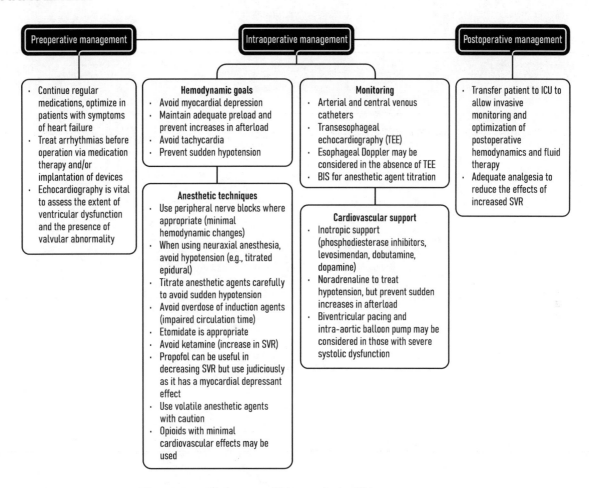

```
Preoperative management          Intraoperative management          Postoperative management
```

**Preoperative management**

- Continue regular medications, optimize in patients with symptoms of heart failure
- Treat arrhythmias before operation via medication therapy and/or implantation of devices
- Echocardiography is vital to assess the extent of ventricular dysfunction and the presence of valvular abnormality

**Hemodynamic goals**

- Avoid myocardial depression
- Maintain adequate preload and prevent increases in afterload
- Avoid tachycardia
- Prevent sudden hypotension

**Anesthetic techniques**

- Use peripheral nerve blocks where appropriate (minimal hemodynamic changes)
- When using neuraxial anesthesia, avoid hypotension (e.g., titrated epidural)
- Titrate anesthetic agents carefully to avoid sudden hypotension
- Avoid overdose of induction agents (impaired circulation time)
- Etomidate is appropriate
- Avoid ketamine (increase in SVR)
- Propofol can be useful in decreasing SVR but use judiciously as it has a myocardial depressant effect
- Use volatile anesthetic agents with caution
- Opioids with minimal cardiovascular effects may be used

**Monitoring**

- Arterial and central venous catheters
- Transesophageal echocardiography (TEE)
- Esophageal Doppler may be considered in the absence of TEE
- BIS for anesthetic agent titration

**Cardiovascular support**

- Inotropic support (phosphodiesterase inhibitors, levosimendan, dobutamine, dopamine)
- Noradrenaline to treat hypotension, but prevent sudden increases in afterload
- Biventricular pacing and intra-aortic balloon pump may be considered in those with severe systolic dysfunction

**Postoperative management**

- Transfer patient to ICU to allow invasive monitoring and optimization of postoperative hemodynamics and fluid therapy
- Adequate analgesia to reduce the effects of increased SVR

SVR, systemic vascular resistance; BIS, bispectral index; ICU, intensive care unit

# HYPERTROPHIC CARDIOMYOPATHY

- Hypertrophy of the left ventricle in the absence of other structural or functional abnormalities
- Inherited disease of the myocardium
- Hypertrophy can be asymmetrical, concentric, midventricular, apical, and can also involve the right ventricle
- Diastolic impairment of the left ventricle
- End-stage: Biventricular systolic dysfunction due to myocardial fibrosis
- 70% of cases have obstructive hypertrophy
- Majority of patients is asymptomatic
- Symptoms of angina and heart failure (dyspnea, chest pain, syncope, arrhythmia)
- Severe complications: Angina pectoris, heart failure, sudden death

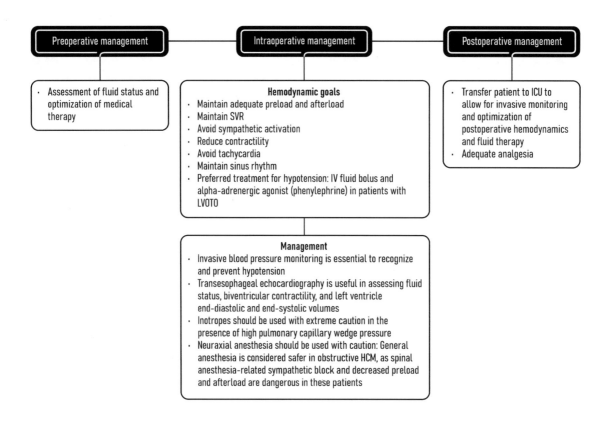

| Preoperative management | Intraoperative management | Postoperative management |
|---|---|---|

**Preoperative management**
- Assessment of fluid status and optimization of medical therapy

**Intraoperative management**

**Hemodynamic goals**
- Maintain adequate preload and afterload
- Maintain SVR
- Avoid sympathetic activation
- Reduce contractility
- Avoid tachycardia
- Maintain sinus rhythm
- Preferred treatment for hypotension: IV fluid bolus and alpha-adrenergic agonist (phenylephrine) in patients with LVOTO

**Management**
- Invasive blood pressure monitoring is essential to recognize and prevent hypotension
- Transesophageal echocardiography is useful in assessing fluid status, biventricular contractility, and left ventricle end-diastolic and end-systolic volumes
- Inotropes should be used with extreme caution in the presence of high pulmonary capillary wedge pressure
- Neuraxial anesthesia should be used with caution: General anesthesia is considered safer in obstructive HCM, as spinal anesthesia-related sympathetic block and decreased preload and afterload are dangerous in these patients

**Postoperative management**
- Transfer patient to ICU to allow for invasive monitoring and optimization of postoperative hemodynamics and fluid therapy
- Adequate analgesia

SVR, systemic vascular resistance; LVOTO, left ventricular outflow tract obstruction; HCM, hypertrophic cardiomyopathy

## RESTRICTIVE CARDIOMYOPATHY

- Impairment of ventricular diastolic function due to fibrotic or infiltrative changes in the myocardium and/or subendocardium
- Primary or secondary (amyloidosis, sarcoidosis, hemochromatosis, ischemic heart disease, hypertension, valvular disease)
- Symptoms of biventricular failure (dyspnea, orthopnea, fatigue, palpitation, edema, chest pain)
- On physical examination, patients may have an audible third heart sound, systolic murmur, raised jugular venous pressure, ascites, and peripheral edema
- Diagnosis: Echocardiography, endomyocardial biopsy, computed tomography, cardiac MRI

## MANAGEMENT

- General anesthesia causes vasodilation, suppresses the myocardium, and reduces venous return. The latter can be exacerbated by intermittent positive ventilation resulting in cardiac arrest.
- Invasive arterial blood pressure monitoring and transesophageal echocardiography are useful in identifying the causes of cardiovascular instability.
- Hemodynamic goals:
  - Maintain adequate preload, SVR, and sinus rhythm
  - Use an anesthetic agent with minimal cardiovascular effect (ketamine or etomidate)

# ARRHYTHMOGENIC RIGHT VENTRICLE CARDIOMYOPATHY

- Structural abnormalities and cardiac dysfunction of the right ventricle, can also involve left ventricle
- Complex genetic condition
- Other causes: Degenerative disease, infection, inflammation
- Usually starts as a localized disease with regional wall abnormalities
- Development of right bundle branch block followed by right ventricular failure between the fourth and fifth decades of life
- Young patients often present with arrhythmia, syncope, cardiac arrest, or sudden death
- 3 clinical phases:
  - Phase 1 (concealed disease): Some structural abnormality in the myocardium, patients can present with sudden cardiac death
  - Phase 2 (overt disease): Established structural abnormality of the myocardium, patients present with arrhythmias and syncope
  - Phase 3 (end-stage disease): Severe structural changes

# MANAGEMENT

- Arrhythmias of both supraventricular and ventricular origins may occur at any time
- Avoid hypovolemia, hypercarbia, acidosis and lighter depth of anesthesia
- Amiodarone is the first-line of medication to treat rhythm disturbances
- Placement of implantable cardioverter defibrillator is beneficial

━━━━━━━━━━━━━━━━━━━━━━━━━━━━ **SUGGESTED READING** ━━━━━━━━━━━━━

- Arbelo E, Protonotarios A, Gimeno JR, et al. 2023 ESC Guidelines for the management of cardiomyopathies: Developed by the task force on the management of cardiomyopathies of the European Society of Cardiology (ESC). European Heart Journal. 2023;44(37):3503-3626. doi:10.1093/eurheartj/ehad194
- Ciarambino T, Menna G, Sansone G, Giordano M. Cardiomyopathies: An Overview. Int J Mol Sci. 2021;22(14):7722.
- Ibrahim IR, Sharma V. Cardiomyopathy and anaesthesia. BJA Education. 2017;17(11):363-9.

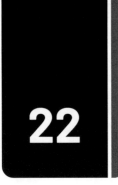

# CORONARY ARTERY DISEASE

## LEARNING OBJECTIVES

- Describe the general pathology of coronary artery disease
- Describe the risk factors for coronary artery disease
- Manage patients with coronary artery disease

## DEFINITION AND MECHANISM

- Coronary artery disease or ischemic heart disease is characterized by obstruction of oxygen supply to the cardiac muscle
- Results in a range of complications, including myocardial infarction, dysrhythmias, heart failure, deteriorating ventricular function, and sudden death
- May also coexist with other cardiac pathologies, including valvular lesions and cardiomyopathies
- Atheromatous disease remains the most common cause
- Ischemia results when myocardial oxygen demand increases beyond supply or when there is a rupture of a plaque which can precipitate thrombosis and result in complete occlusion of a coronary artery

| Risk factors | |
| --- | --- |
| Unmodifiable | Advancing age |
| | Male gender |
| | Family history of premature coronary artery disease |
| | Premature menopause |
| | Ethnicity (e.g., higher in those from the Indian subcontinent) |
| Modifiable | Smoking |
| | Diabetes mellitus |
| | Hypertension |
| | Obesity |
| | Sedentary lifestyle |
| | High cholesterol (specifically a high ratio of low- to high-density lipoprotein) |

# MANAGEMENT

## CORONARY ARTERY DISEASE MANAGEMENT

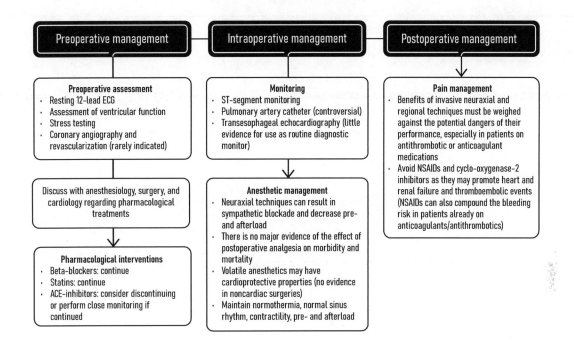

**Preoperative management**

**Preoperative assessment**
- Resting 12-lead ECG
- Assessment of ventricular function
- Stress testing
- Coronary angiography and revascularization (rarely indicated)

Discuss with anesthesiology, surgery, and cardiology regarding pharmacological treatments

**Pharmacological interventions**
- Beta-blockers: continue
- Statins: continue
- ACE-inhibitors: consider discontinuing or perform close monitoring if continued

**Intraoperative management**

**Monitoring**
- ST-segment monitoring
- Pulmonary artery catheter (controversial)
- Transesophageal echocardiography (little evidence for use as routine diagnostic monitor)

**Anesthetic management**
- Neuraxial techniques can result in sympathetic blockade and decrease pre- and afterload
- There is no major evidence of the effect of postoperative analgesia on morbidity and mortality
- Volatile anesthetics may have cardioprotective properties (no evidence in noncardiac surgeries)
- Maintain normothermia, normal sinus rhythm, contractility, pre- and afterload

**Postoperative management**

**Pain management**
- Benefits of invasive neuraxial and regional techniques must be weighed against the potential dangers of their performance, especially in patients on antithrombotic or anticoagulant medications
- Avoid NSAIDs and cyclo-oxygenase-2 inhibitors as they may promote heart and renal failure and thromboembolic events (NSAIDs can also compound the bleeding risk in patients already on anticoagulants/antithrombotics)

## SUGGESTED READING

- Malakar AK, Choudhury D, Halder B, Paul P, Uddin A, Chakraborty S. A review on coronary artery disease, its risk factors, and therapeutics. J Cell Physiol. 2019; 234: 16812–16823.
- Pollard BJ, Kitchen, G. Handbook of Clinical Anaesthesia. Fourth Edition. CRC Press. 2018. 978-1-4987-6289-2.
- Shahjehan RD, Bhutta BS. Coronary Artery Disease. [Updated 2023 Aug 17]. In: StatPearls [Internet]. Treasure Island (FL): StatPearls Publishing; 2024 Jan-. Available from: https://www.ncbi.nlm.nih.gov/books/NBK564304/

# INFECTIVE ENDOCARDITIS: PROPHYLAXIS

## LEARNING OBJECTIVES

- Understand the pathophysiology and risk factors of infective endocarditis
- Understand infective endocarditis prophylaxis strategies
- Anesthetic management of infective endocarditis

## DEFINITION AND MECHANISM

- Infective endocarditis (IE) is a life-threatening infection of the endothelial lining of the heart's chambers and heart valves

## PATHOPHYSIOLOGY

Infection of healthy tissue by highly virulent organisms such as staphylococcus aureus

- Manipulation of the gingiva/infected skin tissue
- Infected central line, chemo ports, PICC lines, other hardware

Transient bacteremia

Attachment of bacteria to the endothelial lining/valves of the heart

- Infection of healthy tissue by highly virulent organisms such as staphylococcus aureus

Note: Formation of a platelet/fibrin complex due to previous endocardial injury

Vegetation growth with possible formation of emboli and subsequent heart failure, ischemic cerebrovascular accident or secondary infections

| Risk factors | |
|---|---|
| High-risk patients | Any prosthetic heart valve<br>History of IE<br>Congenital heart disease (CHD):<br>- Any cyanotic type of CHD<br>- Any CHD repaired with prosthetic material, up to 6 months after the procedure or lifelong |
| Procedure-related risk factors | Incision of infected skin tissue<br>Dental or surgical procedures with manipulation of the gingiva<br>Root canal treatments<br>Root extractions |

# PROPHYLAXIS

- The absolute risk for IE is very low, and while antibiotics are given for the right indication to lower the incidence of IE, they do not prevent all cases of IE
- Antibiotic use poses the risk of anaphylaxis or bacterial resistance
- Consider the pros and cons when giving IE prophylaxis, only use antibiotics for high-risk patients undergoing high-risk procedures

|  | Infected skin tissue | Dental procedure |
|---|---|---|
| No allergy to penicillin or ampicillin | Flucloxacilline: 2 g oral, 30-60 min before procedure Child: 50 mg/kg (max. 1.5 g) | Amoxicillin: 2 g oral, 30-60 min before procedure Child: 50 mg/kg (max. 2 g) |
| Penicillin or ampicillin allergy or treatment with penicillin < 7 days ago | Clindamycin: 600 mg oral, 30-60 min before procedure Child: 20 mg/kg (max. 600 mg) | Clindamycin: 600 mg oral, 30-60 min before procedure Child: 20 mg/kg (max. 600 mg) |

- Use oral antibiotics as the first choice
- Alternatively, use cephalexin 2 g (50 mg/kg IV for children), cefazolin, or ceftriaxone 1 g IV (50 mg/kg IV for children)

# MANAGEMENT

```
                          ┌─────────────────────────┐
                          │  INFECTIVE ENDOCARDITIS  │
                          └─────────────────────────┘
```

| Preoperative management | Intraoperative management | Postoperative management |

### Preoperative management

- Evaluate cardiac function thoroughly, including echocardiography
- Assess for signs of heart failure, embolic phenomena, and systemic infection
- Perform blood cultures to identify causative organisms and guide antibiotic therapy
- Review any history of previous valve surgery or prosthetic valves

### Antibiotic prophylaxis

- Vancomycin: 15-20 mg/kg IV over 1-2 hours before surgery
- Gentamicin: 1 mg/kg IV every 8 hours, adjusted based on renal function
- Ensure timely dosing to maintain therapeutic levels throughout surgery

### Hemodynamic monitoring

- Monitor invasive arterial blood pressure
- Monitor central venous pressure (CVP)
- Consider using a pulmonary artery catheter or transesophageal echocardiography (TEE) for complex cases

### Induction of anesthesia

- Titrate anesthetic agents carefully to avoid hypotension
- Use etomidate 0.2-0.3 mg/kg IV for induction
- Use fentanyl 1-2 mcg/kg IV for analgesia
- Use rocuronium 0.6-1.2 mg/kg IV for muscle relaxation

### Maintenance of anesthesia

- Use a balanced anesthesia technique with a combination of volatile agents, intravenous agents, and opioids
- Maintain anesthesia with sevoflurane or isoflurane
- Infuse propofol 50-150 mcg/kg/min IV if using total intravenous anesthesia (TIVA)
- Infuse fentanyl or remifentanil IV for analgesia
- Monitor fluid status and urine output closely
- Avoid significant fluctuations in blood pressure to reduce the risk of embolization
- Weigh the risk of hemodynamic instability/collapse associated with RSI against the risk of aspiration

### Hemodynamic management

- Use vasopressors and inotropes as needed to maintain cardiac output and organ perfusion
- Infuse norepinephrine 0.02-0.1 mcg/kg/min IV for vasopressor support
- Infuse epinephrine 0.01-0.1 mcg/kg/min IV for inotropic support if needed
- Infuse dobutamine 2-20 mcg/kg/min IV for inotropic support
- Manage fluid balance carefully to avoid both hypovolemia and fluid overload

### Infection control

- Use strict aseptic technique to prevent further infections
- Avoid unnecessary invasive lines and catheters

### Temperature management

- Maintain normothermia using warming blankets or devices to reduce metabolic demand and prevent coagulopathy

### Postoperative management

- Monitor in the ICU for potential complications such as arrhythmias, heart failure, or embolic events
- Continue appropriate antibiotic therapy
- Monitor for signs of recurrent infection or complications related to endocarditis

---

## SUGGESTED READING

- Habib G, Lancellotti P, Antunes MJ, et al. 2015 ESC Guidelines for the management of infective endocarditis: The Task Force for the Management of Infective Endocarditis of the European Society of Cardiology (ESC). Endorsed by: European Association for Cardio-Thoracic Surgery (EACTS), the European Association of Nuclear Medicine (EANM). Eur Heart J. 2015;36(44):3075-3128.
- Hermanns H, Eberl S, Terwindt LE, et al. Anesthesia Considerations in Infective Endocarditis. Anesthesiology. 2022;136(4):633-656.
- Miao H, Zhang Y, Zhang Y, Zhang J. Update on the epidemiology, diagnosis, and management of infective endocarditis: A review. Trends Cardiovasc Med. Published online January 8, 2024.

Intraoperative arrhythmias

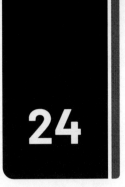

# INTRAOPERATIVE ARRHYTHMIAS

## LEARNING OBJECTIVES

- Define and classify arrhythmias
- Describe the patient, anesthetic, and surgical risk factors for developing intraoperative arrhythmias
- Management of intraoperative arrhythmias

## DEFINITION AND MECHANISM

- Arrhythmias are accelerated, slowed, or irregular heartbeats caused by abnormalities in the electrical impulses of the myocardium
- 60% of patients may experience perioperative arrhythmias
- The majority are benign, but rhythm disturbances can be associated with potentially serious adverse outcomes

## CLASSIFICATION

### Bradyarrhythmia (HR < 60 bpm)

- Sinus arrhythmia: Sinus bradycardia
- Conduction defects
  - AV blocks
    - First-degree AV block
    - Second-degree AV block
    - Third-degree AV block
  - Intraventricular blocks
    - Right bundle branch block
    - Left bundle branch block
  - Fascicular block
    - Left anterior hemiblock
    - Right anterior hemiblock
  - Bifascicular block
  - Trifascicular block

### Tachyarrhythmia (HR > 100 bpm)

- Sinus arrhythmia: Sinus tachycardia
- Supraventricular arrhythmias
  - Premature atrial contraction
  - Supraventricular tachycardia
  - Atrial flutter
  - Atrial fibrillation
- Ventricular arrhythmias
  - Premature ventricular contractions
  - Ventricular tachycardia
  - Ventricular fibrillation
  - Torsade de pointes

## COMPLICATIONS

- Blood clots (i.e., thromboembolism)
- Stroke
- Heart failure
- Sudden death

## RISK FACTORS

### Patient factors

- Preexisting arrhythmias
- Coronary artery disease
- Hypertension
- Congestive heart failure
- Electrolyte disorders (especially potassium, magnesium, and calcium)
- Valvular heart disease
- Obstructive sleep apnea
- Medications:
  - β2-agonists
  - Theophylline
  - Tricyclic antidepressants
- Less common causes:
  - Thyroid disease (i.e., hypothyroidism, hyperthyroidism)
  - Cardiomyopathies (including alcoholic)
  - Myocarditis
  - Trauma (myocardial or intracranial)
  - Connective tissue disorders
  - Smoking
- Drug and solvent abuse

*Anesthetic factors*

- Hypotension or hypertension (e.g., inadequate anesthesia)
- Hypoxia
- Hypercarbia
- Direct laryngoscopy and intubation
- Central nervous pressure lines (irritation by line tip; microshock hazard, advancement of guide wire)
- Medications
  - Volatile anesthetic agents
  - Local anesthetics
  - Suxamethonium
  - Pancuronium
  - Note that multiple medications prolong the QT interval (e.g., volatile agents, macrolide antibiotics, butyrophenone antipsychotics, amiodarone, and ondansetron)
- 4Hs and 4Ts
  - Hypovolemia, hypoxemia, hyper/hypokalemia (electrolyte disorders) metabolic disorders (acidosis), and hypo/hyperthermia
  - Tension pneumothorax, tamponade, toxins/drugs and thromboembolism (pulmonary/cardiac)

*Surgical factors*

- Catecholamines
  - Endogenous (from any surgical stimulus)
  - Exogenous (topical or infiltrated epinephrine or faulty intravascular injection)
- Autonomic stimulation
  - Peritoneal and visceral traction
  - Peritoneal insufflation
  - Trigeminovagal reflexes (oculocardiac reflex)
  - Laryngoscopy, bronchoscopy, esophagoscopy
  - Carotid artery and thyroid surgery
- Direct stimulation of the heart during cardiac or thoracic surgery
- Embolism
  - Thrombus
  - Fat
  - Bone cement
  - Air
  - Carbon dioxide
  - Amniotic fluid
- Other
  - Aortic cross-clamping
  - Limb reperfusion
  - Glycine intoxication
  - TURP syndrome

## TREATMENT GOALS

- Prevent thromboembolism formation
- Control heart rate
- Correct the condition causing the arrhythmia
- Reduce other risk factors for heart disease and stroke

## MANAGEMENT

- Assess and monitor the patient's hemodynamic status continuously
- Ensure the availability of advanced cardiac life support (ACLS) equipment and medications
- Identify and correct reversible causes and note that more than one factor is likely to contribute to the development of intraoperative arrhythmias
- Identify the rhythm and evaluate the significance of arrhythmias in the context of:
  - Coexisting medical problems and their treatment
  - Surgical condition
  - Operative procedure
  - Anesthetic medications and technique
  - Hemodynamic effects of the arrhythmia and the risk of progression to fatal arrhythmias
- Be prepared for potential escalation to defibrillation and/or cardiopulmonary resuscitation (CPR) if arrhythmias progress to cardiac arrest

Intraoperative arrhythmias

## INTRAOPERATIVE ARRHYTHMIAS: MANAGEMENT

### Tachyarrhythmias

- Synchronized direct current (DC) cardioversion is preferred in the already anesthetized patient, especially in case of hemodynamic instability
- Consider antiarrhythmic medications depending on the arrhythmia and patient factors
- Pharmacological options:
  - **Ventricular tachycardia**: Amiodarone 300 mg over 10-60 minutes followed by 900 mg over 24 hours (ideally via central venous access)
  - **Polymorphic ventricular tachycardia (torsades)**: Magnesium 2 mg (8 mmol) over 10 minutes
  - **Supraventricular tachycardia**: Adenosine rapid boluses of 6 mg, (12 mg via a large-bore proximal cannula)
  - **Atrial fibrillation**: β-blockers (e.g., esmolol 50-200 mcg/kg/min infusion), digoxin 500 mcg over 1 hour (± repeat), amiodarone or calcium channel blocker (e.g., Diltiazem)
  - **Atrial flutter**: β-blockers
- Be aware of the negative inotropic effect of many antiarrhythmics
- It can be difficult to distinguish supraventricular tachycardia from ventricular tachycardia in patients with existing conduction abnormalities (e.g., bundle branch block)

| Ventricular tachycardia | Supraventricular tachycardia |
|---|---|
| · VT is primarily based on the presence of a wide QRS complex (≥ 120 ms) with a specific morphology<br>· Axis change from previous ECG<br>· Deep S wave in V6<br>· Fusion beats<br>· Capture beats | · SVT is based on the presence of a narrow QRS complex (< 120 ms)<br>· No axis change and same pattern of bundle branch block as pre-SVT ECG<br>· Conforms to right or left bundle branch block pattern<br>· Dominant R in V1 and Q in V6 |

### Bradyarrhythmias

- Glycopyrrolate or atropine to antagonize the excessive vagal tone (e.g., from peritoneal or ocular traction)
- A complete heart block is unlikely to respond to anticholinergics → requires pacing
- Use positive chronotropic catecholamines (e.g., isoprenaline) as a bridging measure

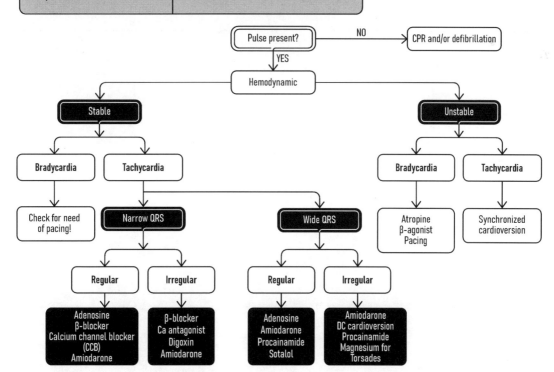

Pulse present? — NO → CPR and/or defibrillation
YES ↓
Hemodynamic

**Stable**
- Bradycardia → Check for need of pacing!
- Tachycardia
  - **Narrow QRS**
    - Regular → Adenosine / β-blocker / Calcium channel blocker (CCB) / Amiodarone
    - Irregular → β-blocker / Ca antagonist / Digoxin / Amiodarone
  - **Wide QRS**
    - Regular → Adenosine / Amiodarone / Procainamide / Sotalol
    - Irregular → Amiodarone / DC cardioversion / Procainamide / Magnesium for Torsades

**Unstable**
- Bradycardia → Atropine / β-agonist / Pacing
- Tachycardia → Synchronized cardioversion

## PREVENTION

- Keep surgical manipulations that can precipitate arrhythmias to a minimum
- An adequate depth of anesthesia may prevent or control intraoperative arrhythmias
- Prevent hypoxia, hypotension, hypovolemia, and hypothermia during surgery

━━━ **SUGGESTED READING** ━━━

- Kim CJ, Lever N, Cooper JO. Antiarrhythmic drugs and anaesthesia: part 1. mechanisms of cardiac arrhythmias. BJA Education. 2023;23(1):8-16. doi:10.1016/j.bjae.2022.11.001
- Noor ZM. Md. Life-Threatening Cardiac Arrhythmias during Anesthesia and Surgery. Cardiac Arrhythmias - Translational Approach from Pathophysiology to Advanced Care. 2021. doi: 10.5772/intechopen.101371.
- Pollard BJ, Kitchen G. Handbook of Clinical Anaesthesia. 4th ed. Taylor & Francis group; 2018. Chapter 30 Management problems, Shelton C.

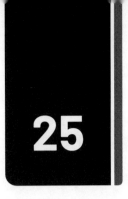

**25**

# MITRAL REGURGITATION

## LEARNING OBJECTIVES

- Describe and classify mitral regurgitation
- Describe the causes and mechanisms of mitral regurgitation
- Manage patients with mitral regurgitation

## DEFINITION AND MECHANISM

- Mitral regurgitation (MR) can be acute or chronic in onset, and primary or secondary in nature
- Primary MR is due to pathology of the valve preventing normal closure
- Secondary MR is caused by left ventricle dysfunction that affects the closing of the mitral valve
- The left atrium dilates as blood is ejected back into it
- Atrial fibrillation is common
- Overload of the pulmonary circulation causes dyspnea
- The LV is volume overloaded, with the dilation of the ventricle further exacerbating MR
- Acute MR:
  - Can be caused by any disruption to the normal mechanism of the valve (growth of vegetations on the leaflets in infective endocarditis, chordae rupture in patients with pre-existing degenerative disease, or papillary muscle due to an ST-elevation myocardial infarction)
  - The left atrium is unable to compensate acutely for the increased pressure caused by blood flowing back into it
  - Patients can present with sudden-onset dyspnea and require rapid stabilization and treatment
- Chronic MR:
  - Primary: Abnormality of the leaflets that prevents them from closing normally
  - Secondary: Anatomy of the valve is normal, but its function is impaired due to left ventricle pathology

## CLASSIFICATION

- Transesophageal echocardiography remains the gold standard for defining the severity of the MR:

|  | Mild | Moderate | Severe |
|---|---|---|---|
| Regurgitant fraction | < 30% | 30–49 | ≥ 50% |
| Regurgitant orifice area | < 0.20 cm² | 0.2–0.39 cm² | ≥ 0.40 cm² |
| Regurgitant volume | < 30 mL/beat | 30–59 mL/beat | ≥ 60 mL/beat |

## TREATMENT

- Medical
  - Acute MR: Filling pressure reduction with nitrates or diuretics and afterload reduction with vasodilators or an intra-aortic balloon pump as bridging to definitive treatment
  - Chronic MR: Treatment is in line with standard heart failure management including β-blockers, angiotensin-converting enzyme inhibitors, and aldosterone antagonists, with diuretics where heart failure is present
- Surgical
  - Primary MR:
    - Surgery is indicated if the MR is severe and acute in nature and if the MR is chronic and causing symptoms, with no contraindications to surgery
    - Valve repair, rather than replacement, is preferred
  - Secondary MR:
    - In symptomatic patients with severe left ventricle failure, the benefits of surgery are controversial unless the underlying condition can be reversed

# MANAGEMENT

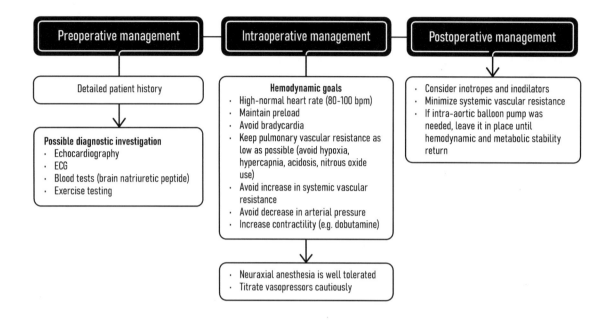

**Preoperative management**

Detailed patient history

**Possible diagnostic investigation**
- Echocardiography
- ECG
- Blood tests (brain natriuretic peptide)
- Exercise testing

**Intraoperative management**

**Hemodynamic goals**
- High-normal heart rate (80-100 bpm)
- Maintain preload
- Avoid bradycardia
- Keep pulmonary vascular resistance as low as possible (avoid hypoxia, hypercapnia, acidosis, nitrous oxide use)
- Avoid increase in systemic vascular resistance
- Avoid decrease in arterial pressure
- Increase contractility (e.g. dobutamine)

- Neuraxial anesthesia is well tolerated
- Titrate vasopressors cautiously

**Postoperative management**
- Consider inotropes and inodilators
- Minimize systemic vascular resistance
- If intra-aortic balloon pump was needed, leave it in place until hemodynamic and metabolic stability return

## SUGGESTED READING

- Apostolidou E, Maslow AD, Poppas A. Primary mitral valve regurgitation: Update and review. Glob Cardiol Sci Pract. 2017 Mar 31;2017(1):e201703.
- Hin J-H, Lee E-H, Choi D-K, Choi I-C. The Effect of Depth of Anesthesia on the Severity of Mitral Regurgitation as Measured by Transesophageal Echocardiography. Journal of Cardiothoracic and Vascular Anesthesia. 2012;26(6):994-998.
- Holmes K, Gibbison B, Vohra HA. Mitral valve and mitral valve disease. BJA Education. 2017;17(1):1-9.

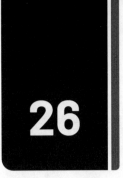

# MITRAL STENOSIS

## LEARNING OBJECTIVES

- Describe the causes and subsequent pathophysiology of mitral stenosis
- Classify the severity of mitral stenosis
- Anesthetic management of mitral stenosis

## DEFINITION AND MECHANISM

- Mitral stenosis occurs when the mitral valve is narrowed and blood cannot flow normally

| Causes | |
| --- | --- |
| Common | Rheumatic fever<br>Degenerative calcification<br>Endocarditis |
| Uncommon | Infiltrating diseases<br>Congenital deformities<br>Diseases that affect multiple systems (e.g., sarcoidosis) |

## SIGNS & SYMPTOMS

- Patients will remain asymptomatic for many years (compensation due to the compliant left atrium dilating and keeping pulmonary venous pressures stable)
- As the disease progresses, compensation is overcome and pulmonary hypertension develops
- Pulmonary edema and dyspnea
- Fatigue
- More frequent lower respiratory tract infections
- Atrial fibrillation, a possible consequence of left atrial dilation, will rapidly progress the pathophysiology

## SEVERITY ASSESSMENT

| | Mild | Moderate | Severe |
| --- | --- | --- | --- |
| Mean pressure decrease | < 5 mmHg | 6–10 mmHg | > 10 mmHg |
| Pressure half-time | < 139 ms | 140–219 ms | ≥ 220 ms |
| Valve area | 1.6–2.0 cm² | 1.5–1.0 cm² | < 1.0 cm² |

# MANAGEMENT

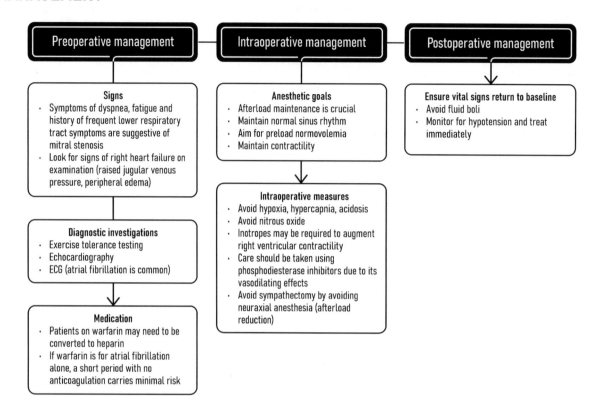

**Preoperative management** → **Intraoperative management** → **Postoperative management**

**Signs**
- Symptoms of dyspnea, fatigue and history of frequent lower respiratory tract symptoms are suggestive of mitral stenosis
- Look for signs of right heart failure on examination (raised jugular venous pressure, peripheral edema)

**Diagnostic investigations**
- Exercise tolerance testing
- Echocardiography
- ECG (atrial fibrillation is common)

**Medication**
- Patients on warfarin may need to be converted to heparin
- If warfarin is for atrial fibrillation alone, a short period with no anticoagulation carries minimal risk

**Anesthetic goals**
- Afterload maintenance is crucial
- Maintain normal sinus rhythm
- Aim for preload normovolemia
- Maintain contractility

**Intraoperative measures**
- Avoid hypoxia, hypercapnia, acidosis
- Avoid nitrous oxide
- Inotropes may be required to augment right ventricular contractility
- Care should be taken using phosphodiesterase inhibitors due to its vasodilating effects
- Avoid sympathectomy by avoiding neuraxial anesthesia (afterload reduction)

**Ensure vital signs return to baseline**
- Avoid fluid boli
- Monitor for hypotension and treat immediately

## SUGGESTED READING

- Harb, S.C., Griffin, B.P. Mitral Valve Disease: a Comprehensive Review. Curr Cardiol Rep 19, 73 (2017).
- Holmes K, Gibbison B, Vohra HA. Mitral valve and mitral valve disease. BJA Education. 2017;17(1):1-9.
- Nishimura RA, Otto CM, Bonow RO, et al. 2014 AHA/ACC guideline for the management of patients with valvular heart disease: a report of the American College of Cardiology/ American Heart Association Task Force on Practice Guidelines. J Am Coll Cardiol 2014; 63:e57.

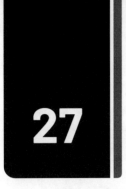

# PULMONARY HYPERTENSION (PH)

**27**

## LEARNING OBJECTIVES

- Describe the definition, clinical classes and treatment of pulmonary hypertension
- Manage patients with pulmonary hypertension

## DEFINITION AND MECHANISM

- Pulmonary hypertension is defined as a mean pulmonary artery pressure (MPAP) > 25 mmHg at rest or 30 mmHg on exercise
- The cause of pulmonary hypertension is of critical importance as it defines subsequent treatment
- Patients are classified into five clinical groups:
  - Group 1: Pulmonary arterial hypertension (PAH): Idiopathic PAH, connective tissue disease-associated PAH, and congenital heart disease (mainly Eisenmenger syndrome) are the most common subgroups; others include aortopulmonary, HIV and drug/toxin-induced PAH
  - Group 2: PH associated with increased pulmonary capillary wedge pressure (post-capillary PH), due to left-sided heart disease
  - Group 3: Lung disease and chronic hypoxia-related PH
  - Group 4: Predominantly chronic thromboembolic PH (CTEPH)
  - Group 5: PH caused by multisystemic disorders or multiple/unknown mechanisms, including sarcoidosis and hematological conditions
- Adequate coupling of the right ventricle to the pulmonary circulation is essential for maintaining cardiac output in patients with PH

## TREATMENT

- Pulmonary vasodilator therapy is predominantly indicated for the treatment of patients with Group 1 PH and Group 4 PH, although the treatment of choice for CTEPH is pulmonary endarterectomy
- Management of PH in patients with Group 2 and 3 PH is focussed on the underlying heart or lung disease
- Transplantation (usually bilateral lung) remains the ultimate treatment option in PAH when other treatments fail

## MANAGEMENT

```
PULMONARY HYPERTENSION (PH) ANESTHETIC MANAGEMENT
```

| Preoperative management | Intraoperative management | Postoperative management |
|---|---|---|

**Preoperative management**

Due to the **high risk of complications**, consider non-surgical or local/regional anesthesia alternatives

↓

Perform planned procedures in centers with PH specialist support

↓

**Preoperative risk assessment**
- Detailed assessment of RV function
- Minimize procedure-related risk factors
- Optimize pulmonary hemodynamics/RV function

↓

Modify and/or escalate pulmonary vasodilator therapy as needed

**Intraoperative management**

**Hemodynamic goals**
- Ensure the right ventricle maintains a sinus rhythm with a heart rate in the upper normal range
- Optimize RV filling
- Maintain RV perfusion & inotropy
- Decrease PVR
- Avoid hypoxia, hypercarbia, acidosis, hypothermia, sympathetic stimulation

**Monitoring**
- Invasive hemodynamic monitoring with measurement of central venous pressures and systemic arterial pressures

**Postoperative management**

Prolonged hemodynamic monitoring for at least 48-72h on ICU/HDU

**Acute PH crisis management**
- Treat hypotension (norepinephrine up to 0.5 µg/kg/min, vasopressin up to 0.04 units/min) without stopping pulmonary vasodilators
- Reduce postoperative PVR (inhaled NO, prostacyclin, iliprost, milrinone, sildenafil)
- Optimize preload, contractility, afterload (dobutamine, dopamine, milrinone)
- Extracorporeal membrane oxygenation to support the RV can be used as a bridge to recovery or transplantation

RV, right ventricle; PVR, pulmonary vascular resistance; ICU, intensive care unit; HDU, high dependency unit.

**SUGGESTED READING**

- Elliot CA, Kiely DG. Pulmonary hypertension. Continuing Education in Anaesthesia Critical Care & Pain. 2006;6(1):17-22.
- Price LC, Martinez G, Brame A, et al. Perioperative management of patients with pulmonary hypertension undergoing non-cardiothoracic, non-obstetric surgery: a systematic review and expert consensus statement. British Journal of Anaesthesia. 2021;126(4):774-790.
- Price L, Brame A, Martinez G, Mukerjee B, Harries C, Kempny A, et al. Perioperative management of patients with Pulmonary Hypertension undergoing Non-Cardiac Surgery. A Systemic Review and UK Consensus Statement. European Respiratory Journal. 2020;56(suppl 64):1467.

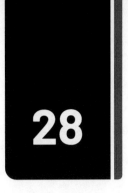

# QT PROLONGATION

**28**

## LEARNING OBJECTIVES

- Describe the underlying mechanisms of QT prolongation
- Manage patients with QT prolongation in the perioperative period
- Treat Torsade de Pointes

## DEFINITION AND MECHANISM

- The QT interval is a measure of the time between the start of the Q wave and the end of the T wave and represents the time taken for ventricular depolarization and repolarization
- QT prolongation is caused by malfunction of cardiac ion channels impairing ventricular repolarization
- This predisposes to the development of the polymorphic ventricular tachycardia torsade de pointes
- May revert spontaneously back to sinus rhythm causing syncope or degenerate to ventricular fibrillation causing sudden death
- Can be congenital (mutations in ion channel genes) or acquired (caused by drugs, neurological injury or metabolic abnormalities)
- The stress of anesthesia and surgery can increase sympathetic tone, provoking Torsade de Pointes in patients with QT prolongation, while some anesthetic medications can further prolong the QT interval

## MANAGEMENT

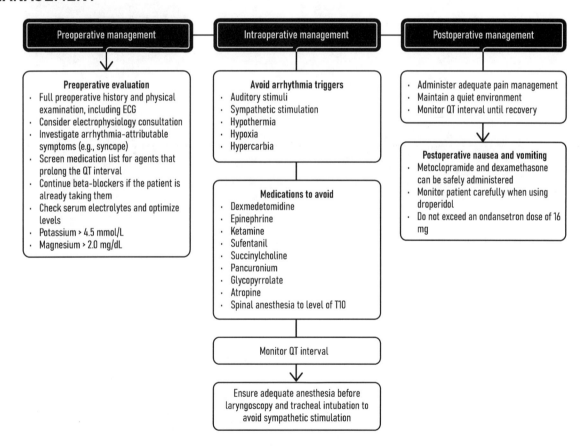

| Preoperative management | Intraoperative management | Postoperative management |
|---|---|---|

**Preoperative evaluation**
- Full preoperative history and physical examination, including ECG
- Consider electrophysiology consultation
- Investigate arrhythmia-attributable symptoms (e.g., syncope)
- Screen medication list for agents that prolong the QT interval
- Continue beta-blockers if the patient is already taking them
- Check serum electrolytes and optimize levels
- Potassium > 4.5 mmol/L
- Magnesium > 2.0 mg/dL

**Avoid arrhythmia triggers**
- Auditory stimuli
- Sympathetic stimulation
- Hypothermia
- Hypoxia
- Hypercarbia

**Medications to avoid**
- Dexmedetomidine
- Epinephrine
- Ketamine
- Sufentanil
- Succinylcholine
- Pancuronium
- Glycopyrrolate
- Atropine
- Spinal anesthesia to level of T10

Monitor QT interval

Ensure adequate anesthesia before laryngoscopy and tracheal intubation to avoid sympathetic stimulation

- Administer adequate pain management
- Maintain a quiet environment
- Monitor QT interval until recovery

**Postoperative nausea and vomiting**
- Metoclopramide and dexamethasone can be safely administered
- Monitor patient carefully when using droperidol
- Do not exceed an ondansetron dose of 16 mg

## TORSADES DE POINTES TREATMENT

**Immediate direct current cardioversion** → *Ventricular fibrillation* → **Immediate defibrillation**

- IV magnesium 2 g over 2 min (30 mg/kg)
- Start infusion of 1-4 g/hr to keep the magnesium levels above 2 mmol/L
- Once the magnesium level is > 3 mmol/L, stop the infusion

Treat hypokalemia: Maintain serum K+ between 4.5 and 5 mmol/L

*Patient continues to have intermittent runs of Torsades de Pointes*

Pharmacologically increase the heart rate with isoproterenol: IV bolus of 10-20mcg or infusion titrated to maintain a heart rate of 100 bpm

**IMPORTANT:** Isoproterenol is contraindicated in patients with congenital QT prolongation because it may prolong the QT interval

Overdrive pacing to 90-110 with a transvenous pacemaker

Stop QT prolonging medications: Antipsychotics, antiemetics, antibiotics, antifungals, antidysrhythmics, antidepressants, antihistamines, antineoplastics

## SUGGESTED READING

- Cohagan B, Brandis D. Torsade de Pointes. [Updated 2022 Aug 8]. In: StatPearls [Internet]. Treasure Island (FL): StatPearls Publishing; 2022 Jan-. Available from: https://www.ncbi.nlm.nih.gov/books/NBK459388/
- Hunter JD, Sharma P, Rathi S. Long QT syndrome. Continuing Education in Anaesthesia Critical Care & Pain. 2008;8(2):67-70.
- Kies SJ, Pabelick CM, Hurley HA, White RD, Ackerman MJ. Anesthesia for patients with congenital long QT syndrome. Anesthesiology. 2005;102(1):204-210.
- O'Hare M, Maldonado Y, Munro J, Ackerman MJ, Ramakrishna H, Sorajja D. Perioperative management of patients with congenital or acquired disorders of the QT interval. Br J Anaesth. 2018;120(4):629-644.

# 29

# RIGHT HEART FAILURE

## LEARNING OBJECTIVES

- Pathogenesis of right heart failure (RHF)
- Treatment of RHF
- Anesthetic management of RHF

## DEFINITION AND MECHANISM

- Right heart failure (RHF) is characterized by dysfunction in the right heart structures, primarily the right ventricle (RV), but also including the tricuspid valve and right atrium
- Impaired vena cava flow, which hampers the right heart's ability to perfuse the lungs at normal central venous pressures, can also lead to RHF
- Additionally, ventricular interdependence, where the function, volume, or pressure in one ventricle directly affects the other, plays a role in RHF when there is left ventricular dysfunction
- Conversely, when the right ventricle (RV) experiences pressure or volume overload, it can negatively impact left ventricular (LV) performance, leading to reduced LV preload and contractility

- Elevated filling pressures on the right side of the heart lead to backward failure and systemic venous congestion
- Backward failure:
  - Negatively affects the hepatic function
  - Causes acute kidney injury and aggravates further fluid retention thereby worsening RHF
- Fundamental management principles involve optimizing rate, rhythm, perfusion, and preload, whilst maintaining contractility and minimizing afterload

## PATHOGENESIS OF RIGHT HEART FAILURE

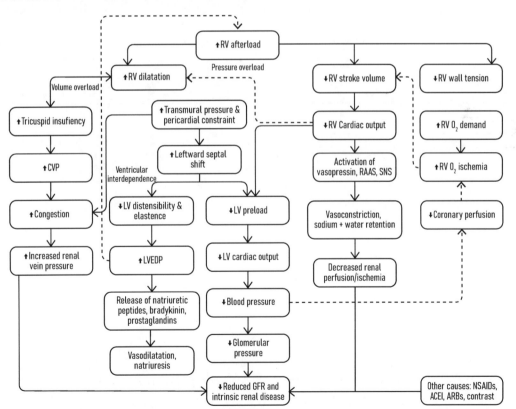

RV, right ventricle; CVP, central venous pressure; LV, left ventricle; LVEDP, left ventricular end-diastolic pressure; GFR, glomerular filtration rate; RAAS, renin-angiotensin-aldosteron system; SNS, sympathetic nervous system; NSAID, non-steroidal anti-inflammatory drugs; ACEI, angiotensin-converting-enzyme inhibitors; ARBs, angiotensin II receptor blockers

# SIGNS & SYMPTOMS

- Breathlessness
- Chest discomfort
- Palpitations
- Swelling
- Elevated jugular venous pressure/jugular venous distention
- Hepatojugular reflux
- Peripheral edema
- Bloating/early satiety/abdominal discomfort
- Hepatosplenomegaly/hepatic pulsation
- Ascites
- Pleural effusion
- A prominent second heart sound (S2)
- Right-sided S3 gallop
- Tricuspid regurgitation murmur
- RV heave
- Paradoxical pulse

# CAUSES

| Decreased RV contractility | RV volume overload | RV pressure overload |
|---|---|---|
| **Acute** | | |
| Sepsis | | Acidosis |
| LVAD support | | Hypoxia |
| Myocarditis | | Acute Respiratory Distress Syndrome |
| Perioperative injury/ischemia (postcardiotomy) | | Positive pressure ventilation |
| Right ventricle myocardial infarction | | Pneumonia ventilation |
| Cardiac tamponade | | Mechanical ventilation |
| **Chronic** | | |
| Right ventricular cardiomyopathy | Left heart disease | |
| Arrhythmogenic right ventricular cardiomyopathy | Single ventricle | Hypoxia |
| Ebstein anomaly | | Pericardial disease |
| | Pulmonary regurgitation | Pulmonary hypertension (PH) |
| | Transposition of the great arteries | Chronic thromboembolic Pulmonary hypertension (PH) |
| | Tricuspid regurgitation (TR) | Pulmonary stenosis |
| | Congenital heart disease with a shunt (ASD or anomalous pulmonary venous return) | Left-sided valvular heart disease |
| | | Restrictive cardiomyopathy |
| | | Chronic obstructive pulmonary disease |
| | | Right ventricular outflow tract obstruction |

Right heart failure

Another important mechanism that leads to RHF is intrinsic RV myocardial disease:

- RV ischemia or infarct
- Infiltrative diseases such as amyloidosis or sarcoidosis
- Arrhythmogenic right ventricular dysplasia (ARVD)
- Cardiomyopathy
- Microvascular disease

RHF may be caused by impaired filling which is seen in the following conditions:

- Constrictive pericarditis
- Tricuspid stenosis
- Systemic vasodilatory shock
- Cardiac tamponade
- Superior vena cava syndrome
- Hypovolemia

## DIAGNOSIS

- Chest X-ray
- ECG
- Echocardiogram
- Blood test (natriuretic peptides)
- MRI/CT
- Cardiac catheterization

## TREATMENT

| Acute RHF | Chronic RHF |
| --- | --- |
| · Volume management<br>  ◦ Diuretics<br>    ▪ Loop diuretics + thiazide diuretic<br>    ▪ Aldosterone antagonists<br>    ▪ Carbonic anhydrase inhibitors<br>  ◦ Renal replacement therapies<br>    ▪ Veno-venous hemofiltration<br>    ▪ Ultrafiltration<br>· Vasoactive therapies<br>  ◦ Afterload reduction<br>    ▪ Non-selective vasodilators including intravenous nitroglycerin and sodium nitroprusside<br>    ▪ Phosphodiesterase-5 inhibitors<br>  ◦ Augment contractility<br>    ▪ Milrinone<br>    ▪ Dobutamine<br>  ◦ Maintain perfusion<br>    ▪ Dopamine<br>    ▪ Norepinephrine<br>    ▪ Epinephrine<br>    ▪ Arginine vasopressin<br>    ▪ Phenylephrine<br>· SGLT2 inhibitors | · Diuretics and sodium restriction<br>  ◦ Combination therapy: loop diuretics with thiazides<br>· Renin-angiotensin-aldosterone system inhibitors, beta-blockers, and hydralazine<br>· Digoxin<br>· Pulmonary vasodilators<br>  ◦ Prostacyclin analogs<br>    ▪ Epoprostenol<br>    ▪ Treprostinil<br>    ▪ Iloprost<br>  ◦ Phosphodiesterase-5 inhibitors<br>  ◦ Endothelin receptor antagonists<br>· Mechanical circulatory support<br>  ◦ ECMO<br>  ◦ RVAD<br>  ◦ LVAD<br>· Transplantation<br>· SGLT2 inhibitors |

Right heart failure

| | Classification | Dose (IV unless stated) | Effects | Advantages | Disdvantages |
|---|---|---|---|---|---|
| Noradrenaline | Vasopressor | 0.02-0.2 µg/kg/min | Vasoconstriction, ↑SVR, ↑myocardial O$_2$ delivery, ↑PVR | Cheap, easy to titrate, familiarity | Arrhythmias, ↑PVR in higher doses |
| Vasopressin | Vasopressor | 1-4 units/min | Vasoconstriction, ↑SVR, pulmonary vasodilatation at low doses via endothelial nitric oxide pathway, ↑ myocardial O$_2$ delivery | Catechol-amine-sparing, less ↑PVR than noradrenaline, easy to titrate | Expensive, bradycardia, splanchnic ischemia |
| Dobutamine | Inodilator | 2.5-10 µg/kg/min | Inotropy, ↑ contractility, ↓SVR, PVR | Easy to titrate, cheap | ↑O$_2$ demand, tachyarrhythmias, systemic hypotension |
| Milrinone | Inodilator | 0.75-0.75 µg/kg/min | Inotropy, ↑ contractility, ↓SVR, PVR | Pulmonary vasodilatation | Systemic hypotension |
| Levosimendan | Inodilator | Loading dose: 6-12 µg/kg/min over 10 min followed by infusion of 0.1 µg/kg/min | ↑Contractility | No effect on myocardial oxygen demand | Expensive, tachycardia, hypotension, headache |
| Sildenafil | Pulmonary vasodilator | 10 mg t.d.s. Oral: 20-100 mg t.d.s | ↓PVR, ↑Contractility | Oral administration for patients with chronic disease | ↓SVR |
| Epoprostenol | Pulmonary vasodilator | 1-2 ng/kg/min Nebulized: 0.2-0.3 ml/min of a 10-20 µg/mil solution | ↓PVR, ↑V/Q mismatch | As efficient as nitric oxide | Systemic hypotension with i.v. administration, flushing, headaches |

Right heart failure

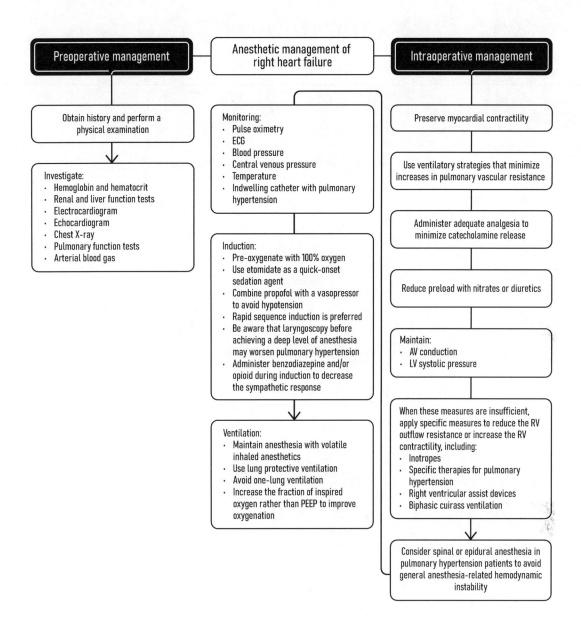

**Anesthetic management of right heart failure**

**Preoperative management**

Obtain history and perform a physical examination

Investigate:
- Hemoglobin and hematocrit
- Renal and liver function tests
- Electrocardiogram
- Echocardiogram
- Chest X-ray
- Pulmonary function tests
- Arterial blood gas

Monitoring:
- Pulse oximetry
- ECG
- Blood pressure
- Central venous pressure
- Temperature
- Indwelling catheter with pulmonary hypertension

Induction:
- Pre-oxygenate with 100% oxygen
- Use etomidate as a quick-onset sedation agent
- Combine propofol with a vasopressor to avoid hypotension
- Rapid sequence induction is preferred
- Be aware that laryngoscopy before achieving a deep level of anesthesia may worsen pulmonary hypertension
- Administer benzodiazepine and/or opioid during induction to decrease the sympathetic response

Ventilation:
- Maintain anesthesia with volatile inhaled anesthetics
- Use lung protective ventilation
- Avoid one-lung ventilation
- Increase the fraction of inspired oxygen rather than PEEP to improve oxygenation

**Intraoperative management**

Preserve myocardial contractility

Use ventilatory strategies that minimize increases in pulmonary vascular resistance

Administer adequate analgesia to minimize catecholamine release

Reduce preload with nitrates or diuretics

Maintain:
- AV conduction
- LV systolic pressure

When these measures are insufficient, apply specific measures to reduce the RV outflow resistance or increase the RV contractility, including:
- Inotropes
- Specific therapies for pulmonary hypertension
- Right ventricular assist devices
- Biphasic cuirass ventilation

Consider spinal or epidural anesthesia in pulmonary hypertension patients to avoid general anesthesia-related hemodynamic instability

## SUGGESTED READING

- Cops J, Mullens W, Verbrugge FH, et al. Selective abdominal venous congestion induces adverse renal and hepatic morphological and functional alterations despite a preserved cardiac function. Sci Rep. 2018;8(1):17757.
- Cops J, Mullens W, Verbrugge FH, et al. Selective abdominal venous congestion to investigate cardiorenal interactions in a rat model. PLoS One. 2018;13(5):e0197687. Published 2018 May 29.
- Gorter TM, van Veldhuisen DJ, Bauersachs J, et al. Right heart dysfunction and failure in heart failure with preserved ejection fraction: mechanisms and management. Position statement on behalf of the Heart Failure Association of the European Society of Cardiology. Eur J Heart Fail. 2018;20(1):16-37.
- Houston BA, Brittain EL, Tedford RJ. Right, Ventricular Failure. N Engl J Med. 2023;388(12):1111-1125.
- Kevin LG. 2007. Right ventricular failure. Continuing Education in Anaesthesia Critical Care & Pain. 7;3:89-94.
- Konstam MA, Kiernan MS, Bernstein D, et al. Evaluation and Management of Right-Sided Heart Failure: A Scientific Statement From the American Heart Association. Circulation. 2018;137(20):e578-e622.
- Murphy, E., Shelley, B., 2018. The right ventricle—structural and functional importance for anaesthesia and intensive care. BJA Education 18, 239–245.
- Murphy, E., Shelley, B., 2019. Clinical presentation and management of right ventricular dysfunction. BJA Education 19, 183–190.
- Price LC, Martinez G, Brame A, et al. Perioperative management of patients with pulmonary hypertension undergoing non-cardiothoracic, non-obstetric surgery: a systematic review and expert consensus statement. Br J Anaesth. 2021;126(4):774-790.

# TRANSPLANTED HEART

**30**

## LEARNING OBJECTIVES

- Describe the hemodynamic implications of a transplanted heart
- Manage patients with a transplanted heart undergoing non-transplant surgery

## DEFINITION AND MECHANISM

- A cardiac transplant is the treatment of choice for many patients with severe cardiac failure who have failed other medical therapy
- A transplanted heart has an absence of sensory, sympathetic, and parasympathetic innervation
- Due to a lack of parasympathetic innervation, vagal tone is lost and the resting heart rate will be 90–110 bpm
- Cardiac output of the transplanted heart is relatively dependent upon preload
- In response to hypovolemia, the cardiac output is increased by increasing the stroke volume rather than the heart rate and contractility, due to insensitivity to neurohormonal stimulation
- A degree of sympathetic and parasympathetic innervation develops with time (3+ years)
- The ECG in 80% of recipients will demonstrate two p-waves due to the posterior portion of the atrial walls being retained from the original heart

## MANAGEMENT

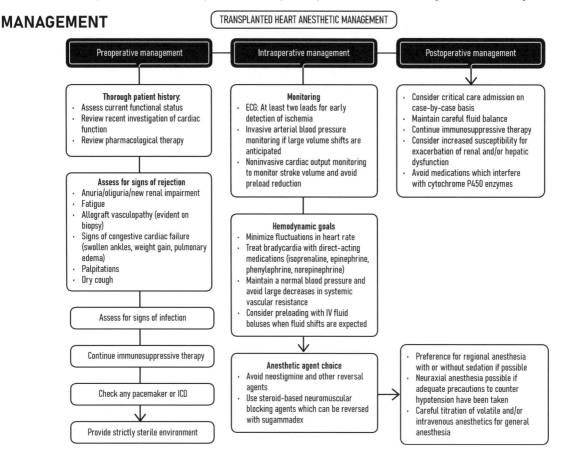

TRANSPLANTED HEART ANESTHETIC MANAGEMENT

**Preoperative management**

**Thorough patient history:**
- Assess current functional status
- Review recent investigation of cardiac function
- Review pharmacological therapy

**Assess for signs of rejection**
- Anuria/oliguria/new renal impairment
- Fatigue
- Allograft vasculopathy (evident on biopsy)
- Signs of congestive cardiac failure (swollen ankles, weight gain, pulmonary edema)
- Palpitations
- Dry cough

Assess for signs of infection

Continue immunosuppressive therapy

Check any pacemaker or ICD

Provide strictly sterile environment

**Intraoperative management**

**Monitoring**
- ECG: At least two leads for early detection of ischemia
- Invasive arterial blood pressure monitoring if large volume shifts are anticipated
- Noninvasive cardiac output monitoring to monitor stroke volume and avoid preload reduction

**Hemodynamic goals**
- Minimize fluctuations in heart rate
- Treat bradycardia with direct-acting medications (isoprenaline, epinephrine, phenylephrine, norepinephrine)
- Maintain a normal blood pressure and avoid large decreases in systemic vascular resistance
- Consider preloading with IV fluid boluses when fluid shifts are expected

**Anesthetic agent choice**
- Avoid neostigmine and other reversal agents
- Use steroid-based neuromuscular blocking agents which can be reversed with sugammadex

**Postoperative management**
- Consider critical care admission on case-by-case basis
- Maintain careful fluid balance
- Continue immunosuppressive therapy
- Consider increased susceptibility for exacerbation of renal and/or hepatic dysfunction
- Avoid medications which interfere with cytochrome P450 enzymes

- Preference for regional anesthesia with or without sedation if possible
- Neuraxial anesthesia possible if adequate precautions to counter hypotension have been taken
- Careful titration of volatile and/or intravenous anesthetics for general anesthesia

## SUGGESTED READING

- Barbara DW, Christensen JM, Mauermann WJ, Dearani JA, Hyder JA. The Safety of Neuromuscular Blockade Reversal in Patients With Cardiac Transplantation. Transplantation. 2016;100(12):2723-2728.
- Herborn J, Parulkar S. Anesthetic Considerations in Transplant Recipients for Nontransplant Surgery. Anesthesiol Clin. 2017;35(3):539-553.
- Pollard BJ, Kitchen, G. Handbook of Clinical Anaesthesia. Fourth Edition. CRC Press. 2018. 978-1-4987-6289-2.

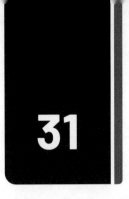

# TRICUSPID REGURGITATION (TR)

**31**

## LEARNING OBJECTIVES

- Recognize common causes of TR
- Describe the signs and symptoms of TR
- Grade the severity of TR cases
- Anesthetic management of TR

## DEFINITION AND MECHANISM

- Tricuspid regurgitation (TR) occurs when the tricuspid valve does not close properly, causing a reversal of blood flow through the valve
- TR can be of primary or secondary origin:
  - Primary (organic) TR: Pathology of the tricuspid valve complex, may be of rheumatic, degenerative, congenital, infectious, traumatic, or iatrogenic origin
  - Secondary (functional) TR: Related to right ventricular dilatation and/or dysfunction, annular dilatation, and leaflet tethering, usually secondary to left-sided valvular heart disease, atrial fibrillation or pulmonary hypertension

## SIGNS & SYMPTOMS

- Often clinically silent and symptoms usually relate to concomitant left-sided valvular heart disease
- General fatigue and reduced exercise capacity
- Upper abdominal pain
- Peripheral lower limb edema
- Systolic jugular distension
- Pulsatile hepatomegaly
- Ascites, liver failure, and cachexia may be observed in end-stage disease
- ECG frequently shows right bundle branch block
- Atrial fibrillation reflects disease evolution

| | Parameters | Mild | Moderate | Severe |
|---|---|---|---|---|
| Qualitative | TV morphology | Normal/abnormal | Normal/abnormal | Abnormal/flail/large coaptation defect |
| | Color flow TR jet | Small, central | Intermediate | Very large central jet or eccentric wall impinging jet |
| | CW signal of TR jet | Faint/parabolic | Dense/parabolic | Dense/triangular with early peaking (peak < 2 m/s in massive TR) |
| Semi-quantitative | VC width (mm) | Not defined | < 7 | > 7 |
| | PISA radius (mm) | ≤ 5 | 6–9 | > 9 |
| | Hepatic vein flow | Systolic dominance | Systolic blunting | Systolic flow reversal |
| | Tricuspid inflow | Normal | Normal | E-wave dominant (≥ 1 m/s) |
| Quantitative | EROA (mm2) | Not defined | < 7 | > 7 |
| | R Vol (ml) | Not defined | Not defined | ≥ 45 |

TV, tricuspid valve; TR jet, tricuspid regurgitation jet; WC, continuous wave Doppler; VC width, vena contracta width; PISA, proximal isovelocity surface area; ERQA, effective regurgitant orifice area; R Vol, regurgitant volume

## KEEP IN MIND

Tricuspid regurgitation is most commonly secondary to other morbidities, which might require further attention

## MANAGEMENT

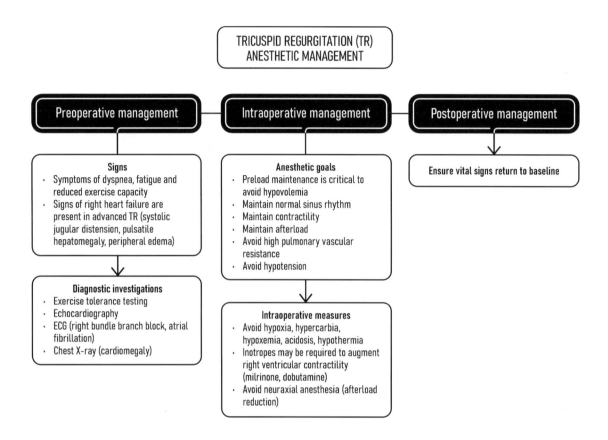

**SUGGESTED READING**

- Antunes MJ, Rodríguez-Palomares J, Prendergast B, De Bonis M, Rosenhek R, Al-Attar N, et al. Management of tricuspid valve regurgitation: Position statement of the European Society of Cardiology Working Groups of Cardiovascular Surgery and Valvular Heart Disease. European Journal of Cardio-Thoracic Surgery. 2017;52(6):1022-30.
- Hahn Rebecca T. Tricuspid Regurgitation. New England Journal of Medicine.
- Henning RJ. Tricuspid valve regurgitation: current diagnosis and treatment. Am J Cardiovasc Dis. 2022 Feb 15;12(1):1-18. PMID: 35291509;

# WOLFF-PARKINSON-WHITE SYNDROME

## LEARNING OBJECTIVES

- Describe the mechanisms & symptoms of Wolff-Parkinson-White Syndrome
- Manage patients with Wolff-Parkinson-White Syndrome

## DEFINITION AND MECHANISM

- Wolff-Parkinson-White Syndrome (WPW) is a congenital abnormality that involves the presence of abnormal electrical conductive circuits between the atria and ventricles, resulting in accessory electrical pathways that bypass the AV node
- Can result in life-threatening arrhythmias

| Signs & symptoms | |
|---|---|
| Electrocardiographic signs | Short PR interval |
| | Prolonged QRS |
| | Initial slurring upstroke ("delta" wave) in the presence of sinus rhythm |
| Clinical symptoms | Palpitations |
| | Episodic lightheadedness |
| | Presyncope |
| | Syncope |
| | Cardiac arrest |

# MANAGEMENT

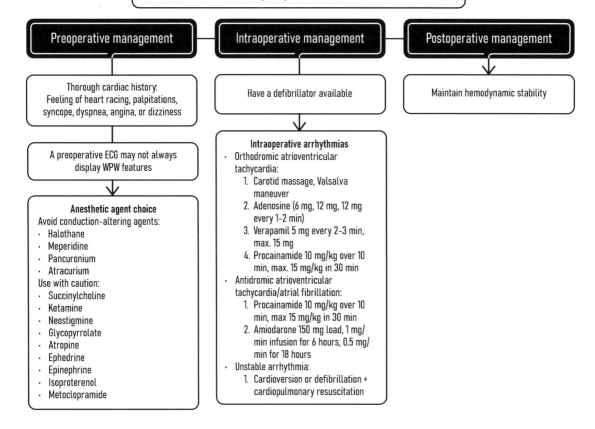

**WOLFF-PARKINSON-WHITE (WPW) SYNDROME ANESTHETIC MANAGEMENT**

**Preoperative management**

Thorough cardiac history:
Feeling of heart racing, palpitations, syncope, dyspnea, angina, or dizziness

A preoperative ECG may not always display WPW features

**Anesthetic agent choice**
Avoid conduction-altering agents:
- Halothane
- Meperidine
- Pancuronium
- Atracurium

Use with caution:
- Succinylcholine
- Ketamine
- Neostigmine
- Glycopyrrolate
- Atropine
- Ephedrine
- Epinephrine
- Isoproterenol
- Metoclopramide

**Intraoperative management**

Have a defibrillator available

**Intraoperative arrhythmias**
- Orthodromic atrioventricular tachycardia:
  1. Carotid massage, Valsalva maneuver
  2. Adenosine (6 mg, 12 mg, 12 mg every 1-2 min)
  3. Verapamil 5 mg every 2-3 min, max. 15 mg
  4. Procainamide 10 mg/kg over 10 min, max. 15 mg/kg in 30 min
- Antidromic atrioventricular tachycardia/atrial fibrillation:
  1. Procainamide 10 mg/kg over 10 min, max 15 mg/kg in 30 min
  2. Amiodarone 150 mg load, 1 mg/min infusion for 6 hours, 0.5 mg/min for 18 hours
- Unstable arrhythmia:
  1. Cardioversion or defibrillation + cardiopulmonary resuscitation

**Postoperative management**

Maintain hemodynamic stability

---

**SUGGESTED READING**

- Bengali R, Wellens HJ, Jiang Y. Perioperative management of the Wolff-Parkinson-White syndrome. J Cardiothorac Vasc Anesth. 2014;28(5):1375-1386.
- Benson DW, Cohen MI. Wolff-Parkinson-White syndrome: lessons learnt and lessons remaining. Cardiology in the Young. 2017;27(S1):S62-S67.
- Chhabra L, Goyal A, Benham MD. Wolff-Parkinson-White Syndrome. [Updated 2023 Aug 7]. In: StatPearls [Internet]. Treasure Island (FL): StatPearls Publishing; 2024 Jan-. Available from: https://www.ncbi.nlm.nih.gov/books/NBK554437/

# CRITICAL CARE

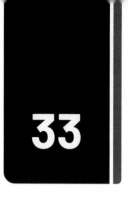

# ABDOMINAL COMPARTMENT SYNDROME (ACS)

**33**

## LEARNING OBJECTIVES

- Difference between intra-abdominal pressure (IAP) and abdominal compartment syndrome (ACS)
- Recognize ACS and the pathophysiological consequences of ACS
- Management of ACS

## DEFINITION AND MECHANISM

- Normal intra-abdominal pressure (IAP) ranges between 0-5 mmHg while in critically-ill patients, an IAP of 5-7 mmHg is considered normal
- Intra-abdominal hypertension is defined as a sustained intra-abdominal pressure (IAP) $\geq$ 12 mmHg
- Abdominal compartment syndrome (ACS) is defined as IAP rising > 20 mmHg thereby leading to new organ dysfunction
- Abdominal perfusion pressure (APP) is calculated as the mean arterial pressure (MAP) minus the IAP
- A patient with ACS is critically ill with high mortality and morbidity

## SIGNS & SYMPTOMS

- Malaise
- Weakness
- Dyspnea
- Abdominal bloating

- Abdominal pain
- Hypoxia
- Hypercarbia
- Oliguria

## ETIOLOGY

**Acute ACS**
- Primary: due to injury or disease in the abdominopelvic region (e.g., pancreatitis, abdominal trauma)
- Secondary: does not originate in the abdomen or pelvis (e.g., fluid resuscitation, sepsis, burns)

**Chronic ACS**
- In association with peritoneal dialysis or chronic ascites

**Artificially raised IAP**
- External compression, for example, prolonged prone positioning for spinal surgery with insufficient provision for abdominal movement

## DIAGNOSIS

- Indirect measurement of IAP using intragastric, intracolonic, intravesical (bladder), or inferior vena cava catheters

| Risk factors | |
|---|---|
| Diminished abdominal wall compliance | Acute respiratory failure, especially with elevated intrathoracic pressure<br>Abdominal surgery with subjectively tight primary closure<br>Major trauma/burns<br>Prone positioning, head of bed elevated > 30°<br>High BMI, central obesity |
| Increased intra-luminal contents | Gastroparesis<br>Ileus<br>Colonic pseudo-obstruction |
| Increased abdominal contents | Hemoperitoneum/pneumoperitoneum<br>Ascites/liver dysfunction |
| Capillary leak/fluid resuscitation | Metabolic acidosis (pH < 7.2)<br>Hypotension<br>Perioperative hypothermia<br>Polytransfusion (> 10 units of blood/24 h)<br>Coagulopathy (platelets < 55,000 mm³, prothrombin time > 15 s, partial thromboplastin time > 2 times normal, or international standardized ratio > 1.5)<br>Massive fluid resuscitation (> 5 L/24 h)<br>Pancreatitis<br>Oliguria<br>Sepsis<br>Trauma<br>Burns<br>Damage control laparotomy |

| Pathophysiological effects of raised IAP | |
|---|---|
| Central nervous system | Increased intracranial pressure |
| Cardiovascular system | Increased systemic vascular resistance<br>Pulmonary vascular resistance<br>Decreased venous return with concomitant venous congestion |
| Gastrointestinal and hepatic system | Decreased celiac, mesenteric, hepatic and portal blood flow<br>Increased edema, bacterial translocation and liver dysfunction |
| Renal system | Increased renal tubular pressure and urinary obstruction<br>Decreased renal blood flow and urine output |
| Respiratory system | Increased ventilation-perfusion mismatch, ventilatory pressure, basal atelectasis and $PaCO_2$<br>Decreased chest wall and pulmonary compliance as well as $PaO_2$ |

# MANAGEMENT

- Patients with two or more risk factors should have IAP monitoring
- Treatment:
  - Regimens lowering IAP
  - Open the abdominal wound and perform a temporary closure of the abdominal wall with mesh or a plastic bag (Bogota bag)
  - Regimens aiming at organ support
- Keep abdominal perfusion pressure (APP) (systemic blood pressure – intra-abdominal pressure) > 60 mmHg

Abdominal compartment syndrome (ACS)

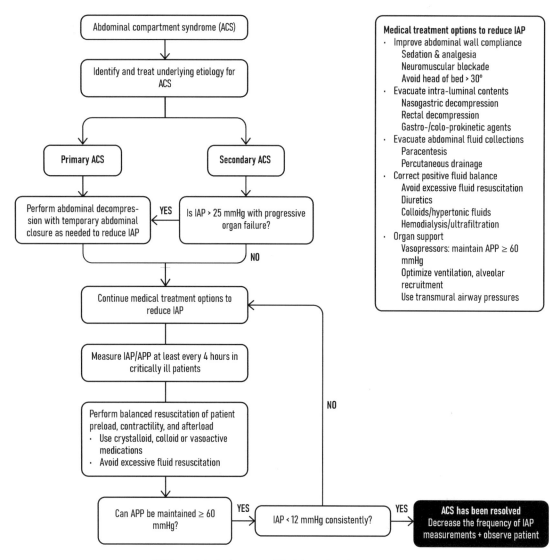

Abdominal compartment syndrome (ACS)

↓

Identify and treat underlying etiology for ACS

Primary ACS | Secondary ACS

Is IAP > 25 mmHg with progressive organ failure?
— YES → Perform abdominal decompression with temporary abdominal closure as needed to reduce IAP
— NO →

Continue medical treatment options to reduce IAP

↓

Measure IAP/APP at least every 4 hours in critically ill patients

↓

Perform balanced resuscitation of patient preload, contractility, and afterload
- Use crystalloid, colloid or vasoactive medications
- Avoid excessive fluid resuscitation

↓

Can APP be maintained ≥ 60 mmHg? — YES → IAP < 12 mmHg consistently? — YES → **ACS has been resolved** Decrease the frequency of IAP measurements + observe patient

NO

**Medical treatment options to reduce IAP**
- Improve abdominal wall compliance
  Sedation & analgesia
  Neuromuscular blockade
  Avoid head of bed > 30°
- Evacuate intra-luminal contents
  Nasogastric decompression
  Rectal decompression
  Gastro-/colo-prokinetic agents
- Evacuate abdominal fluid collections
  Paracentesis
  Percutaneous drainage
- Correct positive fluid balance
  Avoid excessive fluid resuscitation
  Diuretics
  Colloids/hypertonic fluids
  Hemodialysis/ultrafiltration
- Organ support
  Vasopressors: maintain APP ≥ 60 mmHg
  Optimize ventilation, alveolar recruitment
  Use transmural airway pressures

IAP, intra-abdominal pressure; APP, abdominal perfusion pressure.

## KEEP IN MIND

- Consequences of decompression:
  □ Sudden ↓ cardiac output & systemic vascular resistance
  □ Reperfusion: risk of systemic acidosis & hyperkalemia
  □ Possible fatal arrhythmia & arrest
  □ Sudden change in respiratory compliance (avoid overventilation)
- Avoid bradycardia (preload is compromised & cardiac output may be heart rate dependent)
- Maintain high preload particularly once decompressed

## SUGGESTED READING

- Neil Berry, Simon Fletcher, Abdominal compartment syndrome, Continuing Education in Anaesthesia Critical Care & Pain, Volume 12, Issue 3, June 2012, Pages 110–117.
- Mullens W, Abrahams Z, Skouri HN, et al. Elevated intra-abdominal pressure in acute decompensated heart failure: a potential contributor to worsening renal function? J Am Coll Cardiol. 2008;51(3):300-306.

# ACUTE RESPIRATORY DISTRESS SYNDROME (ARDS)

## LEARNING OBJECTIVES

- Recognize ARDS
- Treatment of ARDS
- Anesthetic management of ARDS

## DEFINITION AND MECHANISM

- Acute respiratory distress syndrome (ARDS) is a life-threatening acute onset of respiratory failure
- Characterized by hypoxemia, stiff lungs, alveolar edema, endothelial cell damage, and neutrophil infiltration
- Multiple risk factors trigger the acute onset
- ARDS Berlin definition:

| | |
|---|---|
| Timing | Within 1 week of a known clinical insult or new or worsening respiratory symptoms |
| Chest imaging | Bilateral opacities - not fully explained by effusions, lobar/lung collapse or nodules |
| Origin of edema | Respiratory failure not fully explained by cardiac failure or fluid overload<br>Need objective assessment (e.g., echocardiography) to exclude hydrostatic edema if no risk factor present |
| Oxygenation<br>Mild<br>Moderate<br>Severe | $200$ mmHg $< PaO_2/FiO_2 \leq 300$ mmHg with PEEP or CPAP $\geq 5$ cmH$_2$O<br>$100$ mmHg $< PaO_2/FiO_2 \leq 200$ mmHg with PEEP $\geq 5$ cmH$_2$O<br>$PaO_2/FiO_2 \leq 100$ mmHg with PEEP $\geq 5$ cmH$_2$O |

## SIGNS & SYMPTOMS

- Severe shortness of breath
- Labored and unusually rapid breathing
- Low blood pressure
- Confusion and extreme tiredness

## RISK FACTORS

| Direct | Indirect |
|---|---|
| Pneumonia | Non-pulmonary sepsis |
| Aspiration of gastric contents | Major trauma |
| Inhalation injury | Pancreatitis |
| Pulmonary contusion | Severe burns |
| Pulmonary vasculitis | Non-cardiogenic shock |
| Drowning | Drug overdose |
| | Multiple transfusions or transfusion-related acute lung injury (TRALI) |

# COMPLICATIONS

- Deep vein thrombosis
- Gastrointestinal bleeding
- Barotrauma
- Pneumothorax
- Nosocomial infection
- Delirium
- Pulmonary fibrosis

- Refractory respiratory failure requiring prolonged dependence on mechanical ventilation
- Prolonged stay in ICU
- Need for tracheostomy
- Muscle weakness
- Sepsis
- Ambulatory dysfunction

# TREATMENT

- Supplemental provision of oxygen
- Optimize PEEP: esophageal pressure, power-voltage curves, lung ultrasound
- Protective mechanical ventilation
- Non-conventional therapies: prone position, high-frequency oscillatory ventilation, and extracorporeal membrane oxygenation

- Consider:

- Extracorporeal lung support (ECLS) techniques including extracorporeal membrane oxygenation as possible rescue therapy in patients with severe hypoxemic and hypercapnic respiratory failure
- Steroids: Methylprednisolone
- Neuromuscular blocking agent cisatracurium or inhaled NO as these could improve oxygenation

# MANAGEMENT

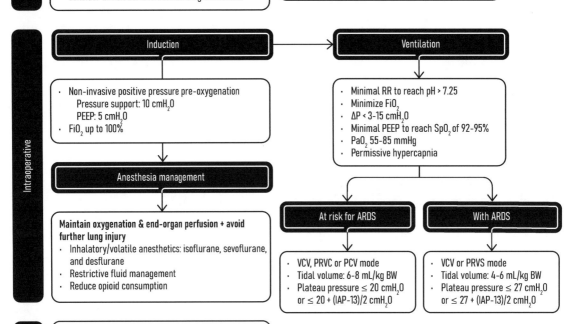

**Preoperative**

**Risk stratification**
- Identification of risk factors for developing ARDS
- Comorbidities
- Early recognition of underlying respiratory infections
- Identification of causative pathogens
- Consider antibiotics and bedside lung ultrasound

**Risk mitigation**
- Discuss surgical procedure and timing
- Decide the type of anesthesia
- Plan admission to the appropriate level of care
- High risk of ARDS postoperatively

**Intraoperative**

**Induction**
- Non-invasive positive pressure pre-oxygenation
    Pressure support: 10 cmH$_2$O
    PEEP: 5 cmH$_2$O
- FiO$_2$ up to 100%

**Ventilation**
- Minimal RR to reach pH > 7.25
- Minimize FiO$_2$
- ΔP < 3-15 cmH$_2$O
- Minimal PEEP to reach SpO$_2$ of 92-95%
- PaO$_2$ 55-85 mmHg
- Permissive hypercapnia

**Anesthesia management**

**Maintain oxygenation & end-organ perfusion + avoid further lung injury**
- Inhalatory/volatile anesthetics: isoflurane, sevoflurane, and desflurane
- Restrictive fluid management
- Reduce opioid consumption

**At risk for ARDS**
- VCV, PRVC or PCV mode
- Tidal volume: 6-8 mL/kg BW
- Plateau pressure ≤ 20 cmH$_2$O or ≤ 20 + (IAP-13)/2 cmH$_2$O

**With ARDS**
- VCV or PRVS mode
- Tidal volume: 4-6 mL/kg BW
- Plateau pressure ≤ 27 cmH$_2$O or ≤ 27 + (IAP-13)/2 cmH$_2$O

**Postoperative**
- Admission to ICU
- Close respiratory monitoring in patients at risk/with ARDS
- Early identification and treatment of PPCs
- Early weaning from ventilation
- Control of pain while minimizing opioids
- Promote mobilization

PPCs, postoperative pulmonary complications; RR, respiratory rate; VCV, volume-controlled ventilation; PRVC, pressure-regulated volume control; PCV, pressure-controlled ventilation; BW, body weight; IAP, intra-abdominal pressure.

# HEMODYNAMIC MANAGEMENT IN ARDS

- Hemodynamic instability is often present in ARDS
- The right ventricle (RV) is most directly affected by positive-pressure mechanical ventilation and ARDS
- Therapeutic strategies should be directed at preventing and treating RV dysfunction
  - Optimize RV preload
  - Optimize RV systolic function
  - Reduce RV afterload
  - Maintain an adequate systemic blood pressure and coronary perfusion
  - Treat underlying disease
- Spectrum of pulmonary vascular dysfunction in acute respiratory distress syndrome (ARDS) and principal treatment strategies:

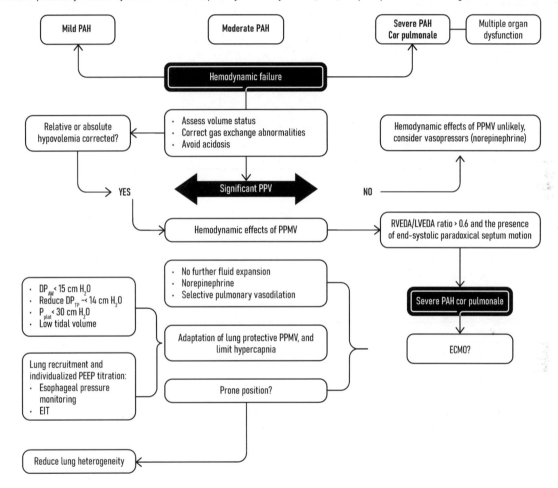

MOD, multiple organ dysfunction; PAH, pulmonary arterial hypertension; NE, norepinephrine; PPV, pulse pressure variation; PPMV, positive-pressure mechanical ventilation; RVEDA, right ventricular end-diastolic area; LVEDA, left ventricular end-diastolic area; DPAW, airway driving pressure; DPTP, transpulmonary driving pressure; PPLAT, plateau pressure; PEEP, positive end-expiratory pressure; EIT, electrical impedance tomography; ECMO, extracorporeal membrane oxygenation.

# SUGGESTED READING

- Battaglini D, Robba C, Rocco PRM, De Abreu MG, Pelosi P, Ball L. Perioperative anaesthetic management of patients with or at risk of acute distress respiratory syndrome undergoing emergency surgery. BMC Anesthesiol. 2019;19(1):153.
- Cortes-Puentes GA, Oeckler RA, Marini JJ. Physiology-guided management of hemodynamics in acute respiratory distress syndrome. Ann Transl Med. 2018;6(18):353.
- DiSilvio B, Young M, Gordon A, Malik K, Singh A, Cheema T. Complications and Outcomes of Acute Respiratory Distress Syndrome. Crit Care Nurs Q. 2019;42(4):349-361.
- Fanelli V, Vlachou A, Ghannadian S, Simonetti U, Slutsky AS, Zhang H. Acute respiratory distress syndrome: new definition, current and future therapeutic options. J Thorac Dis. 2013;5(3):326-334.
- Robert Wise, David Bishop, Gavin Joynt & Reitze Rodseth (2018) Perioperative ARDS and lung injury: for anaesthesia and beyond, Southern African Journal of Anaesthesia and Analgesia, 24:2, 32-39.

# TRANSFUSION OF BLOOD PRODUCTS

## LEARNING OBJECTIVES

- Provide an evidence-based framework for the transfusion of blood products

## DEFINITION AND MECHANISM

- Blood products are any therapeutic substance derived from human blood
- Including whole blood and other blood components for transfusion, and plasma-derived medicinal products

## RECOMMENDATIONS

Massive hemorrhage
- Give red blood cells – fresh frozen plasma – platelets (whole blood derived units) in a 1-1-1 ratio
- Transition to laboratory-guided treatment once hemorrhage control is achieved (as soon as lab results, Visco-elastic tests or conventional lab tests, are available)

Red Blood Cells (RBCs)
- 1 unit of RBCs = 350 mL
- 1 unit will raise hemoglobin by as much as 1 g/dL
- Be restrictive in transfusing RBCs
- Cutoffs for transfusion are:
  - 7 g/dL in hemodynamically stable patients
  - 8 g/dL for orthopedic surgery, 7,5 g/dL for cardiac surgery, and patients with preexisting cardiovascular disease
- There is no benefit in using fresh blood
- Use a single unit policy in stable patients

Platelets
- 1 unit = 1 apheresis unit = 4-6 whole blood derived units
- 1 unit will raise platelets by 30,000–50,000/μL
- Giving more than 2 units is rarely useful
- Transfuse prophylactically at platelet count:
  - < 10,000/μL for patients with hematologic or solid malignancies, undergoing allogeneic hematopoietic stem cell transplantation
  - < 20,000/μL for elective central venous catheter (CVC) placement
  - < 50,000/μL for elective diagnostic lumbar puncture
  - < 50,000/μL for major elective non-neuraxial surgery
  - < 100,000/μL for neuraxial surgery and eye surgery
- Give platelets if thrombocytopenia and active bleeding at platelet count:
  - < 30,000/μL for bleeding WHO grade II
  - < 50,000/μl for bleeding WHO grade III/IV (i.e. massive bleeding)

Fresh Frozen Plasma (FFP)
- 1 unit of FFP derived from whole blood = 250 mL
- FFP contains normal levels of coagulation factors, albumin and immunoglobulins but a variable amount of fibrinogen (1-3 g/L)
- Abnormal coagulation tests (PT/aPTT) are poor predictors of bleeding risk in a non-bleeding patient
- Don't give plasma transfusions to correct minor coagulation test abnormalities in non-bleeding patients
- Standard dose is 15-20 mL/kg and raises clotting factors by as much as 25%
- Give FFP in case of:
  - Massive transfusion
  - Disseminated intravascular coagulation (DIC), liver disease or thrombotic thrombocytopenic purpura (TTP) and active bleeding
  - Specific coagulation factor deficiencies without available coagulation factor concentrate
  - Dilutional coagulopathy but cryoprecipitate or fibrinogen might be needed to sufficiently restore fibrinogen levels

# ADVERSE EVENTS

| RBCs | Platelets | FFP |
|---|---|---|
| Febrile non-hemolytic transfusion reactions (FNHTRs) | FNHTRs | FNHTRs |
| Transfusion associated circulatory overload (TACO) | TACO | TACO |
| Transfusion related acute lung injury (TRALI) | TRALI | TRALI |
| Transfusion transmitted infection (TTI) | TTI | TTI |
| Allergic/anaphylactic reactions | Platelet alloimmunization | Allergic/anaphylactic reactions |
| Acute and delayed hemolytic transfusion reactions | Hemolytic reaction | |
| Transfusion associated graft versus host disease (TA-GVHD) | | |

## SUGGESTED READING

- Storch EK, Custer BS, Jacobs MR, Menitove JE, Mintz PD. Review of current transfusion therapy and blood banking practices. Blood Rev. 2019;38:100593.
- Carson JL, Stanworth SJ, Guyatt G, et al. Red Blood Cell Transfusion: 2023 AABB International Guidelines. JAMA. 2023;330(19):1892-1902.
- Holcomb JB, Tilley BC, Baraniuk S, et al. Transfusion of plasma, platelets, and red blood cells in a 1:1:1 vs a 1:1:2 ratio and mortality in patients with severe trauma: the PROPPR randomized clinical trial. JAMA. 2015;313(5):471-482.

# BURNS

## LEARNING OBJECTIVES

- Describe the main challenges of caring for a patient with major burns
- Explain the ways for optimizing intravenous fluid therapy to avoid under- and over-resuscitation
- Anesthetic management of patients with burns

## DEFINITION AND MECHANISM

- A burn is an injury to the skin or other organic tissue primarily caused by heat, cold, radiation, radioactivity, electricity, friction, or contact with chemicals
- Thermoregulation, blood loss, and coagulopathy are key considerations for the anesthesiologist during surgery for major burns
- Burns around the mouth or singed hair inside the nose may indicate that burns to the airways have occurred

## SIGNS AND SYMPTOMS

Skin burns:
- Discomfort, pressure, or pain
- Coloring of the skin: red, pink, white or black
- Blisters

Airway burns:
- Shortness of breath
- Hoarseness
- Stridor
- Wheezing

## CLASSIFICATION

- First degree: epidermal or superficial burn
  - Simple erythema involving damage to the epidermis
  - Excluded from the calculation of the surface area involved
- Second degree: partial thickness
- Third degree: full thickness

## COMPLICATIONS

- Bacterial infection
- Sepsis
- Hypovolemia
- Hypothermia
- Hypoperfusion
- Airway problems:
  - Obstruction of airway
  - Infection
  - Pneumonia
- Burn shock (deprivation of oxygenated blood to organs)
- Multiorgan failure
  - Acute respiratory distress syndrome
  - Acute kidney injury
- Scars
- Bone and joint problems
- Compartment syndrome

## Systemic effects

| | |
|---|---|
| Respiratory effects | Bronchospasm<br>Acute Respiratory Distress Syndrome |
| Cardiovascular effects | Hypovolemia<br>Myocardial depression<br>↓ Cardiac output<br>Burns shock up to 48h |
| Vascular effects | ↑ Capillary permeability<br>Na+ and proteins leak into interstitium<br>Tissue edema |
| Peripheral and splanchnic vasoconstriction | Acute kidney injury (AKI)<br>Ileus<br>GI stress ulceration |
| Fluid resuscitation | Tissue edema<br>Pulmonary edema<br>Abdominal compartment syndrome |
| Systemic inflammatory response to injury | Hypothalamix-pituitary-adrenal axis activation<br>↑ antidiuretic hormone<br>Sympathetic nervous system activation<br>↑ renin-angiotensin-aldosterone system<br>Hypercoagulability<br>Hypoalbuminemia |
| Hypermetabolic phase from 48h up to 1 year | ↑ Catecholamines, cortisol, glucagon<br>↓ Insulin<br>↑ Hepatic gluconeogenesis, glycogenolysis, lipolysis, proteolysis<br>Hyperdynamic circulation<br>Hyperthermia<br>Increased $O_2$ consumption<br>Weight loss<br>Muscle weakness<br>Immunosupression<br>Impaired wound healing |

# MANAGEMENT

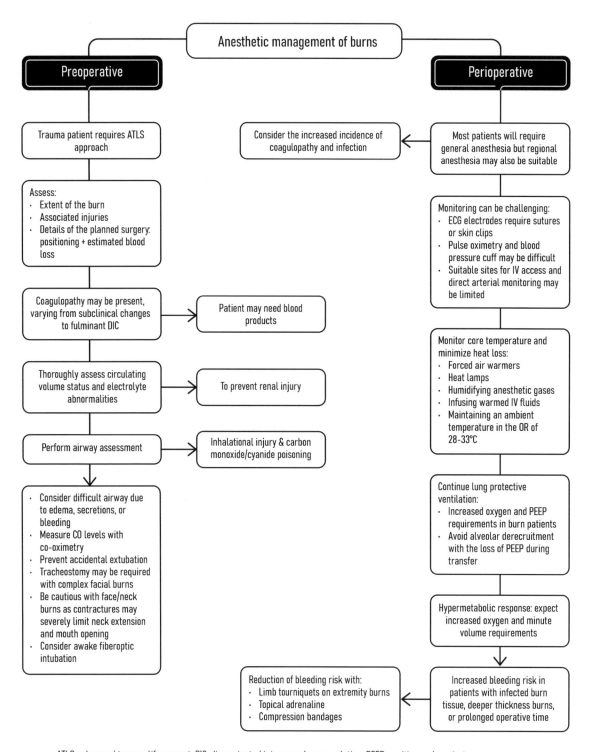

**Anesthetic management of burns**

**Preoperative**

Trauma patient requires ATLS approach

Assess:
- Extent of the burn
- Associated injuries
- Details of the planned surgery: positioning + estimated blood loss

Coagulopathy may be present, varying from subclinical changes to fulminant DIC → Patient may need blood products

Thoroughly assess circulating volume status and electrolyte abnormalities → To prevent renal injury

Perform airway assessment → Inhalational injury & carbon monoxide/cyanide poisoning

- Consider difficult airway due to edema, secretions, or bleeding
- Measure CO levels with co-oximetry
- Prevent accidental extubation
- Tracheostomy may be required with complex facial burns
- Be cautious with face/neck burns as contractures may severely limit neck extension and mouth opening
- Consider awake fiberoptic intubation

**Perioperative**

Most patients will require general anesthesia but regional anesthesia may also be suitable → Consider the increased incidence of coagulopathy and infection

Monitoring can be challenging:
- ECG electrodes require sutures or skin clips
- Pulse oximetry and blood pressure cuff may be difficult
- Suitable sites for IV access and direct arterial monitoring may be limited

Monitor core temperature and minimize heat loss:
- Forced air warmers
- Heat lamps
- Humidifying anesthetic gases
- Infusing warmed IV fluids
- Maintaining an ambient temperature in the OR of 28-33°C

Continue lung protective ventilation:
- Increased oxygen and PEEP requirements in burn patients
- Avoid alveolar derecruitment with the loss of PEEP during transfer

Hypermetabolic response: expect increased oxygen and minute volume requirements

Increased bleeding risk in patients with infected burn tissue, deeper thickness burns, or prolonged operative time → Reduction of bleeding risk with:
- Limb tourniquets on extremity burns
- Topical adrenaline
- Compression bandages

ATLS, advanced trauma life support; DIC, disseminated intravascular coagulation; PEEP, positive end-expiratory pressure

# ICU MANAGEMENT

ICU management of burns

## Fluid resuscitation

Appropriate fluid resuscitation in first 24-48h

Parkland formula: 2-4 mL x BW x %TBSA burned

- From the time burn sustained
- ½ in first 8 h, ½ in subsequent 16 h
- Subtract any fluid already given
- Use warm, isotonic balanced crystalloid (Hartmann's solution)

Colloid rescue: 4.5% human albumin solution addition

Target is an hourly urine output of 0.5-1 mL/kg

Check peripheral perfusion, serum lactate, acid-base balance, hematocrit

## Thermoregulation

Minimize heat loss

Prevent temperature > 40°C → multiorgan failure

1. Debulking dressings
2. Administer antipyretics such as paracetamol
3. Apply ice to non-burned areas
4. Infusion of cooled IV fluids
5. Irrigate bladder and stomach with cold fluids
6. Consider invasive procedures such as intravascular heat exchange catheters or extracorporeal circuits

## Nutrition

BMR increases significantly (x 2 with burns > 40% TBSA)

Start enteral nutrition immediately after the injury

Consider postpyloric feeding if gastric stasis is present to reduce aspiration risk

Parenteral nutrition is rarely required, but be cautious of infection, overfeeding, and erratic blood glucose control

Assess caloric needs with indirect calorimetry or formula

## Infection

Due to loss of skin coupled + relative immunosuppression

High morbidity and mortality rates after major burns

Common pathogens: S. aureus, Streptococcus, Enterococcus, Pseudomonas aeruginosa, Acinetobacter, E. coli

Specific criteria to diagnose sepsis in burn patients:
1. T > 39°C or < 36.5°C
2. HR > 110 beats/min
3. Ventilatory frequency > 25 bpm
4. Thrombocytopenia < 100 x 109 /L
5. Hyperglycemia > 11.1 mmol/L or insulin infusion dose requirement > 7 units/h
6. Intolerance of enteral feed

## Pain management

Structure approach to managing background, breakthrough, and procedural pain

Pharmacological treatment:
- Regional anesthesia
- Opioids
- NSAIDs
- Ketamine
- Gabapentinoids
- Dexmedetomidine

BW, body weight; TBSA, total body surface area; BMR, basal metabolic rate; HR, heart rate; NSAIDs, non-steroidal anti-inflammatory drugs.

Burns

# PARKLAND FORMULA

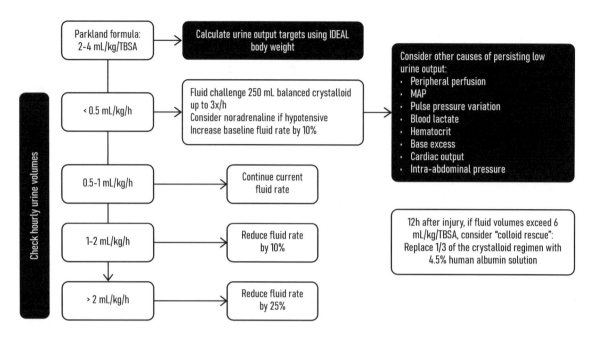

TBSA, total body surface area; MAP, mean arterial pressure.

**SUGGESTED READING**

- McCann C, Watson A, Barnes D. Major burns: Part 1. Epidemiology, pathophysiology and initial management. BJA Educ. 2022;22(3):94-103.
- Mgovern C, Puxty K, Paton L. Major burns: part 2. Anaesthesia, intensive care and pain management. BJA Educ. 2022;22(4):138-145.

# CRUSH INJURIES

## LEARNING OBJECTIVES

- The course and symptoms of crush injuries/crush syndrome
- Anesthetic management of crush injuries

## DEFINITION AND MECHANISM

- Crush injuries are the result of physical trauma from prolonged compression of the torso, limb(s), or other parts of the body
- Muscles are grossly swollen, hard, cold, insensitive, and necrotic
- Extended entrapment with compression may cause:
  - Crush syndrome
  - Traumatic rhabdomyolysis
  - Compartment syndrome
- Rhabdomyolysis is characterized by skeletal muscle disintegration and the release of myoglobin and other proteins and electrolytes into the circulation:
  - Magnesium, phosphate, acids, creatine phosphokinase, and lactate dehydrogenase
  - ↑ Potassium → cardiac arrhythmias
  - Sodium, calcium, and fluids → raised muscle volume and tension
  - Nitric Oxide (NO) → muscle vasodilatation and aggravation of hypotension
- Myoglobinuria and hypovolemia may lead to acute kidney injury
  - Tubular obstruction
  - Direct and ischemic tubular injury
  - Intrarenal vasoconstriction
- Disseminated intravascular coagulation may rarely happen with severe rhabdomyolysis
- Ultimately, patients go into shock affecting respiratory gas exchange due to lung edema

## SIGNS AND SYMPTOMS

- Petechiae
- Blisters
- Muscle bruising
- Superficial injuries
- Myalgia
- Muscle paralysis
- Sensory deficit
- Fever
- Cardiac arrhythmia

- Pneumonia
- 'Tea or cola' colored urine
- Oliguria
- Renal failure
- Nausea
- Vomiting
- Agitation
- Delirium

# MANAGEMENT

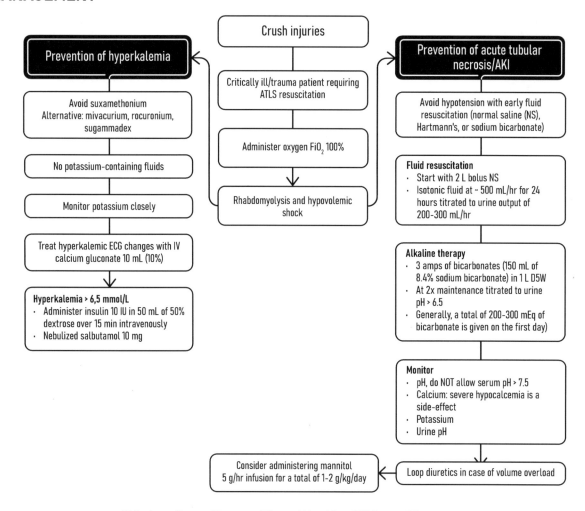

ATLS, advanced trauma life support; AKI, acute kidney injury; D5W, dextrose 5% in water.

## SUGGESTED READING

- James Williams, MBBCh FRCA FFICM, Chris Thorpe, MBBS FRCA FFICM, Rhabdomyolysis, Continuing Education in Anaesthesia Critical Care & Pain, Volume 14, Issue 4, August 2014, Pages 163-166.
- Pollard BJ, Kitchen, G. Handbook of Clinical Anaesthesia. Fourth Edition. CRC Press. 2018. 978-1-4987-6289-2.
- Rajagopalan S. Crush Injuries and the Crush Syndrome. Med J Armed Forces India. 2010;66(4):317-320.

# DROWNING

**38**

- Drowning is a type of suffocation induced by the submersion of the mouth and nose in a liquid
- The third leading cause of unintentional death
- 360,000 drowning victims annually worldwide
- Submersion time is the strongest predictor of outcome
- Patients require a trauma/advanced trauma life support (ATLS) approach
- Problem: survival after cardiac arrest from drowning-related asphyxia is rare
  □ 100% mortality = submersion > 25 min, resuscitation > 25 min, pulseless on arrival to ER, unconscious at the scene and on arrival to ED
- Most survivors sustain severe central nervous system injury

## MECHANISMS OF INJURY

- Hypoxia due to inhalation of fluid in the lungs, potentially leading to cardiac arrest
- Hypothermia:
  □ Coagulopathy
  □ Arrhythmias
  □ Hypovolemia
  □ Rewarming technique
  □ Electrolyte abnormalities
- Coagulopathy:
  □ Arrhythmias
  □ Hypovolemia
  □ Rewarming technique
  □ Electrolyte abnormalities

# MANAGEMENT

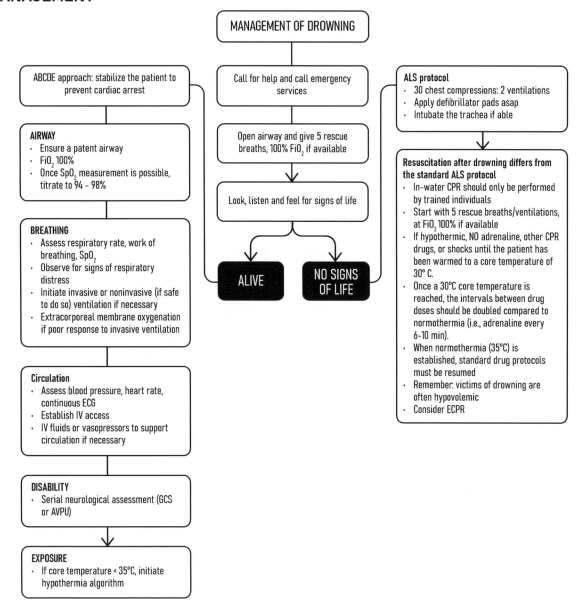

**MANAGEMENT OF DROWNING**

**ABCDE approach:** stabilize the patient to prevent cardiac arrest

**AIRWAY**
- Ensure a patent airway
- $FiO_2$ 100%
- Once $SpO_2$ measurement is possible, titrate to 94 - 98%

**BREATHING**
- Assess respiratory rate, work of breathing, $SpO_2$
- Observe for signs of respiratory distress
- Initiate invasive or noninvasive (if safe to do so) ventilation if necessary
- Extracorporeal membrane oxygenation if poor response to invasive ventilation

**Circulation**
- Assess blood pressure, heart rate, continuous ECG
- Establish IV access
- IV fluids or vasopressors to support circulation if necessary

**DISABILITY**
- Serial neurological assessment (GCS or AVPU)

**EXPOSURE**
- If core temperature < 35°C, initiate hypothermia algorithm

Call for help and call emergency services

Open airway and give 5 rescue breaths, 100% $FiO_2$ if available

Look, listen and feel for signs of life

**ALIVE**

**NO SIGNS OF LIFE**

**ALS protocol**
- 30 chest compressions: 2 ventilations
- Apply defibrillator pads asap
- Intubate the trachea if able

**Resuscitation after drowning differs from the standard ALS protocol**
- In-water CPR should only be performed by trained individuals
- Start with 5 rescue breaths/ventilations, at $FiO_2$ 100% if available
- If hypothermic, NO adrenaline, other CPR drugs, or shocks until the patient has been warmed to a core temperature of 30° C.
- Once a 30°C core temperature is reached, the intervals between drug doses should be doubled compared to normothermia (i.e., adrenaline every 6-10 min).
- When normothermia (35°C) is established, standard drug protocols must be resumed
- Remember: victims of drowning are often hypovolemic
- Consider ECPR

GCS, Glasgow Coma Scale; AVPU, Alert-Voice-Pain-Unresponsive; ECPR, Extracorporeal cardiopulmonary resuscitation.

## SUGGESTED READING

- Lott C, Truhlář A, Alfonzo A, et al. European Resuscitation Council Guidelines 2021: Cardiac arrest in special circumstances. Resuscitation. 2021;161:152-219.

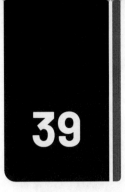

# INHALATION INJURY

## LEARNING OBJECTIVES

- Definition, classification, and management of inhalation injury

---

## DEFINITION AND MECHANISM

- Refers to damage to the respiratory tract or lung tissue from heat, smoke, or chemical irritants carried into the airway during inspiration
- The term is often used synonymously with smoke inhalation injury

## CLASSIFICATION AND CAUSES

| | Cause | Effect |
|---|---|---|
| Upper airway injury | Hot air<br>Steam | Laryngeal obstruction<br>Bronchospasm |
| Tracheobronchial injury | Chemicals in smoke<br>Inhalation of noxious gases (e.g., chlorine) or liquids (e.g., acid)<br>Direct airway fire (e.g., intraoperative)<br>Aspiration | Mucosal slough<br>Infection<br>Bronchiolar plugging<br>Atelectasis<br>Bronchospasm |
| Parenchymal injury | Irritant gases | Pneumonia<br>Pulmonary edema<br>Alveolar capillary defect |
| Systemic toxicity | CO poisoning<br>Hydrogen cyanide | |

## SIGNS AND SYMPTOMS

- Voice changes
- Hoarseness
- Stridor
- Cough
- Respiratory distress
- Decreased level of consciousness or confusion
- Agitation
- Clinical hypoxemia ($SpO_2$ < 94%)
- Dizziness
- Nausea
- Vomiting

# MANAGEMENT

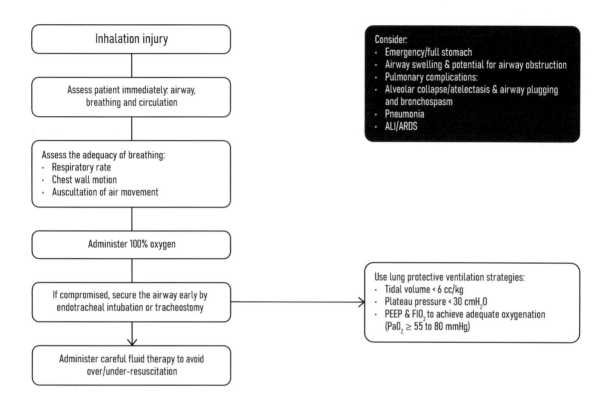

**Inhalation injury**

↓

Assess patient immediately: airway, breathing and circulation

↓

Assess the adequacy of breathing:
· Respiratory rate
· Chest wall motion
· Auscultation of air movement

↓

Administer 100% oxygen

↓

If compromised, secure the airway early by endotracheal intubation or tracheostomy  →  Use lung protective ventilation strategies:
· Tidal volume < 6 cc/kg
· Plateau pressure < 30 cmH$_2$O
· PEEP & FIO$_2$ to achieve adequate oxygenation (PaO$_2$ ≥ 55 to 80 mmHg)

↓

Administer careful fluid therapy to avoid over/under-resuscitation

**Consider:**
· Emergency/full stomach
· Airway swelling & potential for airway obstruction
· Pulmonary complications:
· Alveolar collapse/atelectasis & airway plugging and bronchospasm
· Pneumonia
· ALI/ARDS

# KEEP IN MIND

General burn considerations:
• Hypovolemic shock
• Hypo- or hyperthermia
• Rhabdomyolysis
• Cardiac depression
• Disseminated intravascular coagulation, consumptive coagulopathy

# SUGGESTED READING

• Bittner EA, Shank E, Woodson L, Martyn JA. Acute and perioperative care of the burn-injured patient. Anesthesiology. 2015;122(2):448-464.
• Preea Gill, FRCA, Rebecca V Martin, FRCA FFICM, Smoke inhalation injury, BJA Education, Volume 15, Issue 3, June 2015, Pages 143-148.

Inhalation injury

# ORGAN DONATION

## LEARNING OBJECTIVES

- Specify the adverse effects on organs after the diagnosis of death
- Describe the active management of the donor's physiology to optimize the quality of organs donated
- Outline the associated anesthesia interventions

## DEFINITION AND MECHANISM

- Organ donation and transplantation is removing an organ from one person (the donor) and surgically placing it in another (the recipient) whose organ has failed
- Death can be diagnosed by somatic, circulatory, and neurological criteria
- DBD: Donation after Brain Death
  - At least 2 physicians must declare brain death

- DCD: Donation after Cardiac Death
  - A DCD donor has suffered a severe non-recoverable brain insult
  - DCD donor's death is declared based on cardiopulmonary criteria after withdrawal of life support
  - Organ procurement can only start 5 minutes after death is declared

### *Active management of potential organ donors*

| Parameter | Target |
|---|---|
| Heart rate | 60-120 beats/min |
| Arterial pressure | Systolic pressure > 100 mmHg<br>Mean pressure $\geq$ 70 mmHg |
| Central venous pressure | 6-10 mmHg |
| Urine output | 0.5-3 mL/kg/h |
| Electrolytes | Serum sodium 130-150 mmol/L<br>Normal potassium, calcium, magnesium, phosphate<br>Glucose 4-8 mmol/L |
| Blood gases | pH 7.35-7.45<br>$PaCO_2$ 4.7-6 kPa<br>$PaO_2 \geq$ 10.7 kPa<br>$SPO_2$ saturation > 95% |
| Pulmonary capillary wedge pressure | 6-10 mmHg |
| Cardiac index | 2.4 L/min/m² |
| Systemic vascular resistance | 800-1200 dynes/sec/cm⁵ |

# MANAGEMENT

- Trauma and potential for multi-organ involvement
- Pulmonary/cardiac contusion

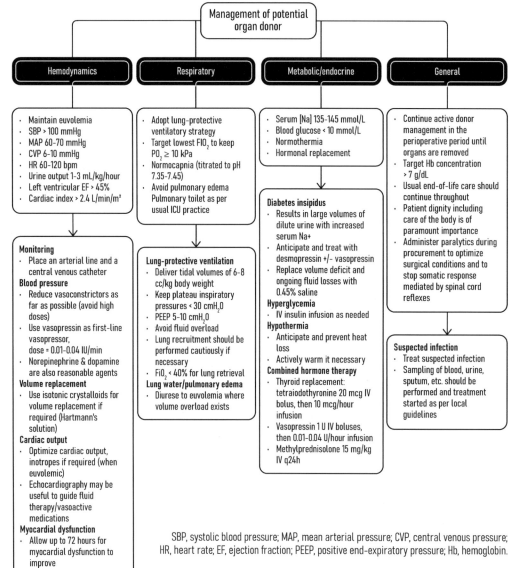

**Management of potential organ donor**

## Hemodynamics

- Maintain euvolemia
- SBP > 100 mmHg
- MAP 60-70 mmHg
- CVP 6-10 mmHg
- HR 60-120 bpm
- Urine output 1-3 mL/kg/hour
- Left ventricular EF > 45%
- Cardiac index > 2.4 L/min/m²

**Monitoring**
- Place an arterial line and a central venous catheter

**Blood pressure**
- Reduce vasoconstrictors as far as possible (avoid high doses)
- Use vasopressin as first-line vasopressor, dose = 0.01-0.04 IU/min
- Norepinephrine & dopamine are also reasonable agents

**Volume replacement**
- Use isotonic crystalloids for volume replacement if required (Hartmann's solution)

**Cardiac output**
- Optimize cardiac output, inotropes if required (when euvolemic)
- Echocardiography may be useful to guide fluid therapy/vasoactive medications

**Myocardial dysfunction**
- Allow up to 72 hours for myocardial dysfunction to improve

## Respiratory

- Adopt lung-protective ventilatory strategy
- Target lowest $FIO_2$ to keep $PO_2 \geq 10$ kPa
- Normocapnia (titrated to pH 7.35-7.45)
- Avoid pulmonary edema Pulmonary toilet as per usual ICU practice

**Lung-protective ventilation**
- Deliver tidal volumes of 6-8 cc/kg body weight
- Keep plateau inspiratory pressures < 30 cmH₂O
- PEEP 5-10 cmH₂O
- Avoid fluid overload
- Lung recruitment should be performed cautiously if necessary
- $FiO_2$ < 40% for lung retrieval

**Lung water/pulmonary edema**
- Diurese to euvolemia where volume overload exists

## Metabolic/endocrine

- Serum [Na] 135-145 mmol/L
- Blood glucose < 10 mmol/L
- Normothermia
- Hormonal replacement

**Diabetes insipidus**
- Results in large volumes of dilute urine with increased serum Na+
- Anticipate and treat with desmopressin +/- vasopressin
- Replace volume deficit and ongoing fluid losses with 0.45% saline

**Hyperglycemia**
- IV insulin infusion as needed

**Hypothermia**
- Anticipate and prevent heat loss
- Actively warm it necessary

**Combined hormone therapy**
- Thyroid replacement: tetraiodothyronine 20 mcg IV bolus, then 10 mcg/hour infusion
- Vasopressin 1 U IV boluses, then 0.01-0.04 U/hour infusion
- Methylprednisolone 15 mg/kg IV q24h

## General

- Continue active donor management in the perioperative period until organs are removed
- Target Hb concentration > 7 g/dL
- Usual end-of-life care should continue throughout
- Patient dignity including care of the body is of paramount importance
- Administer paralytics during procurement to optimize surgical conditions and to stop somatic response mediated by spinal cord reflexes

**Suspected infection**
- Treat suspected infection
- Sampling of blood, urine, sputum, etc. should be performed and treatment started as per local guidelines

SBP, systolic blood pressure; MAP, mean arterial pressure; CVP, central venous pressure; HR, heart rate; EF, ejection fraction; PEEP, positive end-expiratory pressure; Hb, hemoglobin.

## SUGGESTED READING

- Balogh J. Srikar J, Diaz G, Williams GW, Moguilevitch M. The role of anesthisiologists in organ donation. Transplantation reports. 2022;7(4).
- Corbett S, Trainor D, Gaffney A. Perioperative management of the organ donor after diagnosis of death using neurological criteria. BJA Educ. 2021;21(5):194-200.
- McKeown DW, Bonser RS, Kellum JA. Management of the heartbeating brain-dead organ donor. Br J Anaesth. 2012 Jan;108 Suppl 1:i96-107.

# PREGNANT TRAUMA PATIENTS

## LEARNING OBJECTIVES

- Discuss the potential for obstetric complications after trauma
- Outline the complex management challenges of trauma during pregnancy

## DEFINITION AND MECHANISM

- Trauma is the leading cause of non-obstetric mortality and affects 7% of all pregnancies
- The most common traumatic injuries are motor vehicle crashes, assaults, falls, or partner violence
- Major trauma has been associated with 7% of maternal and 80% of fetal mortality
- Placental abruption is the most common cause of fetal death:
    - First trimester: the thick-walled uterus is protected from trauma by the pelvic girdle
    - Second trimester: the fetus is protected by relatively abundant amniotic fluid volume
    - Third trimester: the thin-walled uterus is exposed to blunt and penetrating abdominal trauma
- Pregnant trauma patients should be approached and managed like any other trauma patient using a standard ABCD approach
- Clinical decision-making is complicated by:
    - The needs of both mother and fetus must be considered
    - Anatomical and physiological changes in pregnancy can mask or mimic injury
    - Life-threatening obstetric complications can occur even after seemingly minor trauma and may require urgent delivery of the fetus
    - Consider that fetal injury may predominate of that of the mother
- Establishing maternal stability may not be possible without obstetric intervention

## COMPLICATIONS

- Fetomaternal hemorrhage
- Placental abruption
- Uterine rupture
- Preterm labor
- Spontaneous miscarriage
- Pelvic fracture

## INJURY SEVERITY SCORE

- The same injury severity score applies to pregnant women as non-pregnant women

## Physiological changes of pregnancy

| System | Changes | Implications |
|---|---|---|
| Pulmonary system | ↑ Tidal volume<br>The respiratory rate is unchanged<br>↓ FRC<br>↑ Oxygen consumption<br>↑ Minute ventilation<br>↓ Arterial $CO_2$ tension<br>↓ Thoracic compliance<br>Elevated diaphragm | Apply supplementary oxygen to avoid hypoxia<br>Consider desaturation<br>Bag mask ventilation may be difficult<br>Place chest drains higher (3rd or 4th intercostal space) |
| Airway | ↑ Airway edema<br>↑ Vascular engorgement<br>↑ Tissue friability<br>↑ Breast size and neck adiposity<br>↑ Aspiration risk | Difficult intubation<br>Consider cricoid pressure<br>insert early NGT |
| Cardiovascular system | ↑ Plasma volume (40-50%)<br>↑ Heart rate (15-25%)<br>↑ Cardiac output (50%)<br>↓ SVR (20%) | Increased blood volume may initially mask the shock<br>Supine hypotension due to IVC compression may reduce CO |
| Hematological changes | Hypercoagulability<br>Anemia<br>Thrombocytopenia<br>↑ Factors VII, VIII, IX, X, XII, von Willebrand, and fibrinogen<br>↓ aPTT, PT, and INR | All Rhesus-negative mothers should receive anti-D within 72 hours of injury<br>Consider rhesus status when initiating blood product transfusion |
| Renal system | ↑ Renal blood flow<br>↑ Glomerular filtration rate (60%)<br>↓ Serum creatinine and bicarbonate | |
| Gastrointestinal system | ↓ Esophageal sphincter tone<br>Cephalad displacement of the stomach<br>↑ Intra-gastric pressure<br>Delayed gastric emptying | Perform early gastric decompression with NGT<br>The bladder becomes an intra-abdominal organ after 1st trimester<br>Other abdominal organs are displaced by the uterus |

FRC, functional residual capacity; SVR, systemic vascular resistance; aPTT, activated partial thromboplastin time; PT, prothrombin time; INR, international normalised ratio; NGT, nasogastric tube; IVC, inferior vena cava; CO, cardiac output.

Pregnant trauma patients

# MANAGEMENT

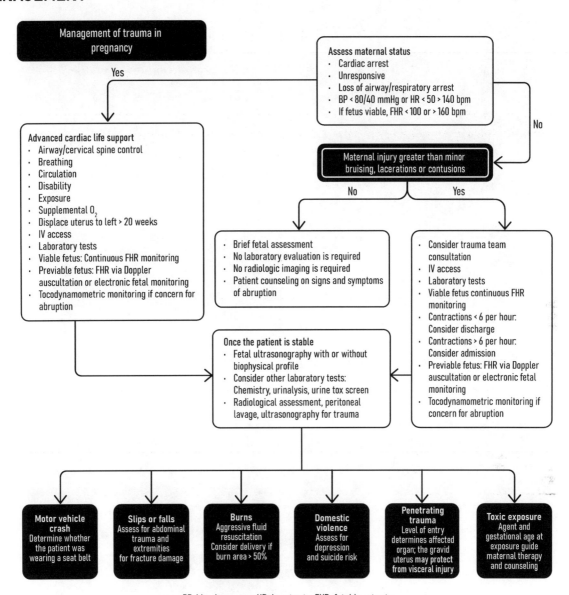

**Management of trauma in pregnancy**

**Assess maternal status**
- Cardiac arrest
- Unresponsive
- Loss of airway/respiratory arrest
- BP < 80/40 mmHg or HR < 50 > 140 bpm
- If fetus viable, FHR < 100 or > 160 bpm

Yes

No

**Advanced cardiac life support**
- Airway/cervical spine control
- Breathing
- Circulation
- Disability
- Exposure
- Supplemental O$_2$
- Displace uterus to left > 20 weeks
- IV access
- Laboratory tests
- Viable fetus: Continuous FHR monitoring
- Previable fetus: FHR via Doppler auscultation or electronic fetal monitoring
- Tocodynamometric monitoring if concern for abruption

**Maternal injury greater than minor bruising, lacerations or contusions**

No

Yes

- Brief fetal assessment
- No laboratory evaluation is required
- No radiologic imaging is required
- Patient counseling on signs and symptoms of abruption

- Consider trauma team consultation
- IV access
- Laboratory tests
- Viable fetus continuous FHR monitoring
- Contractions < 6 per hour: Consider discharge
- Contractions > 6 per hour: Consider admission
- Previable fetus: FHR via Doppler auscultation or electronic fetal monitoring
- Tocodynamometric monitoring if concern for abruption

**Once the patient is stable**
- Fetal ultrasonography with or without biophysical profile
- Consider other laboratory tests: Chemistry, urinalysis, urine tox screen
- Radiological assessment, peritoneal lavage, ultrasonography for trauma

**Motor vehicle crash**
Determine whether the patient was wearing a seat belt

**Slips or falls**
Assess for abdominal trauma and extremities for fracture damage

**Burns**
Aggressive fluid resuscitation Consider delivery if burn area > 50%

**Domestic violence**
Assess for depression and suicide risk

**Penetrating trauma**
Level of entry determines affected organ; the gravid uterus may protect from visceral injury

**Toxic exposure**
Agent and gestational age at exposure guide maternal therapy and counseling

BP, blood pressure; HR, heart rate; FHR, fetal heart rate.

### AIRWAY AND SPINAL IMMOBILIZATION

Consider:
- Tissue edema
- Difficult laryngoscopy
- Airway trauma
- Facial burns
- Perform early intubation in case of airway problems
- Position the patient carefully with a 30° head-up tilt to improve FRC
- Preoxygenate the patient
- Remove the cervical collar and provide manual-in-line stabilization to allow for effective laryngoscopy

Perform rapid sequence induction
- Tailor induction drugs and neuromuscular blocking agents to the individual circumstances
- Avoid nasal or blind airway interventions

Apply apneic oxygenation technique:
- Provide 10 cmH₂O continuous positive airway pressure via a tightly fitted face mask
- Supplemental oxygen flow through a nasal cannula
- Perform a tracheostomy in case of a failed intubation

### BREATHING

- Be aware of the rapid development of maternal hypoxemia
- Provide high-concentration oxygen supplementation
- Position the patient carefully with a 30° head-up tilt to improve FRC
- Aim for a $PaCO_2$ of 4.0 kPa if mechanically ventilated
- Immediately perform thoracic decompression in case of hemodynamic instability and severe respiratory compromise secondary to a hemopneumothorax
- Place thoracostomy tubes one or two spaces above the usual intercostal space to avoid iatrogenic injury

### CATASTROPHIC HEMORRHAGE

- Note that > 1.5 L of blood may be lost before signs of hypovolemia present during the third trimester
- Identify bleeding sources with the systematic examination, bedside investigation, CT, or ultrasound
- Be aware of pelvic fractures and apply pelvic binders immediately
- Perform fetal assessment and monitoring after 20 weeks of gestation
- Consider the appropriateness of a restrictive fluid replacement strategy
- Consider delivery of the fetus to manage the bleeding and provide a viable fetus
- Treat hemorrhagic shock with O-negative blood transfusion until group and Rh status are determined
- If blood is not immediately available, small boluses of warmed crystalloid can be used
- Correct hypocalcemia and hyperkalemia during massive transfusion
- Tranexamic acid (1 g IV) is safe during pregnancy
- Avoid vasopressor use
- Perform frequent point-of-care and coagulation tests
- Individualized clotting factor and fibrinogen replacement strategy and aim for:
  - Fibrinogen > 2/L
  - Activated partial thromboplastin time and prothrombin time ratios < 1.5
  - Platelets > 100 x 109/L
- Avoid hypothermia to avoid coagulopathy and further bleeding by using warming devices
- Administer 12 mg betamethasone IM between 24-34 weeks of gestation to promote fetal lung maturity in case of imminent delivery and repeat in 24 hours

### CIRCULATION

Provide aortocaval relief by manual uterine displacement or left lateral tilt the patient in gestations > 20 weeks
Insert two large-bore cannulas immediately
Provide intraosseous access or central venous access if IV access is difficult
Perform blood tests:
- Cross-match
- Full blood count
- Urea and electrolytes
- Liver function tests
- Coagulation screen
- Arterial blood gas
- Acid-base balance
- Thromboelasticity assays
- Hemoglobin

Insert an arterial line if compromised cardiorespiratory function is expected
Perform the Kleihauer-Betke blood test to investigate the degree of fetomaternal hemorrhage after uteroplacental injury
Monitor the patient by tocodynamometry:
- Minor trauma: minimum 4 hours
- Major trauma: minimum 24 hours if:
- At least six uterine contractions have occured
- Nonreassuring fetal heart rate patterns
- Vaginal bleeding
- Significant uterine tenderness
- Severe maternal injury
- Positive Kleihauer-Betke test result

FRC, functional residual capacity.

### MATERNAL CARDIAC ARREST

- Perform immediate left lateral uterine displacement to allow for more effective cardiac compressions:
  - By left lateral tilting the maternal body 25-30 degrees
  - Or by manual uterine displacement
- Manage according to standard advanced cardiac life support (ACLS)
  - Perform early intubation
  - Remove all uterine and fetal monitors
- Perform a perimortem cesarean delivery within 4 min of arrest

### NEUROLOGICAL DISABILITY

- Asses LOC and pupillary reactions
- Supplement oxygen delivery to prevent secondary insult
- Perform head-up tilt
- Maintain adequate MAP and oxygenation
- Avoid venous congestion in the neck
- Control $PaCO_2$
- In case of intracranial hypertension and associated brain herniation:
  - Maternal hyperventilation is required
  - Allow hypocapnia and alkalosis but this may be at the expense of fetal oxygenation
- In case of spinal cord injury:
  - Correct placement of cervical collar might be impossible due to neck edema, adipose tissue, or large breasts
  - Perform manual in-line stabilization
  - Remove spinal boards asap
- Monitor blood glucose to prevent hyper- or hypoglycemia

LOC, level of consciousness; MAP, mean arterial pressure.

Discharge criteria:

- Resolution of contractions
- A reassuring fetal heart tracing
- Intact membranes
- No vaginal bleeding
- No uterine tenderness
- Administer Rh immune globulin therapy to all Rh-negative patients unless the injury is remote from the uterus

## MANAGEMENT

- Cesarean delivery
- Challenges in obstetrics anesthesiology
- Non-obstetric surgery

## SUGGESTED READING

- Huls CK, Detlefs C. Trauma in pregnancy. Semin Perinatol. 2018;42(1):13-20.
- Irving, T., Menon, R., Ciantar, E., 2021. Trauma during pregnancy. BJA Education 21, 10–19.
- Jain V, Chari R, Maslovitz S, et al. Guidelines for the Management of a Pregnant Trauma Patient. J Obstet Gynaecol Can. 2015;37(6):553-574.

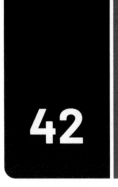

# SEPSIS

## LEARNING OBJECTIVES

- Definition of sepsis
- Diagnostic features of sepsis
- Management of sepsis

## DEFINITION AND MECHANISM

- Sepsis is a dysregulated systemic response to infection that is associated with organ dysfunction
- Quick sequential organ failure assessment (qSOFA) criteria:
  - Altered mental status (GCS score < 15)
  - Systolic blood pressure < 100 mmHg
  - Respiratory rate > 22 breaths per min
- Septic shock is defined as low blood pressure due to sepsis that does not improve after fluid replacement
- Characterized by high morbidity and mortality (30-50% of affected patients)
- Septic patients are at risk for secondary injuries
- Bacteria, fungi, and viruses can all cause sepsis

## SIGNS AND SYMPTOMS

- Fever or hypothermia
- Increased heart rate
- Increased breathing rate
- Confusion
- Hypotension
- Sweating
- Edema
- Low urine output

## RISK FACTORS

- Age > 65 years
- Newborns and infants
- Pregnancy
- Medical conditions such as diabetes, obesity, cancer, and kidney disease
- A weakened immune system
- Patients hospitalized for other medical reasons
- Severe injuries, such as large burns or wounds
- Patients with catheters, IVs, or breathing tubes

## DIAGNOSTIC FEATURES

| Organ system | Alteration or dysfunction |
|---|---|
| Neurological | Delirium<br>Altered mental status<br>Ischemia<br>Formation of blood clots in small blood vessels<br>Microabscesses<br>Multifocal necrotizing leukoencephalopathy |
| Cardiovascular | Vasodilation<br>Hypovolemia<br>Cardiac dysfunction<br>Systolic and diastolic dysfunction |
| Pulmonary | Tachypnea<br>Poor gas exchange<br>Acute Respiratory Distress Syndrome |
| Gastrointestinal | Ileus<br>Hyperbilirubinemia |
| Kidney | Oliguria<br>Elevated plasma urea and creatinine<br>Volume overload |
| Hepatic | Disruption of blood clotting<br>Elevated unconjugated serum bilirubin levels |
| Hematological | Perioperative anemia<br>Thrombocytopenia<br>Coagulopathy<br>Disseminated Intravascular Coagulation (DIC) |
| Endocrine and metabolic | Hyperglycemia<br>Sick euthyroid syndrome<br>Elevated lactate |
| Infectious disease | Leucocytosis<br>Elevated inflammatory mediators |

# TREATMENT

- Aggressive source control, resuscitation, and antibiotic therapy are the mainstays of management
- Be aware of subtle changes such as hyperglycemia, ileus, mental status changes, and potential sources of infections

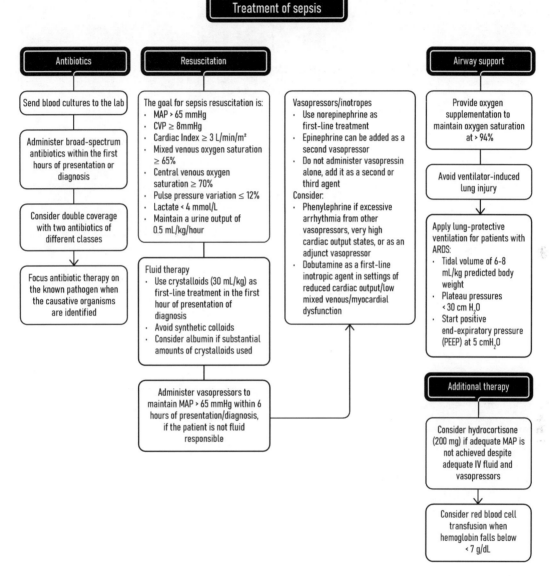

MAP, mean arterial pressure; CVP, central venous pressure; ARDS, acute respiratory distress syndrome

# MANAGEMENT

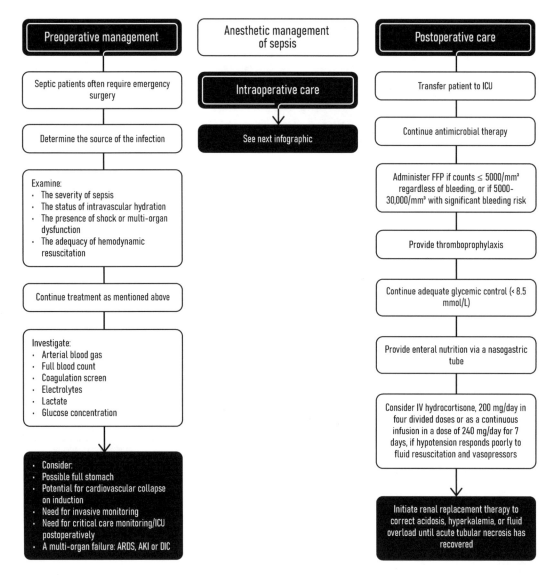

**Preoperative management**

Septic patients often require emergency surgery

Determine the source of the infection

Examine:
- The severity of sepsis
- The status of intravascular hydration
- The presence of shock or multi-organ dysfunction
- The adequacy of hemodynamic resuscitation

Continue treatment as mentioned above

Investigate:
- Arterial blood gas
- Full blood count
- Coagulation screen
- Electrolytes
- Lactate
- Glucose concentration

- Consider:
- Possible full stomach
- Potential for cardiovascular collapse on induction
- Need for invasive monitoring
- Need for critical care monitoring/ICU postoperatively
- A multi-organ failure: ARDS, AKI or DIC

**Anesthetic management of sepsis**

**Intraoperative care**

See next infographic

**Postoperative care**

Transfer patient to ICU

Continue antimicrobial therapy

Administer FFP if counts ≤ 5000/mm³ regardless of bleeding, or if 5000-30,000/mm³ with significant bleeding risk

Provide thromboprophylaxis

Continue adequate glycemic control (< 8.5 mmol/L)

Provide enteral nutrition via a nasogastric tube

Consider IV hydrocortisone, 200 mg/day in four divided doses or as a continuous infusion in a dose of 240 mg/day for 7 days, if hypotension responds poorly to fluid resuscitation and vasopressors

Initiate renal replacement therapy to correct acidosis, hyperkalemia, or fluid overload until acute tubular necrosis has recovered

ARDS, acute respiratory distress syndrome; AKI, acute kidney injury; DIC, disseminated intravascular coagulation; FFP, fresh frozen plasma.

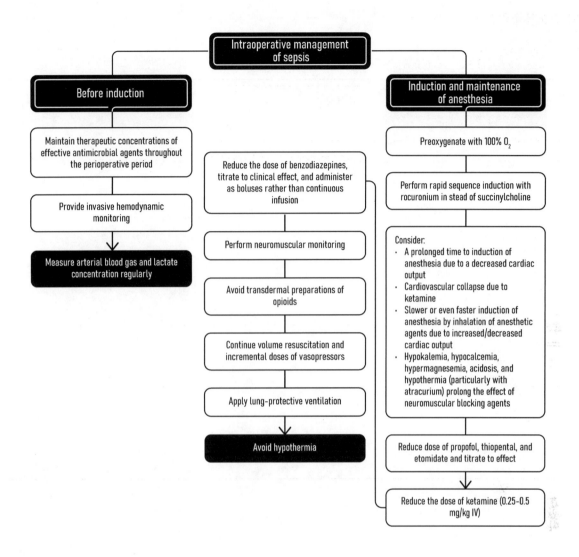

**Intraoperative management of sepsis**

**Before induction**

Maintain therapeutic concentrations of effective antimicrobial agents throughout the perioperative period

Provide invasive hemodynamic monitoring

Measure arterial blood gas and lactate concentration regularly

Reduce the dose of benzodiazepines, titrate to clinical effect, and administer as boluses rather than continuous infusion

Perform neuromuscular monitoring

Avoid transdermal preparations of opioids

Continue volume resuscitation and incremental doses of vasopressors

Apply lung-protective ventilation

Avoid hypothermia

**Induction and maintenance of anesthesia**

Preoxygenate with 100% $O_2$

Perform rapid sequence induction with rocuronium in stead of succinylcholine

Consider:
- A prolonged time to induction of anesthesia due to a decreased cardiac output
- Cardiovascular collapse due to ketamine
- Slower or even faster induction of anesthesia by inhalation of anesthetic agents due to increased/decreased cardiac output
- Hypokalemia, hypocalcemia, hypermagnesemia, acidosis, and hypothermia (particularly with atracurium) prolong the effect of neuromuscular blocking agents

Reduce dose of propofol, thiopental, and etomidate and titrate to effect

Reduce the dose of ketamine (0.25-0.5 mg/kg IV)

## SUGGESTED READING

- Ammar, M.A., Ammar, A.A., Wieruszewski, P.M. et al. Timing of vasoactive agents and corticosteroid initiation in septic shock. Ann. Intensive Care 12, 47 (2022).
- Charlton, M., Thompson, J.P., 2019. Pharmacokinetics in sepsis. BJA Education 19, 7–13.
- Gyawali B, Ramakrishna K, Dhamoon AS. Sepsis: The evolution in definition, pathophysiology, and management. SAGE Open Med. 2019;7:2050312119835043.
- Eissa D, Carton EG, Buggy DJ. Anaesthetic management of patients with severe sepsis. Br J Anaesth. 2010;105(6):734-743.
- Keeley A, Hine P, Nsutebu EThe recognition and management of sepsis and septic shock: a guide for non-intensivistsPostgraduate Medical Journal 2017;93:626-634.
- Nunnally, M.E., 2016. Sepsis for the anaesthetist. British Journal of Anaesthesia 117, 44–51.

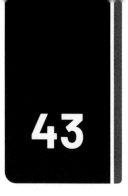

# TRAUMA

## LEARNING OBJECTIVES

- Assessment of the injury severity score of trauma
- Immediate treatment of trauma
- Anesthetic management of trauma

## DEFINITION AND MECHANISM

- Defined as a body wound resulting from a sudden physical injury from impact, violence, or accident
- Minor, serious, life-threatening, or potentially life-threatening injuries
- Blunt or penetrating wound
- The severity of trauma is classified according to the injury type, the physical location of the injury, and how many injuries there are
- Immediately life-threatening injuries:
  - Airway obstruction
  - Tension pneumothorax
  - Open pneumothorax
  - Cardiac tamponade
  - Massive hemothorax
  - Flail chest
- Delayed/hidden injuries:
  - Thoracic aortic disruption
  - Tracheobronchial disruption
  - Myocardial contusion
  - Traumatic diaphragmatic tear
  - Esophageal disruption
  - Pulmonary contusion and lacerations

## COMPLICATIONS

- Hemorrhage
- Infection
- Sepsis
- Multi-organ failure

## INJURY SEVERITY SCORE

- Individual body regions are assigned an abbreviated injury scale (AIS) score
- The three most severely injured body regions then have their score squared and added together to produce the AIS score
- The total score is labeled "injury severity scale" and a total of 75 or more is considered unsurvivable

| Abbreviated injury scale | Injury |
|---|---|
| 1 | Minor |
| 2 | Moderate |
| 3 | Serious |
| 4 | Severe |
| 5 | Critical |
| 6 | Unsurvivable |

## IMMEDIATE TREATMENT

- Cardiovascular reuscitation
- Cervical collars:
  - May increase secondary neurological injury, intracranial pressure
  - May worsen intubation conditions
- Secure the airway
  - Use video laryngoscopy if a cneck collar is present
- Proactive early treatment to counter the 'lethal triad' of acidosis, hypothermia, and coagulopathy
  - Warm the OR
  - Warmed IV line
  - Rapid infuser with warming capability
- Permissive hypotension and establishment of a massive transfusion protocol
- Early treatment of anticipated coagulopathy with blood products
- Other injuries, considerable pain, or distal ischemia may complicate the management

# MANAGEMENT

- Fracture reduction requires general or regional anesthesia
- Proximal fracture reduction or joint relocation performed under GA may require a small dose of a neuromuscular blocker to facilitate manipulation

- Manipulation under anesthesia (MUA)
  - Relocation of dislocated joints
  - Correct fracture deformity
  - Improve mobility of fixed joints
  - Improve mobility after arthroplasty:
    - Internal fixation
    - Distal long bone fracture plating
    - Intramedullary nailing procedures
    - External fixation

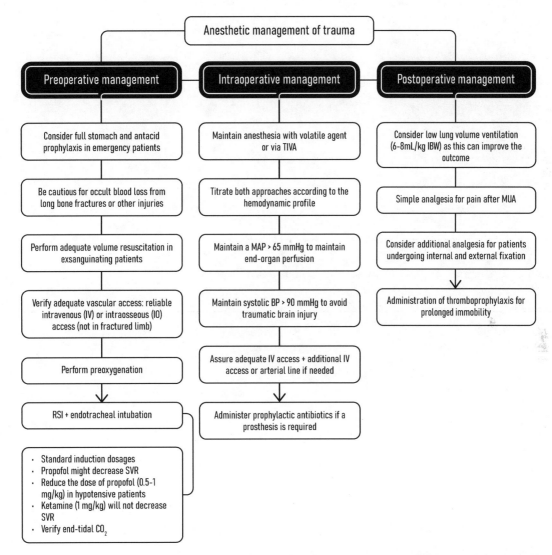

RSI, rapid sequence intubation; SVR, systemic vascular resistance; TIVA, total intravenous anesthesia; MAP, mean arterial pressure; BP, blood pressure; MUA, manipulation under anesthesia.

# SUGGESTED READING

- Pollard BJ, Kitchen, G. Handbook of Clinical Anaesthesia. Fourth Edition. CRC Press. 2018. 978-1-4987-6289-2.
- Tobin JM, Barras WP, Bree S, et al. Anesthesia for Trauma Patients. Mil Med. 2018;183(suppl_2):32-35.
- Uday Jain, Maureen McCunn, Charles E. Smith, Jean-Francois Pittet; Management of the Traumatized Airway. Anesthesiology 2016; 124:199-206.

# EMERGENCIES

# ADVANCED LIFE SUPPORT

**44**

## LEARNING OBJECTIVES

- Recognize anesthetic complications associated with cardiac arrest
- Recognize cardiac arrest
- Treat cardiac arrest associated with anesthesia

## DEFINITION AND MECHANISM

- Advanced life support is a set of life-saving protocols and skills that extend basic life support to further support the circulation and provide an open airway and adequate ventilation (breathing)
- Advanced life support is used to provide urgent treatment for cardiac emergencies such as cardiac arrest, stroke, myocardial infarction, and other conditions
- Should only be performed by paramedics and healthcare providers who have undergone certified training course

## SIGNS OF CARDIAC ARREST

- ECG with pulseless rhythm
  - Ventricular tachycardia
  - Ventricular fibrillation
  - Severe bradycardia
  - Asystole
- Loss of:
  - Carotid pulse > 10 seconds
  - End-tidal $CO_2$ on capnograph
  - Arterial line tracing
  - Pulse oximeter signal

## ANESTHETIC COMPLICATIONS ASSOCIATED WITH PERIOPERATIVE CARDIAC ARREST

- Intravenous anesthetic overdose
- Inhalation anesthetic overdose
- Neuraxial block with high-level sympathectomy
- Local anesthetic systemic toxicity
- Malignant hyperthermia
- Drug administration errors

# MANAGEMENT OF CARDIAC ARREST ASSOCIATED WITH ANESTHESIA

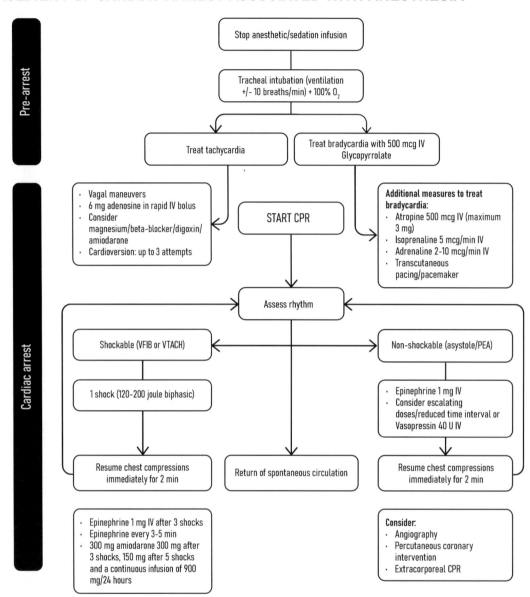

**Pre-arrest**

Stop anesthetic/sedation infusion

Tracheal intubation (ventilation +/- 10 breaths/min) + 100% $O_2$

Treat tachycardia

Treat bradycardia with 500 mcg IV Glycopyrrolate

- Vagal maneuvers
- 6 mg adenosine in rapid IV bolus
- Consider magnesium/beta-blocker/digoxin/amiodarone
- Cardioversion: up to 3 attempts

START CPR

**Additional measures to treat bradycardia:**
- Atropine 500 mcg IV (maximum 3 mg)
- Isoprenaline 5 mcg/min IV
- Adrenaline 2-10 mcg/min IV
- Transcutaneous pacing/pacemaker

**Cardiac arrest**

Assess rhythm

Shockable (VFIB or VTACH)

Non-shockable (asystole/PEA)

1 shock (120-200 joule biphasic)

- Epinephrine 1 mg IV
- Consider escalating doses/reduced time interval or Vasopressin 40 U IV

Resume chest compressions immediately for 2 min

Return of spontaneous circulation

Resume chest compressions immediately for 2 min

- Epinephrine 1 mg IV after 3 shocks
- Epinephrine every 3-5 min
- 300 mg amiodarone 300 mg after 3 shocks, 150 mg after 5 shocks and a continuous infusion of 900 mg/24 hours

**Consider:**
- Angiography
- Percutaneous coronary intervention
- Extracorporeal CPR

CPR, cardiopulmonary resuscitation; VFIB, ventricular fibrillation; VTACH, ventricular tachycardia; PEA, pulseless electrical activity.

Advanced life support

## POST RESUSCITATION CARE

- Apply invasive monitoring
- Finalize surgical plan and transport patient to ICU
- Perform a full history and examination
- Consider therapeutic hypothermia

## KEEP IN MIND

- Defibrillation is only possible if there is a shockable rhythm (i.e., ventricular fibrillation, ventricular tachycardia) occurs
- Bradycardia and hypotension under general anesthesia are relatively common
- Cardiac arrest in the perioperative setting is relatively rare and knowing when to initiate CPR can be difficult
- CPR should be established immediately and treatment will depend on the rhythm seen on ECG monitoring

**SUGGESTED READING**

- McEvoy MD, Thies KC, Einav S, et al. Cardiac Arrest in the Operating Room: Part 2-Special Situations in the Perioperative Period [published correction appears in Anesth Analg. 2018 May;126(5):1797]. Anesth Analg. 2018;126(3):889-903.
- Moitra VK, Gabrielli A, Maccioli GA, O'Connor MF. Anesthesia advanced circulatory life support. Can J Anaesth. 2012 Jun;59(6):586-603. doi: 10.1007/s12630-012-9699-3.
- Moitra VK, Einav S, Thies KC, et al. Cardiac Arrest in the Operating Room: Resuscitation and Management for the Anesthesiologist: Part 1. Anesth Analg. 2018;126(3):876-888.
- Panchal AR, Bartos JA, Cabañas JG, et al. Part 3: Adult Basic and Advanced Life Support: 2020 American Heart Association Guidelines for Cardiopulmonary Resuscitation and Emergency Cardiovascular Care. Circulation. 2020;142(16_suppl_2):S366-S468.
- Pollard BJ, Kitchen, G. Handbook of Clinical Anaesthesia. Fourth Edition. CRC Press. 2018. 978-1-4987-6289-2.
- Soar J, Böttiger BW, Carli P, et al. European Resuscitation Council Guidelines 2021: Adult advanced life support [published correction appears in Resuscitation. 2021 Oct;167:105-106]. Resuscitation. 2021;161:115-151.

# AIRWAY FIRE

## LEARNING OBJECTIVES

- Recognize an airway fire
- Management of an airway fire

## DEFINITION AND MECHANISM

- An airway fire is defined as a fire occurring in a patient's airway
- May or may not include a fire in the attached breathing circuit
- All airway fires require three components known as the "fire triad":
  - Oxidizers: Oxygen and nitrous oxide
  - Ignition source: electrosurgical devices, lasers, heated probes, burrs and drills, fiberoptic scopes, and defibrillator paddles or pads
  - Fuel: tracheal tubes, sponges, drapes, gauzes, alcohol-containing solutions, oxygen masks, nasal cannulae, patient's hair, dressings, gowns, gloves, or packaging materials

## PREVENTION

- Determine if the procedure is high-risk
- Agree upon a team plan and team roles for preventing and managing a fire
- Notify the surgeon of the presence of an increase in an oxidizer-enriched atmosphere
- Before an ignition source is activated:
  - Announce the intended use of an ignition source
  - Reduce the oxygen concentration to a minimum value needed to avoid hypoxia
  - Stop the use of nitrous oxide
- Avoid using ignition sources near oxidizer-enriched environments
- Configure the drapes to avoid oxidizer pooling or accumulation
- Allow flammable skin-prepping solutions to dry completely
- Sponges and gauzes should be moistened if used near ignition sources
- Airway laser procedures: use laser-resistant cuffed tubes and fill the cuff with saline tinted with methylene blue to identify a cuff puncture by the laser

# MANAGEMENT

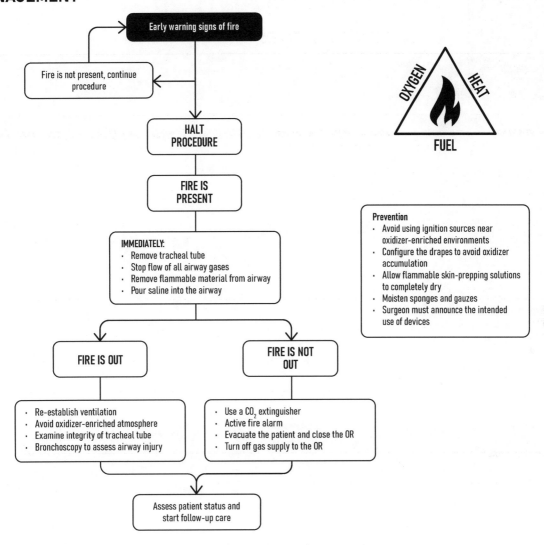

**Early warning signs of fire**

Fire is not present, continue procedure

**HALT PROCEDURE**

**FIRE IS PRESENT**

**IMMEDIATELY:**
- Remove tracheal tube
- Stop flow of all airway gases
- Remove flammable material from airway
- Pour saline into the airway

**FIRE IS OUT**
- Re-establish ventilation
- Avoid oxidizer-enriched atmosphere
- Examine integrity of tracheal tube
- Bronchoscopy to assess airway injury

**FIRE IS NOT OUT**
- Use a $CO_2$ extinguisher
- Active fire alarm
- Evacuate the patient and close the OR
- Turn off gas supply to the OR

Assess patient status and start follow-up care

OXYGEN — HEAT — FUEL

**Prevention**
- Avoid using ignition sources near oxidizer-enriched environments
- Configure the drapes to avoid oxidizer accumulation
- Allow flammable skin-prepping solutions to completely dry
- Moisten sponges and gauzes
- Surgeon must announce the intended use of devices

## KEEP IN MIND

The following supplies should be immediately available in the operating room:

- Several containers of sterile saline
- A $CO_2$ fire extinguisher
- Replacement tracheal tubes, guides, facemasks
- Rigid laryngoscope blades including a rigid fiberoptic laryngoscope
- Replacement airway breathing circuits and lines
- Replacement drapes, sponges

## SUGGESTED READING

- Akhtar N, Ansar F, Baig MS, Abbas A. Airway fires during surgery: Management and prevention. J Anaesthesiol Clin Pharmacol. 2016;Jan-Mar;32(1):109-11.
- Apfelbaum JL, Caplan RA, Barker SJ, et al. Practice advisory for the prevention and management of operating room fires: an updated report by the American Society of Anesthesiologists Task Force on Operating Room Fires. Anesthesiology. 2013;118(2):271-290.
- Cowles CE Jr, Culp WC Jr. Prevention of and response to surgical fires. BJA Educ. 2019;19(8):261-266.

Airway fire

# ANAPHYLAXIS

## LEARNING OBJECTIVES

- Recognize signs and symptoms of anaphylaxis
- Define the grade and management of anaphylaxis

## DEFINITION AND MECHANISM

- Anaphylaxis is a severe and potentially life-threatening allergic reaction that develops suddenly and requires immediate medical attention
- The most common anaphylactic reactions are to foods, insect stings, medications, and latex
- Tissues in different parts of the body release histamine and other substances, which causes the airway to tighten

## SIGNS AND SYMPTOMS

- Sweating
- Rash/hives
- Nausea
- Vomiting or diarrhea
- Wheezing/shortness of breath due to airway constriction or swollen throat
- Fainting with loss of consciousness
- Angiedema
- Hypotension
- Tachycardia

## ANAPHYLAXIS GRADES

| | Dermal | Abdominal | Respiratory | Cardiovascular |
|---|---|---|---|---|
| Grade I | Erythema<br>Urticaria<br>Angioedema | | | |
| Grade II | Erythema<br>Urticaria<br>Angioedema | Nausea<br>Cramping | Bronchospasm | Moderate hypotension<br>Tachycardia |
| Grade III | Erythema<br>Urticaria<br>Angioedema | Nausea<br>Vomiting<br>Diarrhea | Severe<br>bronchospasm | Life-threatening hypotension<br>Tachycardia or bradycardia with or<br>without intraoperative arrhythmias |
| Grade IV | Erythema<br>Urticaria<br>Angioedema | Vomiting<br>Defecation<br>Diarrhea | Respiratory arrest | Cardiac arrest |

# MANAGEMENT

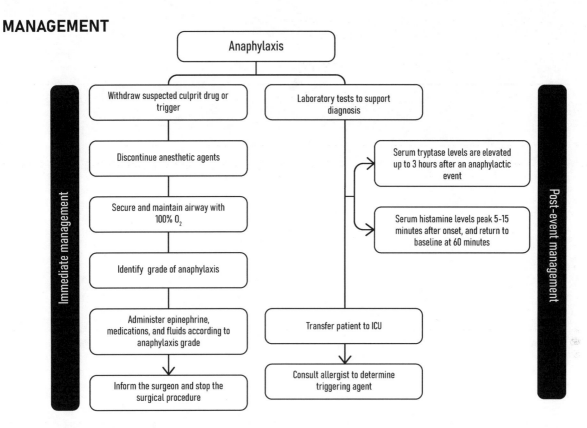

## TREATMENT OF ANAPHYLAXIS GRADES

| | Intravenous epinephrine | Intravenous fluids (crystalloids) |
|---|---|---|
| Grade II | Start with 20 μg bolus IV<br>Inadequate response after 2 minutes: escalate to 50 μg and repeat every 2 minutes<br>If no IV access: administer 300 μg IM | 500 mL rapid bolus<br>Review response<br>Repeat as needed |
| Grade III | 50 μg bolus or 100 μg bolus IV if inadequate response to other vasopressors or bronchodilators<br>Inadequate response at 2 min: escalate to 200 μg and repeat every 2 minutes | 1 L rapid bolus<br>Review response<br>Repeat as needed up to 30 mL/kg |
| Grade IV | 500 μg IM/IV over 3 minutes followed by a continuous infusion (4–10 μg/min)<br>Repeat as per ALS guidelines<br>Suggest ECM if systolic < 50 mmHg or end-tidal $CO_2$ < 3 kPa (20 mmHg) | |
| Refractory anaphylaxis: inadequate response > 10 min after symptom onset | Double epinephrine dose<br>If response after more than three boluses of epinephrine IV is inadequate, add epinephrine infusion 0.05–0.1 μg/kg/min<br><br>Hypotension - consider adding:<br>Vasopressin 1–2 IU with or without infusion 2 IU/h<br>Glucagon 1–2 mg (if on beta-adrenergic receptor blockers)<br>Norepinephrine infusion 0.05–0.5 μg/kg/min<br>Suggest ECLS: where available<br><br>Bronchospasm - add: inhaled or IV bronchodilators (β2-agonist such as salbutamol or albuterol) | |

ALS, advanced life support; ECLS, extracorporeal life support; ECM, external cardiac massage.

Anaphylaxis

## SUGGESTED READING

- Dewachter P, Mouton-Faivre C, Emala CW. Anaphylaxis and anesthesia: controversies and new insights. Anesthesiology. 2009;111(5):1141-1150.
- Garvey LH, Dewachter P, Hepner DL, et al. Management of suspected immediate perioperative allergic reactions: an international overview and consensus recommendations. Br J Anaesth. 2019;123(1):e50-e64.

Anaphylaxis

# BRONCHOSPASM

## LEARNING OBJECTIVES

- Recognize the signs and symptoms of bronchospasm
- Manage and prevent bronchospasm

**DEFINITION AND MECHANISM**

- Bronchospasm or a bronchial spasm is a sudden constriction of the muscles in the walls of the bronchioles
- It is caused by the release (degranulation) of substances from mast cells or basophils under the influence of anaphylatoxins

## SIGNS AND SYMPTOMS

- Wheezing
- Prolonged expiration
- ↑ Peak inspiratory pressure
- ↓ Exhaled tidal volume
- ↓ Oxygen saturation
- A delayed rise in end-tidal $CO_2$ on capnograph
- Hypotension
- Moderate tachycardia
- ↑ Resistance
- ↓ Lung compliance

## CAUSES

- Bronchospasm is a reversible reflex spasm of the smooth muscle in the bronchi, is vagally mediated and is more common in asthmatics
- Histamine, released due to stimuli such as cold air, smoking, upper respiratory tract infection, or inhaled irritants, provokes bronchospasm
- Bronchospasm during the perioperative period may be caused by anaphylaxis, tracheal intubation, or drugs (i.e., morphine or atracurium)

## MANAGEMENT

### Preoperative managment
- Supplemental oxygen
- Inhaled β2-agonists
- Intravenous steroids

## BRONCHOSPASM DURING ANESTHESIA

SUSPICION OF BRONCHOSPASM

- Switch to 100% oxygen
- Ventilate by hand
- Stop administration of suspected agents: β-blockers, NSAIDs, neostigmine, antibiotics, neuromuscular blockers, latex
- Call for help

FIRST-LINE DRUG THERAPY

**β2-agonist: Salbutamol**
- Metered dose inhaler: 6-8 puffs repeated as necessary
- Nebulized: 5 mg repeated as necessary
- IV: 250 mcg slow IV, followed by 5 mcg/min up to 20 mcg/min

SECOND-LINE DRUG THERAPY

| | |
|---|---|
| Anticholinergics | Ipratropium bromide: 4-8 puffs or 0.5 mg nebulized 6 hourly |
| Magnesium sulphate | 50 mg/kg IV over 20 min (max 2 g) |
| Hydrocortisone | 200 mg IV 6 hourly |
| Steroids | Methylprednisolone: 125 mg IV<br>Dexamethasone: 8 mg IV |
| Bronchodilating anesthetics | Ketamine bolus 10-20 mg, infusion 1-3 mg/kg/hour |
| Epinephrine | Nebulized: 5 mL 1:1000<br>IV: 10 mcg to 100 mcg, titrated to response |

IMMEDIATE MANAGEMENT

**Prevent hypoxemia & reverse bronchoconstriction**
- Deepen anesthesia: volatiles > ketamine (only bronchodilating agent) > propofol
- Consider alternative causes of high airway pressure: endobronchial intubation, kinked circuitry, excessive tidal volume, small diameter tracheal tube, obesity, etc.
- Check tube position and exclude blocked/misplaced tube
- Exclude laryngospasm and consider aspiration in non-intubated patients
- Avoid dynamic hyperinflation with appropriate ventilation: longer expiratory time, low/normal respiratory rates, permissive hypercapnia

SECONDARY MANAGEMENT

**Provide ongoing therapy and address underlying cause**
- Optimize mechanical ventilation (Titrate peep according to the PEEPi)
- Consider aborting the surgery
- Request & review chest X-ray
- Transfer patient to ICU
- Apply ECMO with severe bronchospasm and refractory to all other treatments

## PREVENTION

- Perform a thorough assessment of the patient before surgery
- Careful medication history should be taken with particular reference to drug sensitivities
- Encourage the patient to stop smoking preoperatively
- Wheezing, cough increased sputum production, shortness of breath, and diurnal variability in peak expiratory flow rate (PEFR) indicate poor control
- Recent or frequent exacerbations or admission to the hospital may be an indication to postpone non-essential surgery

## KEEP IN MIND

The risk of bronchospasm is reduced by:

- Pretreatment with an inhaled/nebulized β-agonist, 30 minutes prior to surgery
- Induction of anesthesia with propofol
- An adequate depth of anesthesia before airway instrumentation

## SUGGESTED READING

- Pascale Dewachter, Claudie Mouton-Faivre, Charles W. Emala, Sadek Beloucif, Bruno Riou; Case Scenario: Bronchospasm during Anesthetic Induction. Anesthesiology 2011; 114:1200
- Pollard BJ, Kitchen, G. Handbook of Clinical Anaesthesia. Fourth Edition. CRC Press. 2018. 978-1-4987-6289-2.
- Vojdani S. Bronchospasm During Induction of Anesthesia: A Case Report and Literature Review. Galen Med J. 2018 May 19;7:e846.
- Westhorpe RN, Ludbrook GL, Helps SC. Crisis management during anaesthesia: bronchospasm. Qual Saf Health Care. 2005;14(3):e7.

# COMPARTMENT SYNDROME

## LEARNING OBJECTIVES

- Pathophysiology of compartment syndrome
- Management of compartment syndrome

## DEFINITION AND MECHANISM

- Compartment syndrome is an orthopedic emergency and occurs when the pressure within a compartment increases
- It is essentially soft tissue ischemia, generally associated with trauma, fracture with subsequent casting, prolonged malpositioning during surgery, or reperfusion injury
- Because various osseofascial compartments have a relatively fixed volume, excess fluid or external constriction increases pressure within the compartment and decreases tissue perfusion
- The tissue hypoperfusion results in tissue hypoxia impeding cellular metabolism
- If prolonged, permanent myoneural tissue damage occurs
- As tissue pressure increases, extrinsic venous luminal pressure is exceeded, resulting in vein collapse
- Normal compartment pressure should be within 12-18 mmHg, a pressure above 18 mmHg is considered abnormal
- It is generally agreed that compartmental pressures greater than 30 mmHg require emergent intervention because ischemia is imminent
- Hypoxic injury causes cells to release free radicals, which increases endothelial permeability, leading to a vicious cycle of continued fluid loss, further increasing tissue pressure and injury

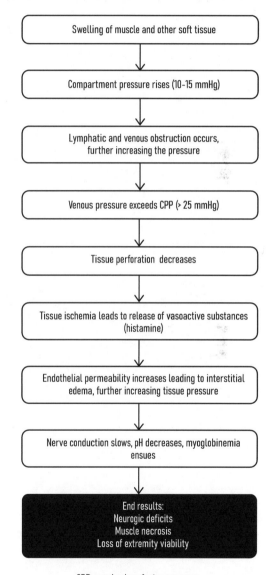

CPP, cerebral perfusion pressure.

# SIGNS AND SYMPTOMS

| | Acute compartment syndrome | Chronic compartment syndrome |
|---|---|---|
| Characteristics | • Occurs gradually, usually during and immediately after repetitive exercise<br>• Usually passes within minutes of stopping the activity<br>• Happens suddenly, usually after a fracture or severe injury<br>• A medical emergency that requires urgent treatment<br>• Can lead to permanent muscle damage if not treated quickly | • Occurs gradually, usually during and immediately after repetitive exercise<br>• Usually passes within minutes of stopping the activity<br>• Is not a medical emergency and does not cause permanent damage |
| Signs and symptoms | • Intense pain, especially when the muscle is stretched, which seems much worse than would normally be expected for the injury<br>• Tenderness in the affected area<br>• Tightness in the muscle<br>• Paresthesia<br>• Numbness or weakness | • Cramping pain during exercise, most often in the legs<br>• Swelling or a visibly bulging muscle<br>• A tingling sensation<br>• The affected area turning pale and cold<br>• In severe cases, difficulty moving the affected body part |

# ETIOLOGY OF ACUTE COMPARTMENT SYNDROME

| Conditions that increase the compartment volume | Conditions that lead to a reduction in the volume of tissue compartments |
|---|---|
| • Direct soft tissue trauma with or without a long bone fracture<br>• Closed tibial shaft fractures and closed forearm fractures<br>• Soft tissue crush injuries<br>• Open fractures, which should theoretically decompress the adjacent compartments<br>• Hemorrhage: vascular injury, coagulopathy<br>• Anticoagulation therapy<br>• Revascularization of a limb after ischemia<br>• High-energy trauma, such as from a high-speed motor vehicle accident or crush injury<br>• Increased capillary permeability after burns<br>• Infusions or high-pressure injections<br>• Extravasations of arthroscopic fluid<br>• Reperfusion after prolonged periods of ischemia<br>• Anabolic steroid use<br>• Decreased serum osmolarity (e.g., nephritic syndrome)<br>• Strenuous exercise, especially in previously sedentary people | • Tight circumferential dressings<br>• Closure of fascial defects<br>• Cast or splint, especially if placed before removal of the surgical tourniquet<br>• Prolonged limb compression, as in Trendelenburg and lateral decubitus positions<br>• Excessive traction to fractured limbs |

# COMPLICATIONS OF ACUTE COMPARTMENT SYNDROME

- Tissue necrosis
- Volkmann's contractures
- Neurological deficits
- Gangrene
- Chronic regional pain syndrome
- Rhabdomyolysis with subsequent acute kidney injury

# DIAGNOSIS

- Based on clinical signs and symptoms
- Pain out of proportion to the injury, especially with passive stretch of the muscles in the suspicious compartment or limb
- A palpable tense extremity compared with the uninjured limb
- Paresthesia – late clinical sign
- Paresis – even later clinical sign
- Measure compartment pressure
- Maintain adequate pain control with the lowest possible dose in an attempt to avoid a delayed diagnosis of compartment syndrome

# MANAGEMENT

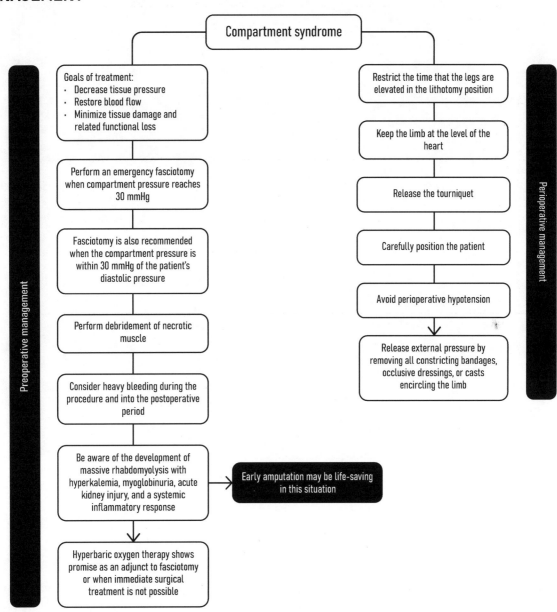

**Compartment syndrome**

**Preoperative management**

Goals of treatment:
- Decrease tissue pressure
- Restore blood flow
- Minimize tissue damage and related functional loss

Perform an emergency fasciotomy when compartment pressure reaches 30 mmHg

Fasciotomy is also recommended when the compartment pressure is within 30 mmHg of the patient's diastolic pressure

Perform debridement of necrotic muscle

Consider heavy bleeding during the procedure and into the postoperative period

Be aware of the development of massive rhabdomyolysis with hyperkalemia, myoglobinuria, acute kidney injury, and a systemic inflammatory response → Early amputation may be life-saving in this situation

Hyperbaric oxygen therapy shows promise as an adjunct to fasciotomy or when immediate surgical treatment is not possible

**Perioperative management**

Restrict the time that the legs are elevated in the lithotomy position

Keep the limb at the level of the heart

Release the tourniquet

Carefully position the patient

Avoid perioperative hypotension

Release external pressure by removing all constricting bandages, occlusive dressings, or casts encircling the limb

# REGIONAL ANESTHESIA AND COMPARTMENT SYNDROME

- Be cautious with regional anesthesia, as it may obscure signs and symptoms of acute compartment syndrome
- Avoid neuroaxial or peripheral regional techniques that result in dense blocks of long duration
- Single-shot or continuous peripheral nerve blocks using lower concentrations of local anesthetic agents without adjuncts are considered safe as they are not associated with delays in diagnosis

========================= SUGGESTED READING =========================

- Nathanson, M.H., Harrop-Griffiths, W., Aldington, D.J., Forward, D., Mannion, S., Kinnear-Mellor, R.G.M., Miller, K.L., Ratnayake, B., Wiles, M.D., Wolmarans, M.R., 2021. Regional analgesia for lower leg trauma and the risk of acute compartment syndrome. Anaesthesia 76, 1518–1525.
- Farrow C, Bodenham A, Troxler M. 2011. Acute limb compartment syndromes. Continuing Education in Anaesthesia Critical Care & Pain. 11;1:24-28.
- https://www.nysora.com/topics/sub-specialties/acute-compartment-syndrome-limb-implications-regional-anesthesia/

# DELAYED EMERGENCE

**49**

## LEARNING OBJECTIVES

- Identify the causes leading to delayed emergence
- Explain the risk factors associated with an increased risk of delayed emergence
- Manage delayed emergence

## DEFINITION AND MECHANISM

- Failure to regain consciousness or alertness following general anesthesia after surgery
- The transition from unconsciousness to complete wakefulness occurs along a normal trajectory, although slowed down
- Alternatively, the awakening trajectory proceeds abnormally, possibly leading to emergence delirium
- Most cases of delayed return of consciousness are rapidly treatable

## CAUSES

| | |
|---|---|
| Pharmacodynamic causes | Genetic variations<br>Hypothermia<br>Drug interaction<br>Serotonin syndrome<br>Neuromuscular blockers<br>Heroin or opioid toxicity<br>IV anesthetic agents (Total intravenous anesthesia (TIVA))<br>Central anticholinergic syndrome<br>Cement implantation syndrome<br>Toxicity of the local anesthetic if anesthesia is combined (i.e., GA with a PNB block or GA with local aneshtesia administered by the surgeon) |
| Metabolic alterations | Hypoglycemia<br>Hyperglycemia<br>Hyponatremia<br>Hypernatremia<br>Metabolic acidosis<br>Malignant hyperthermia<br>Dialysis disequilibrium syndrome |
| Neurological rare causes | Hypoperfusion/ischemia<br>Intracranial hemorrhage<br>Venous thromboembolism<br>Seizures<br>Myxedema coma<br>Functional coma<br>Brainstem stroke<br>Fat embolism |
| Psychiatric rare causes | Conversion disorder |

# RISK FACTORS

| Patients conditions | Older age<br>Body habitus<br>Gender | |
|---|---|---|
| Preexisting clinical conditions | Psychological disorders<br>Neurologic conditions<br>Cardiac diseases<br>Hypertension<br>Pulmonary diseases<br>Chronic kidney disease | Liver diseases<br>Hypothyroidism<br>Drug or alcohol abuse<br>Metabolic alterations<br>Smoking |
| Intraoperative conditions | Drugs (e.g., heroin or opioid toxicity)<br>Metabolic alterations (intraoperative)<br>Hip surgery<br>Cardiac surgery<br>Vascular surgery<br>Open greater than endovascular surgery<br>Emergency surgery | Increased surgical duration<br>Hypotension<br>Shock<br>Arrhythmias<br>Hypothermia/hyperthermia<br>Blood transfusion<br>Systemic toxicity of local anesthetics |
| Chronic pharmacotherapy | Benzodiazepines<br>Barbiturates<br>Anticholinergics<br>Antidepressants<br>Antipsychotics<br>Herbal medications | |

# DIAGNOSTIC STEPS

- Vital signs (including temperature)
- Neuromuscular monitor
- Neurologic exam (pupils, cranial nerves, reflexes, response to pain)
- Fingerstick glucose
- Arterial blood gas with electrolytes

## Differential diagnosis

| Drug effects | Residual anesthetic (volatile, propofol, barbiturates, ketamine)<br>Excess narcotics<br>Inadequate reversal or no reversal of muscle relaxation<br>Pseudocholinesterase deficiency<br>Alcohol or street drugs<br>Herbal medicines (valerian root, St. John's wort)<br>Infection |
|---|---|
| Infection | Encephalitis<br>Meningitis<br>Sepsis |
| Metabolic disorders | Hypercarbia<br>Hypoxemia<br>Metabolic acidosis<br>Acidosis<br>Hypoglycemia/Hyperglycemia<br>Hyponatremia/Electrolyte abnormalities<br>Hypothermia/Malignant hyperthermia<br>Uremia<br>Hepatic encephalopathy<br>Osmolality problems<br>Myxedema coma |
| Neurologic disorders | New ischemic event<br>Subarachnoid hemorrhage<br>Seizures or postictal state<br>Increased intracranial pressure or preexisting obtundation<br>Perioperative stroke (ischemic or hemorrhagic)<br>Hydrocephalus<br>Diffuse anoxic injury<br>Pneumocephalus<br>Cerebral hyperperfusion syndrome |

Delayed emergence

# MANAGEMENT

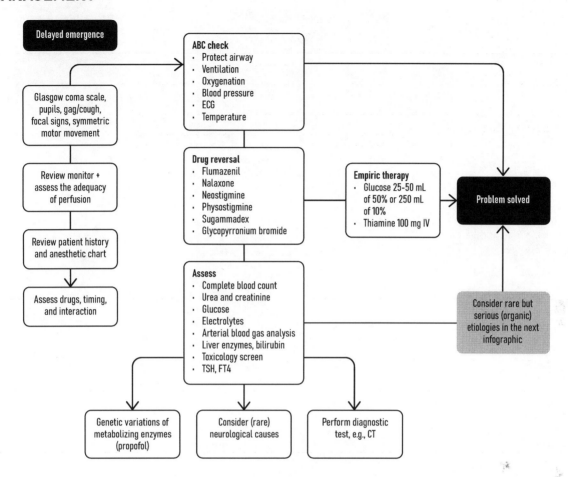

**Delayed emergence**

**Glasgow coma scale, pupils, gag/cough, focal signs, symmetric motor movement**

**Review monitor + assess the adequacy of perfusion**

**Review patient history and anesthetic chart**

**Assess drugs, timing, and interaction**

**ABC check**
- Protect airway
- Ventilation
- Oxygenation
- Blood pressure
- ECG
- Temperature

**Drug reversal**
- Flumazenil
- Nalaxone
- Neostigmine
- Physostigmine
- Sugammadex
- Glycopyrronium bromide

**Empiric therapy**
- Glucose 25-50 mL of 50% or 250 mL of 10%
- Thiamine 100 mg IV

**Problem solved**

**Assess**
- Complete blood count
- Urea and creatinine
- Glucose
- Electrolytes
- Arterial blood gas analysis
- Liver enzymes, bilirubin
- Toxicology screen
- TSH, FT4

**Consider rare but serious (organic) etiologies in the next infographic**

**Genetic variations of metabolizing enzymes (propofol)**

**Consider (rare) neurological causes**

**Perform diagnostic test, e.g., CT**

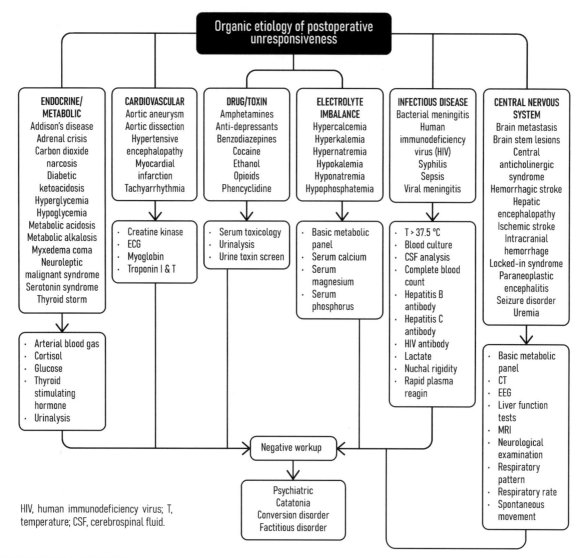

**Organic etiology of postoperative unresponsiveness**

**ENDOCRINE/ METABOLIC**
Addison's disease
Adrenal crisis
Carbon dioxide narcosis
Diabetic ketoacidosis
Hyperglycemia
Hypoglycemia
Metabolic acidosis
Metabolic alkalosis
Myxedema coma
Neuroleptic malignant syndrome
Serotonin syndrome
Thyroid storm

- Arterial blood gas
- Cortisol
- Glucose
- Thyroid stimulating hormone
- Urinalysis

**CARDIOVASCULAR**
Aortic aneurysm
Aortic dissection
Hypertensive encephalopathy
Myocardial infarction
Tachyarrhythmia

- Creatine kinase
- ECG
- Myoglobin
- Troponin I & T

**DRUG/TOXIN**
Amphetamines
Anti-depressants
Benzodiazepines
Cocaine
Ethanol
Opioids
Phencyclidine

- Serum toxicology
- Urinalysis
- Urine toxin screen

**ELECTROLYTE IMBALANCE**
Hypercalcemia
Hyperkalemia
Hypernatremia
Hypokalemia
Hyponatremia
Hypophosphatemia

- Basic metabolic panel
- Serum calcium
- Serum magnesium
- Serum phosphorus

**INFECTIOUS DISEASE**
Bacterial meningitis
Human immunodeficiency virus (HIV)
Syphilis
Sepsis
Viral meningitis

- T > 37.5 °C
- Blood culture
- CSF analysis
- Complete blood count
- Hepatitis B antibody
- Hepatitis C antibody
- HIV antibody
- Lactate
- Nuchal rigidity
- Rapid plasma reagin

**CENTRAL NERVOUS SYSTEM**
Brain metastasis
Brain stem lesions
Central anticholinergic syndrome
Hemorrhagic stroke
Hepatic encephalopathy
Ischemic stroke
Intracranial hemorrhage
Locked-in syndrome
Paraneoplastic encephalitis
Seizure disorder
Uremia

- Basic metabolic panel
- CT
- EEG
- Liver function tests
- MRI
- Neurological examination
- Respiratory pattern
- Respiratory rate
- Spontaneous movement

**Negative workup**

Psychiatric
Catatonia
Conversion disorder
Factitious disorder

HIV, human immunodeficiency virus; T, temperature; CSF, cerebrospinal fluid.

## ADDITIONAL FACTS

- Recent studies indicate that induction and awakening are asymmetric processes
- Neural circuits that mediate induction do not completely overlap those that mediate emergence for anesthesia

## SUGGESTED READING

- Cascella M, Bimonte S, Di Napoli R. Delayed Emergence from Anesthesia: What We Know and How We Act. Local Reg Anesth. 2020 Nov 5;13:195-206.
- Khanna, Gautam Cernovsky, Jan et al. Bone cement and the implications for anaesthesia. Continuing Education in Anaesthesia, Critical Care and Pain, Volume 12, Issue 4, 213 - 216.
- Rafizadeh S, Kerry-Gnazzo AR, DeWalt K. An Unresponsive Patient in Postanesthesia Care Unit: A Case Report of an Unusual Diagnosis for a Common Problem. A A Pract. 2020 Aug;14(10):e01293.
- Thomas E, Martin F, Pollard B. Delayed recovery of consciousness after general anaesthesia. BJA Educ. 2020 May;20(5):173-179.
- Yonekura H, Murayama N, Yamazaki H, Sobue K. A Case of Delayed Emergence After Propofol Anesthesia: Genetic Analysis. A A Case Rep. 2016 Dec 1;7(11):243-246.

Delayed emergence

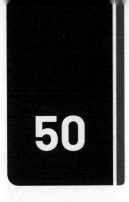

# DENTAL LUXATION, FRACTURE, OR AVULSION

## 50

### LEARNING OBJECTIVES

- Management of dental emergencies resulting from airway management to maximize the chances of saving the tooth

## DEFINITION AND MECHANISM

- Tooth luxation occurs when trauma disrupts the tissues, ligaments, and bone that hold the tooth in place
- Can also affect the tooth's nerves and blood supply
- Tooth avulsion occurs when the tooth is completely dislodged from its socket
- Avulsed teeth are dental emergencies and require immediate treatment

## SIGNS AND SYMPTOMS

- Teeth that are mobile or completely dislodged from the jaw due to airway management

## RISK FACTORS

- Bad dental hygiene
- Difficult intubation
- Laryngoscopy by an inexperienced operator

# MANAGEMENT

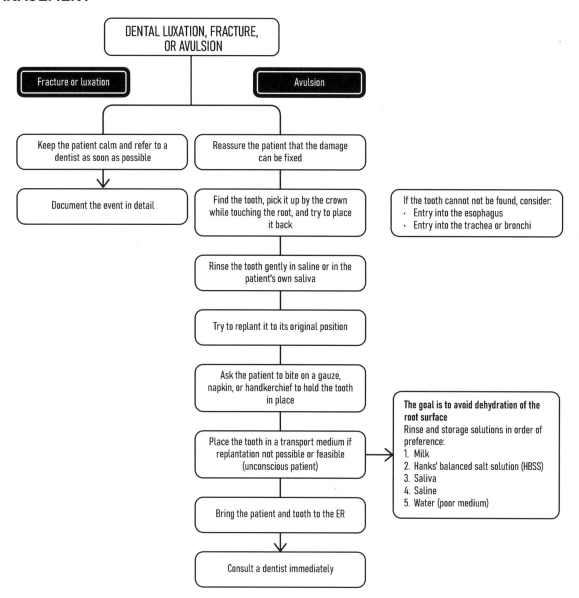

**DENTAL LUXATION, FRACTURE, OR AVULSION**

**Fracture or luxation**

- Keep the patient calm and refer to a dentist as soon as possible
- Document the event in detail

**Avulsion**

- Reassure the patient that the damage can be fixed
- Find the tooth, pick it up by the crown while touching the root, and try to place it back
- Rinse the tooth gently in saline or in the patient's own saliva
- Try to replant it to its original position
- Ask the patient to bite on a gauze, napkin, or handkerchief to hold the tooth in place
- Place the tooth in a transport medium if replantation not possible or feasible (unconscious patient)
- Bring the patient and tooth to the ER
- Consult a dentist immediately

If the tooth cannot not be found, consider:
- Entry into the esophagus
- Entry into the trachea or bronchi

**The goal is to avoid dehydration of the root surface**
Rinse and storage solutions in order of preference:
1. Milk
2. Hanks' balanced salt solution (HBSS)
3. Saliva
4. Saline
5. Water (poor medium)

## SUGGESTED READING

- Bourguignon C, Cohenca N, Lauridsen E, et al. International Association of Dental Traumatology guidelines for the management of traumatic dental injuries: 1. Fractures and luxations. Dent Traumatol. 2020;36(4):314-330.
- Fouad AF, Abbott PV, Tsilingaridis G, Cohenca N, Lauridsen E, Bourguignon C, et al. International Association of Dental Traumatology guidelines for the management of traumatic dental injuries: 2. Avulsion of permanent teeth. Dent Traumatol. 2020;36(4):331-42.

# EXTRAVASATION INJURIES

**51**

## LEARNING OBJECTIVES

- Identify the risk factors associated with extravasation injuries
- Recognize the differential diagnosis of extravasation injuries
- Manage and prevent extravasation injuries
- Recognize warning signs of extravasation injuries

## DEFINITION AND MECHANISM

- The unintentional injection or leakage of fluid in the perivascular or subcutaneous space
- Resulting from solution cytotoxicity, osmolality, vasoconstrictor properties, infusion pressure, and regional anatomical peculiarities
- May cause significant tissue necrosis resulting in the amputation of an extremity

## RISK FACTORS

- Preexisting cutaneous, vascular, or lymphatic pathophysiology
- Fragile or mobile veins
- Site of injection
- Toxicity of the drug
- Amount of agent extravasated
- Duration of tissue exposure
- Decreased vigilance of doctor or patient

## DIFFERENTIAL DIAGNOSIS

- Propofol, ondansetron, rocuronium, and cyclizine can all cause discomfort or pain on injection
- Venous spasms may occur and can lead to localized skin blanching

## THREE CATEGORIES OF ANESTHETIC/ICU AGENTS CAUSING EXTRAVASATION INJURY

| 1) Hyperosmolar agents | 2) Acids / alkalis | 3) Vascular regulators |
|---|---|---|
| Calcium chloride | Aminophylline | Epinephrine |
| Calcium gluconate | Amiodarone | Dobutamine |
| Glucose > 10% | Amphotericin | Dopamine |
| Magnesium sulphate 20% | Co-trimoxazole | Metaraminol |
| Mannitol 10% and 20% | Diazepam | Norepinephrine |
| Parenteral nutrition | Erythromycin | Prostaglandin |
| Potassium chloride | Phenytoin | Vasopressin |
| Sodium bicarbonate | Thiopental | |
| Sodium chloride > 0.9% | Vancomycin | |
| X-ray contrast media | | |

# MANAGEMENT

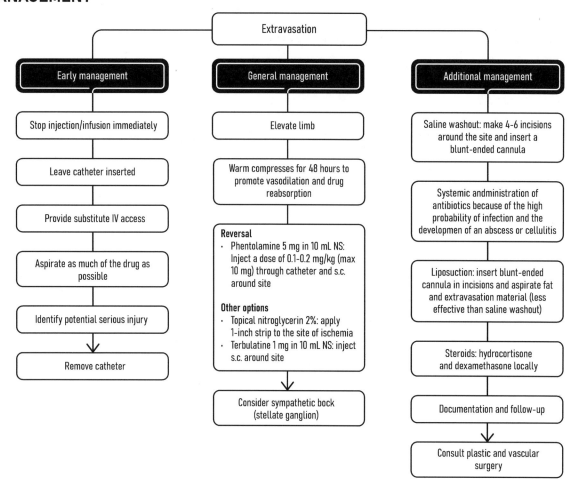

**Extravasation**

**Early management**
- Stop injection/infusion immediately
- Leave catheter inserted
- Provide substitute IV access
- Aspirate as much of the drug as possible
- Identify potential serious injury
- Remove catheter

**General management**
- Elevate limb
- Warm compresses for 48 hours to promote vasodilation and drug reabsorption

**Reversal**
- Phentolamine 5 mg in 10 mL NS: Inject a dose of 0.1-0.2 mg/kg (max 10 mg) through catheter and s.c. around site

**Other options**
- Topical nitroglycerin 2%: apply 1-inch strip to the site of ischemia
- Terbulatine 1 mg in 10 mL NS: inject s.c. around site

- Consider sympathetic bock (stellate ganglion)

**Additional management**
- Saline washout: make 4-6 incisions around the site and insert a blunt-ended cannula
- Systemic andministration of antibiotics because of the high probability of infection and the developmen of an abscess or cellulitis
- Liposuction: insert blunt-ended cannula in incisions and aspirate fat and extravasation material (less effective than saline washout)
- Steroids: hydrocortisone and dexamethasone locally
- Documentation and follow-up
- Consult plastic and vascular surgery

# PREVENTION

- Avoid IVs in the hand/wrist as the most appropriate site is considered to be the forearm
- Careful insertion of peripheral venous catheters
- Flush the catheter with sterile saline
- Apply a suitable dressing to prevent movement of the catheter and avoid unreassuring IVs
- Inspect the catheterization site regularly
- Regulated delivery of IV fluids from continuous infusion pumps
- Hyperosmolar fluids, acidic or alkaline solutions, or infusates with irritant or vesicant properties should be given through central venous lines, if possible, or should be diluted or neutralized
- For slow infusion of high-risk drugs, a central line or peripherally inserted central catheter (PICC) line should be used
- Keep antidotes and the worksheet in the room with the patient
- 10 mg of phentolamine mesylate can be added to each liter of solution containing norepinephrine (the vasopressor effect of norepinephrine is not affected)

## ═══ SUGGESTED READING ═══

- Adeyinka A, Pierre L. Fat Embolism. [Updated 2022 Oct 31]. In: StatPearls [Internet]. Treasure Island (FL): StatPearls Publishing; 2024 Jan-. Available from: https://www.ncbi.nlm.nih.gov/books/NBK499885/
- Al-Benna S, O'Boyle C, Holley J. Extravasation injuries in adults. ISRN Dermatol. 2013 May 8;2013:856541.
- Lake C, Beecroft CL. Extravasation injuries and accidental intra-arterial injection, Continuing Education in Anaesthesia Critical Care & Pain, Volume 10, Issue 4, August 2010, Pages 109-113.
- Schummer W, Schummer C, Bayer O, Müller A, Bredle D, Karzai W. Extravasation Injury in the Perioperative Setting. Anesthesia & Analgesia: March 2005 - Volume 100 - Issue 3 - p 722-727.

# FAT EMBOLISM SYNDROME

## LEARNING OBJECTIVES

- Recognize fat embolism syndrome (FES)
- Describe the presenting clinical features in patients with suspected FES
- Explain the management of FES, including the limited drug treatments

## DEFINITION AND MECHANISM

- The presence of fat globules within the lung parenchyma or peripheral microcirculation
- Causes direct tissue damage as well as the induction of a systemic inflammatory response
- Results in pulmonary, cutaneous, neurological, and retinal symptoms
- Estimated to occur in 1-10% of patients
- Mortality is 10-20%

## SIGNS AND SYMPTOMS

| | |
|---|---|
| Respiratory | Tachypnea<br>Hypoxemia<br>Acute respiratory distress syndrome (ARDS) |
| Neurological | Confusion<br>Seizures<br>Altered level of consciousness<br>Focal neurological deficits |
| Dermatological | Petechial rash |
| Systemic | Fever |
| Cardiovascular | Tachycardia<br>Hypotension<br>Intraoperative arrhythmias<br>Myocardial ischemia<br>Pulmonary hypertension (PH)<br>Right-sided heart failure |
| Ophthalmic | Purtscher's retinopathy (cotton wool exudates, macular edema, and hemorrhage) |
| Renal | Oliguria<br>Proteinuria<br>Lipiduria<br>Hematuria |
| Hepatic | Jaundice |
| Hematological | Perioperative anemia<br>Thrombocytopenia<br>Coagulopathy<br>Fat macroglobulinemia |

## CAUSES

- Trauma to long bone/pelvis
- Prosthetic joint replacement
- Liposuction
- Bone marrow harvest or transplant
- Bone tumor lysis
- Acute pancreatitis
- Hepatic necrosis and fatty liver
- Acute sickle cell crisis
- Major soft tissue injury
- Recent orthopedic procedure
- Recent lipid infusion
- Severe burns
- Prolonged cardiopulmonary resuscitation

## DIAGNOSIS

- One major and 4 minor of Gurd's diagnostic criteria are proposed, together with fat macroglobulinemia, as sufficient to diagnose fat embolism syndrome
- Perform an MRI of the brain and a CT scan of the lungs

## GURD'S DIAGNOSTIC CRITERIA

| Diagnosis | Criteria |
|---|---|
| Major criteria | Respiratory insufficiency<br>Cerebral involvement<br>Petechial rash |
| Minor criteria | Tachycardia<br>Fever<br>Jaundice<br>Retinal changes<br>Renal changes<br>↓ Hemoglobin<br>Thrombocytopenia<br>↑ Erythrocyte sedimentation rate<br>Fat globulus in sputum |
| Laboratory findings | ↓ in hematocrit at 24 to 48 hours<br>Thrombocytopenia<br>Fat globulus in blood and urine<br>Fat macroglobulinemia raised free<br>fatty acids and triglyceride in serum |

## DIFFERENTIAL DIAGNOSIS

- A differential diagnosis is performed depending on the predominant manifestations
- Pulmonary embolism
- Air embolism
- Hemorrhagic shock
- Cerebrovascular accident
- Aspiration pneumonia
- Pulmonary edema
- Meningitis
- Encephalitis
- Lung contusion

## MANAGEMENT

- Respiratory support: intubation/ventilation, indications for respiratory support:
  - Sustained $SaO_2$ < 90% and $PaO_2$ < 8 kPa on oxygen
  - Respiratory rate of > 35 breaths/min
- Hemodynamic support:
  - Maintain a systolic blood pressure > 90 mmHg
  - Avoid hypovolemia with fluid resuscitation and vasopressors
  - Apply invasive monitoring
  - Provide central venous access, including for invasive monitoring of central venous pressure
  - Transesophageal echocardiogram (TEE)
- Early surgical stabilization of fractures
- Perform operative correction rather than traction alone
- Limit the intraosseous pressure during an orthopedic procedure

## PHARMACOLOGICAL TREATMENT

- Corticosteroids may reduce the risk of a fat embolism in patients with long bone fractures of the lower limbs
- Heparin clears lipemic serum by stimulating lipase activity, thereby reducing pulmonary complications
- Albumin use is considered potentially therapeutic in its ability to bind free fatty acids

## SUGGESTED READING

- Luff D, Hewson DW. Fat embolism syndrome. BJA Educ. 2021;21(9):322-328.
- Pollard BJ, Kitchen, G. Handbook of Clinical Anaesthesia. Fourth Edition. CRC Press. 2018. 978-1-4987-6289-2.

Fat embolism syndrome

# FULL STOMACH

## LEARNING OBJECTIVES

- Outline the risks of having a full stomach in combination with anesthesia
- Describe the factors that delay gastric emptying
- Anesthetic management of a patient with a full stomach

## DEFINITION AND MECHANISM

- In anesthesia, the term "full stomach" applies to patients that have recently ingested foods and/or have pharmacologic, metabolic, anatomic, or hormonal conditions, which impair gastric emptying
- A full stomach and any reduction in the functional integrity of the lower esophageal sphincter (LES) predispose a patient to regurgitation
- The active process of vomiting and the passive process of regurgitation of gastric contents are more hazardous in a patient with a full stomach
- No patient can ever be assumed to have a completely empty stomach

General anesthesia suppresses the upper airway reflexes that prevent pulmonary aspiration of active or passively regurgitated gastric contents
- Aspiration of solid material can cause a mechanical obstruction with subsequent lung collapse, pneumonia, or abscess formation
- Aspiration of liquid (> 25 mL, pH < 2.5) can cause bronchospasm, pneumonitis, bronchopneumonia, and acute respiratory distress syndrome

Strategies to reduce the risk of pulmonary aspiration
- Minimize residual gastric volumes → fasting (stomach is considered "empty" within 6 hours after food and milky drinks, 4 hours after breast milk, and 2 hours after water)
- Rapidly secure the anesthetized airway

Emergency patients are more likely to have a full stomach as
- Presenting pathology causes a mechanical obstruction (e.g., laparotomy for small bowel obstruction)
- Surgery is urgent and cannot wait for the full fasting time
- The surgical pathology results in pain and anxiety

## RISK FACTORS

Factors delaying gastric emptying
- Mechanical obstruction of the gastrointestinal tract
- Ileus
- Following surgical manipulation of the bowel (postoperative)
- Recent trauma
- Electrolyte imbalance
- Peritonitis
- Pain
- Fear and anxiety
- Third trimester of pregnancy
- Drugs
- Alcoholism, state of intoxication

# MANAGEMENT

- Any emergency patient should be treated as a "full stomach" and appropriate management should be chosen.

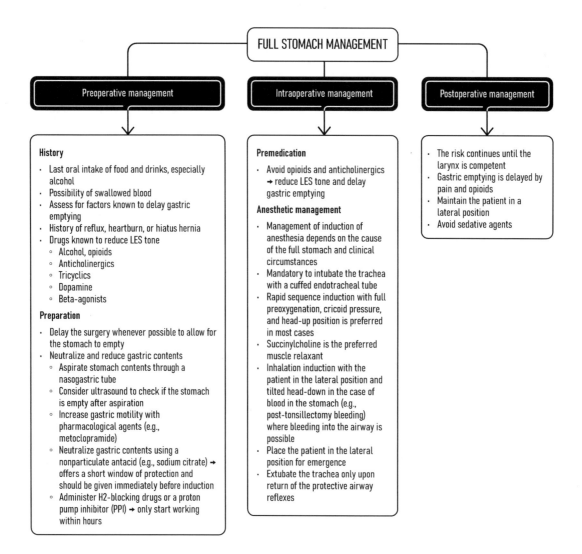

**FULL STOMACH MANAGEMENT**

**Preoperative management**

**History**

- Last oral intake of food and drinks, especially alcohol
- Possibility of swallowed blood
- Assess for factors known to delay gastric emptying
- History of reflux, heartburn, or hiatus hernia
- Drugs known to reduce LES tone
  - Alcohol, opioids
  - Anticholinergics
  - Tricyclics
  - Dopamine
  - Beta-agonists

**Preparation**

- Delay the surgery whenever possible to allow for the stomach to empty
- Neutralize and reduce gastric contents
  - Aspirate stomach contents through a nasogastric tube
  - Consider ultrasound to check if the stomach is empty after aspiration
  - Increase gastric motility with pharmacological agents (e.g., metoclopramide)
  - Neutralize gastric contents using a nonparticulate antacid (e.g., sodium citrate) → offers a short window of protection and should be given immediately before induction
  - Administer H2-blocking drugs or a proton pump inhibitor (PPI) → only start working within hours

**Intraoperative management**

**Premedication**

- Avoid opioids and anticholinergics → reduce LES tone and delay gastric emptying

**Anesthetic management**

- Management of induction of anesthesia depends on the cause of the full stomach and clinical circumstances
- Mandatory to intubate the trachea with a cuffed endotracheal tube
- Rapid sequence induction with full preoxygenation, cricoid pressure, and head-up position is preferred in most cases
- Succinylcholine is the preferred muscle relaxant
- Inhalation induction with the patient in the lateral position and tilted head-down in the case of blood in the stomach (e.g., post-tonsillectomy bleeding) where bleeding into the airway is possible
- Place the patient in the lateral position for emergence
- Extubate the trachea only upon return of the protective airway reflexes

**Postoperative management**

- The risk continues until the larynx is competent
- Gastric emptying is delayed by pain and opioids
- Maintain the patient in a lateral position
- Avoid sedative agents

## SUGGESTED READING

- Perry JJ, Lee JS, Sillberg VA, Wells GA. Rocuronium versus succinylcholine for rapid sequence induction intubation. Cochrane Database Syst Rev. 2008;(2):CD002788. Published 2008 Apr 16.
- Pollard BJ, Kitchen G. Handbook of Clinical Anaesthesia. 4th ed. Taylor & Francis group; 2018. Chapter 4 Gastrointestinal tract, Jackson MJ.

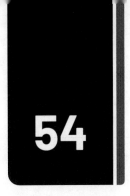

# HIGH OR TOTAL SPINAL ANESTHESIA

## LEARNING OBJECTIVES

- Describe the contributing factors to high spinal anesthesia
- Apply preventative measures for high spinal anesthesia
- Describe the symptoms of high spinal anesthesia
- Manage cases of high spinal anesthesia

## DEFINITION AND MECHANISM

- High spinal anesthesia is a complication of central neuraxial techniques that include spinal and epidural anesthesia
- It is defined as a spread of local anesthetic affecting the spinal nerves above T4
- The effects are of variable severity depending on the maximum level that is involved but can include cardiovascular and/or respiratory compromise
- In total spinal anesthesia, there is an intracranial spread of local anesthetic resulting in loss of consciousness

## CONTRIBUTING FACTORS

- Local anesthetic dose
- Positioning of patient
- Preexisting epidural block
- Unrecognized dural puncture and intrathecal injection
- Accidental subdural block
- Accidental intradural space
- A complication of blocking the brachial plexus due to interscalene brachial plexus block

## PREVENTION

- **Epidural analgesia/anesthesia:**
  - Use low concentrations of local anesthetic for labor analgesia
  - Prior to top-up:
    - Assess block (to guide top-up dosage)
    - Aspirate the epidural catheter with a 2 mL syringe to rule out intrathecal or intravenous placement
  - Consider giving large volumes of local anesthetic in divided doses (clinical urgency may preclude this)

- **Spinal anesthesia:**
  - Consider the level (and therefore local anesthetic dose) required for surgery
  - Patient position: block height can be manipulated for up to 30 min when using hyperbaric ("heavy") anesthetics – if using head down position to establish the block, remember to remove it as soon as possible
  - Patient characteristics: consider dose reduction in short or morbidly obese patients
  - Technique:
    - Consider the effects of the speed of injection
    - Avoid excessive barbotage
  - If performing a spinal following an epidural, a dose reduction may be necessary depending on the existing level of block (reductions to 1-1.5 mL of local anesthetic have been suggested following a failed epidural top-up); there is no clear consensus on this

- **Epidural and spinal anesthesia:**
  - Don't inject during a contraction/cough/Valsalva maneuver as this can increase the cephalad spread of local anesthetic
  - The use of the Oxford wedge is recommended to prevent the cephalad spread of local anesthetic (and to optimize airway positioning in the event of requiring general anesthesia)

## SYMPTOMS

| Spinal level | Area(s) affected | Symptoms |
|---|---|---|
| T1-T4 | Cardiac sympathetic fibers blocked | Hypotension<br>Bradycardia |
| C6-C8 | Hands and arms | Paresthesia or numbness in hands/arms<br>Weakness of hands/arms<br>Shortness of breath (accessory respiratory muscles affected) |
| C3-5 | Diaphragm and shoulders | Shoulder weakness – respiratory compromise imminent<br>Hypoventilation and/or desaturation<br>Respiratory arrest |
| Intracranial spread | Brain stem | Slurred speech<br>Sedation<br>Loss of consciousness |

## MANAGEMENT

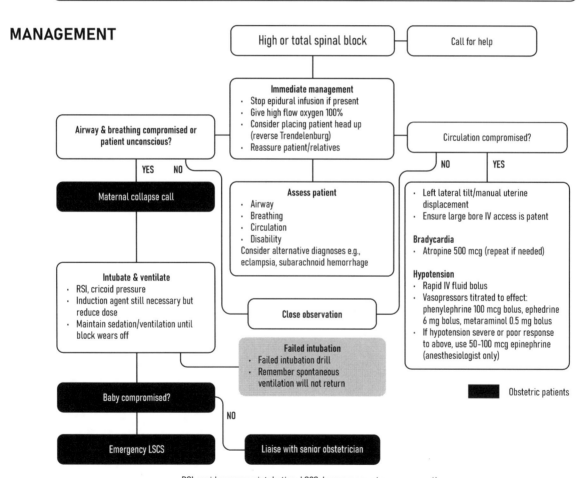

RSI, rapid sequence intubation; LSCS, lower segment cesarean section.

## SUGGESTED READING

- Sivanandan S., Surendran A. (2019) Management of total spinal block in obstetrics. Update in Anaesthesia, 34: 22-25.
- Reeve J. (2017) NHS Foundation trust clinical guideline: High Regional Block (including Total Spinal Anaesthesia).

High or total spinal anesthesia

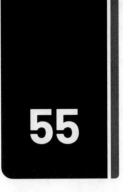

# HYPERTENSION

## LEARNING OBJECTIVES

- Define the stages of hypertension
- Discuss the perioperative management of patients with hypertension
- Describe the acute and long-term treatment of hypertension

## DEFINITION AND MECHANISM

- Hypertension is defined as a systolic blood pressure (BP) > 130 mmHg
- Episodes of hypertension are relatively common during anesthesia and are reported by nearly one-third of adult patients
- Whether it is ultimately harmful to the patient depends on its degree, cause, and duration, and on the patient's condition

## SIGNS AND SYMPTOMS

Hypertension rarely has noticeable symptoms, however, the following signs and symptoms can be associated with hypertension:
- Headaches
- Shortness of breath
- Nosebleeds
- Blurred vision
- Chest pain
- Dizziness

## STAGES

| Stage | Systolic blood pressure (mmHg) | Diastolic blood pressure (mmHg) |
|---|---|---|
| Prehypertension | 120 - 129 | 60 - 79 |
| Stage 1 hypertension | 130 - 139 | 80 - 89 |
| Stage 2 hypertension | > 140 | > 90 |
| Hypertensive crisis | ≥ 180 | ≥ 120 |

# CAUSES

| | |
|---|---|
| Preexisting hypertension | Control BP prior to surgery < 160 mmHg systolic and < 100 mmHg diastolic |
| Side effects of agents | Ketamine, ergometrine, desflurane anesthesia (> 1.0 MAC) |
| Inadequate anesthesia/analgesia | Adjust administration |
| Inadequate ventilation | $CO_2$ retention causes catecholamine release |
| Interaction of agents | For example monoamine oxygenase inhibitors + vasopressors or opioids |
| Tourniquet pain | |
| Preeclampsia | Treat with magnesium sulfate and hypotensive agents |
| Pheochromocytoma | If suspected, a small bolus dose of phentolamine (1–5 mg) usually gives a significant fall in BP <br> If systolic BP falls more than 35 mmHg, a pheochromocytoma is likely <br> Administer alpha-blockers in addition to beta-blockers |
| Rare causes | Fluid overload <br> Aortic cross-clamping <br> Hyperthyroidism/thyroid storm <br> Malignant hyperthermia <br> Increased intracranial pressure <br> Interference with the carotid body, brainstem, or spinal cord <br> Bladder distension <br> Alcohol withdrawal syndrome or addictive drug withdrawal <br> Autonomic hyperreflexia |

# COMPLICATIONS OF INTRAOPERATIVE HYPERTENSION

- Myocardial ischemia (especially subendocardial), myocardial infarction, or heart failure
- Hemorrhage from the operation site
- Rupture of an existing aneurysm
- Encephalopathy, cerebral edema, or cerebral hemorrhage
- May precipitate acute renal failure

# MANAGEMENT

- Inform the surgeon and consider halting the surgical procedure if possible
- Cycle BP, scan monitors for HR, ECG rhythm, $EtCO_2$, and temperature
- Check if the patient is adequately oxygenated and ventilated
- Deepen the anesthetic
- Examine the patient:
  □ Pupils (high intracranial pressure (ICP))
  □ Diaphoresis & flushing (carcinoid, pheochromocytoma, hyperthyroidism)
  □ Rigidity (malignant hyperthermia, serotonin syndrome)
  □ Bladder distension
  □ Hot (thyroid storm, malignant hyperthermia, serotonin syndrome)
- If severe and life-threatening (e.g., MAP > 150 mmHg with signs of myocardial ischemia), immediate therapy is warranted
- Otherwise, seek the cause and treat this cause
- If there is no likely cause, nonspecific therapy may need to be instituted

## ACUTE TREATMENT

| Agent | Example | Action and dose |
|-------|---------|-----------------|
| Vasodilators | Anesthetic agents<br>Isoflurane<br>Sevoflurane<br>Propofol | Easy to titrate |
| | Hydralazine | Arteriolar dilator<br>Peak action after 20 min following 5-10 slow IV (maximal dose of 30 mg)<br>Slow IV push every 20 minutes |
| | Nitroglycerine | Arterial and venous dilator<br>Dose: 10-200 mcg/min IV<br>Start infusion at 10 mcg/min |
| | Labetalol | Combined alpha and beta blockade<br>Dose: 10-50 mg slow IV, repeated after 5 min if necessary<br>Maximal dose of 200 mg |
| | Sodium nitroprusside | Arterial dilator with a very rapid response<br>Dose: continuous IV: 0.5-1.5 mcg/kg/min starting dose<br>Increase every 5 min in 500 ng/kg/min graduations according to response<br>Large doses may cause cyanide poisoning |
| Beta blockers | Atenolol | Reduces vascular tone<br>Cardioselective<br>Dose: 2.5 mg slow IV, repeated after 5 min if necessary |
| | Esmolol | Reduces vascular tone<br>Rapid onset with a short half-life of about 9 min<br>Dose: 50-200 mcg/kg/min infusion<br>Start infusion at 50 mcg/kg/min |
| | Nicardipine (Rydene) | Arterial dilator<br>Dose: 0.1 mg/mL |
| Alpha blockers | Phentolamine | Vasodilator<br>Relaxes vascular tone<br>Dose: 1-5 mg IV |

## MANAGEMENT

| Agent | Example | Action and dose |
|-------|---------|-----------------|
| Thiazide diuretics | Bendrofluazide<br>Indapamide | Blocks $Na^+$ channels<br>Complications: electrolyte disturbances |
| Loop diuretics | Furosemide | Inhibit $Na^+$, $K^+$ and $Cl^-$ uptake |
| Aldosterone antagonists | Spironolactone | Inhibit $Na^+$ reabsorption and $K^+$ secretion |
| Osmotic diuretics | Mannitol | Increase osmotic pressure and inhibit water and solute reabsorption |
| Carbonic anhydrase inhibitors | Acetazolamide | Inhibits carbonic anhydrase thereby inhibiting $HCO_3^-$ and reduces $Na^+$ reabsorption |
| Sodium channel blockers | Triamterene | Directly inhibit $Na^+$ reabsorption and $K^+$ secretion |
| Beta blockers | Atenolol<br>Propranolol<br>Esmolol | Slow heart rate<br>Improved ventricular filling<br>Complications: lethargy, nausea, and general malaise |
| ACE inhibitors | Perindopril<br>Enalapril | Block angiotensin-converting enzyme (ACE)<br>Complications: cough and deterioration of renal function |
| A2 inhibitors | Candesartan<br>Losartan | Block angiotensin 2 |
| Calcium channel blockers | Nifedipine | Vasodilation |

Hypertension

## POSTOPERATIVE CARE

- Continue to monitor the patient
- Provide adequate analgesia
- Administer oxygen titrated to $SpO_2$ of 94%–98% (reduce myocardial ischemia)
- Patient may need investigations to exclude complications (e.g., myocardial infarction) or to identify the cause

## KEEP IN MIND

- Postoperative hypertension can occur in up to 20% of patients after surgery
- Is associated with adverse outcomes such as myocardial injury, bleeding, stroke, or arrhythmias
- Systolic BP > 180 mmHg is a high risk for postoperative hypertension

**SUGGESTED READING**

- Pollard BJ, Kitchen, G. Handbook of Clinical Anaesthesia. Fourth Edition. CRC Press. 2018. 978-1-4987-6289-2.
- Tait A, Howell SJ. Preoperative hypertension: perioperative implications and management. BJA Educ. 2021;21(11):426-432.
- Yancey R. Anesthetic Management of the Hypertensive Patient: Part I. Anesth Prog. 2018;65(2):131-138.
- Yancey R. Anesthetic Management of the Hypertensive Patient: Part II. Anesth Prog. 2018;65(3):206-213.

Hypertension

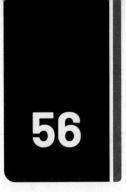

**56**

# HYPOGLYCEMIA

## LEARNING OBJECTIVES

- Recognize signs and symptoms of hypoglycemia
- Manage and prevent hypoglycemia

## DEFINITION AND MECHANISM

- Hypoglycemia is a fall in blood sugar (glucose) to levels below normal, typically below 70 mg/dL or 3.9 mmol/L
- Hypoglycemia during general anesthesia is rarely reported in the general population
- May cause cerebral damage

## SIGNS AND SYMPTOMS

- Diaphoresis is a marked sign of hypoglycemia
- Other symptoms are usually masked under anesthesia
- In the awake patient, hypoglycemia is characterized by neuroglycopenic and adrenergic symptoms

| Neuroglycopenic symptoms | Adrenergic symptoms |
|---|---|
| Dizziness | Tachycardia |
| Blurred vision | Palpitations |
| Headache | Diaphoresis |
| Unusual behavior | Clamminess |
| Confusion | Feeling shaky or trembling |
| Altered mental status (like being drunk) | Hunger |
| Seizures | Nausea |
| Loss of consciousness | Tingling sensation |
| Coma | Pale skin color |
| | Easily irritated, tearful, anxious, or moody |

Hypoglycemia

# MANAGEMENT AND PREVENTION

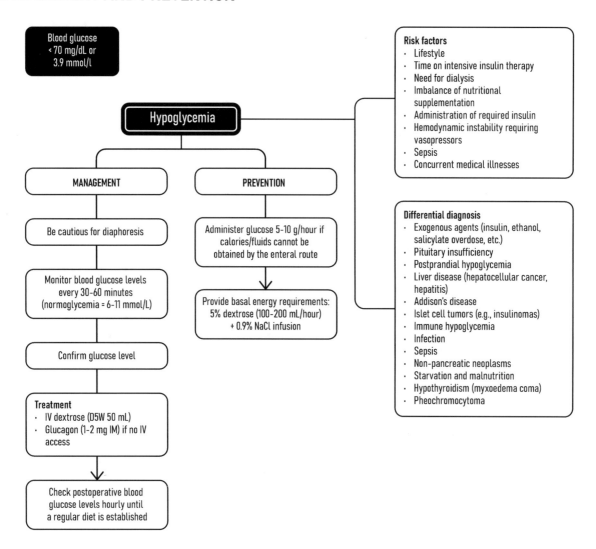

Blood glucose
< 70 mg/dL or
3.9 mmol/l

**Hypoglycemia**

**MANAGEMENT**

Be cautious for diaphoresis

Monitor blood glucose levels
every 30-60 minutes
(normoglycemia = 6-11 mmol/L)

Confirm glucose level

Treatment
· IV dextrose (D5W 50 mL)
· Glucagon (1-2 mg IM) if no IV
  access

Check postoperative blood
glucose levels hourly until
a regular diet is established

**PREVENTION**

Administer glucose 5-10 g/hour if
calories/fluids cannot be
obtained by the enteral route

Provide basal energy requirements:
5% dextrose (100-200 mL/hour)
+ 0.9% NaCl infusion

**Risk factors**
· Lifestyle
· Time on intensive insulin therapy
· Need for dialysis
· Imbalance of nutritional
  supplementation
· Administration of required insulin
· Hemodynamic instability requiring
  vasopressors
· Sepsis
· Concurrent medical illnesses

**Differential diagnosis**
· Exogenous agents (insulin, ethanol,
  salicylate overdose, etc.)
· Pituitary insufficiency
· Postprandial hypoglycemia
· Liver disease (hepatocellular cancer,
  hepatitis)
· Addison's disease
· Islet cell tumors (e.g., insulinomas)
· Immune hypoglycemia
· Infection
· Sepsis
· Non-pancreatic neoplasms
· Starvation and malnutrition
· Hypothyroidism (myxoedema coma)
· Pheochromocytoma

## KEEP IN MIND

• Monitor blood glucose levels closely in starved patients with a history of significant alcohol intake as anesthesia masks cognitive dysfuntion

## SUGGESTED READING

• Ackland, Gareth L. PhD, FRCA; Smith, Megan MBBS; Mglennan, Alan P. FRCA. Acute, Severe Hypoglycemia Occurring During General Anesthesia in a Nondiabetic Adult. Anesthesia & Analgesia: August 2007 - Volume 105 - Issue 2 - p 553-554.
• Kalra S, Bajwa SJ, Baruah M, Sehgal V. Hypoglycaemia in anesthesiology practice: Diagnostic, preventive, and management strategies. Saudi J Anaesth. 2013;7(4):447-452.
• Pollard BJ, Kitchen, G. Handbook of Clinical Anaesthesia. Fourth Edition. CRC Press. 2018. 978-1-4987-6289-2.

Hypoglycemia

# HYPOTENSION

## LEARNING OBJECTIVES

- Discuss the perioperative management of patients with hypotension
- Describe the management of hypotension

## DEFINITION AND MECHANISM

- Frequently used definitions are:
  - A systolic arterial pressure (SAP) < 80 mmHg
  - A mean arterial pressure (MAP) < 65 mmHg
  - A decrease of 10-60% in baseline MAP or SAP
- Caused by excessive vasodilation or insufficient constriction of arterioles
- Due to decreased sympathetic nervous system output or increased parasympathetic activity

## SIGNS AND SYMPTOMS

- Cold, clammy skin
- Decrease in skin color (pallor)
- Rapid, shallow breathing
- Weak and rapid pulse

## CAUSES

- Vasodilation
- Intravascular hypovolemia
- Anaphylaxis
- Sepsis/systemic inflammatory response syndrome (SIRS)
- Anesthetic agent overdose or swap
- Low cardiac output
- High intrathoracic pressure
- Impairment of sympathetic nervous system
- Compromised baroreflex regulation

## RISK FACTORS

- Older age
- High ASA class
- Male sex
- Lower preinduction SAP
- General anesthesia with propofol
- Combination of general and regional anesthesia
- Duration of surgery
- Emergency surgery
- Antihypertensive medications (ACE inhibitors, A2 receptor antagonists, beta blockers or alpha-2 agonists)

# MANAGEMENT

## Hypotension during anesthesia

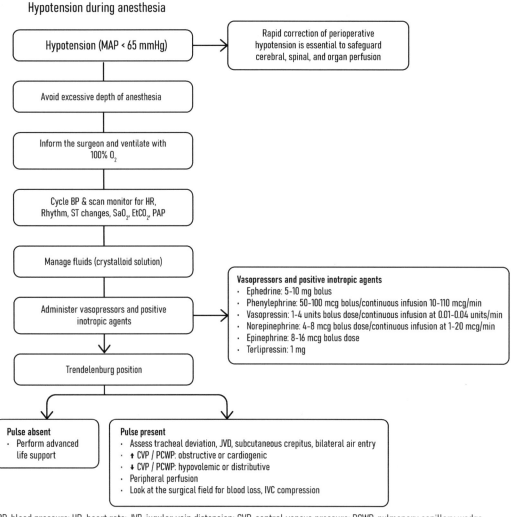

BP, blood pressure; HR, heart rate; JVD, jugular vein distension; CVP, central venous pressure; PCWP, pulmonary capillary wedge pressure; IVC, inferior vena cava.

## POSTOPERATIVE COMPLICATIONS

- Myocardial injury
- Myocardial infarction
- Cardiogenic shock
- Acute kidney injury
- Delirium
- Stroke
- Death

## SUGGESTED READING

- Guarracino, F., Bertini, P. Perioperative hypotension: causes and remedies. J Anesth Analg Crit Care 2, 17 (2022).
- Kouz K, Hoppe P, Briesenick L, Saugel B. Intraoperative hypotension: Pathophysiology, clinical relevance, and therapeutic approaches. Indian J Anaesth. 2020;64(2):90-96.
- Lonjaret L, Lairez O, Minville V, Geeraerts T. Optimal perioperative management of arterial blood pressure. Integr Blood Press Control. 2014;7:49-59.
- Weinberg L, Li SY, Louis M, et al. Reported definitions of intraoperative hypotension in adults undergoing non-cardiac surgery under general anaesthesia: a review. BMC Anesthesiol. 2022;22(1):69.

# HYPOVOLEMIA

## 58

## LEARNING OBJECTIVES

- Description of hypovolemia
- Treatment and perioperative management of hypovolemia
- Management of a hypovolemic shock

## DEFINITION AND MECHANISM

- Also known as volume depletion or volume contraction, is a state of abnormally low extracellular fluid volume
- The maintenance of an adequate fluid balance is key to preserving homeostasis
- Caused by either a loss of both sodium and water or a decrease in blood volume
- Hypovolemia refers to the loss of extracellular fluid and should not be confused with dehydration
- Untreated hypovolemia or excessive and rapid losses of volume may lead to hypovolemic shock
- Immediate treatment for hypovolemia is necessary to prevent life-threatening organ damage, shock, or death

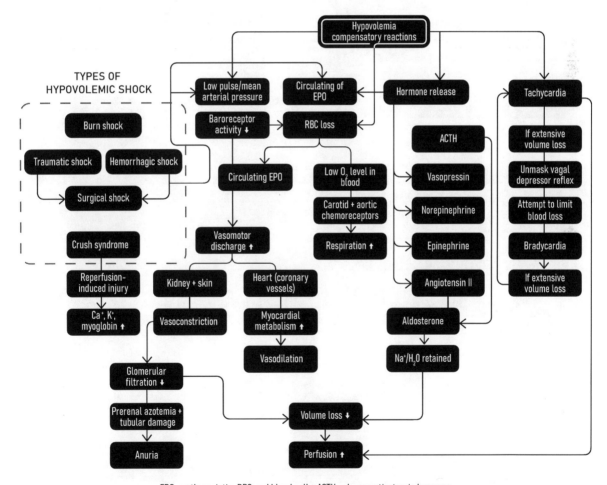

EPO, erythropoietin; RBC, red blood cells; ACTH, adrenocorticotropic hormone.

Hypovolemia

## SIGNS AND SYMPTOMS

- Dizziness
- Headache
- Weakness
- Thirst
- Fatigue
- Muscle cramps
- Urinary retention or the color of the urine is darker than normal

## HYPOVOLEMIC SHOCK:

- Tachycardia
- Hypotension
- Pale or cold skin
- Cyanosis
- Confusion
- Difficulty breathing or rapid breathing
- Excessive sweating
- Oliguria
- Abdominal and chest pain
- Cold hands and feet

## STAGES OF HYPOVOLEMIC SHOCK

| Blood loss | Blood pressure | Heart rate | Respiratory rate | Mental status | Skin | Capillary refill | Urine output |
|---|---|---|---|---|---|---|---|
| **Stage 1** | | | | | | | |
| Up to 15% (750 mL) | Normal (maintained by vasoconstriction) | Normal | Normal | Normal | Pale | Normal | Normal |
| **Stage 2** | | | | | | | |
| 15-30% (750-1500 mL) | Increased diastolic BP | Slight tachycardia (> 100 bpm) | Increased (> 20) | Slight anxiety, restless | Pale, cool, clammy | Delayed | 20-30 mL/h |
| **Stage 3** | | | | | | | |
| 30-40% (1500-2000mL) | Systolic BP < 100 | Tachycardia (> 120 bpm) | Tachypnea (> 30) | Altered, confused | Increased diaphoresis | Delayed | 20 mL/h |
| **Stage 4** | | | | | | | |
| Over 40% (> 2000 mL) | Systolic BP < 70 | Extreme tachycardia (> 140bpm) with weak pulse | Extreme tachypnea | Decreased loss of consciousness (LOC), lethargy, coma | Extreme diaphoresis; mottling possible | Absent | Negligible |

## CAUSES OF HYPOVOLEMIC SHOCK

| Renal | Extrarenal | Anesthesia-associated relative hypovolemia |
|---|---|---|
| Diuretic excess<br>Mineralocorticoid deficiency<br>Ketonuria<br>Osmotic diuresis<br>Cerebral salt wasting syndrome<br>Salt-wasting nephropathies | Gastrointestinal losses: vomiting and diarrhea<br>Skin losses: excessive sweating and burns<br>Respiratory losses: hyperventilation<br>Build-up of fluid in third spaces:<br>· Acute pancreatitis<br>· Intestinal obstruction<br>· Increased vascular permeability<br>· Hypoalbuminemia<br>Internal bleeding<br>Trauma | Decreased central sympathetic output<br>Decreased cardiovascular reflex responses<br>Decreased baroreceptor reflex activity<br>Decreased vascular smooth muscle (VSM) contractile response or sensitivity to neurohumoral and adrenoceptor agonists (e.g., norepinephrine)<br>Depressed mechanisms regulating VSM cytosolic $Ca^{2+}$<br>Reduced VSM intracellular $Ca^{2+}$ concentration<br>Reduced VSM L-type calcium channel ion transport<br>Reduced VSM myofilament sensitivity to calcium<br>Activation of $K^+ATP$ channels |

## COMPLICATIONS

- Shock
- Ischemic stroke
- Myocardial infarction
- Liver failure
- Acute renal failure
- Multi-organ failure
- Death

## DIAGNOSIS

- Physical exam
- Central venous catheter
- Arterial line
- Blood tests: urea and electrolytes, basic metabolic panel, full blood count, glucose, blood type, and screen
- Pulse, body temperature, and blood pressure
- Kidney function tests
- Ultrasound
- Echocardiogram

## TREATMENT

- Fluid replacement depends on the type of fluid that has been lost:
  - Blood transfusion
  - Fresh frozen plasma
  - Other coagulation factors
  - Crystalloid solution: lactated Ringer's solution → fill both the interstitial and intravascular spaces
  - Colloids (plasma substitutes): human serum albumin (5% and 25%), dextran, gelatin, hydroxyethyl starch (HES) → stay within the intravascular space
  - Treating underlying illness, wounds, or burns
  - Restore electrolyte balance

## PERIOPERATIVE MANAGEMENT

- Minimize preoperative fasting times
- Encourage unrestricted intake of clear fluids until 2 h before elective surgery
- Assess fluid responsiveness in hemodynamically unstable adults throughout the perioperative period with passive leg raising followed by measurement of blood pressure or (ideally) stroke volume
- Administer IV fluid with an overall positive fluid balance of 1–2 L at the end of surgery
- In case of major abdominal surgery, provide an average crystalloid fluid infusion rate of 10-12 mL/kg/h during surgery and 1.5 mL/kg/h in the 24-h postoperative period
- Ensure that intravascular volume status is optimized before adding vasopressor therapy
- Measure fluid responsiveness in higher-risk patients having major surgery using an advanced hemodynamic monitor
- Apply a goal-directed hemodynamic strategy, and if needed, introduce a vasopressor or inotrope
- Aim for the early transition from IV to oral fluid therapy after surgery
- Be aware that anesthesia can also lead to relative hypovolemia
  - Identify and treat relative hypovolemia

## DIFFERENTIAL DIAGNOSIS

- Pregnancy
- Sepsis
- Hypoglycemia
- Anaphylaxis
- Anemia
- Heart failure
- Bradycardia
- Valvular pathology

- Monitor:
  - Heart rate and rhythm
  - Arterial pressure/CVP
  - Pulse oximetry
  - End-tidal carbon dioxide
  - Inhalant anesthetic concentrations
  - Arterial blood gases
  - Lactate
- Selection of a fluid management strategy:
  - Minimally/moderately invasive surgery: 1-2 L of a balanced electrolyte procedure administered over a period of 30-120 minutes
  - Major invasive procedures:
    - Restrictive strategy: Replace only fluid lost during the procedure (approximately 3 mL/kg/h) if anticipated blood loss is < 500 mL and/or without fluid shifts
    - Goal-directed therapy (GDT): For procedures with an anticipated blood loss > 500 mL and/or fluid shifts use GDT with invasive dynamic hemodynamic parameters
  - Avoid liberal or fixed-volume approaches that lead to the administration of large volumes of crystalloid solution, tissue edema, and associated adverse outcomes

# MANAGEMENT

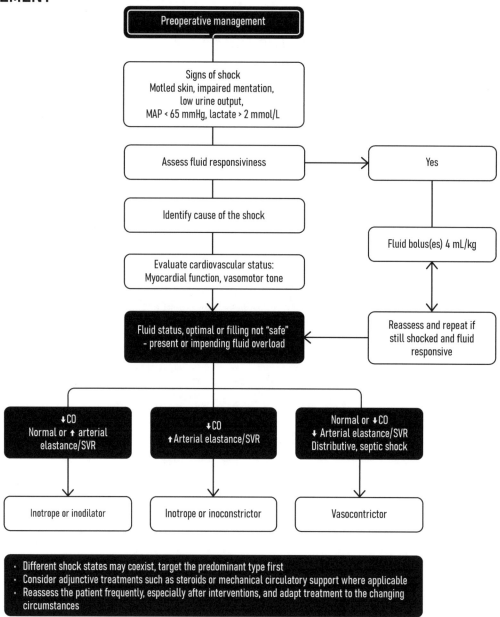

SVR, systemic vascular resistance; CO, cardiac output.

## SUGGESTED READING

- Al-Khafaji, A., Webb, A. 2004. Fluid resuscitation. Continuing Education in Anaesthesia Critical Care & Pain. 4;4:127-131.
- Joshi, G. 2022. Intraoperative fluid management. Up to date. https://www.uptodate.com/contents/intraoperative-fluid-management#H254311346
- Jha, A., Zilahi, G., Rhodes, A., 2021. Vasoactive therapy in shock. BJA Education 21, 270–277.
- Noel-Morgan J, Muir WW. Anesthesia-Associated Relative Hypovolemia: Mechanisms, Monitoring, and Treatment Considerations. Front Vet Sci. 2018;5:53.
- Timothy E. Miller, Paul S. Myles; Perioperative Fluid Therapy for Major Surgery. Anesthesiology 2019; 130:825-832.

Hypovolemia

# HYPOXEMIA

## LEARNING OBJECTIVES

- Recognize hypoxemia
- Differential diagnosis of hypoxemia
- Management of hypoxemia

## DEFINITION AND MECHANISM

- A decrease in the partial pressure of oxygen in the blood
- Severe when oxygen saturation falls below 90%
- Acute hypoxemia will eventually cause circulatory arrest due to myocardial hypoxia with:
  - Irreversible cardiac damage
  - Loss of consciousness within 10 seconds
  - Irreversible brain damage within 4-5 minutes

## SIGNS AND SYMPTOMS

- Shortness of breath
- Increased breathing rate
- Headache
- Coughing
- Tachycardia
- Use of chest and abdominal muscles to breath
- Cyanosis
- Hemoptysis

## DIAGNOSIS

- Pulse oximetry
- Arterial blood gas test
- Six-minute walk test

| Differential diagnosis | |
|---|---|
| Equipment failure | |
| Hypoventilation | Low TV or RR<br>Ventilator dyssynchrony<br>Circuit leak<br>Obstructed ETT |
| Ventilation-perfusion mismatch | Bronchospasm<br>Mainstem intubation<br>Pulmonary edema<br>Aspiration<br>Atelectasis<br>Pneumothorax<br>Pleural effusion |
| Right-to-left shunt | Intracardiac shunting |
| Diffusion impairment | Pulmonary edema<br>Pneumonia |
| Low PO$_2$ | Increased dead space<br>Pulmonary embolism<br>Reduced cardiac output |
| Increased metabolic O$_2$ demand | Malignant hyperthermia<br>Sepsis<br>Neuroleptic malignant syndrome |

TV, tidal volume; RR, respiratory rate; ETT, endotracheal tube.

# MANAGEMENT

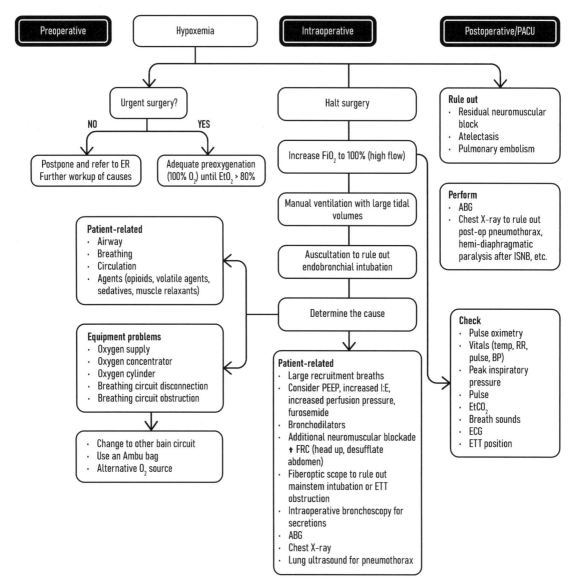

ABG, arterial blood gas; ISNB, interscalene brachial plexus nerve block; RR, respiratory rate; BP, blood pressure; ETT, endotracheal tube; PEEP, positive end-expiratory pressure; FRC, functional residual capacity.

**SUGGESTED READING**

- Pollard BJ, Kitchen, G. Handbook of Clinical Anaesthesia. Fourth Edition. CRC Press. 2018. 978-1-4987-6289-2.
- Rozé H, Lafargue M, Ouattara A. Case scenario: Management of intraoperative hypoxemia during one-lung ventilation. Anesthesiology. 2011;114(1):167-174.

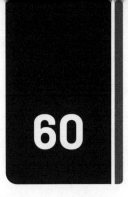

# INCREASED AIRWAY PRESSURE

**60**

## LEARNING OBJECTIVES

- Differential diagnosis and management of increased airway pressure in a mechanically ventilated patient

## DEFINITION AND MECHANISM

- Airway pressures that exceed the safe limit for ventilation, typically > 30 mmHg plateau pressure, could make ventilation difficult or cause barotrauma
- Can be constantly elevated in a given patient due to underlying conditions or can increase suddenly due to a wide variety of causes

## SIGNS AND SYMPTOMS

- High plateau and peak airway pressures
- Distorted capnography
- Inadequate tidal volumes
- Hemodynamic instability

## DIFFERENTIAL DIAGNOSIS

"Man versus machine"

- Anesthesia machine
  - Machine malfunction
  - Kinked breathing circuit
  - Physical obstruction of the circuit (water or an occluded filter)
  - Dislodgement, kinking, or obstruction of the endotracheal tube
  - Incorrectly positioned endotracheal tube
- Patient
  - Inadequate depth of anesthesia
  - Decrease in pulmonary compliance:
    - Fibrosis
    - Pneumothorax
    - Atelectasis
    - Pulmonary edema
  - Decrease in chest wall compliance
    - Obesity
    - Ascites
    - Abdominal distension
    - Kyphoscoliosis
    - Pharmacological (opiates, neuromuscular blocking drugs)
  - Malignant hyperthermia
  - Broncho or laryngospasm (anesthesiologic emergency!)

# MANAGEMENT

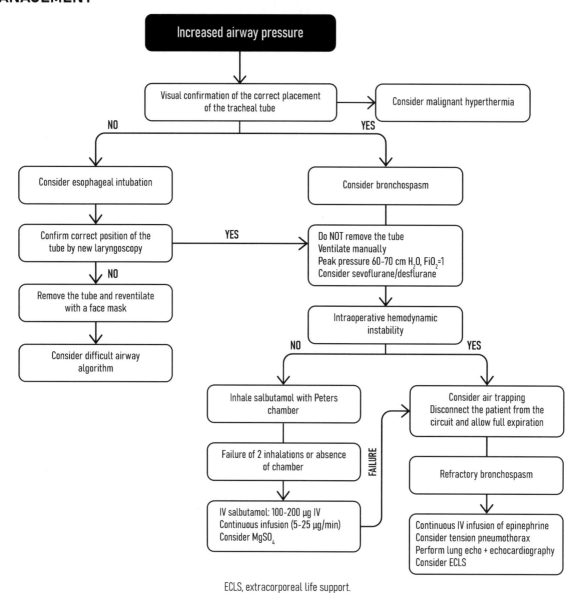

ECLS, extracorporeal life support.

## SUGGESTED READING

- Gouel-Cheron A, Neukirch C, Kantor E, et al. Clinical reasoning in anaphylactic shock: addressing the challenges faced by anaesthesiologists in real time: A clinical review and management algorithms. Eur J Anaesthesiol. 2021;38(11):1158-1167.
- Woods BD, Sladen RN. Perioperative considerations for the patient with asthma and bronchospasm. Br J Anaesth. 2009;103 Suppl 1:i57-i65.

# INCREASED INTRACRANIAL PRESSURE

## LEARNING OBJECTIVES

- Describe the causes of and risk factors for increased intracranial pressure
- Identify increased intracranial pressure
- Manage increased intracranial pressure

## DEFINITION AND MECHANISM

- Increased intracranial pressure (ICP) commonly occurs in patients with traumatic brain injury and subarachnoid hemorrhage
- It is the most frequent cause of morbidity and mortality in these patients
- Brain tumors can also increase ICP
- Increased ICP can impair cerebral perfusion pressure, cerebral blood flow, and cerebral oxygenation, resulting in ischemia, edema, and further increases in ICP
- Can impede surgical access to deep lesions requiring brain retraction
- Can predispose to or exacerbate brain retraction injury
- Can complicate dural closure

## SIGNS AND SYMPTOMS

- Before craniotomy:
  - Hypertension
  - Bradycardia
  - Irregular respiratory pattern
  - Cushing reflex: the triad of hypertension, bradycardia and irregular respiratory pattern

- After craniotomy:
  - Tense dura
  - Brain swelling out of the dural opening
  - Difficult brain retraction
- Quantitative measurements:
  - ICP Monitoring (Continuous)
  - External Ventricular Drain (EVD)
  - Intraparenchymal Pressure Monitor
  - ICP Measurement (Intermittent)
  - Epidural Pressure Transducer
  - Subdural/Subarachnoid Bolt

## RISK FACTORS

- Subdural ICP > 10 mmHg
- Peritumoral edema
- Mean arterial blood pressure > 140 mmHg
- Intraoperative hypotension with systolic blood pressure < 90 mmHg
- Glioblastoma
- Metastasis
- Difficult brain retraction

## CAUSES

- Intracranial
  - Tumor
  - Infarct
  - Trauma
  - Hemorrhage
  - Hydrocephalus
  - Abscess/infection
  - Parenchymal edema
  - Idiopathic

- Extracranial
  - Airway obstruction
  - Hypoxia/hypercarbia
  - Hypertension exceeding cerebral autoregulatory capacity
  - Hypotension causing cerebral hypoperfusion and reflex vasodilation
  - Venous hypertension from outflow obstruction
  - Volatile anesthetics
  - Nitroglycerin
  - Sodium nitroprusside
  - Vomiting, coughing, pain, shivering, and seizure activity during awake craniotomy

# MANAGEMENT

### Reduce cerebral blood volume

- Increase venous drainage by elevating the head and placing it in a neutral position
- Suppress arterial inflow by cerebral vasoconstriction (e.g., by hyperventilation)
- Avoid inhalational anesthetics in patients with intracranial hypertension
- Ideally, use propofol as the anesthetic agent
- Barbiturates, benzodiazepines, and etomidate can decrease ICP
- Avoid large boluses of opioids
- Avoid nitrous oxide
- Therapeutic hypothermia

### Reduce brain tissue volume

- Hypertonic saline
- Mannitol (use cautiously in patients with renal dysfunction)
- Target osmolarity < 320 mOsm/L

### Reduce CSF volume

- Acetazolamide
- Topiramate

### Intracranial invasive methods

- Resect tumor (evacuate hematoma) if a mass is the cause of increased ICP
- Resect damaged or normal non-eloquent brain tissue
- Gyrus rectus resection
- Anterior temporal lobectomy
- Cerebellar tissue resection (avoid deep nuclei and medial parenchyma)

### Extracranial invasive methods

- Dural expansion (duraplasty, scarify dura, section falx, do not replace bone flap, increase craniectomy size, or perform bilateral craniectomy)
- Decompressive craniectomy
- Hinge craniotomy

### CSF drainage

- Lumbar or external ventricular drain
- Fenestration of cisternal compartments
- Arachnoid dissection with CSF drainage

ICP, intracranial pressure; CSF, cerebrospinal fluid.

# SUGGESTED READING

- Desai VR, Sadrameli SS, Hoppe S, Lee JJ, Jenson A, Steele WJ, et al. Contemporary Management of Increased Intraoperative Intracranial Pressure: Evidence-Based Anesthetic and Surgical Review. World Neurosurgery. 2019;129:120-9.
- Ragland J, Lee K. Critical Care Management and Monitoring of Intracranial Pressure. J Neurocrit Care. 2016;9(2):105-12.
- Tameem A, Krovvidi H. Cerebral physiology. Continuing Education in Anaesthesia Critical Care & Pain. 2013;13(4):113-8.

Increased intracranial pressure

# LARYNGOSPASM

## LEARNING OBJECTIVES

- Describe the mechanism and risk factors of laryngospasm
- Prevent laryngospasm
- Recognize and treat laryngospasm

## DEFINITION AND MECHANISM

- Laryngospasm is the sustained closure of the vocal cords resulting in partial or complete loss of the airway
- Primitive protective airway reflex to prevent tracheobronchial aspiration after an irritating stimulus
- Problematic prolongation of this initial reflex can occur under general anesthesia, often during intubation or extubation
- Can rapidly result in hypoxemia and bradycardia
- Overall incidence ~1%
- Incidence up to 25% in patients undergoing tonsillectomy and adenoidectomy

## SIGNS AND SYMPTOMS

- Respiratory stridor
- Paradoxical respiratory movements
- Suprasternal and supraclavicular retractions
- Rapidly decreasing oxygen saturation
- Excessive chest movements but no movement of the reservoir bag and no capnogram reading
- Bradycardia
- Negative pressure pulmonary edema
- Cardiac arrest
- Pulmonary aspiration
- Arrhythmias

## RISK FACTORS

| Patient-related | Surgery-related | Anesthesia-related |
|---|---|---|
| Obesity | Nasal, oral, or pharyngeal surgeries (adenoidectomy and tonsillectomy) | Laryngeal mask/Guedel airway device |
| Young age | Gastrointestinal endoscopy | Extubation |
| Active and passive smoking | Bronchoscopy | Suction catheter |
| ASA IV | Appendectomy | Light anesthesia plan |
| Gastroesophageal reflux | Anal or cervical dilation | Blood/secretions in the airway |
| Obstructive sleep apnea | Mediastinoscopy | Regurgitation |
| Upper airway infection | Inferior urologic surgery | Desflurane |
| Hypocalcemia | Skin transplant | Ketamine and thiopental induction |
| Asthma | Nociception | Nasogastric tube |
| Difficult airway | Surgical stimulus | Inexperience of anesthesiologist |
|  | Movement | Failed intubation |
|  | Recurrent laryngeal nerve damage | Laryngoscopy |
|  | Esophageal stimulation |  |
|  | Iatrogenic removal of parathyroid glands |  |

# PREVENTION

- Anesthetic technique
  - Ensure adequate depth
  - Inhalation induction with non-irritant agent (e.g., sevoflurane)
  - IV induction with propofol is less problematic
  - Extubate either in a deep plane of anesthesia or fully awake, but not in-between
    - "Deep" extubation: Suction the airway
    - Key clinical criteria and considerations for making deep extubation possible
      * Patient selection
      * Adequate depth of anesthesia
      * Muscle relaxant reversal
      * Surgical considerations (e.g., non-airway surgery, minimal bleeding and secretions)
      * Continuous monitoring and readiness for reintubation
      * The importance of postoperative care
    - Awake extubation: Once facial grimacing, adequate tidal volume, a regular respiratory pattern, coughing, and preferably eye opening have returned, use "no touch" technique: Pharyngeal suctioning and lateral positioning while anesthetized, followed by avoidance of any stimulation until eye opening when extubation is performed
    - Extubation during forced positive pressure inflation decreases laryngeal adductor excitability, decreasing the risk of laryngospasm
- Pharmacological prevention
  - Magnesium 15 mg/kg IV intraoperatively
  - Lidocaine topically 4 mg/kg or IV 1.5-2 mg/kg (further research needed)

# MANAGEMENT

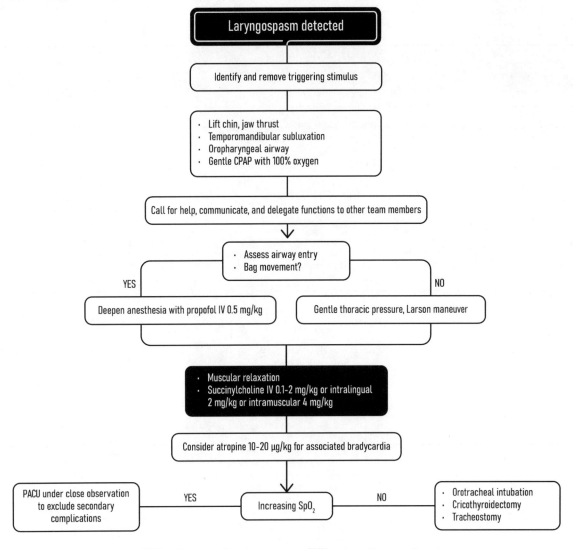

CPAP, continuous positive airway pressure; PACU, postoperative care unit.

## SUGGESTED READING

- Benham-Hermetz J, Mitchell V. Safe tracheal extubation after general anaesthesia. BJA Educ. 2021;21(12):446-454.
- Gavel G, Walker RWM. Laryngospasm in anaesthesia. Continuing Education in Anaesthesia Critical Care & Pain. 2014;14(2):47-51.
- Silva CR, Pereira T, Henriques D, Lanca F. Comprehensive review of laryngospasm. WFSA Resource Library. https://resources.wfsahq.org/uia/volume-35/comprehensive-review-of-laryngospasm/. Published July 8, 2020. Accessed February 2, 2023.
- Visvanathan T, Kluger MT, Webb RK, Westhorpe RN. Crisis management during anaesthesia: laryngospasm. Qual Saf Health Care. 2005;14(3):e3.

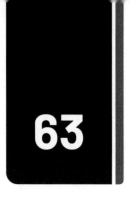

# 63

# LOCAL ANESTHETIC SYSTEMIC TOXICITY (LAST)

## LEARNING OBJECTIVES

- Describe the mechanisms of LAST
- Recognize the symptoms of LAST
- Manage LAST occurrence

## DEFINITION AND MECHANISM

- Local anesthetic systemic toxicity (LAST) is a life-threatening adverse event that may occur after the administration of local anesthetics through a variety of routes
- A supratherapeutic plasma concentration of local anesthetics has several adverse effects on the central nervous and cardiovascular systems

## MECHANISMS OF LAST

> Local anesthetic (LA) are generally safe and effective in therapeutic doses for tissue infiltration, fascial planes, or near a nerve/plexus of nerves. However, supratherapeutic plasma levels of LAs can result in **Local anesthetic systemic toxicity (LAST)**.

### PLASMA CONCENTRATION FACTORS

**High plasma concentration of LAs:**
- Partial venous/arterial injection
- Intravascular injection
- Rapid vascular absorption from the highly vascularized injection site

**Plasma levels of LA:** Proportional to the rate of systemic absorption from the site of therapy.

**Rate of absorption:**
- Varies among tissues
- Depends on the size of the absorptive surface
- Depends on vascularization of the tissue planes where the injection is made
- ↑ Doses = ↑ plasma levels of LAs, independent of the injection site

### LA: MECHANISMS ON THE CELLULAR LEVEL

- **Inhibitory action** on nerve conduction by inhibiting the movement of ions through voltage-gated ionotropic channels at the level of the cell membrane
- **Primary therapeutic target:** Voltage-gated sodium channel where inhibition alters the transmission of sensory and motor signals in axons
- **Also:** LAs inhibit voltage-gated $Ca^{2+}$ channels, $K^+$ channels, the Na-K ATPase, and other channels and enzymes
- **Non-ionized vs ionized molecules:** The inhibition occurs from the intracellular side and requires LAs to cross the lipid bilayer first as unbound, non-ionized free molecules
- **At lower concentrations:** LAs block protein kinase signaling induced by tumor necrosis factor alpha (TNF-α)
- **At higher concentrations:** LAs can inhibit other channels, enzymes, and receptors, including the carnitine-acylcarnitine translocase in the mitochondria

### LA & CARDIAC TOXICITY

- **Cardiovascular toxicity:** Caused by the combination of electrophysiologic and contractile dysfunction

- **CAUTION:** Bupivacaine = lipophilic and greater affinity for the voltage-gated sodium channels, resulting in its uniquely high cardiotoxic profile

- **More on bupivacaine:** Cardiac toxicity can occur at lower serum concentrations because it can accumulate in the mitochondria and cardiac tissue at a ratio of about 6:1 (or greater) relative to plasma

## SIGNS AND SYMPTOMS

- Central nervous symptoms precede cardiovascular symptoms
- Neurological signs/symptoms range between excitation (early) and depression (late)
- Early LAST: Excitatory manifestations
- Neurological symptoms: Seizures (70%), agitation (10%), loss of consciousness (7%)
- Prodromal (early) symptoms: Perioral paresthesia, metallic taste, tinnitus
- ± 40% of cases present as a sudden, rapid-onset seizure, progressing to cardiac arrest
- High dose of LA or inadvertent IV injection: Prodromal (early) central nervous symptoms may be absent and the first manifestation could be cardiovascular toxicity (11%)
- Cardiovascular toxicity: Heart conduction anomalies, decreased cardiac contractility, decreased systemic vascular resistance
- Early-onset ECG changes: Increased PR and QTc, QRS abnormalities (bundle branch blocks), and increased ST intervals with/without refractory brady-/tachyarrhythmias

- Depression of spontaneous pacemaker activity can rapidly lead to high-degree AV blocks or asystole
- Cardiogenic shock and refractory hypotension may follow as a result of decreased cardiac contractility and vasomotor control disturbances, caused by peripheral vascular ion-channel alterations

## KEEP IN MIND

- LAST can occur immediately at the time of injection (usually accidental intravascular injection) or up to an hour after it (due to delayed tissue absorption)
- Continue monitoring for 30-45 min after injection of large volumes or toxic doses of LAs
- Monitor patients with any signs of LAST for 2-6 hours because cardiovascular depression due to LAs can persist or recur after treatment

## MANAGEMENT

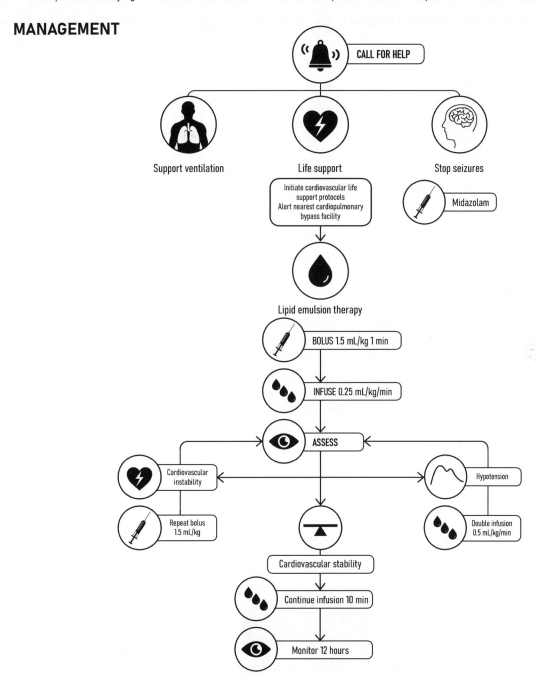

Local anesthetic systemic toxicity (LAST)

**64**

# MALIGNANT HYPERTHERMIA

## LEARNING OBJECTIVES

- Describe the risk factors for malignant hyperthermia
- Describe the symptoms of malignant hyperthermia
- Manage malignant hyperthermia and its consequences

## DEFINITION AND MECHANISM

- Malignant hyperthermia (MH) is a severe and potentially life-threatening condition typically triggered by exposure to certain anesthetic agents and muscle relaxants
- It is characterized by a hypermetabolic state of the skeletal muscle, leading to a rapid increase in body temperature and severe muscle contractions
- Malignant hyperthermia is caused by genetic defects, most commonly in the RYR1 gene (more rarely affected genes include CACNA1S and STAC3)
- Caused by an increase in metabolic rate driven by an increase in intracellular calcium levels in muscle tissue
- Can be triggered when exposed to potent inhalation anesthetics and/or succinylcholine

## SIGNS AND SYMPTOMS

- Unexplained, unexpected increase in $EtCO_2$
- Unexplained, unexpected increase in heart rate
- Unexplained, unexpected increase in temperature
- Decreased urine output
- Muscle spasms
- Masseter muscle rigidity

## RISK FACTORS

Patients that have a higher risk of MH when exposed to triggering agents:

- Any close relative has a confirmed susceptibility to MH
- The patient or a close relative has a history of an event that is suspected to be MH during anesthesia
- The patient or a close relative has a history of rhabdomyolysis, which can be triggered by exercise in extreme heat and humidity or when taking a statin drug
- Patients with another genetic muscle disorder (e.g., Duchenne muscular dystrophy)
- Patients with idiopathic hyperCKemia
- Patients with otherwise unexplained exertional heat illness

## MANAGEMENT

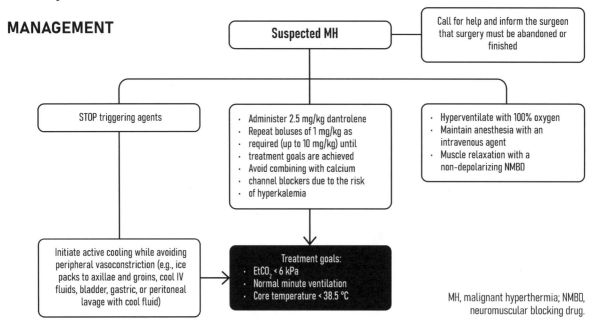

MH, malignant hyperthermia; NMBD, neuromuscular blocking drug.

## SUPPORTIVE MANAGEMENT

- Hyperkalemia may require administration of calcium chloride, sodium bicarbonate, and/or insulin with glucose
- Treat arrhythmias with magnesium, amiodarone, or beta-blockers. Avoid calcium channel blockers as they interact with dantrolene, potentiating myocardial depression.
- Disseminated intravascular coagulation may require blood product transfusion
- Rhabdomyolysis may result in acute kidney injury; measure creatine kinase, and institute forced alkaline diuresis
- Transfer the patient to the ICU once sufficiently stable

## FOLLOW-UP

- The diagnosis of MH is confirmed by muscle biopsy and in vivo contracture testing at specialist centers
- The patient and their family members must be followed-up and counseled regarding future anesthetics
- An alert should be documented in the patient notes and the patient should consider wearing an alert bracelet or carrying an alert card to notify medical staff of their condition in case of future emergencies

## KEEP IN MIND

- Taking a personal and family history of anesthetic problems is a mandatory part of the preoperative assessment for all patients requiring general or regional anesthesia
- Activated charcoal filters should be available at all anesthetizing locations
- Patients at increased risk of developing MH must not be exposed to potent inhalation anesthetics or succinylcholine

## ■ SUGGESTED READING ■

- Gupta, Pawan K, and Philip M Hopkins. "Diagnosis and Management of Malignant Hyperthermia." BJA Education, vol. 17, no. 7, July 2017, pp. 249–254, 10.1093/bjaed/mkw079.
- Hopkins PM, Girard T, Dalay S, et al. Malignant hyperthermia 2020: Guideline from the Association of Anaesthetists. Anaesthesia. 2021;76(5):655-664.

# PERIOPERATIVE BLEEDING

**65**

## LEARNING OBJECTIVES

- Describe the causes of perioperative bleeding
- Optimize patients at risk of perioperative bleeding
- Manage perioperative bleeding

--- DEFINITION AND MECHANISM ---

- Perioperative bleeding is a complex surgical complication with a range of causes
- Usually characterized by a site of bleeding and confined exclusively to the operative site
- Can evolve into pathologic thrombosis

## CAUSES

- Blood loss
- Hemodilution
- Acquired platelet dysfunction
- Coagulation factor consumption in extracorporeal circuits
- Activation of fibrinolytic, fibrinogenolytic, and inflammatory pathways
- Hypothermia
- Anticoagulant use
- Platelet inhibitor use
- Congenital coagulopathies

## INTERPLAY BETWEEN COAGULATION, ANTICOAGULATION, FIBRINOLYTIC SYSTEM

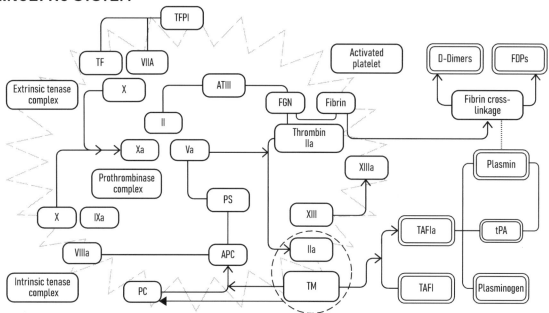

Together, TM and IIa complex activate PC indicated by the circle and arrow.
Plasmin inhibits the fibrin cross-linkage indicated by the dotted inhibition line.

TF, tissue factor; PC, protein C; PS, protein S; TFPI(a), tissue factor pathway inhibitor (activated); ATIII, antithrombin III; FCN, fibrinogen; TM, thrombomodulin; FDPs, fibrin degradation products; tPA, tissue plasminogen activator; TAFI, thrombin-activatable fibrinolysis inhibitor.

Perioperative bleeding

**Coagulation:**

- Factors Xa and Va convert prothrombin to thrombin through the activation of factor X via intrinsic (factor IXa, VIIIa) and extrinsic tenase (Xase complexes)
- Thrombin cleaves fibrinogen into fibrin
- Fibrin polymerization is facilitated by the activation of factor XIII which forms cross-links leading to clot stabilization
- Prothrombin complex concentrate (PCC) administration targets factors II, VII, IX, and X for repletion
- Factor VIIa is targeted for repletion with the administration of recombinant factor VIIa (rFVIIa)

**Anticoagulation:**

- Anticoagulants negatively modulate clot formation
- Antithrombin III (ATIII) modulates factor IIa (primarily) and factor Xa (secondarily)
- ATIII-dependent inhibition of factor IXa, XIa, and VIIa-TF complex occurs to a lesser extent
- Other important anticoagulants include TFPI-modulation of Tissue Factor and factor VIIa, and Activated Protein C (APC)
  - APC activates protein S and inhibits factor Va, weakening the prothrombinase complex and impairing thrombin generation
  - Upstream, APC inhibits factor VIIIa of the intrinsic Xase complex
- Factor IIa complexes with Thrombomodulin (TM) to activate PC
- The thrombin-thrombomodulin complex activates TAFI, which reduces plasminogen activation to plasmin, thus reducing fibrinolysis but not completely preventing plasmin production
- Plasmin is the primary driver of fibrinolysis and results:
  - In clot destabilization
  - Degradation of fibrin cross-linkage
  - Production of fibrin degradation products (D-dimers)
- Plasmin primarily acts on fibrin and does not directly trigger platelet activation. TAFI inhibits fibrinolysis by modifying fibrin to be less susceptible to plasmin

# PREOPERATIVE OPTIMIZATION

---

**PREOPERATIVE ANEMIA**

- Assess patients at risk of bleeding for anemia well before surgery
- Anemia correction: 1-2 weeks for parenteral stimulation of erythropoiesis and uncomplicated causes of anemia, 3-8 weeks for oral correction of iron deficiency anemia and complex causes of anemia
- Postpone surgery in noncancer patients with preoperative anemia scheduled for elective major surgery
- Identify the cause of anemia if present
- Iron deficiency anemia: Weight-based doses of iron supplementation if not contraindicated (IV > oral)
- Erythropoietin-stimulating agents when other causes were excluded/treated
- Avoid preoperative RBC transfusion to mask mild to moderate anemia
- Consider RBC transfusion when comprehensive hematological therapy fails
- Early noninvasive hemoglobin monitoring may speed up detection and correction of preoperative anemia
- If autologous blood donation is performed: Concomitant treatment with iron and/or erythropoietin-stimulating agents

---

**COMORBIDITIES INVOLVING IMPAIRED HOMEOSTASIS**

- Desmopressin treatment in high-risk uremic patients during invasive procedures and for managing acute bleeding
- Consider conjugated estrogen therapy in uremic platelet dysfunction
- Fibrinogen level assessment in patients with advanced liver disease
- Viscoelastic hemostatic assay to reduce allogeneic blood product transfusion in cirrhotic patients
- Consider thrombopoietin receptor agonists in cirrhotic patients with severe thrombocytopenia scheduled for high-risk procedures
- Individualized thromboprophylaxis strategy in patients with chronic liver disease who are not auto-anticoagulated
- Do not correct elevated INR before invasive procedures, with the exception of intracranial pressure monitor insertion

---

**CHRONIC MEDICATION ASSOCIATED WITH IMPAIRED HEMOSTASIS**

- Individualized perioperative management of selective serotonin reuptake inhibitor treatment
- Individualized preoperative management of antiepileptic agents (e.g., valproic acid)
- Discontinue Ginkgo biloba at least two weeks before surgery to reduce the risk of perioperative bleeding

---

**INHERITED BLEEDING DISORDERS**

- Bleeding assessment tools to detect and predict perioperative bleeding risk
- Manage in cooperation with a hematologist
- Individualized preoperative hemostatic correction based on specific disorder, type of surgery, and individual factors
- Replacement/substitution therapy with factor concentrates for major bleeding/surgery in patients with von Willebrand disease (VWD) or hemophilia A/B
- rFVIIq or aPCCs for hemophilia patients with inhibitors
- No routine perioperative platelet transfusion in patients with inherited platelet disorders
- DDAVP as a first-line treatment for minor bleeding/surgery in patients with VWD or mild hemophilia A after a trial test and in the absence of contraindications
- Perioperative antifibrinolytics as adjunct therapy in patients with hemophilia or VWD
- Consider antifibrinolytic agents as perioperative hemostatic monotherapy in patients with hemophilia or VWD undergoing minor mucosal or dental procedures and in patients with inherited platelet defects
- Consider rFVIIa in patients with Glanzmann thrombasthenia
- rFVIIa in perioperative bleeding caused by inherited factor VII deficiency

---

RBC, red blood cell; rFVIIa, recombinant activated factor VII; aPCC, activated prothrombin complex concentrate; DDAVP, desmopressin; INR, international normalized ratio.

# PERIOPERATIVE BLEEDING: ANTITHROMBOTIC AGENTS

## ANTIPLATELET AGENTS

- Continue aspirin for secondary prevention in most surgical settings, especially cardiac surgery
- Discontinue aspirin when prescribed for primary prevention 5-7 days before surgery
- Do not initiate aspirin preoperatively in patients with risk factors for vascular complications naïve of any antiplatelet treatment, except for carotid endarterectomy
- Aspirin may be interrupted for very high-risk procedures in patients chronically treated with aspirin for secondary prevention of cardiovascular events, except those with coronary stents
- Carefully discuss timing and dose of first administration of postoperative anticoagulants and resumption of aspirin
- Consider platelet transfusion (0.7 x 1011 per 10 kg body weight) for intra- or postoperative bleeding related to aspirin
- Continue aspirin at least 4 weeks after bare metal stent implantation and 3-12 months after drug-eluting stent implantation, unless the risk is unacceptably high
- Postpone surgery at least 5 days after cessation of ticagrelor and clopidogrel and 7 days in the case of prasugrel if feasible
- Resume antiplatelet agent therapy as soon as possible postoperatively
- Resume P2Y12 inhibitors early (24-72h after surgery)
- Avoid perioperative use of NSAIDs in patients on dual antiplatelet therapy, coxibs use is possible
- Have a multidisciplinary team decide on the perioperative use of antiplatelet agents in urgent and semi-urgent surgery
- Postpone noncardiac elective surgery until completion of the full course of dual antiplatelet therapy
- Perform urgent/semi-urgent surgery under aspirin/clopidogrel or aspirin/prasugrel combination therapy if possible
- Consider platelet transfusion in perioperative bleeding related to clopidogrel or prasugrel

## HEPARIN, FONDAPARINUX, VITAMIN K ANTAGONISTS

- Treat severe bleeding associated with IV unfractionated heparin (UFH) with IV protamine (1 mg per 100 IU UFH given in the preceding 2-3h), or with continuous IV protamine guided by anti-Xa activity if unresponsive to this dose
- Treat severe bleeding associated with subcutaneous LMWH with IV protamine (1 mg per 100 anti-Fxa units of LMWH administered), if unresponsive, measure anti-Xa activity
- Consider rFVIIa to treat severe bleeding associated with subcutaneous fondaparinux
- Do not interrupt vitamin K antagonists (VKA) for low-risk procedures
- For procedures requiring INR < 1.5, the time from last VKA intake should be 3-5 days
- Consider: If the INR is still elevated (e.g., > 1.5) the day before surgery, administering 2.5-5 mg of oral vitamin K can help normalize it. However, the dose may need adjustment based on the initial INR value
- Avoid bridging with LMWH or UFH in patients with high thromboembolic risk (e.g., mechanical heart valves, recent VTE, or atrial fibrillation with high stroke risk)
- Resume VKA within 24h after surgery, administer a prophylactic dose of a LMWH until the target INR is observed in the two following measurements
- Postoperative bridging with therapeutic LMWH may be appropriate for high-risk patients but should generally be started 24-48 hours post-surgery, depending on bleeding risk and surgical site
- Administer four-factor PCC 25-50 IU factor IX/kg + 5-10 mg IV vitamin K in bleeding patients with VKA-induced coagulopathy
- If PCC is not available, transfusion of plasma 15-20 mL/kg + 5-10 IV vitamin K

## DIRECT ORAL ANTICOAGULANTS

- Assess creatinine clearance in patients on direct oral anticoagulants (DOACs)
- DOACs can be given up to the day of surgery in patients undergoing low-risk procedures
- For rivaroxaban, apixaban, and edoxaban, halt treatment 3 days before surgery for moderate-to-high-risk procedures, pending a creatinine clearance > 30 mL/min
- For dabigatran, halt treatment 3 days before surgery if creatinine clearance > 50 mL/min and 5 days if creatinine clearance is 30-50 mL/min
- Consider idarucizumab in severe bleeding patients treated with dabigatran
- Prothrombin complex concentrate (PCC) is generally used for reversal of vitamin K antagonists and may not be the first choice for DOACs. For anti-Xa agents like rivaroxaban and apixaban, specific reversal agents (e.g., andexanet alfa) are preferred. PCC may be considered in the absence of specific reversal agents.
- Restart DOACs ~6h after surgery without LMWH administration after low-risk procedures, when hemostasis is achieved
- Give prophylactic doses of LMWH or DOACs postoperatively whenever thromboprophylaxis is requested and resume the full therapeutic dose of DOAC up to 72h postoperatively when surgical hemostasis is achieved

NSAID, non-steroidal anti-inflammatory drug; LMWH, low molecular weight heparin; INR, international normalized ratio; PCC, prothrombin complex concentrate

# COVID-19 COAGULOPATHY

- Avoid major elective surgery in patients with COVID-19 coagulopathy
- VHA-guided, goal-directed procoagulant treatment of perioperatively acquired coagulopathic bleeding avoiding overcorrection
- Perioperative drug monitoring of LMWH used as a standard anticoagulant in COVID-19 critical illness; if anti-Xa activity > 0.3 IU/mL in clinical bleeding, consider reversal agents or dose adjustments based on anti-Xa activity
- A restrictive red blood cell transfusion strategy as in non-COVID-19 patients
- In patients recovered from COVID-19 and free of post-COVID-19 symptoms, manage severe perioperative bleeding as in non-COVID-19 patients
- Administer postoperative thromboprophylaxis as early as possible
- A restrictive red blood cell, plasma, and platelet transfusion strategy in the critically ill
- Use a goal-directed coagulation therapy algorithm in the presence of ongoing bleeding, considering altered laboratory tests and VHA in critical illness

Perioperative bleeding

- If ongoing bleeding is unresponsive to multimodal coagulation therapy or there are wound healing defects in the critically ill, monitor FXIII and correct deficiency
- A restrictive systemic administration of TXA in case of fibrinolytic shutdown in critical illness
- Initiate thromboprophylaxis after bleeding as soon as the bleeding risk is overbalanced by the risk of thromboembolic complications

# PERIOPERATIVE BLEEDING CONTROL

- Perioperative bleeding is a major complication during and after surgery
- Massive transfusion protocols (MTPs)
- Defined as receiving ≥ 10 or more red blood cell units in 24h
  □ Include blood components or whole blood + coagulation factor concentrates, prothrombin complex concentrates (PCCs), and fibrinogen
- Bleeding management is guided by coagulation monitoring:
  □ Conventional coagulation tests: platelet counts, prothrombin time, and fibrinogen level
  □ Viscoelastic testing (VET)
- Hemostatic support is used to optimize hemostasis
- Surgical correction of site-specific bleeding

## Fibrinogen

- A critical hemostatic factor for clot formation
- Converted into insoluble fibrin by thrombin and cross-linked by factor XIII
- Replete fibrinogen to a level of 1.5-2 g/L during bleeding using fibrinogen concentrates or cryoprecipitate

## Ionized calcium

- Critical for coagulation
- Rapid infusion of citrated blood products administered during MTPs acutely lowers ionized calcium and inhibits calcium-dependent coagulation factors
- Maintain normocalcemia during resuscitation

## Prothrombin complex concentrates (PCCs) and factor concentrates

- PCCs contain factors II, VII, IX, and X and variable levels of protein C, S, and antithrombin
- Developed for vitamin K antagonist reversal
- Increasingly used for perioperative bleeding management to correct perioperative coagulopathy
- Be aware of the potential thrombotic risks
- Other factor concentrates include recombinant FVIIa and factor XIII

## Tranexamic acid (TXA)

- Routinely administered
- Early administration is beneficial in severely injured patients
- Consider the potential for increased thromboembolic risk in severe traumatic brain injury and gastrointestinal bleeding
- Plasma transfusion
- Contains fresh-frozen plasma (FFP) or solvent-detergent plasma (SDP)
- Plasma does not correct clotting times
- May minimize during massive volume resuscitation
- Note that plasma transfusion is associated with transfusion-related acute lung injury (TRALI), circulatory overload, bacterial contamination, and hypersensitivity reactions

## Platelets

- Critical for hemostasis
- Red blood cells (RBCs) are initially administered in MTPs, followed by plasma and platelets
- Consider the use of cold-stored platelets as they have extended storage times

## Red blood cells (RBCs)

- Change into a polyhedral shape when incorporated into a forming clot to maximize clot strength
- Interact with platelets, fibrinogen, von Willebrand factor, and FXIII to optimize clot formation

## Coagulation support

- The goal of coagulation support during perioperative bleeding management is to promote clot formation
- Components of primary clot formation:
  □ Fibrinogen
  □ Fibrinogen concentrate
  □ Cryoprecipitate (contains more FXIII than most of the fibrinogen concentrates)
  □ Platelets: supplemented by platelet transfusion and activated by calcium supplementation
- Secondary coagulation process: promotion of thrombin and fibrin formation to further stabilize clot formation
  □ Calcium
  □ Plasma transfusion
  □ Prothrombin complex concentrate administration
- Coagulation process:
  □ By thrombin-activated FXIII crosslinks fibrin monomers to create a fibrin polymer network
  □ Red blood cells become deformed to fit into the clot and they interact with other clotting factors to stabilize the clot
  □ Plasma transfusion, next to coagulation factor supplementation, also protects glycocalyx release and limits excessive clot formation
  □ TXA acid binds lysine groups of plasminogen to limit the transversion of plasminogen into plasmin to reduce the fibrinolysis reaction

# TRANSFUSION PROTOCOL

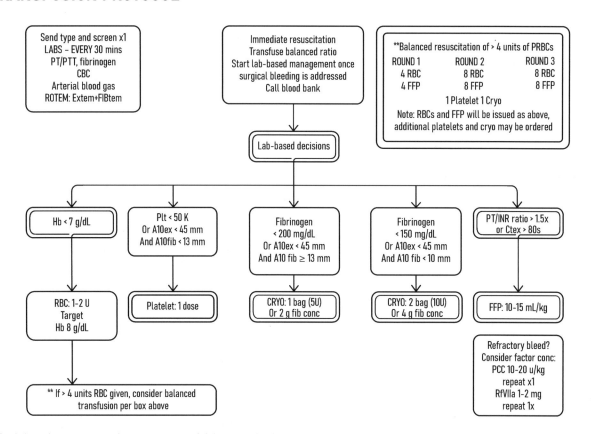

Send type and screen x1
LABS – EVERY 30 mins
PT/PTT, fibrinogen
CBC
Arterial blood gas
ROTEM: Extem+FIBtem

Immediate resuscitation
Transfuse balanced ratio
Start lab-based management once
surgical bleeding is addressed
Call blood bank

**Balanced resuscitation of > 4 units of PRBCs

| ROUND 1 | ROUND 2 | ROUND 3 |
|---------|---------|---------|
| 4 RBC | 8 RBC | 8 RBC |
| 4 FFP | 8 FFP | 8 FFP |

1 Platelet 1 Cryo

Note: RBCs and FFP will be issued as above,
additional platelets and cryo may be ordered

Lab-based decisions

Hb < 7 g/dL

Plt < 50 K
Or A10ex < 45 mm
And A10fib < 13 mm

Fibrinogen
< 200 mg/dL
Or A10ex < 45 mm
And A10 fib ≥ 13 mm

Fibrinogen
< 150 mg/dL
Or A10ex < 45 mm
And A10 fib < 10 mm

PT/INR ratio > 1.5x
or Ctex > 80s

RBC: 1-2 U
Target
Hb 8 g/dL

Platelet: 1 dose

CRYO: 1 bag (5U)
Or 2 g fib conc

CRYO: 2 bag (10U)
Or 4 g fib conc

FFP: 10-15 mL/kg

** If > 4 units RBC given, consider balanced
transfusion per box above

Refractory bleed?
Consider factor conc:
PCC 10-20 u/kg
repeat x1
RfVIIa 1-2 mg
repeat 1x

Our balanced ratio recommendations are presented if the patient has been transfused four units of blood and intraoperative hemorrhage is ongoing. CBC, complete blood count; Cryo, cryoprecipitate; FFP, fresh frozen plasma; Hgb, hemoglobin; RBC, red blood cell; PLT, platelet count; T & S, type and screen; PCC, prothrombin complex concentrates

# MANAGEMENT

## PERIOPERATIVE BLEEDING: MANAGEMENT I

### CARDIOVASCULAR SURGERY

- Postpone non-emergency cardiac surgery at least 5 days after discontinuation of ticagrelor or clopidogrel and 7 days after prasugrel
- Consider platelet function testing to guide the decision on timing of surgery in patients who have recently received P2Y12 inhibitors
- Avoid bridging oral antiplatelet therapy with LMWH
- Consider bridging P2Y12 inhibitors with glycoprotein IIb/IIIa inhibitors or cangrelor in high ischemic patients
- Aspirin or P2Y12 inhibitors may be administered in the early postoperative period
- Prophylactic administration of TXA (or EACA) before cardiopulmonary bypass
- Administer TXA or EACA IV at low doses
- Consider topical TXA if systemic TXA is contraindicated
- Monitor heparin upon withdrawal from CPB
- If bleeding is accompanied by hypofibrinogenemia, administer FFP
- Consider rFVIIa for patients with bleeding that remains intractable after conventional hemostatic therapy
- Use standardized hemostatic algorithms
- Use point-of-care hemostatic testing
- Consider hemo-adsorption in patients on ticagrelor or rivaroxaban undergoing emergency cardiac/aortic surgery on CPB
- Use acute normovolemic hemodilution in patients with normal/high initial Hb concentration
- Use red cell salvage for blood conservation

### LIVER RESECTION

- Maintain a low central venous pressure and restrictive fluid administration
- Intraoperative hypovolemic phlebotomy or infrahepatic inferior vena cava clamping in selected patients
- Consider maintaining a high stroke volume variation (10-20%)
- During the liver resection phase, ventilate with low airway pressures
- Consider terlipressin infusion during hepato-pancreato-biliary surgery
- Use improved surgical hemostatic devices and topical hemostatic agents
- Consider preoperative continuation of aspirin monotherapy
- Consider TXA in cirrhotic patients

### ORTHOPEDIC SURGERY

- Give prophylactic TXA in patients with a relevant risk for bleeding
- Give EACA if TXA is not available
- Treat hip fractures within 48h to avoid global perioperative complications
- The osteosynthesis technique of proximal endomedullary nailing may reduce blood loss in trochanteric femur fracture
- Maintain restrictive transfusion thresholds while managing hip fractures
- Monitor FXIII and correct deficiency in cases of ongoing bleeding as part of a goal-directed coagulation therapy
- Employ intraoperative and postoperative cell salvage in high-risk procedures

### ORTHOTOPIC LIVER TRANSPLANTATION

- Employ a strategy for lowering portal pressure during the dissection and liver resection phases and VHA-guided transfusion protocols
- Consider perioperative VHA to predict blood loss and transfusion requirements
- Use VHA monitoring with assessment of fibrinogen for guiding fibrinogen replacement
- Treat fibrinolysis with TXA but do not use prophylactically
- In significant bleeding patients without fibrinogen deficiency, administer PCC in low doses guided by VHA
- Restrict fibrinogen concentrate only to patients with documented hypofibrinogenemia
- Only use rFVIIa as a rescue therapy for uncontrolled bleeding
- Use cell salvage and autotransfusion with leukodepletion filters

### OTHER VISCERAL SURGERY

- Consider TXA in percutaneous nephrolithotomy and prostate surgery
- Use CT or angiography for the diagnosis of late bleeding after pancreatectomy, and use endovascular interventional therapy as the primary treatment
- Cell salvage is not contraindicated in cancer surgery, provided that blood aspiration close to the tumor site is avoided and leukodepletion filters are used

LMWH, low molecular weight heparin; TXA, tranexamic acid; EACA, epsilon-aminocaproic acid; CPB, cardiopulmonary bypass; Hb, hemoglobin; PCC, prothrombin complex concentrate; FFP, fresh frozen plasma; rFVIIa, recombinant activated factor VII; FXIII, factor XIII; VHA, viscoelastic hemostatic assay

# PERIOPERATIVE BLEEDING: MANAGEMENT II

### ACUTE UPPER GASTROINTESTINAL BLEEDING

- Primary prophylaxis in cirrhotic patients with high-risk esophageal varices: Beta-blockers, variceal band ligation, sclerotherapy, beta-blockers + nitrates
- Have a multimodal protocol available
- Early interventional endoscopy with vasoactive medication (somatostatin, terlipressin, octreotide)
- When initial medical and endoscopic therapy fail: Transjugular intrahepatic portosystemic shunt or surgical shunts
- Consider early transjugular intrahepatic portosystemic shunt placement in selected high-risk cirrhotic patients with acute upper gastrointestinal bleeding following intial hemostasis using pharmacological management and endoscopic band ligation
- Secondary prophylaxis of variceal bleeding: Beta-blockers + endoscopic therapy with band ligation
- Use a restrictive transfusion policy aiming for a Hb level of 7-8 g/dL in hemodynamically stable patients
- Employ endoscopic therapy combined with high-dose proton pump inhibitors in non-variceal upper gastrointestinal bleeding

### GYNECOLOGICAL (NON-PREGNANT) SURGERY

- Consider normovolemic hemodilution as an alternative approach in gynecological cancer to reduce allogeneic transfusion
- Cell salvage may reduce allogeneic transfusion
- Administer preoperative IV iron in anemic gynecological cancer patients receiving chemotherapy
- IV iron to correct preoperative anemia in women with menorrhagia
- Administer EPO with iron in gynecological patients with IDA
- Administer TXA for reduction of perioperative bleeding in abdominal, laparoscopic, robotic or hysteroscopic myomectomy, and hysterectomy (tailor the dose and use of TXA to the type and surgy and patient condition)

### OBSTETRIC SURGERY

- Manage postpartum hemorrhage with a multidisciplinary team
- Use an escalating postpartum hemorrhage management protocol including uterotonic drugs, surgical and/or endovascular interventions and procoagulant drugs
- Early recognition of postpartum hemorrhage is essential
- Treat patients with known placenta accreta spectrum disorders with a multidisciplinary team
- Implement PBM programs in parturients
- Cell salvage is well tolerated, with precautions against rhesus isoimmunization
- IV iron supplementation in anemic patients
- Assess fibrinogen levels in parturients with bleeding
- Include obstetrical conditions associated with PPH in coagulopathy risk assessment
- Use VHA-guided hemostatic treatment
- Use fibrinogen replacement in ongoing postpartum hemorrhage with hypofibrinogenemia
- Use a VHA-guided intervention protocol in severe postpartum hemorrhage
- Administer TXA (1 g IV) as soon as possible (within 3h) in postpartum hemorrhage
- Consider TXA before high-risk cesarean section and vaginal deliveries or cases of antepartum bleeding

### NEUROSURGICAL BLEEDING

- Use PCC for reversal of VKA-associated non-traumatic intracranial bleeding
- Intracranial surgery can be safely performed in the presence of low-dose aspirin
- Antiplatelet agents (APAs) like clopidogrel or aspirin do not typically respond well to platelet transfusions or DDAVP for reversal
- For significant bleeding associated with antiplatelet medications,prothrombin complex concentrates or specific reversal agents (e.g., idarucizumab for dabigatran), might be more appropriate depending on the medication involved
- Bleeding prophylaxis in elective intracranial and spine surgery: IV TXA bolus with or without infusion, from induction of anesthesia until the end of surgery

Hb, hemoglobin; EPO; erythropoietin; IDA, iron deficiency anemia; TXA, tranexamic acid; PBM, patient blood management; RBC, red blood cell; PPH, peripartum hemorrhage; VHA, viscoelastic hemostatic assay; rFVIIa, recombinant activated factor VII; PCC, prothrombin complex concentrate; DDAVP, desmopressin

# PERIOPERATIVE BLEEDING: MANAGEMENT III

## PEDIATRIC SURGERY

- Use VHA-guided interventions to help transfusion in neonates and children undergoing cardiac and non-cardiac surgery
- Base the decision for transfusion of RBCs on the clinical status of the child and the risks and benefits of transfusion in addition to laboratory values
- Do not perform a transfusion of the child is hemodynamically stable and has a Hb concentration of at least 7 g/dL
- Administer fibrinogen concentrate to bleeding patients diagnosed with hypofibrinogenemia
- In patients with a high bleeding risk undergoind non-cardiac surgery: Prophylactic administration of antifibrinolytics

## INTRAOPERATIVE TRANSFUSION TRIGGERS AND VOLUME MANAGEMENT

- Target Hb concentration during active bleeding: 7-9 g/dL
- In patients with a superior vena cava catheter in place, use central venous oxygen saturation or arteriovenous oxygen difference surrogates for the oxygen delivery to consumption ratio to provide a personalized approach to identify patients who may benefit from transfusion
- Repeated measurements of a combination of Hct/Hb, serum lactate, and base deficit to monitor tissue perfusion, tissue oxygenation, and the dynamics of blood loss during acute bleeding
- Extend these tests by measurements of cardiac output, dynamic variables of volume status (stroke volume variation, pulse pressure variation), $CO_2$ gap, and central venous oxygen saturation or the combination of these
- Replace extracellular fluid losses with isotonic crystalloids in a timely and protocol-based manner
- Compared with crystalloids, macro-hemodynamic and micro-hemodynamic stabilization can be achieved with less volume of iso-oncotic colloids, and less tissue edema
- Infusion of colloids in patients with severe bleeding can aggravate dilutional coagulopathy by additional effects on fibrin polymerization and platelet aggregation
- Use balanced solutions for crystalloids and as a basic solute for iso-oncotic preparations

## INTRA- AND POSTOPERATIVE ANEMIA MANAGEMENT

- In the early treatment phase of uncontrolled massive elective surgery bleeding, perform a massive transfusion (6 to 10 units) with a high ratio (1:1) of plasma to RBCs
- Switch to a goal-directed transfusion strategy (based on Hb and/or physiological RBC transfusion triggers, coagulation factor substitution and platelet transfusion triggers) as soon as possible
- Monitor Hb concentrations for anemia detection prior to, during, and after high-bleeding-risk surgery and in situations where silent bleeding, massive blood loss, and fluid shifts are suspected
- Monitor Hb levels after severe perioperative bleeding during the first postoperative days
- When severe bleeding and volume shifts are expected and/or occurring, consider continuous non-invasive Hb monitoring for trend analyses and for reducing blood sampling for invasive laboratory measurement of Hb concentration, especially in children
- In postoperative anemia with Hb at least 10 g/dL, test for iron deficiency and administer IV iron at weight-based dosing if ferritin < 100 µg/L or ferritin < 300 µg/L and transferrin saturation < 20%
- In postoperative anemia with Hb < 10 g/dL, timely IV iron administration at weight-based dosing after considering contraindications
- Consider additional treatment with an ESA
- In postoperative anemia with Hb < 6-8 g/dL or falling below physiological RBC transfusion triggers, perform an aggressive RBC transfusion with often more unit at a time, especially if the patient is symptomatic or has significant ongoing bleeding
- For postoperative iron administration: IV > oral
- IV iron formulations allowing higher maximal single doses (e.g., isomaltoside, carboxymaltose) may be more effective than those with low licensed maximum single doses (e.g., sucrose)

VHA, viscoelastic hemostatic assay; RBC, red blood cell; Hb, hemoglobin; Hct, hematocrit; ESA, erythropoietin-stimulating agent

# SUGGESTED READING

- Ghadimi K, Levy JH, Welsby IJ. Perioperative management of the bleeding patient. Br J Anaesth. 2016;117(suppl 3):iii18-iii30.
- Kietaibl S, Ahmed A, Afshari A, Albaladejo P, Aldecoa C, Barauskas G, et al. Management of severe peri-operative bleeding: Guidelines from the European Society of Anaesthesiology and Intensive Care: Second update 2022. European Journal of Anaesthesiology | EJA. 2023;40(4).

# PERIOPERATIVE MYOCARDIAL INFARCTION/INJURY (PMI)

**66**

## LEARNING OBJECTIVES

- Describe the risk factors for PMI
- Give prophylactic treatment to high-risk patients
- Manage PMI cases

## DEFINITION AND MECHANISM

- Postoperative myocardial infarction/injury (PMI) is a common complication after non-cardiac surgery
- PMI is defined as the increase of troponin caused by ischemia within 30 days after surgery

## PATHOPHYSIOLOGY

- Type I MI: Plaque destruction followed by coronary atherosclerotic thrombosis
- Type II MI: Imbalance in myocardial oxygen supply and demand resulting in ischemia

## RISK FACTORS

| | |
|---|---|
| Patient-specific | Previous coronary artery disease<br>Age > 70 years<br>Male sex<br>Renal failure<br>Diabetes<br>Peripheral artery disease<br>Emergency or redo surgery<br>Severe LV dysfunction (LVEF < 35%) or cardiogenic shock |
| Intraoperative | Open surgery<br>Prolonged intraoperative time with hypotension<br>Intraoperative heart rate of > 110 or < 55 BPM<br>Tachycardia<br>Intraoperative transfusions<br>Perioperative vasopressors |
| Postoperative | Postoperative bleeding<br>Sepsis<br>Hypoxia<br>Sustained tachycardia<br>Hypotension<br>Severe anemia |

LVEF, left ventricular ejection fraction; BPM, beats per minute.

## PROPHYLAXIS

- β-adrenergic blockers
- Calcium channel blockers
- α2 agonists
- Statins
- Aspirin
- Coronary revascularization (requires further investigation)
- Anemia corrections

# MANAGEMENT

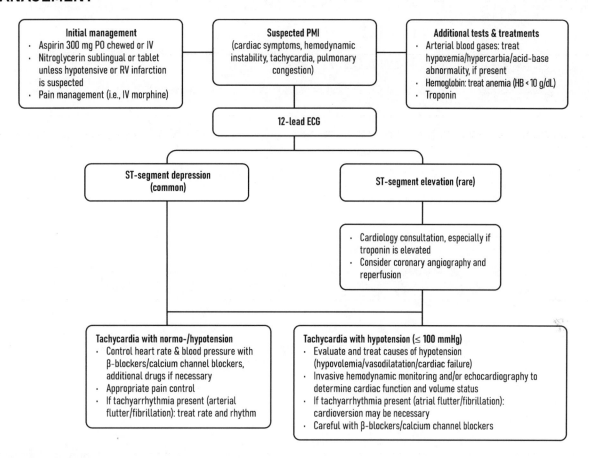

**Initial management**
- Aspirin 300 mg PO chewed or IV
- Nitroglycerin sublingual or tablet unless hypotensive or RV infarction is suspected
- Pain management (i.e., IV morphine)

**Suspected PMI**
(cardiac symptoms, hemodynamic instability, tachycardia, pulmonary congestion)

**Additional tests & treatments**
- Arterial blood gases: treat hypoxemia/hypercarbia/acid-base abnormality, if present
- Hemoglobin: treat anemia (HB < 10 g/dL)
- Troponin

**12-lead ECG**

**ST-segment depression (common)**

**ST-segment elevation (rare)**
- Cardiology consultation, especially if troponin is elevated
- Consider coronary angiography and reperfusion

**Tachycardia with normo-/hypotension**
- Control heart rate & blood pressure with β-blockers/calcium channel blockers, additional drugs if necessary
- Appropriate pain control
- If tachyarrhythmia present (arterial flutter/fibrillation): treat rate and rhythm

**Tachycardia with hypotension (≤ 100 mmHg)**
- Evaluate and treat causes of hypotension (hypovolemia/vasodilatation/cardiac failure)
- Invasive hemodynamic monitoring and/or echocardiography to determine cardiac function and volume status
- If tachyarrhythmia present (atrial flutter/fibrillation): cardioversion may be necessary
- Careful with β-blockers/calcium channel blockers

# KEEP IN MIND

- Careful perioperative monitoring for ischemia, along with a proactive approach to treating and preventing tachycardia, while avoiding hypotension, reduced cardiac output, and cardiac decompensation, can help prevent PMI
- Coronary intervention is rarely indicated as the first line of treatment
- Antithrombotic therapy may exacerbate bleeding

━━ **SUGGESTED READING** ━━

- Gao L, Chen L, He J, et al. Perioperative Myocardial Injury/Infarction After Non-cardiac Surgery in Elderly Patients. Front Cardiovasc Med. 2022;9:910879.
- Landesberg G, Beattie WS, Mosseri M, Jaffe AS, Alpert JS. Perioperative myocardial infarction. Circulation. 2009;119(22):2936-2944.
- Nashef S., Roques F., Michel P., et al. European system for cardiac operative risk evaluation. Eur J Cardiothorac Surg 1999; 16:9-13

# POSTOPERATIVE VISUAL LOSS (POVL)

## LEARNING OBJECTIVES

- Describe the symptoms & risk factors of POVL
- Prevent POVL
- Manage POVL

## DEFINITION AND MECHANISM

- Postoperative visual loss (POVL) is an uncommon complication primarily associated with cardiac, spine, and head and neck surgery that can have a potentially severe impact on quality of life
- Most cases of POVL occur after spinal surgery and while there are many different etiologies, pressure on the eye due to improper head positioning has a very high risk for POVL

## ETIOLOGY

| Common | Retinal artery occlusion:<br>- Central retinal artery occlusion (CRAO)<br>- Branch retinal artery occlusion (BRAO)<br>Ischemic optic neuropathy (ION)<br>Cerebral vision |
|---|---|
| Less common | Cortical blindness<br>Corneal abrasion<br>Cortical blindness secondary to visual field stroke<br>Transient ischemic attack (TIA)<br>Acute glaucoma<br>Expansion of intraocular vitrectomy gas bubble (nitrous oxide)<br>Transurethral resection of the prostate (TURP) glycine toxicity |

POVL, postoperative visual loss.

## RISK FACTORS

- Male sex
- Obesity
- Diabetes
- Hypertension
- Atherosclerosis
- Hyperlipidemia
- Smoking
- Sleep apnea
- Hypercoagulability
- Use of vasopressors

- Hemodilution
- Low cup-to-disc ratio
- Use of the Wilson frame
- Longer anesthetic duration
- Prone positioning
- Perioperative anemia & hypotension
- Blood loss
- Type of surgery (highest risk in spinal fusion)
- Erectile dysfunction medication

## PREVENTION

- Preoperative evaluation & identification of risk factors
- Preoperative discontinuation of erectile dysfunction medications
- Attention to intraoperative positioning (avoidance of direct ocular pressure)
- Hemodynamic and respiratory monitoring and management
- Postoperative visual evaluation following high-risk procedure
- Monitoring of hemoglobin during long procedures & procedures associated with high blood loss

## MANAGEMENT

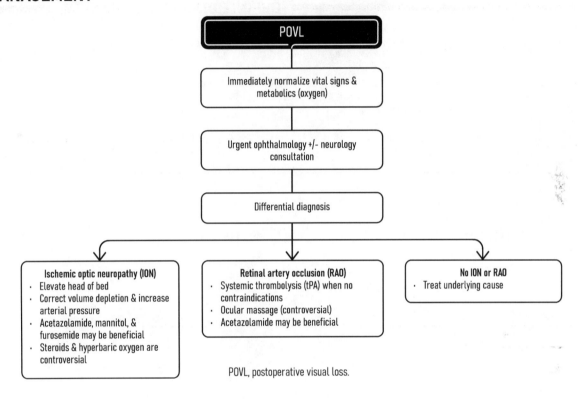

POVL, postoperative visual loss.

## SUGGESTED READING

- Brunk AJ, Ehrhardt KP, Green JB, Mothersele SM, Kaye AD. Postoperative Visual Loss: Anatomy, Pathogenesis, and Anesthesia Considerations. In: Fox IIICJ, Cornett EM, Ghali GE, editors. Catastrophic Perioperative Complications and Management: A Comprehensive Textbook. Cham: Springer International Publishing; 2019. p. 19-29.
- Fleisher, L.A. and Rosenbaum, S.H. (2018) Complications in Anesthesia. Philadelphia, PA: Elsevier.
- Frost EA. Visual loss after anesthesia different causes: different solutions–a review. Middle East J Anaesthesiol. 2010;20(5):639-648.
- Kitaba A, Martin DP, Gopalakrishnan S, Tobias JD. Perioperative visual loss after nonocular surgery. J Anesth. 2013;27(6):919-926.
- Lee LA. Perioperative visual loss and anesthetic management. Curr Opin Anaesthesiol. 2013;26(3):375-381.
- Mac Grory B, Schrag M, Biousse V, et al. Management of Central Retinal Artery Occlusion: A Scientific Statement From the American Heart Association [published correction appears in Stroke. 2021 Jun;52(6):e309]. Stroke. 2021;52(6):e282-e294.
- Roth S. Perioperative visual loss: what do we know, what can we do? British Journal of Anaesthesia. 2009;103:i31-i40.

Postoperative visual loss (POVL)

# SEIZURES

## LEARNING OBJECTIVES

- Definition of seizures
- Treatment of seizures

## DEFINITION AND MECHANISM

- Defined as a sudden, uncontrolled burst of electrical activity in the brain and is characterized by changes in behavior, movements, feelings, and levels of consciousness
- Outward effects vary from:
  - Uncontrolled shaking movements involving much of the body with loss of consciousness (tonic-clonic seizure)
  - Shaking movements involving only part of the body with variable levels of consciousness (focal seizure)
  - Or a subtle momentary loss of awareness (absence of seizure)
- Loss of bladder control may occur during the seizure
- After the active portion of a seizure, there is typically a period of confusion called the postictal period, before a normal level of consciousness returns
- Seizures can be provoked (see causes) or unprovoked (without a known cause) and may be stress, sleep deprivation or flash lights
- Most seizures last from 30 seconds to two minutes
- Any seizure lasting longer than five minutes should be treated as status epilepticus and is a medical emergency
- Epilepsy is characterized by recurrent (2 or more) seizures which means that having a single seizure does not mean that a patient also has epilepsy
- Approximately 8–10% of people will experience an epileptic seizure during their lifetime

## SIGNS AND SYMPTOMS

- Temporary confusion
- A staring spell
- Jerking movements of the arms and legs that can't be controlled
- Loss of consciousness or awareness
- Cognitive or emotional changes

**Classification**
- Generalized epilepsy
  - Tonic-clonic
  - Absence
  - Myoclonic
  - Clonic
  - Tonic
  - Atonic
  - Simple
  - Complex
  - Evolving to generalized
- Mixed seizures (focal and generalized)
- Unclassified

## CAUSES

| Metabolic | Dehydration |
|---|---|
| | Hypoxemia |
| | Hypercarbia |
| | Hyponatremia |
| | Hypernatremia |
| | Hypoglycemia |
| | Hyperosmolar nonketotic hyperglycinemia |
| | Hypocalcemia |
| | Hypomagnesemia |
| | Uremia |
| | Hepatic encephalopathy |
| | Porphyria |
| | Dialysis disequilibrium syndrome |
| Structural | Carcinoma |
| | Arteriovenous malformation |
| | Abscess |
| | Intracranial tumor |
| | Cerebral edema |
| | Stroke |

| | |
|---|---|
| Medications | Medication or drug overdoses: antidepressants, antipsychotics, cocaine intoxication, insulin, local anesthetic systemic toxicity (LAST) Alcohol withdrawal syndrome Delirium tremens |
| Infections | Encephalitis Meningitis Sepsis |
| Other | Hypertension (hypertensive encephalopathy) Preeclampsia Amniotic fluid embolism Hyperthermia Head trauma Celiac disease Shunt Multiple sclerosis Concussion Febrile seizures Dementia Stress Epilepsy |

## DIAGNOSIS

- Physical examination
- Blood test
- Lumbar puncture
- EEG
- CT, MRI

## MANAGEMENT

- See management of epilepsy
- See management of status epilepticus

## TREATMENT

- Place the person experiencing a seizure in the recovery position
- Maintain airway, breathing, and circulation
- If needed, hand ventilate with 100% $O_2$ but DO NOT hyperventilate
- Administer anticonvulsant if seizure lasts more than 2 min:
  - Benzodiazepines (first-line treatment)
    - Midazolam 0.05 mg/kg or 1 mg at a time, titrate to effect
    - Diazepam 0.1-0.4 mg/kg IV, 0.04-0.2 mg/kg PR
    - Lorazepam 1-2 mg at a time, titrate to effect
  - Propofol 0.5 mg/kg at a time, titrate to effect
  - Phenytoin 20 mg/kg total loading dose at a rate of 50 mg/min, watch for hypotension & arrhythmias
  - Barbiturates:
    - Phenobarbital 20 mg/kg infused at a rate of 50 mg/min
    - Thiopental 25-100 mg dose
    - Pentobarbital 10 mg/kg infused at a rate of up to 100 mg/min
    - Valproic acid IV 30 mg/kg over 15 min
- Ongoing anti-epileptic medications are only recommended after a second seizure has occurred
- Intubate in case of no response to medication and respiratory compromise

## SUGGESTED READING

- Carter, E.L., Adapa, R.M., 2015. Adult epilepsy and anaesthesia. BJA Education 15, 111–117.
- DE WAELE, LIESBETH, Paul Boon, Berten Ceulemans, Bernard Dan, Anna Jansen, Benjamin Legros, Patricia Leroy, Francoise Delmelle, Michel Ossemann, Sylvie De Raedt, Katrien Smets, Patrick Van de Voorde, Helene Verhelst, and Lieven Lagae. 2013. First Line Management of Prolonged Convulsive Seizures in Children and Adults: Good Practice Points. Acta Neurologica Belgica. 113 (4): 375–380.
- Gratrix A, Enright S. 2005. Epilepsy in anaesthesia and intensive care. Continuing Education in Anaesthesia Critical Care & Pain. 5;4:118-121.

# STATUS EPILEPTICUS

## LEARNING OBJECTIVES

- Describe the overall mechanisms and common causes of status epilepticus
- Describe the signs of status epilepticus
- Prevent status epilepticus
- Manage status epilepticus

## DEFINITION AND MECHANISM

- Status epilepticus is defined as more than 30 minutes of either 1) continuous seizure activity or 2) two or more sequential seizures without full recovery of consciousness between seizures
- Cerebral damage is more likely if the seizure is prolonged
- There are lots of different types of seizures and not all of them involve obvious convulsive activity
- Epilepsy can occur at any age but is commonly diagnosed in those aged below 20 or over 65 years
- First stage is characterized by an increase in:
  □ Cerebral metabolism
  □ Blood flow
  □ Glucose and lactate concentration
- Compensatory mechanisms:
  □ Massive catecholamine release
  □ Raised cardiac output
  □ Hypertension
  □ Increased central venous pressure

- After 30-60 min, compensatory mechanisms fail, resulting in:
  □ Hypoxemia
  □ Hypoglycemia
  □ Increased intracranial pressure
  □ Cerebral edema
  □ Hyponatremia
  □ Potassium imbalance
  □ Evolving metabolic acidosis
  □ Consumptive coagulopathy
  □ Rhabdomyolysis
  □ Multi-organ failure

## ETIOLOGY

Acute
- CNS hemorrhage
- Stroke
- Metabolic abnormalities
- Hypoxia
- Systemic infection
- Anoxia
- Trauma
- Traumatic brain injury
- Drug overdose
- CNS infection

Chronic
- Inheritance tendency
- Low concentration of anti-epileptic drugs
- Structural changes to the brain (trauma) or space occpying lesions (tumor, stroke)
- Alcohol misuse (adults)
- Idiopathic

## SIGNS & SYMPTOMS

Status epilepticus can present in several forms:

- Convulsive: unresponsiveness and tonic, clonic, or tonic-clonic movements of the extremities
- Non-convulsive: prolonged seizure activity evidenced by epileptiform discharges on EEG, change in behavior or cognition in some patients
- Electrographic: commonly used for comatose patients who show electrographic evidence of prolonged seizure activity

## DIAGNOSIS

- Based on history and clinical examination
- Often present either actively convulsing or minimal time between clustered seizures

## PREVENTION

- Seizure detection based on EEG and immediate treatment
- In patients with a history of well-controlled epilepsy, avoid disruption of antiepileptic medication perioperatively

## MANAGEMENT

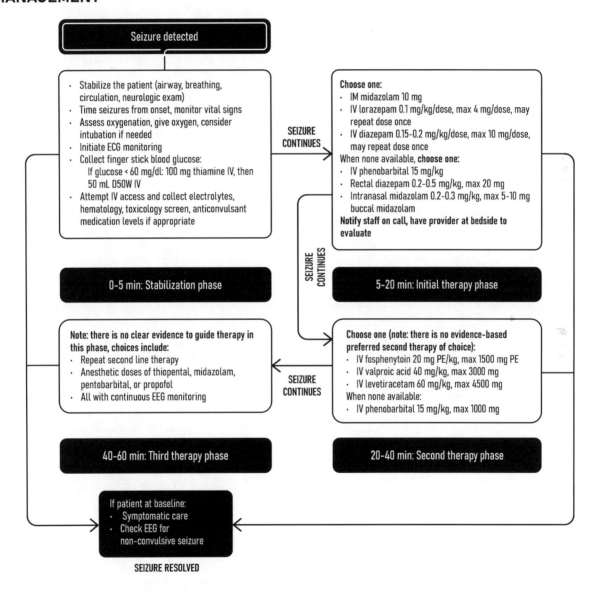

# STATUS EPILEPTICUS MEDICATIONS: OVERVIEW

**Rescue benzodiazepines**

| Medication | Dose range (max dose) | Comments |
|---|---|---|
| IV lorazepam | 0.05-0.1 mg/kg/dose (2-4 mg) | May repeat dose once |
| Rectal diazepam | 0.2-0.5 mg/kg (20 mg) | Age 6 months - 5 years: 0.5 mg/kg<br>Age 6-12 years: 0.3 mg/kg<br>Age 12+ years: 0.2 mg/kg |
| Nasal midazolam | 0.2-0.3 mg/kg (5-10 mg) | < 40 kg: 0.2-0.3 mg/kg<br>< 40 kg: give 10 mg (max dose), half the dose in each nostril |
| IM midazolam | 0.2-0.3 mg/kg (5-10 mg) | < 13 kg: 0.2-0.3 mg/kg<br>13-40 kg: give 5 mg<br>> 40 kg: give 10 mg (max dose) |
| IV diazepam | 0.15-0.3 mg/kg (10 mg) | Shorter duration compared to lorazepam<br>Higher risk for respiratory depression |

**Tier 2 medications**

| Medication | Dose range (max dose) | Comments |
|---|---|---|
| Fosphenytoin | 20 mg PE/kg (1500 mg) | Drug levels quickly available for titration<br>Avoid if known generalized epilepsy or Dravet syndrome<br>Beware of hypotension and bradycardia<br>Tissue extravasation is potentially dangerous |
| Levetiracetam | 60 mg/kg (4500 mg) | Also effective for myoclonic seizures |
| Valproic acid | 40 mg/kg (3000 mg) | Effective in juvenile myoclonic epilepsy, myoclonic status, and absence status<br>Caution in patients with liver dysfunction and select metabolic diseases (e.g., POLG1) |
| Phenobarbital | 10-20 mg/kg (1000 mg) | Drug of choice in newborns<br>Beware of hypotension and respiratory depression<br>May use in adults if previously used with status due to missed or held doses |
| Lacosamide | 5-10 mg/kg (400 mg) | Caution with cardiac issues, can prolong PR interval<br>Use if previously used and status due to missed or held doses |

## SUGGESTED READING

- Betjemann JP, Lowenstein DH. Status epilepticus in adults. Lancet Neurol. 2015;14(6):615-624.
- Glauser T, Shinnar S, Gloss D, et al. Evidence-Based Guideline: Treatment of Convulsive Status Epilepticus in Children and Adults: Report of the Guideline Committee of the American Epilepsy Society. Epilepsy Curr. 2016;16(1):48-61.
- Perks A, Cheema S, Mohanraj R. Anaesthesia and epilepsy. BJA: British Journal of Anaesthesia. 2012;108(4):562-71.

Status epilepticus

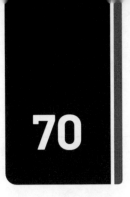

# TENSION PNEUMOTHORAX

## LEARNING OBJECTIVES

- Describe the mechanism and causes of tension pneumothorax
- Diagnose tension pneumothorax
- Manage tension pneumothorax

## DEFINITION AND MECHANISM

- Pneumothorax is the collapse of the lung when air accumulates between the parietal and visceral pleura inside the chest
- Air outside the lung inside the thoracic cavity creates pressure on the lung and can lead to its collapse
- Can be traumatic or iatrogenic

- Tension pneumothorax: Shift in mediastinal structures, results from air under positive pressure trapped in the pleural space through a one-way valve system
- Rare, life-threatening condition
- Commonly occurs in intensive care unit ventilated patients

## CAUSES

| | |
|---|---|
| Iatrogenic | Central venous catheterization in the subclavian or internal jugular vein<br>Lung biopsy<br>Barotrauma due to positive pressure ventilation<br>Percutaneous tracheostomy<br>Thoracentesis<br>Pacemaker insertion<br>Bronchoscopy<br>Cardiopulmonary resuscitation<br>Intercostal nerve block |
| External trauma | Penetrating or blunt trauma<br>Rib fracture<br>Diving or flying |
| Other | Idiopathic spontaneous pneumothorax<br>Open pneumothorax<br>Conversion of spontaneous pneumothorax to tension |

## SIGNS & SYMPTOMS

- Sharp pleuritic pain that can radiate to the ipsilateral back or shoulder
- Increased respiratory rate
- Dyspnea
- Retractions
- Decreased or absent breath sounds, reduced tactile fremitus, hyperresonant percussion sounds, and possibly asymmetrical lung expansion upon lung auscultation

- Signs of hemodynamic instability with hypotension and tachycardia
- Cyanosis
- Jugular vein distension
- Subcutaneous emphysema
- In severe cases: acute respiratory failure, cardiac arrest

## DIAGNOSIS

- Patient hemodynamically unstable and in acute respiratory failure: Bedside ultrasound, stabilize patient, and assess airway, breathing, and circulation
- Patient hemodynamically stable: Chest X-ray:
  - Effacement of lung markings distal to the edge of the visceral pleura
  - Complete ipsilateral lung collapse

  - Mediastinal shift away from the pneumothorax
  - Subcutaneous emphysema
  - Tracheal deviation to the contralateral side
  - Flattening of the hemidiaphragm on the ipsilateral side
- Diagnosis unclear on chest X-ray: Chest CT

# MANAGEMENT

- Patient with chest trauma
  - Assess airway, breathing, and circulation
  - Cover penetrating chest wound with an airtight occlusive bandage and clean plastic sheeting
  - Administer 100% supplemental oxygen
  - Avoid positive pressure ventilation initially
  - Positive pressure ventilation is possible after a chest tube is placed
- Hemodynamically unstable patient
  - Immediate needle decompression
  - Chest X-ray after needle decompression
  - Place chest tube
  - If needle decompression fails: Video-assisted thoracoscopic surgery or thoracotomy
- Hemodynamically stable patient

Diagnostic imaging can be performed prior to treatment

# KEEP IN MIND

- Cardiac tamponade can clinically mimic tension pneumothorax
- Patients with high peak inspiratory pressure are at greater risk of tension pneumothorax
- There is a high suspicion of tension pneumothorax when the patient becomes hemodynamically unstable or goes into cardiac arrest
- If a chest tube is malpositioned or becomes plugged, the pneumothorax can reoccur
- Administer local anesthesia or adequate analgesia/sedation in stable patients

## SUGGESTED READING

- Jalota Sahota R, Sayad E. Tension Pneumothorax. [Updated 2022 Nov 28]. In: StatPearls [Internet]. Treasure Island (FL): StatPearls Publishing; 2022 Jan-. Available from: https://www.ncbi.nlm.nih.gov/books/NBK559090/
- MacDuff A, Arnold A, Harvey J. Management of spontaneous pneumothorax: British Thoracic Society pleural disease guideline 2010. Thorax. 2010;65(Suppl 2):ii18.
- Paramasivam E, Bodenham A. Air leaks, pneumothorax, and chest drains. Continuing Education in Anaesthesia Critical Care & Pain. 2008;8(6):204-9.

Tension pneumothorax

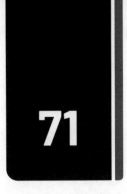

# TRANSFUSION REACTIONS

## LEARNING OBJECTIVES

- Describe the different types of transfusion reactions
- Recognize the signs of the different types of transfusion reactions
- Take preventative measures against transfusion reactions
- Manage the occurrence of transfusion reactions

---

## DEFINITION AND MECHANISM

- Transfusion reactions are the most frequent adverse event associated with the administration of blood products, occurring in up to one in 100 transfusions
- There are several types of adverse reactions:
  - Allergic/anaphylactic reactions
  - Acute hemolytic reactions
  - Delayed hemolytic reactions
  - Febrile non-hemolytic reactions
  - Hyperhemolytic reactions
  - Hypotensive reactions
  - Massive transfusion-associated reactions
  - Post-transfusion purpura
  - Septic reactions
  - Transfusion-associated circulatory overload
  - Transfusion-associated graft versus host disease
  - Transfusion-associated necrotizing enterocolitis
  - Transfusion-related acute lung injury

## SIGNS & SYMPTOMS

TRANSFUSION REACTIONS:
SIGNS & SYMPTOMS

**Increase in temperature**

- Incremental increase < 1 °C above baseline, no other new symptoms → Possible febrile non-hemolytic reaction
- Incremental increase ≥ 1 °C above baseline, or incremental increase < 1 °C with any other new symptoms (chills or rigors, hypotension, nausea or vomiting) → Possible bacterial contamination
  → Possible hemolysis

**Allergic symptoms**

- Mild hives, rash, or skin itching only → Urticaria
- Hives, rash, itching, and/or any other new symptoms (throat, eye, and tongue swelling, etc.) → Possible allergic reaction

**Respiratory symptoms**

- Bronchospasm, dyspnea, tachypnea and hypoxemia, copious frothy pink-tinged fluid (from endotracheal tube) → Possible anaphylaxis, transfusion associated circulatory overload, septic transfusion reaction, or transfusion-related acute lung injury

**All other symptoms**

- Chills, rigors, hypotension, nausea or vomiting, feeling of impending doom, back or chest pain, intravenous site pain, cough, dyspnea, hypoxia → Possible anaphylaxis, hemolytic transfusion reaction, fluid overload, or transfusion-related acute lung injury

# PREVENTION

- Comprehensive training of staff
- Close adherence to blood handling and administration policies
- Laboratory testing
- Prospective monitoring and planning
- A restrictive transfusion strategy to avoid unnecessary transfusions
- Every person should check a blood product twice before administering it to the patient

# MANAGEMENT

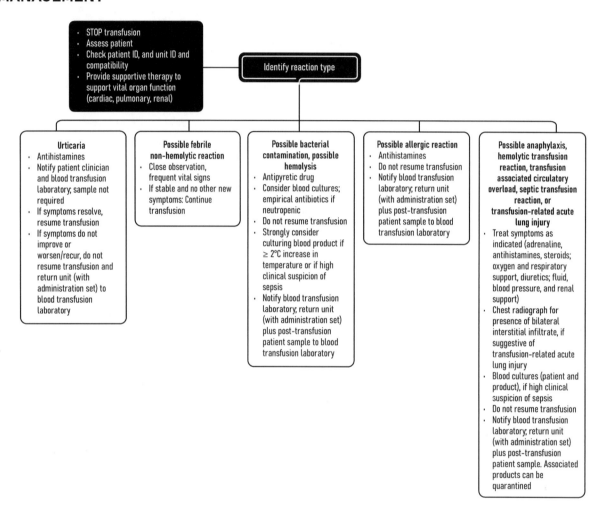

**STOP transfusion**
- **Assess patient**
- **Check patient ID, and unit ID and compatibility**
- **Provide supportive therapy to support vital organ function (cardiac, pulmonary, renal)**

**Identify reaction type**

**Urticaria**
- Antihistamines
- Notify patient clinician and blood transfusion laboratory; sample not required
- If symptoms resolve, resume transfusion
- If symptoms do not improve or worsen/recur, do not resume transfusion and return unit (with administration set) to blood transfusion laboratory

**Possible febrile non-hemolytic reaction**
- Close observation, frequent vital signs
- If stable and no other new symptoms: Continue transfusion

**Possible bacterial contamination, possible hemolysis**
- Antipyretic drug
- Consider blood cultures; empirical antibiotics if neutropenic
- Do not resume transfusion
- Strongly consider culturing blood product if ≥ 2°C increase in temperature or if high clinical suspicion of sepsis
- Notify blood transfusion laboratory; return unit (with administration set) plus post-transfusion patient sample to blood transfusion laboratory

**Possible allergic reaction**
- Antihistamines
- Do not resume transfusion
- Notify blood transfusion laboratory; return unit (with administration set) plus post-transfusion patient sample to blood transfusion laboratory

**Possible anaphylaxis, hemolytic transfusion reaction, transfusion associated circulatory overload, septic transfusion reaction, or transfusion-related acute lung injury**
- Treat symptoms as indicated (adrenaline, antihistamines, steroids; oxygen and respiratory support, diuretics; fluid, blood pressure, and renal support)
- Chest radiograph for presence of bilateral interstitial infiltrate, if suggestive of transfusion-related acute lung injury
- Blood cultures (patient and product), if high clinical suspicion of sepsis
- Do not resume transfusion
- Notify blood transfusion laboratory; return unit (with administration set) plus post-transfusion patient sample. Associated products can be quarantined

## SUGGESTED READING

- Delaney M, Wendel S, Bercovitz RS, et al. Transfusion reactions: prevention, diagnosis, and treatment. Lancet. 2016;388(10061):2825-2836.

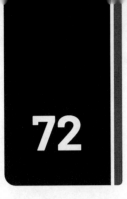

# 72

# VENOUS AIR EMBOLISM (VAE)

## LEARNING OBJECTIVES

- Describe common causes of VAE and high-risk procedures
- Prevent VAE
- Manage VAE

## DEFINITION AND MECHANISM

- Venous air embolism (VAE) is caused by the ingress of gas into the venous system, most commonly air
- Rare iatrogenic complication in a wide range of clinical scenarios involving line placement, trauma, barotrauma, and several types of surgical procedures including cardiac, vascular, and neurosurgery
- Traditionally, surgery and trauma were the most significant causes of air embolism; now, endoscopy, angiography, tissue biopsy, thoracocentesis, hemodialysis, and central/peripheral venous access comprise a greater proportion
- May cause end-organ ischemia or infarction
- May cause direct endothelial injury leading to the release of inflammatory mediators, activation of the complement cascade, and in situ thrombus formation

## SIGNS & SYMPTOMS

- The presentation of VAE is dependent on the rate and volume of air entrained; signs include:

Respiratory Symptoms:
  - Apnea
  - Hypoxia
  - Tachypnea
  - Breathing difficulties
  - Shortness of breath
  - Chest pain
  - Pulmonary edema may develop later

Cardiovascular Symptoms:
  - Cardiopulmonary collapse
  - Tachycardia
  - Hypotension
  - 'Mill wheel' murmur on cardiac auscultation
  - $ETCO_2$ falls
  - ECG abnormalities such as tachyarrhythmias, atrioventricular block, signs of right ventricular strain, ST-segment elevation or depression, nonspecific T wave changes
  - Arterial oxygen saturation falls

Neurological Symptoms:
  - Altered mental status
  - Decreased conscious level
  - Focal neurological deficits
  - Light-headedness, vertigo
  - Sense of impending death
- Transesophageal echocardiography is the most reliable monitor to detect VAE

## PREVENTION

- Patient positioning: avoid the sitting position and Trendelenburg position during the insertion of central venous catheters, try to prevent a negative gradient between the open site veins and the right atrium (increasing right atrial pressure via leg elevation and using the "flex" option on the operating table control)
- Holding ventilation when placing tunnel catheters
- Removal of temporary catheter synchronized with active exhalation/Valsalva maneuver or positive end-expiratory pressure
- Avoid nitrous oxide

Venous air embolism (VAE)

# MANAGEMENT

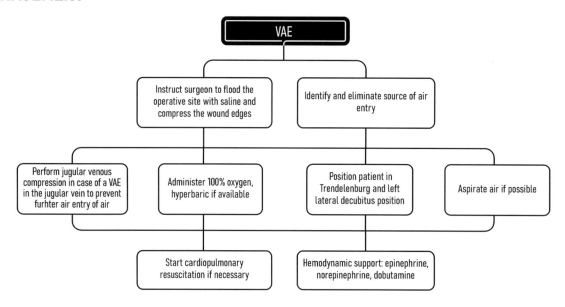

VAE, venous air embolism.

## SUGGESTED READING

- Chuang DY, Sundararajan S, Sundararajan VA, Feldman DI, Xiong W. Accidental Air Embolism. Stroke. 2019;50(7):e183-e186.
- McCarthy CJ, Behravesh S, Naidu SG, Oklu R. Air Embolism: Diagnosis, Clinical Management and Outcomes. Diagnostics (Basel). 2017;7(1):5. Published 2017 Jan 17.
- Mirski MA, Lele AV, Fitzsimmons L, Toung TJ. Diagnosis and treatment of vascular air embolism. Anesthesiology. 2007;106(1):164-177.
- Webber S, Andrzejowski J, Francis G. Gas embolism in anaesthesia. BJA CEPD Reviews. 2002;2(2):53-7.

# VENOUS THROMBOEMBOLISM (VTE)

## LEARNING OBJECTIVES

- Describe the mechanisms and risk factors for (VTE)
- Prevent perioperative VTE
- Diagnose and manage venous VTE

## DEFINITION AND MECHANISM

- Venous thromboembolism (VTE) is a major cause of morbidity and mortality in both hospital and community settings
- Most preventable cause of mortality in hospitalized patients
- Encompasses deep vein thrombosis (DVT) and pulmonary embolism (PE)
- DVT occurs when red blood cells, fibrin, platelets, and leukocytes form a mass within an intact deep vein

- Signs & symptoms are nonspecific and only occur in up to 50% of patients
- PE occurs in about a third of patients with a DVT
- Adequate perioperative thromboprophylaxis is essential to prevent perioperative VTE

## RISK FACTORS

- Three main factors that cause thrombosis:
  - Alterations in blood flow (stasis and turbulence)
  - Vascular endothelial injury
  - Alterations in the blood coagulability
  - These are know as the Virchow triad
- Risk factors:

| Stasis-endothelial injury | Thrombophilias | Medical conditions | Medications | Other |
|---|---|---|---|---|
| Indwelling venous device | Activated protein C resistance | Malignancy (solid tumor and myeloproliferative disorders) | Oral contraceptive use (combined only) | Increasing age |
| Surgery (abdominal, pelvic, orthopedic most commonly) | Factor V Leiden | Pregnancy, postpartum | Hormone replacement therapy | Smoking |
| Major trauma, burns | Prothrombin gene mutation G20210A | Myocardial infarction | Chemotherapy (including tamoxifen) | |
| Prolonged travel | Hyperhomocysteinemia | Congestive heart failure | | |
| Paralysis (including anesthesia for > 30 min) | Anticardiolipin antibodies | Obesity | | |
| Varicose veins | Lupus anticoagulant | Inflammatory bowel disease | | |
| | Elevated factor VIII level | Nephrotic syndrome | | |
| | Protein C deficiency | History of VTE | | |
| | Protein S deficiency | Heparin-induced thrombocytopenia | | |
| | Dysfibrinogenemia | Paroxysmal nocturnal hemoglobinuria | | |
| | Dysplasminogenemia | | | |
| | Antithrombin deficiency | | | |

VTE, venous thromboembolism.

Venous thromboembolism

# PATHOPHYSIOLOGY

- Venous thrombi typically develop at a site of vascular trauma, around intravascular catheters, or in areas of reduced blood flow (e.g., venous valves)
- Accumulation of fibrin and platelets causes rapid growth in the direction of blood flow
- Endogenous fibrinolysis results in partial or complete resolution of the thrombus
- Any residual thrombus may result in incomplete recanalization of the vein, potentially narrowing the lumen and causing valve incompetence
- Extensive collateral network may develop

# DIAGNOSIS

- DVT
  - Duplex ultrasonography
  - D-dimer blood test
  - Contrast venography
  - MRI
- PE
  - Computed tomographic pulmonary angiography
  - Ventilation-perfusion scan
  - Pulmonary angiography
  - MRI

# PREVENTION

### PREOPERATIVE RISK ASSESSMENT

- Perform a thorough multidisciplinary risk assessment for each patient
- Patients at increased risk: Significantly reduced mobility ≥ 3 days, procedure > 90 min, acute surgical admission with inflammatory or intra-abdominal condition
- Assess for bleeding risk before giving pharmacological VTE prophylaxis

### MECHANICAL PROPHYLAXIS

- Anti-embolism stockings (do not use if the patient has peripheral vascular disease, arteriosclerosis, severe peripheral neuropathy, massive leg edema, or pulmonary edema, edema secondary to congestive heart failure, acute stroke)
- Intermittent pneumatic compression
- Foot impulse devices

### REGIONAL ANESTHESIA

- Lower limb neuraxial block, single shot or continuous

### PHARMACOLOGICAL PROPHYLAXIS

- Unfractionated heparin (usually inconvenient compared to low molecular weight heparins)
- Low molecular weight heparins (use with caution in severe renal failure)
- Warfarin (monitor every 3 days until stable, then weekly)
- Direct factor Xa inhibitors
- Aspirin (not recommended in recent major international guidelines)
- Danaparoid (platelet monitoring required)
- Fondaparinux
- Lepirudin (used in patients with suspeced or confirmed heparin-induced thrombocytopenia)
- Dextrans (not routinely recommended)

### PHYSIOTHERAPY AND NURSING

- Mechanical calf and foot venous compression
- Bed exercise
- Early mobilization

# MANAGEMENT

- Preferred DVT treatment: Low molecular weight heparins
- Maintain anticoagulation for 3-6 months for VTE secondary to transient risk factors and > 12 months for recurrent VTE
- Thrombolytics in severe cases
- When anticoagulation fails: Inferior vena cava filter
- Thrombectomy/embolectomy (rarely required)

# SUGGESTED READING

- Gordon RJ, Lombard FW. Perioperative Venous Thromboembolism: A Review. Anesthesia & Analgesia. 2017;125(2).
- Barker RC, Marval P. Venous thromboembolism: risks and prevention. Continuing Education in Anaesthesia Critical Care & Pain. 2011;11(1):18-23.
- National Clinical Guideline Centre - Acute and Chronic Conditions (UK). Venous Thromboembolism: Reducing the Risk of Venous Thromboembolism (Deep Vein Thrombosis and Pulmonary Embolism) in Patients Admitted to Hospital. London: Royal College of Physicians (UK); 2010. (NICE Clinical Guidelines, No. 92.) 2, Summary of recommendations. Available from: https://www.ncbi.nlm.nih.gov/books/NBK116536/

# ENDOCRINOLOGY

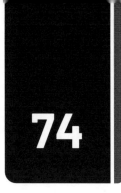

# ACROMEGALY

## LEARNING OBJECTIVES

- Describe acromegaly
- Recognize signs and symptoms of acromegaly
- Anesthetic management of a patient with acromegaly

## DEFINITION AND MECHANISM

- Acromegaly is a chronic, progressive, hormone hypersecretion syndrome caused by an excess of growth hormone (GH) after the growth plates have closed (i.e., puberty)
- The hypersecretion of GH is the result of oversecretion of growth hormone-releasing hormone (GHRH) from the hypothalamus or oversecretion of the hormone itself from a pituitary adenoma

## SIGNS AND SYMPTOMS

| Affected area | Signs & symptoms |
| --- | --- |
| Face | Increase in size of skull and supraorbital ridges; enlarged lower jaw; increase in spacing between teeth/malocclusion |
| Hands and feet | Spade-shaped; carpal tunnel syndrome |
| Mouth/tongue | Macroglossia; thickened pharyngeal and laryngeal soft tissues; thickened vocal cords; reduction in the size of the laryngeal aperture; obstructive sleep apnea |
| Soft tissue | Thick skin; doughlike feel to palm |
| Skeleton | Vertebral enlargement; osteoporosis; kyphosis |
| Cardiovascular | Hypertension; cardiomegaly; impaired left ventricular function |
| Endocrine | Impaired glucose tolerance; diabetes |
| Other | Arthropathy; proximal myopathy |

## COMPLICATIONS

- Diabetes mellitus type 2
- Hypertension
- Hypercholesterolemia
- Cardiomyopathy
- Pulmonary dysfunction

- Obstructive sleep apnea
- Osteoarthritis
- Goiter (enlargement of the thyroid gland)
- Colon polyps

# TREATMENT

- **Surgery:** Preferred treatment; to remove the pituitary tumor
- **Drugs:**
  - **Somatostatin analogs:** Drugs that reduce GH production
  - **Dopamine agonists:** Drugs to lower hormone levels
  - **GH receptor antagonists:** Drugs to block the action of GH
- **Radiation therapy:** Both used alone or in combination with surgery or drugs

# MANAGEMENT

Four grades of airway involvement have been described in acromegaly:

| Grade | Airway involvement |
|-------|--------------------|
| 1 | No significant involvement |
| 2 | Nasal and pharyngeal mucosa hypertrophy but normal cords and glottis |
| 3 | Glottic involvement including glottic stenosis or vocal cord paresis |
| 4 | Combination of grades 2 and 3: Glottic and soft tissue abnormalities |

- Laryngoscopy and tracheal intubation prove to be more difficult due to a combination of macrognathia, macroglossia, and expansion of the upper airway soft tissues
- Tracheostomy is recommended for grades 3 and 4, however, fiberoptic laryngoscopy is a safe alternative
- Tracheal intubation is feasible with standard techniques (i.e., external laryngeal pressure and the use of a gum elastic bougie or airway exchange catheter)
- Awake fiberoptic intubation is the technique of choice in case of anticipated difficult intubation in these patients
- Preoperative transthoracic echocardiography is useful to assess left ventricular size and performance, and to estimate pulmonary pressures due to associated cardiopulmonary complications

# KEEP IN MIND

- About one-quarter of acromegalic patients have an enlarged thyroid, which may compress the trachea
- Preoperative assessments help the anesthesiologist to understand the possibility of difficulties with airway management and tracheal intubation
- Difficult airway
  - Macroglossia and enlarged epiglottis: Difficult bag-mask ventilation and direct laryngoscopy
  - Recurrent laryngeal nerve palsy, narrow glottic opening, subglottic narrowing (stridor)
  - Nasal turbinate enlargement: Caution with nasal intubation and consider a smaller endotracheal tube

# SUGGESTED READING

- Menon R, Murphy PG, Lindley AM. Anaesthesia and pituitary disease. Continuing Education in Anaesthesia Critical Care & Pain. 2011;11(4):133-137.
- Smith M, Hirsch NP. Pituitary disease and anaesthesia. Br J Anaesth. 2000;85(1):3-14.
- Seidman PA, Kofke WA, Policare R, Young M. Anaesthetic complications of acromegaly. Br J Anaesth. 2000;84(2):179-182.

# ADRENOCORTICAL INSUFFICIENCY

## LEARNING OBJECTIVES

- Describe adrenocortical insufficiency
- Recognize the symptoms and signs of acute adrenal insufficiency
- Anesthetic management of a patient with adrenocortical insufficiency

## DEFINITION AND MECHANISM

- The adrenal glands of patients with adrenocortical insufficiency do not produce adequate levels of steroid hormones (i.e., glucocorticoids [cortisol], mineralocorticoids [aldosterone], and androgens]
- These hormones play an important role in blood pressure homeostasis, electrolyte and fluid balance, and metabolism

| Type | Mechanism |
|------|-----------|
| Primary adrenal insufficiency (Addison's disease) | Deficient glucocorticoid secretion by the adrenal glands. The adrenal glands are directly affected, thus mineralocorticoid production is also reduced. |
| Secondary adrenal insufficiency | Deficient adrenocorticotropin hormone (ACTH) secretion by the pituitary gland and subsequent decreased adrenal stimulation. The adrenal glands are not directly affected, thus mineralocorticoid production is minimally impacted. |
| Tertiary adrenal insufficiency | Deficient corticotropin-releasing hormone (CRH) secretion by the hypothalamus, causing a downstream reduction in ACTH production and subsequently decreased adrenal stimulation. The adrenal glands are not directly affected, thus mineralocorticoid production is minimally impacted. |

## SIGNS AND SYMPTOMS

- **Acute condition (Addisonian crisis):** Abdominal pain, vomiting, dehydration, and hypotension (particularly postural)
- **Chronic condition:** Insidious onset with fatigue, anorexia, weight loss, and postural hypotension (salt and water loss)
- Increased pigmentation
- Hypoglycemia
- Hyponatremia
- Hyperkalemia
- Raised serum urea
- Disorientation
- Weakness
- Dizziness
- Cardiovascular collapse
- Muscle and joint pain
- Nausea, vomiting, diarrhea

## COMPLICATIONS

- **Addisonian crisis:** Life-threatening situation resulting in hypotension, hypoglycemia, and hyperkalemia requiring emergency treatment (i.e., IV hydrocrotisone, fluid support an ion correction). It may result from undiagnosed or untreated Addison's disease combined with sudden stress on the body (i.e., injury, infection, or illness).
- Autoimmune Addison's disease may be associated with other **autoimmune diseases** (e.g., pernicious anemia and Grave's disease)

# TREATMENT

- Physiological replacement doses of corticosteroids for all types of adrenocortical insufficiency
- Adrenal crisis (acute) treatment
  - IV fluids
  - IV glucocorticoids (i.e., (methyl) prednisolone, dexamethasone or other) and mineralocorticoids
  - Supportive measures and correction of any additional issues (e.g., electrolyte abnormalities)
- Chronic adrenal insufficiency treatment
  - Oral glucocorticoids (i.e., hydrocortisone, prednisone, methylprednisolone, or dexamethasone) to replace cortisol
  - Oral mineralocorticoids (i.e., fludrocortisone) to replace aldosterone, if primary adrenocortical insufficiency
  - Oral androgens (i.e., dehydroepiandrosterone) to replace androgens, if necessary

*Symptoms of long-term steroid therapy*
- Hypertension
- Skin atrophy
- Myopathy
- Arthritis
- Osteoporosis
- Coronary artery disease
- Secondary diabetes mellitus
- Suppressed immune response
- Impaired wound healing

# ANESTHETIC CONSIDERATIONS

- Potential life-threatening situation: Shock, dehydration, hypotension
- Physiological considerations
  - **Cardiovascular:** Impaired myocardial contractility, arrhythmias secondary to hyperkalemia
  - **Volume status:** Dehydration (2-3 L)
  - **Electrolyte imbalance:** Hyperkalemia, hyponatremia (decreased level of consciousness, seizures), and hypoglycemia (decreased level of consciousness, seizures)
- Pharmacologic considerations
  - Reduced circulating catecholamines (consider vasopressin for hypotension)
  - Succinylcholine-induced hyperkalemia

Adrenocortical insufficiency

# MANAGEMENT

**ADRENOCORTICAL INSUFFICIENCY**

## Preoperative management

- Routine laboratory investigations: Electrolytes, fasting blood glucose, full blood count, creatinine, urea
- Screen for hypothyroidism and diabetes mellitus
- Chest X-ray for signs of pulmonary or cardiac disease and ECG
- Stabilize circulation, correct fluid deficits and electrolyte disturbances, and initiate glucocorticoid therapy

## Intraoperative management

- Prevent perioperative cardiovascular collapse
  - Steroid supplementation
    - Hydrocortisone 100 mg IV q6-8h for 24 hours then taper to maintenance of 15-20 mg PO qAM and 5-10 mg PO qPM
    - Add maintenance fludrocortisone 0.05-0.2 mg PO daily if aldosterone-deficient (primary adrenal insufficiency) when tapering hydrocortisone
  - Volume resuscitation
  - Correction of electrolyte abnormalities
- Cautiously perform induction with small doses of hypnotic repeated at delayed intervals to allow for increased sensitivity, hypovolemia, and prolonged circulatory times
- Infusion of vasoconstrictors (e.g., norepinephrine, vasopressin) and inotropic agents may be required
- Continuous infusion of crystalloid solutions to correct preoperative fluid deficits and replace perioperative losses
- Colloids to replace blood loss if necessary

## Postoperative management

- Patients with latent (poorly controlled) adrenocortical insufficiency might require a transfer to the ICU
- Patients with untreated manifest adrenocortical insufficiency or Addisonian crisis presenting for emergency surgery have to be managed postoperatively at the ICU
- Invasive hemodynamic monitoring
- Balance fluid intake and output
- Correct electrolyte abnormalities
- Monitor renal function
- Continue corticosteroid therapy

Adrenocortical insufficiency

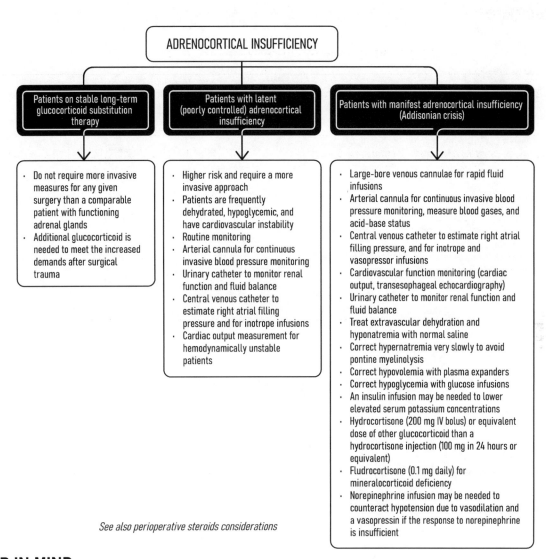

```
                        ┌─────────────────────────────────┐
                        │  ADRENOCORTICAL INSUFFICIENCY   │
                        └─────────────────────────────────┘
```

**Patients on stable long-term glucocorticoid substitution therapy**

- Do not require more invasive measures for any given surgery than a comparable patient with functioning adrenal glands
- Additional glucocorticoid is needed to meet the increased demands after surgical trauma

*See also perioperative steroids considerations*

**Patients with latent (poorly controlled) adrenocortical insufficiency**

- Higher risk and require a more invasive approach
- Patients are frequently dehydrated, hypoglycemic, and have cardiovascular instability
- Routine monitoring
- Arterial cannula for continuous invasive blood pressure monitoring
- Urinary catheter to monitor renal function and fluid balance
- Central venous catheter to estimate right atrial filling pressure and for inotrope infusions
- Cardiac output measurement for hemodynamically unstable patients

**Patients with manifest adrenocortical insufficiency (Addisonian crisis)**

- Large-bore venous cannulae for rapid fluid infusions
- Arterial cannula for continuous invasive blood pressure monitoring, measure blood gases, and acid-base status
- Central venous catheter to estimate right atrial filling pressure, and for inotrope and vasopressor infusions
- Cardiovascular function monitoring (cardiac output, transesophageal echocardiography)
- Urinary catheter to monitor renal function and fluid balance
- Treat extravascular dehydration and hyponatremia with normal saline
- Correct hypernatremia very slowly to avoid pontine myelinolysis
- Correct hypovolemia with plasma expanders
- Correct hypoglycemia with glucose infusions
- An insulin infusion may be needed to lower elevated serum potassium concentrations
- Hydrocortisone (200 mg IV bolus) or equivalent dose of other glucocorticoid than a hydrocortisone injection (100 mg in 24 hours or equivalent)
- Fludrocortisone (0.1 mg daily) for mineralocorticoid deficiency
- Norepinephrine infusion may be needed to counteract hypotension due to vasodilation and a vasopressin if the response to norepinephrine is insufficient

## KEEP IN MIND

- Stress of surgery, infection, or trauma can cause adrenocortical insufficiency to decompensate and lead to an Addisonian crisis
- Prolonged steroid therapy can suppress the HPA axis without causing symptoms → symptoms manifest if the steroids are withheld or the dose is not adapted to increased requirements
- Patients on corticosteroid substitution therapy require a perioperative increase of the dose to compensate for the increased requirements posed by the trauma of surgery
- Patients with untreated adrenocortical insufficiency should not be scheduled for elective surgery until corticosteroid therapy has been given for a sufficient length of time
- Patients with untreated manifest adrenocortical insufficiency or Addisonian crisis presenting for emergency surgery are high-risk patients and require invasive intraoperative monitoring

## SUGGESTED READING

- Pollard BJ, Kitchen G. Handbook of Clinical Anaesthesia. 4th ed. Taylor & Francis group; 2018. Chapter 6 Endocrine system.
- Davies MJ, Hardman JG. Anaesthesia and adrenocortical disease. Continuing Education in Anaesthesia. Critical Care & Pain. 2005;5(4):122-126.

# ALCOHOL WITHDRAWAL SYNDROME

## LEARNING OBJECTIVES

- Recognize signs and symptoms of alcohol withdrawal syndrome and delirium tremens
- Manage and treat alcohol withdrawal syndrome and delirium tremens

## DEFINITION AND MECHANISM

- Alcohol withdrawal syndrome (AWS) is a set of symptoms that occur following a reduction in alcohol use after a period of excessive use
- Symptoms can be suppressed by alcohol intake and are more common in the postoperative period
- AWS starts typically after 6-24 hours without alcohol and is most pronounced at 24-36 hours, however, can be delayed for up to 5 days
- AWS results from neurological changes after long-term alcohol use:
  - Ethanol binds to postsynaptic GABA-A receptors, thereby enhancing their inhibitory effect
  - The resulting chronic excitatory suppression leads to an increased brain synthesis of excitatory neurotransmitters such as norepinephrine, 5-hydroxytryptamine, and dopamine
  - The brain is flooded with increased levels of excitatory neurotransmitters when the inhibitory effects of ethanol are withdrawn
- Delirium tremens is a rapid onset of confusion due to alcohol withdrawal
- Delirium tremens occurs in 5% of patients experiencing withdrawal
- Mortality rate of delirium tremens is 10% (due to hypotension, dysrhythmias or seizures)

## SIGNS AND SYMPTOMS

| AWS | Delirium tremens |
|---|---|
| Tremors | Shaking |
| Nightmares | Shivering |
| Hallucinations | Tachycardia |
| Gastric upset | Sweating |
| Nausea | Hallucinations |
| Vomiting | Hyperthermia |
| Hyperreflexia | Nausea |
| Anxiety | Vomiting |
| Agitation | Seizures |
| Mild confusion | Agitation |
| Insomnia | Aggression |
| Autonomic nervous system hyperactivity | Tachycardia |
| (tachycardia, hypertension, cardiac dysrhythmia) | Hypertension or hypotension |
| | Grand mal seizures |

| Medical disorders associated with alcoholism | |
|---|---|
| Central nervous system | Wernicke–Korsakoff syndrome<br>Peripheral neuropathy<br>Autonomic dysfunction |
| Cardiovascular system | Cardiomyopathy<br>Heart failure<br>Hypertension<br>Arrhythmias (e.g. AF, SVT, VT) |
| Gastrointestinal | Alcoholic liver disease<br>Pancreatitis<br>Gastritis<br>Oesophageal and bowel carcinoma |
| Metabolic | Hyperlipidemia<br>Obesity<br>Hypoglycemia<br>Hypokalemia<br>Hypomagnesemia<br>Hyperuricemia |
| Hematological | Macrocytosis<br>Anemia<br>Thrombocytopenia<br>Leucopenia |
| Musculoskeletal | Myopathy<br>Osteoporosis<br>Osteomalacia |

## TREATMENT

Prophylactic treatment before the onset of AWS symptoms
- Benzodiazepines or clomethiazole
- Oral or enterally applied alcohol administration (0.5 g/kg body weight/day)
- Adjuncts such as alpha2-agonists

Benzodiazepines are the first-line treatment for AWS and delirium tremens

| Class | Example | Duration of action | Route of administration | Dose |
|---|---|---|---|---|
| Benzodiazepines | Chlordiazepoxide | Long | p.o. | Prophylaxis: 5-25 mg<br>Treatment: 50-100 mg |
| | Lorazepam | Short | p.o./IV | Prophylaxis: 0.5-2 mg<br>Treatment: 1-8 mg |
| | Diazepam | Long | p.o. | Prophylaxis: 2.5-10 mg<br>Treatment: 10-40 mg |
| Other agents | Clomethiazole | | p.o. | Prophylaxis: 9-12 capsules in 24h |
| | Haloperidol | | p.o./IV/IM | Treatment: 0.5-20 mg |
| | Clonidine | | IV | Treatment: 0.1 (bolus) -1 mg (titrated dose) / 0.1-4 µg/kg/h |

Alcohol withdrawal syndrome

- Be aware that the required doses for severe AWS can vary substantially within the first 24h
- Clomethiazole is not advised in critically ill patients due to bronchial secretion and a elevated risk of pneumonia
- Non-benzodiazepine agents should be used in conjunction with benzodiazepines
- Beta-adrenergic blockers and centrally acting alpha-adrenergic agonists (clonidine, dexmedetomidine) achieve symptomatic control but they do not reduce the incidence of delirium or seizures
- Haloperidol (for severe agitation or hallucinations) may increase the risk of seizures and cardiac conduction abnormalities as it increases QTc

- Consider anticonvulsant agents such as carbamazepine, sodium valproate, and topiramate

General treatment
- Correct metabolic (potassium, magnesium, and thiamine) and hemodynamic derangements
- Correct fluid and blood product deficits
- General supportive care (early nutrition)
- Severe cases will need ICU admission & propofol infusion/dexmedetomidine & possible intubation
- Offer psychosocial support: counseling and detoxification/rehab

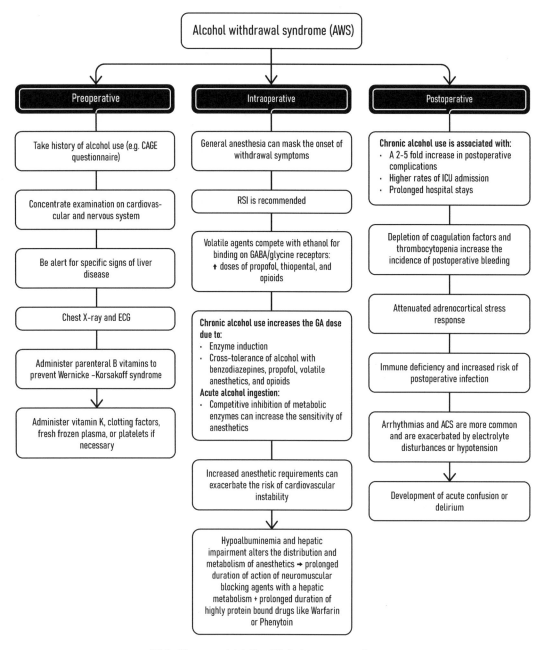

RSI, Rapid sequence intubation; ACS, Acute coronary syndrome

Alcohol withdrawal syndrome

## KEEP IN MIND

As the severity of withdrawal symptoms can vary greatly, a scale such as the Clinical Institute Withdrawal Assessment for Alcohol scale (CIWA-Ar) is useful for:
- Monitoring the effectiveness of prophylactic treatment or fixed-schedule treatment regimens
- Guiding administration in symptom-triggered treatment regimens

## SUGGESTED READING

- Chapman, Richard & Plaat, Felicity. (2009). Alcohol and anaesthesia. Continuing Education in Anaesthesia, Critical Care & Pain. 9. 10-13.
- Ungur A, L, Neumann T, Borchers F, Spies C: Perioperative Management of Alcohol Withdrawal Syndrome. Visc Med 2020;36:160-166.

Alcohol withdrawal syndrome

# ANOREXIA NERVOSA

## LEARNING OBJECTIVES

- Describe the physiological changes associated with anorexia nervosa
- Manage anorexia nervosa patients in the perioperative period

## DEFINITION AND MECHANISM

- Anorexia nervosa is a psychiatric disorder characterized by an intense fear of gaining weight and a distorted perception of weight, resulting in an abnormally low body weight

| System | Changes |
|---|---|
| Cardiovascular | Hypotension, bradycardia, mitral valve prolapse, impaired myocardial contractility, cardiomyopathy, ECG changes (risk of arrhythmias) |
| Respiratory | Metabolic alkalosis, decreased lung compliance, aspiration pneumonia, pneumothorax, and pneumo-mediastinum |
| Renal | Proteinuria, reduced glomerular filtration rate, $\downarrow Na^+$, $\downarrow K^+$, $\downarrow Mg^{2+}$, $\downarrow Cl^-$, $\downarrow H^+$, $\downarrow Ca^{2+}$, $\downarrow PO_4^{2-}$ |
| Gastrointestinal | Enlarged salivary glands, dental caries, periodontitis, Mallory-Weiss tears, esophageal strictures, esophagitis, gastritis, gastric dilatation/infarction/perforation, $\downarrow$ gastric emptying time, risk of refeeding syndrome, fatty liver, hepatomegaly, cirrhosis, $\uparrow$ amylase, abnormal liver function tests |
| Endocrine | $\downarrow FSH$, $\downarrow LH$, $\downarrow GnRH$, $\uparrow cortisol$, $\uparrow GH$, $\downarrow glucose$, $\downarrow insulin$ $\downarrow T3$, $\downarrow T4$, $\leftrightarrow TSH$, impaired thermoregulation |
| Immunological | Leucopenia, thrombocytopenia, hemolytic anemia |
| Hematological | Bone marrow hypoplasia |
| Neurological | White and gray matter changes, $\downarrow$ cognitive function, coma EEG abnormalities, seizures, neuropathy, $\uparrow$ pain threshold |
| Musculoskeletal | Myalgia, myopathy, rhabdomyolysis, osteopenia, osteoporosis, stress fractures |
| Dermatological | Laguno hair, Russell's sign, poor wound healing |

FSH, follicle-stimulating hormone; LH, luteinizing hormone; GnRH, gonadotropin-releasing hormone; GH, growth hormone; T3, triiodothyronine; T4, thyroxine; TSH, thyroid stimulating hormone.

# MANAGEMENT

| Preoperative | Intraoperative | Postoperative |
|---|---|---|

### Assessment
- Thorough anamnesis, specifically question self-induced vomiting, laxative/diuretic/alcohol and illicit drug use
- Blood analysis: Full blood count, urea and electrolytes, phosphate, magnesium, liver function tests, calcium, and serum glucose
- Electrocardiogram (ECG) for all patients
- Echocardiography if the patient has anamnestic or physical signs suggestive for myocardial dysfunction
- Rehydrate all patients and correct and recheck electrolyte abnormalities before the procedure

### Considerations
- Consider all patients with anorexia nervosa to have a full stomach, due to delayed gastric emptying
- Place a nasogastric tube if gastric dilation is suspected to reduce the risk of aspiration, however, note that the tube may interfere with the sphincters and create a trajectory for reflux + the tube could induce vomiting
- Perform a rapid sequence induction for every patient
- Carefully position the patient as they often have frail skin, bones and increased susceptibility to nerve injury

### Considerations
- Avoid hypothermia
- Hypocalcemia and hypokalemia can prolong the action of nondepolarizing neuromuscular blockers
- The relative amount of free drug in the plasma will increase, due to hypoalbuminemia
- A lower basal metabolic rate and reduced renal function can lead to decreased drug metabolism and clearance

### Monitoring
- Body temperature
- Neuromuscular monitoring

### Considerations
- The risk of arrhythmias secondary to the reversal of neuromuscular block is increased
- Only extubate when the patient is awake and therefore laryngeal reflexes are fully intact

## SUGGESTED READING

- Denner AM, Townley SA. Anorexia nervosa: perioperative implications. Continuing Education in Anaesthesia Critical Care & Pain. 2009;9(2):61-4.

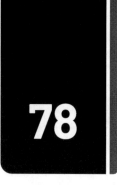

# CARCINOID

## LEARNING OBJECTIVES

- Describe carcinoid and carcinoid syndrome
- Recognize the symptoms and signs of carcinoid and carcinoid syndrome
- Anesthetic management of a patient with carcinoid

## DEFINITION AND MECHANISM

- A carcinoid is a slow-growing neuroendocrine tumor derived from enterochromaffin or Kulchitsky cells
- Carcinoid tumors usually begin in the gastrointestinal tract (i.e., stomach, appendix, small intestine, colon, or rectum), or in the lungs
- Carcinoid syndrome (± 20% of patients with carcinoid tumors) results from the direct release of vasoactive amines (e.g., serotonin and histamine) and peptides into the systemic circulation, usually from hepatic metastases associated with midgut (jejunum, ileum, appendix, and cecum) carcinoids

## SIGNS AND SYMPTOMS

Some tumors do not cause any signs or symptoms. When they do occur, signs and symptoms are usually vague and depend on the tumor's location.

| Location | Signs & symptoms |
|---|---|
| Gastrointestinal (GI) tract | Abdominal pain<br>Diarrhea<br>Nausea, vomiting, and bowel obstruction<br>Rectal bleeding<br>Rectal pain<br>Skin flushing |
| Lungs | Chest pain<br>Wheezing<br>Dyspnea<br>Diarrhea<br>Skin flushing<br>Weight gain<br>Pink or purple marks on the skin (looking like stretch marks) |

*Clinical manifestations of carcinoid syndrome*

| Sign/symptom | Frequency | Characteristics | Involved mediators |
|---|---|---|---|
| Flushing | 85-90% | Foregut: long-lasting purple face and neck<br>Midgut: short-lasting, pink/red<br>Severe flushing associated with hypotension and tachycardia | Kallikrein, 5-hydroxytryptophan (5-HTP; chemical precursor and metabolic intermediate in the biosynthesis of serotonin), histamine, substance P, prostaglandins (PGs) |
| GI hypermotility | 70-80% | Secretory diarrhea, nausea, vomiting | Gastrin, 5-HTP, histamine, PGs, vasoactive intestinal peptides (VIPs) |
| Abdominal pain | 35% | Progressive | Small bowel obstruction, hepatomegaly, ischemia |
| Right-sided heart failure | 30% | Dyspnea | 5-HTP, substance P |
| Left-sided heart failure | 10% | Dyspnea | 5-HTP, substance P |
| Telangiectasia | 25% | Face | Unknown |
| Bronchospasm | 15% | Wheezing | Histamine, 5-HTP |
| Pellagra | 5% | Dermatitis, diarrhea, dementia | Niacin deficiency |

Carcinoid

# RISK FACTORS

- **Age:** Older adults
- **Sex:** Female gender
- **Family history:** History of multiple endocrine neoplasia, type 1 (MEN 1)

# COMPLICATIONS

The cells of carcinoid tumors can secrete hormones and other chemicals, causing a range of complications including:

- **Carcinoid syndrome:** Causes skin flushing, chronic diarrhea, and difficulty breathing (i.e., bronchospasm), among other signs and symptoms (see table above)
- **Carcinoid heart disease:** Carcinoid tumors may secrete hormones causing thickening of the endocardium of the cardiac chambers, valves, and blood vessels, leading to leaky heart valves and heart failure (i.e., typically right-sided heart failure)
- **Other endocrine disorders:** Carcinoid tumors can also secrete growth hormone and adrenocorticotropin-releasing hormone, respectively leading to acromegaly and Cushing's syndrome

# TREATMENT

- **Surgery:** When detected early, possible to dissect completely
- **Medications:** To block the excess hormone secretion by the tumor and reduce the signs and symptoms, and to slow tumor growth
- **Chemotherapy:** Recommended for advanced tumors that cannot be removed surgically
- **Targeted drug therapy:** Usually combined with chemotherapy for advanced tumors
- **Treatment for tumors with metastases to the liver:** Surgery to remove part of the liver, hepatic artery embolization (blocking blood flow to the liver), and using heat (i.e., radiofrequency ablation) and/or cold (i.e., cryoablation) to kill cancer cells

# MANAGEMENT

### PREOPERATIVE MANAGEMENT

- Full preoperative work-up including cardiac investigations for carcinoid heart disease
- Correct electrolyte abnormalities, dehydration, and preexisting protein abnormalities
- **Appropriate monitoring:** Arterial pressures, central venous pressures

### PREOPERATIVE MEDICATIONS

- Octreotide: 100-1000 µgm as bolus, then 100-1000 µgm/hr infusion (titrated to effect)
- Antihistamines: H1 antagonists (i.e., diphenhydramine, loratadine, etc); H2 antagonists (i.e., ranitidine, famotidine)
- Anxiolytics: Benzodiazepines (i.e., midazolam, diazepam, etc)

### INTRAOPERATIVE MANAGEMENT

- **Octreotide:** Continue infusion at 100-1000 µgm/hr with boluses when indicated
- Avoid drugs that have a potential for histamine release (e.g., morphine, pethidine, codeine, atracurium, mivacurium)
- Effective blunting of the pressor response to intubation and maintenance of depth of anesthesia
- Prepare for periods of potential carcinoid crisis
- **Management of carcinoid crisis hemodynamic instability**
  - Bolus doses of octreotide: 100-1000 µgm
  - Use of crystalloids or colloids to expand intravascular space while avoiding right ventricular overload or strain
  - Use of vasoconstrictors (i.e., phenylephrine, metaraminol, noradrenaline (low doses))
  - Adrenaline has the potential to cause more release of vasoactive peptides but this is inconsistently seen and has been used in resuscitation
- Monitor fluid balance, temperature and blood glucose levels

### POSTOPERATIVE MANAGEMENT

- Continue octreotide infusion and wean over days
- Monitor in a high dependency or ICU setting: 48 hours of invasive monitoring, analgesia, and fluid management
- Ensure good pain control with regional techniques, neuraxial block, or patient-controlled analgesia (PCA)

## KEEP IN MIND

- The goal is to prevent, recognize, and treat perioperative carcinoid crises
- Triggers include histamine-releasing drugs, vasoactive drugs, succinylcholine; tumor manipulation; and hypovolemia, hypoxia, hypothermia, hypercarbia
- Treatment of perioperative bronchospasms include octreotide, steroids, histamine blockade (diphenhydramine), and Atrovent
- Avoid beta-agonists, theophylline, and epinephrine to treat perioperative bronchospasms

**SUGGESTED READING**

- Kaltsas G, Caplin M, Davies P, et al. ENETS Consensus Guidelines for the Standards of Care in Neuroendocrine Tumors: Pre- and Perioperative Therapy in Patients with Neuroendocrine Tumors. Neuroendocrinology. 2017;105(3):245-254.
- Powell B, Al Mukhtar A, Mills GH. Carcinoid: the disease and its implications for anaesthesia. Continuing Education in Anaesthesia Critical Care & Pain. 2011;11(1):9-13.
- Mancuso K, Kaye AD, Boudreaux JP, et al. Carcinoid syndrome and perioperative anesthetic considerations. J Clin Anesth. 2011;23(4):329-341.

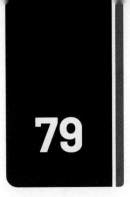

# CUSHING'S SYNDROME

**79**

## LEARNING OBJECTIVES

- Describe Cushing's syndrome
- Recognize the symptoms and signs of Cushing's syndrome
- Anesthetic management of a patient with Cushing's syndrome

## DEFINITION AND MECHANISM

- Cushing's syndrome is a collection of signs and symptoms due to prolonged exposure to glucocorticoids (i.e., cortisol)
- Cushing's disease is a specific type of Cushing's syndrome caused by a pituitary tumor leading to excessive production of adrenocorticotropic hormone (ACTH)
  → excessive ACTH stimulates the adrenal cortex to produce high levels of cortisol

## CAUSES

### Exogenous

- Patients taking prescribed glucocorticoids (e.g., prednisone) to treat other diseases (i.e., asthma and rheumatoid arthritis) or for immunosuppression after organ transplants = **iatrogenic Cushing's syndrome**
- Adrenal glands may gradually atrophy due to lack of stimulation by ACTH, which's production is reduced by the glucocorticoid medication
- Resolves when the patient stops the glucocorticoid medication

### Endogenous

- Derangement of the body's system to secrete cortisol
- Hormone-secreting tumors of the adrenal glands or pituitary
- **Pituitary Cushing's:** Benign pituitary adenoma secretes ACTH = **Cushing's disease**
- **Adrenal Cushing's:** Excess cortisol production by adrenal glands tumors, hyperplastic adrenal glands, or adrenal glands with nodular adrenal hyperplasia
- Tumors (e.g., small cell lung cancer) outside the pituitary-adrenal system can also produce ACTH = **ectopic or paraneoplastic Cushing's disease**

## SIGNS AND SYMPTOMS

- Moon face
- Central obesity with buffalo hump
- Thin skin that bruises easily
- Purple striae on the abdomen and thighs
- Proximal muscle wasting
- Thin extremities
- Osteoporosis
- Hypertension
- Left ventricular hypertrophy
- Hyperglycemia
- Impaired glucose tolerance and diabetes mellitus type II
- Metabolic alkalosis
- Hypokalemia
- Poor wound healing
- Menstrual irregularities

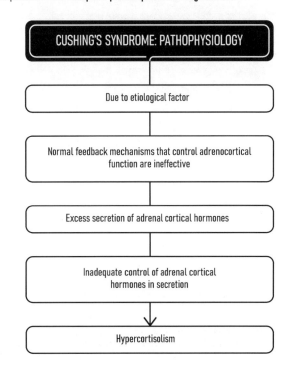

Cushing's syndrome

# TREATMENT

- Transsphenoidal microadenomectomy and radiotherapy for pituitary-dependent Cushing's disease
- Adrenal adenoma or carcinoma requires surgical removal of the affected gland
- Hypercortisolism can be controlled with adrenal enzyme inhibitors, such as ketoconazole, metyrapone, mitotane, or aminoglutethimide, given alone or in combination → drugs to inhibit release and synthesis of glucocorticoids

# MANAGEMENT

## Preoperative considerations

- **Airway evaluation:** Mallampati score, mouth opening, neck extension, thyromental and sternomental distances, and Wilson score
- **Careful cardiovascular evaluation:** ECG, echo
- **Careful respiratory evaluation:** X-ray, blood gases, pulmonary function test (PFT)
- **Stabilize glycemia:** Stop oral therapy and start insulin regimen

| Regular insulin | Type 1 DM (male) | Type 1 DM (female) | Type 2 (DM) |
|---|---|---|---|
| Initial bolus infusion | 0.05-0.1 U/kg 1 U/h | 0.05-0.1 U/kg 0.5 U/h | 0.05-0.1 U/kg 1 U/h |

- **Correct acid-base and electrolytes imbalances:** Spironolactone, potassium
- Continue antihypertensive drugs until the morning of surgery except for the angiotensin-converting enzyme inhibitors (i.e., captopril, enalapril, lisinopril, enalaprilat, and ramipril) and angiotensin II receptor blocks (i.e., valsartan)
- Discontinue clopidogrel 5-7 days before surgery, except in coronary-stent patients (risk of stent occlusion)
- Continue glucocorticoid inhibitors (i.e., ketoconazole, metyrapone, mitotane, or aminoglutethimide)
- **Prevent perioperative venous thromboembolism and pulmonary embolism:** LMWH (i.e., enoxaparin, dalteparin) or fondaparinux
- Avoid deep preoperative sedation → **Premedication drugs:** Midazolam 1 mg IV

## Intraoperative considerations

- **Positioning and taping:** Careful and gentle positioning to avoid fractures
- **Standard monitoring:** Non-invasive blood pressure, temperature, end-tidal carbon dioxide, pulse oximetry, and ECG
- **Invasive monitoring:** Invasive blood pressure via arterial catheter cannulation and Swan-Ganz pulmonary artery catheter (if necessary)
- **Venous access:** Large bore peripheral and central venous catheters
- Maintain the glucose blood level within normal values (i.e., 120-180 mg/dL) → insulin regimen

| Glucose blood level (mg/dL) | Infusion rate change (U/h) |
|---|---|
| ≤ 70 | Reassessment within 30 min |
| 70-120 | ↓ 0.3 |
| 121-180 | No change |
| 181-240 | ↑ 0.3 |
| 241-300 | ↑ 0.6 |
| ≥ 300 | ↑ 1 |

- **Prevent gastric aspiration:** Metoclopramide 10 mg, ranitidine 50 mg IV, and sodium citrate 30 mL P.O.
- **Induction of anesthesia and endotracheal intubation:** Rapid induction sequence
- **Blunt sympathetic response (i.e., hypertension and arrhythmias) during induction:** Opioids, lidocaine, clonidine, and esmolol
- **Avoid ketamine** because of its sympathetic effects
- Extubate if the patient is alert, warm, hemodynamically stable, and fully reversed from muscle relaxants

Cushing's syndrome

### Postoperative considerations

- **Prevent respiratory complications (i.e., atelectasis, hypoxemia):** Effective postoperative pain relief, early mobilization, and respiratory exercises
- **Postoperative acute pain treatment:** Systemic analgesic drugs (i.e., patient-controlled analgesia pumps or epidural analgesia)
- Routinely check cortisol, glucose, and electrolytes blood levels
- Continue replacement of cortisol, guided by cortisol blood levels
- Use insulin regimen to maintain the glucose blood level within recommended levels
- Continue antihypertensive drugs based on the patient's hemodynamic status

## KEEP IN MIND

- The anesthesiologist has to deal with difficult ventilation and intubation, hemodynamic disturbances, volume overload and hypokalemia, glucose intolerance, diabetes, maintain the blood cortisol level, and prevent glucocorticoid deficiency in the perioperative period

## ■ SUGGESTED READING ■

- Domi R, Sula H, Kaci M, Paparisto S, Bodeci A, Xhemali A. Anesthetic considerations on adrenal gland surgery. J Clin Med Res. 2015;7(1):1-7.
- Melanie Davies, FRCA, Jonathan Hardman, DM FRCA, Anaesthesia and adrenocortical disease, Continuing Education in Anaesthesia Critical Care & Pain, Volume 5, Issue 4, August 2005, Pages 122–126, https://doi.org/10.1093/bjaceaccp/mki033

# DIABETES INSIPIDUS

## LEARNING OBJECTIVES

- Describe diabetes insipidus
- Recognize the symptoms and signs of diabetes insipidus
- Anesthetic management of a patient with diabetes insipidus

## DEFINITION AND MECHANISM

- Diabetes insipidus (DI) is a disorder of urinary concentration caused by a temporary or chronic deficiency of, or insensitivity to, antidiuretic hormone (ADH) or vasopressin
- The condition renders the kidneys unable to effectively autoregulate water balance, resulting in polyuria, polydipsia, and electrolyte abnormalities (e.g., hypernatremia, hypokalemia)

## CLASSIFICATION

- **Central DI or ADH deficiency:** Reduced ADH secretion due to damage to the pituitary gland or hypothalamus or genetics
- **Nephrogenic DI or ADH resistance:** Normal ADH secretion, but the kidneys are unable to properly respond to ADH due to an inherited genetic disorder or chronic kidney disease
- **Gestational DI:** A very rare condition that occurs during pregnancy when an enzyme made by the placenta destroys ADH
- **Primary polydipsia (dipsogenic DI):** Damage to the hypothalamic thirst center causes excessive fluid intake leading to polyuria

## SIGNS AND SYMPTOMS

| Adults | Children | Infants |
|---|---|---|
| Polyuria | Anorexia | Irritability |
| Polydipsia | Growth defects | Chronic dehydration |
| Nocturia | Enuresis | Growth retardation |
| Craving for ice water | Sleep disturbance | Neurologic disturbance |
| | Fatigue | Hyperthermia |

### Clinical findings

- **If the thirst mechanism is intact:** Hydronephrosis and bladder distension due to excessive urinary volume
- **If there is no access to free water or damage to the hypothalamic thirst center:** Hypernatremia, dehydration, hypertonic encephalopathy, obtundation, coma, seizure, subarachnoid hemorrhage, and intracerebral hemorrhage

## COMPLICATIONS

**Dehydration, which may cause:**

- Dry mouth
- Changes in skin elasticity
- Thirst
- Fatigue

**Electrolyte imbalance, resulting in:**

- Weakness
- Nausea
- Vomiting
- Loss of appetite
- Muscle cramps
- Confusion

# PATHOPHYSIOLOGY

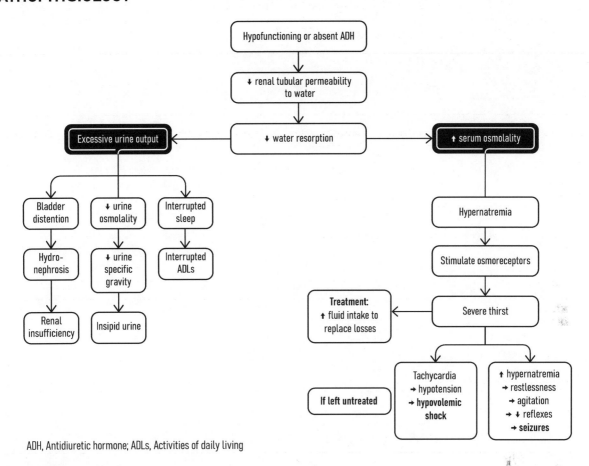

ADH, Antidiuretic hormone; ADLs, Activities of daily living

# TREATMENT

- There is no cure ➜ treatments aim to relieve thirst, decrease urine output, and prevent dehydration

- **Central and gestational DI:** Desmopressin (DDAVP)
- **Nephrogenic DI:** Treat the underlying cause or use thiazide, aspirin, or ibuprofen
- **Primary polydipsia:** Decrease fluid intake

# MANAGEMENT

- **Hypernatremia:** ↑ MAC requirements
- Treat hypernatremia by estimating the water deficit and replacing it with free water:
  - □ Water deficit = total body water x (Serum Na [ ]/140-1)
- **Volume depletion:** Resuscitate with normal saline initially
- **Central DI:** DDAVP 1-2 µg IV BID
- **Nephrogenic DI:** Hydrochlorothiazide/Amiloride

Diabetes insipidus

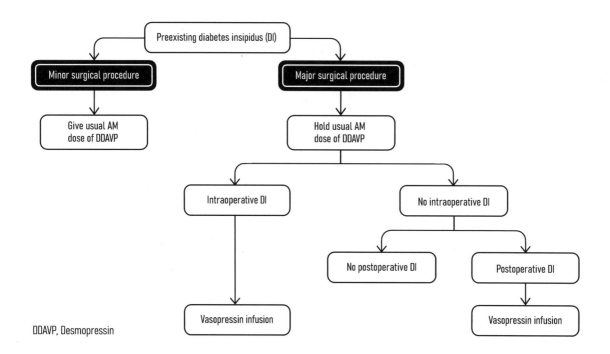

DDAVP, Desmopressin

## KEEP IN MIND

- Avoid rapid overcorrection if chronic hypernatremia (goal: < 10 mEq/day)
- Be careful of cerebral edema, water intoxication, and volume overload

━━ **SUGGESTED READING** ━━

- Mutter CM, Smith T, Menze O, Zakharia M, Nguyen H. Diabetes Insipidus: Pathogenesis, Diagnosis, and Clinical Management. Cureus. 2021;13(2):e13523.
- Dharshan AC, Kohli-Seth R. Chapter 117. Diabetes Insipidus. In: Atchabahian A, Gupta R. eds. The Anesthesia Guide. Mgraw Hill; 2013. Accessed January 17, 2023.

# DIABETIC KETOACIDOSIS

**81**

## LEARNING OBJECTIVES

- Describe diabetic ketoacidosis
- Recognize the symptoms and signs of diabetic ketoacidosis
- Anesthetic management of a patient with diabetic ketoacidosis

## DEFINITION AND MECHANISM

- Diabetic ketoacidosis (DKA) is a potentially life-threatening complication of diabetes mellitus
- DKA results from a relative or absolute insulin deficiency with an excess of hyperglycemic hormones (i.e., glucagon, catecholamines, cortisol, and growth hormone) leading to hyperglycemia because of increased gluconeogenesis, accelerated glycogenolysis, and impaired glucose use by peripheral tissues
- DKA leads to lipolysis and the synthesis of ketoacids to use as fuel
- Ketoacids trigger metabolic acidosis and polyuria, leading to severe dehydration
- DKA occurs most often in patients with type 1 diabetes, but can also occur in patients with type 2 diabetes (rare)
- Triggers include infection or inflammation (e.g., pneumonia, UTI, foot ulcer, abdominal [appendicitis, cholecystitis, pancreatitis]), inadequate insulin administration, myocardial infarction, stroke, certain medications (e.g., steroids, cocaine), pregnancy, and trauma

## SIGNS AND SYMPTOMS

- Polydipsia
- Polyuria
- Nausea and vomiting
- Abdominal pain
- Weakness and fatigue
- Deep, rapid gasping breathing (Kussmaul breathing)
- Fruity breath/ fruity odor/ acetone breath
- Confusion
- Hyperglycemia
- Ketonuria

## RISK FACTORS

- Patients with type 1 diabetes
- Patients who often miss insulin doses

## COMPLICATIONS

Most common complications are related to the treatment of DKA with fluids and electrolytes

- Hypoglycemia
- Hypokalemia
- Cerebral edema

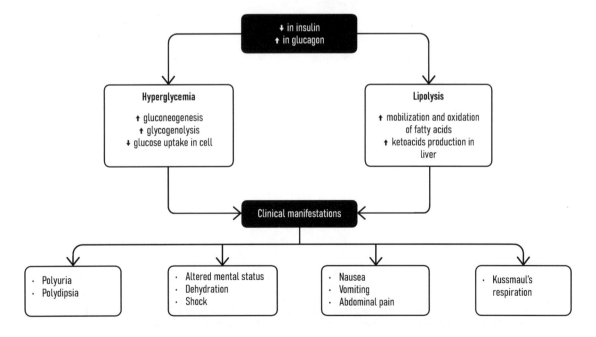

# TREATMENT

Patients with DKA receive emergency treatment in the hospital, including:

- IV insulin to lower ketones
- Fluids to prevent dehydration
- Electrolyte replacement: Sodium, potassium, and chloride
- Antibiotics if an infection is also present

# MANAGEMENT

### Fluids
- The average fluid deficit in DKA is 6 L
- Start with 500-1500 mL of colloid bolus if clinically hypovolemic (hypotension, tachycardia)
- Initial bolus should be normal saline (NS; 0.9% saline) bolus 10-15 mL/kg
- Change to ½ NS with 20 mEq/L potassium after that
- Replace ongoing intraoperative blood and fluid losses as usually
- Change fluid to D5W with ½ NS if blood sugar drops to 250 mg/dL and the anion gap is still present → allows insulin administration to reduce ketone without causing hypoglycemia

### Insulin
- Regular insulin 10 U IV bolus followed with an infusion at (blood glucose/150) U/h
- Do not stop insulin if glucose < 90, rather increase IV glucose administration
- Consider changing to SC insulin when the patient resumes P.O. alimentation

### Electrolytes
- Follow electrolytes closely every 4-6 h (every 2 h at the very beginning) until the anion gap closed
- **Potassium:**
  - 10-15 mEq/h for at least the first 4 h
  - Irrespective of the initial potassium level, for a goal of 4–5 mEq/L
  - Potassium will shift back to the intracellular compartment because of insulin and lead to hypokalemia if uncorrected
- **Phosphate:** 1-2 mg/dL
- **Magnesium:** 2 mEq/L

### Acidosis
- Typically, will correct itself with insulin treatment
- Administer bicarbonate only if pH < 7.0 or hemodynamic instability (rare)

### Triggering factors
- Diagnose and treat accordingly

### Other
- Consider thromboprophylaxis depending on the risk

# PREVENTION

- Manage diabetes
- Monitor blood sugar levels
- Adjust the insulin dose as needed
- Check the ketone level
- Be prepared to act quickly

# KEEP IN MIND

- DKA is a life-threatening medical emergency characterized by the biochemical triad of ketonemia, hyperglycemia, and acidemia
- Bedside monitoring of capillary ketones, glucose, blood gases, and electrolytes is used to make the initial diagnosis and guide management
- Balanced electrolyte solutions resolve acidosis faster, but contain insufficient potassium to justify their safe use except in critical care
- Continuation of long-acting insulins may reduce complications during the transition from IV to SC insulin
- Early involvement of diabetic specialist teams is required

# SUGGESTED READING

- Levy N, Penfold NW, Dhatariya K. Perioperative management of the patient with diabetes requiring emergency surgery. BJA Education. 2017;17(4):129-136.
- Hallet A, Modi A, Levy N. Developments in the management of diabetic ketoacidosis in adults: implications for anaesthetists. BJA Education. 2016;16(1):8-14.
- Patel K, Kohli-Seth R. Chapter 210. Diabetic Ketoacidosis. In: Atchabahian A, Gupta R. eds. The Anesthesia Guide. Mgraw Hill; 2013. Accessed January 17, 2023.

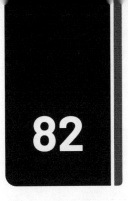

# DIABETES MELLITUS TYPE 2

## LEARNING OBJECTIVES

- Anesthetic management of a patient with diabetes mellitus type 2
- Physiological changes due to diabetes mellitus

---

## DEFINITION AND MECHANISM

- Diabetes mellitus type 2 is a consequence of peripheral resistance to insulin action
- It is characterized by insulin resistance (hepatic, extrahepatic, or both) probably due to a decreased stimulation of glycogen synthesis in the muscle by insulin, related to impaired glucose transport
- Insulin secretion and/or insulin action are thought to be deficient with excessive hepatic glucose production
- It is frequently associated with dysfunction in pancreatic β-cells responsible for insulin secretion
- The age of onset is variable, however, it is usually a disease of adults with slow onset
- Ketoacidosis is uncommon

## PHYSIOLOGICAL CHANGES

| Musculoskeletal system | Stiff joint syndrome (SJS) |
|---|---|
| Renal | Diabetic nephropathy |
| Neurological system | Increased risk of cerebrovascular accident (CVA)<br>Nerve fibers at risk for ischemic injury<br>Peripheral neuropathies |
| Autonomic neuropathy | Diabetic autonomic neuropathy<br>Resting tachycardia<br>Orthostatic hypotension<br>Intestinal constipation<br>Gastroparesis<br>Bladder dysfunction<br>Impaired neurovascular function<br>Loss of autonomic response to hypoglycemia |
| Cardiovascular system | Hypertension<br>Coronary artery disease<br>Silent myocardial ischemia<br>Systolic and diastolic heart failure<br>Congestive heart failure<br>Peripheral vascular disease |
| Retinal | Diabetic retinopathy |

**Management of diabetes mellitus type 2**
- Diet
- Exercise
- Medications:
  - Sulphonylureas (e.g., gliclazide)
  - Biguanides (e.g., metformin)
  - Thiazolidinediones (e.g., pioglitazone, rosiglitazone)
  - Meglinitides (e.g., repaglinide, nateglinide)
  - Alpha-glucosidase inhibitors (e.g., acarbose, miglitol)
  - Incretin mimetics:
    - GLP-1 agonists (e.g., Exenatide, liraglutide)
    - DPP-4 inhibitors (e.g., sitagliptin and vildagliptin)
  - SGLT2 inhibitors (e.g., canagliflozin, dapagliflozin, empagliflozin)

# MANAGEMENT
## PREOPERATIVE ASSESSMENT

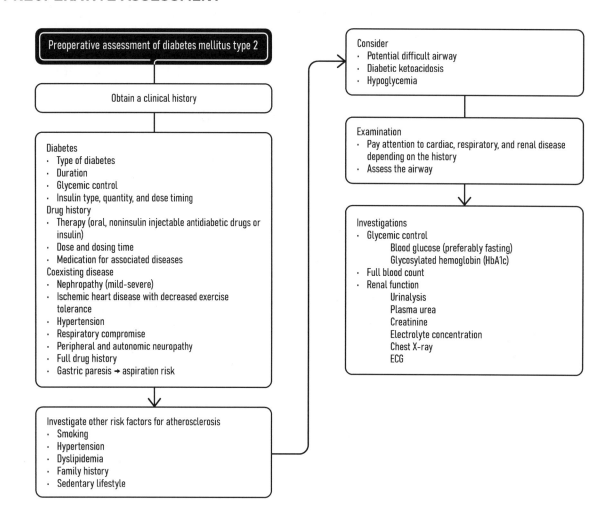

**Preoperative assessment of diabetes mellitus type 2**

Obtain a clinical history

Diabetes
- Type of diabetes
- Duration
- Glycemic control
- Insulin type, quantity, and dose timing

Drug history
- Therapy (oral, noninsulin injectable antidiabetic drugs or insulin)
- Dose and dosing time
- Medication for associated diseases

Coexisting disease
- Nephropathy (mild-severe)
- Ischemic heart disease with decreased exercise tolerance
- Hypertension
- Respiratory compromise
- Peripheral and autonomic neuropathy
- Full drug history
- Gastric paresis → aspiration risk

Investigate other risk factors for atherosclerosis
- Smoking
- Hypertension
- Dyslipidemia
- Family history
- Sedentary lifestyle

Consider
- Potential difficult airway
- Diabetic ketoacidosis
- Hypoglycemia

Examination
- Pay attention to cardiac, respiratory, and renal disease depending on the history
- Assess the airway

Investigations
- Glycemic control
  Blood glucose (preferably fasting)
  Glycosylated hemoglobin (HbA1c)
- Full blood count
- Renal function
  Urinalysis
  Plasma urea
  Creatinine
  Electrolyte concentration
  Chest X-ray
  ECG

# PERIOPERATIVE MANAGEMENT

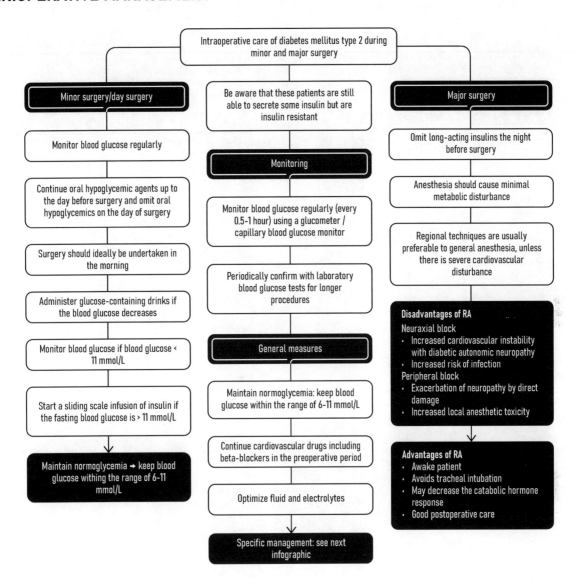

Intraoperative care of diabetes mellitus type 2 during minor and major surgery

**Minor surgery/day surgery**

Monitor blood glucose regularly

Continue oral hypoglycemic agents up to the day before surgery and omit oral hypoglycemics on the day of surgery

Surgery should ideally be undertaken in the morning

Administer glucose-containing drinks if the blood glucose decreases

Monitor blood glucose if blood glucose < 11 mmol/L

Start a sliding scale infusion of insulin if the fasting blood glucose is > 11 mmol/L

Maintain normoglycemia ➜ keep blood glucose withing the range of 6-11 mmol/L

Be aware that these patients are still able to secrete some insulin but are insulin resistant

**Monitoring**

Monitor blood glucose regularly (every 0.5-1 hour) using a glucometer / capillary blood glucose monitor

Periodically confirm with laboratory blood glucose tests for longer procedures

**General measures**

Maintain normoglycemia: keep blood glucose within the range of 6-11 mmol/L

Continue cardiovascular drugs including beta-blockers in the preoperative period

Optimize fluid and electrolytes

Specific management: see next infographic

**Major surgery**

Omit long-acting insulins the night before surgery

Anesthesia should cause minimal metabolic disturbance

Regional techniques are usually preferable to general anesthesia, unless there is severe cardiovascular disturbance

**Disadvantages of RA**
Neuraxial block
· Increased cardiovascular instability with diabetic autonomic neuropathy
· Increased risk of infection
Peripheral block
· Exacerbation of neuropathy by direct damage
· Increased local anesthetic toxicity

**Advantages of RA**
· Awake patient
· Avoids tracheal intubation
· May decrease the catabolic hormone response
· Good postoperative care

Diabetes mellitus type 2

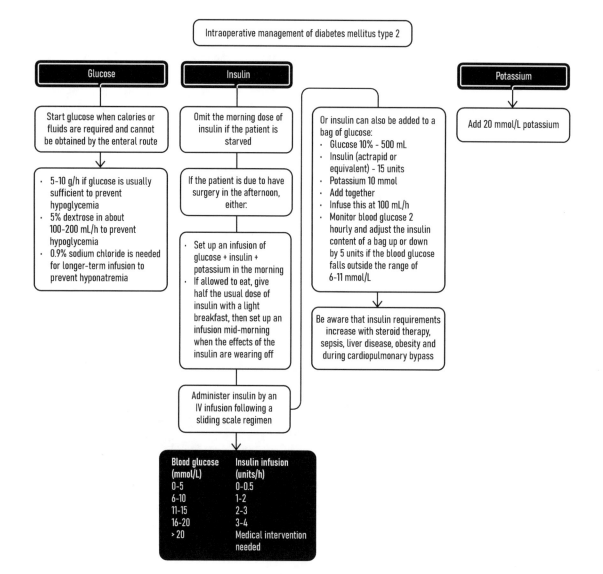

**Intraoperative management of diabetes mellitus type 2**

**Glucose**

Start glucose when calories or fluids are required and cannot be obtained by the enteral route

- 5-10 g/h if glucose is usually sufficient to prevent hypoglycemia
- 5% dextrose in about 100-200 mL/h to prevent hypoglycemia
- 0.9% sodium chloride is needed for longer-term infusion to prevent hyponatremia

**Insulin**

Omit the morning dose of insulin if the patient is starved

If the patient is due to have surgery in the afternoon, either:

- Set up an infusion of glucose + insulin + potassium in the morning
- If allowed to eat, give half the usual dose of insulin with a light breakfast, then set up an infusion mid-morning when the effects of the insulin are wearing off

Administer insulin by an IV infusion following a sliding scale regimen

| Blood glucose (mmol/L) | Insulin infusion (units/h) |
| --- | --- |
| 0-5 | 0-0.5 |
| 6-10 | 1-2 |
| 11-15 | 2-3 |
| 16-20 | 3-4 |
| > 20 | Medical intervention needed |

Or insulin can also be added to a bag of glucose:
- Glucose 10% - 500 mL
- Insulin (actrapid or equivalent) - 15 units
- Potassium 10 mmol
- Add together
- Infuse this at 100 mL/h
- Monitor blood glucose 2 hourly and adjust the insulin content of a bag up or down by 5 units if the blood glucose falls outside the range of 6-11 mmol/L

Be aware that insulin requirements increase with steroid therapy, sepsis, liver disease, obesity and during cardiopulmonary bypass

**Potassium**

Add 20 mmol/L potassium

## POSTOPERATIVE CARE

- Check blood glucose levels hourly until a normal diet is established
- Monitor plasma potassium every 3-4 hours, or more frequently if clinically indicated
- Administer appropriate analgesia
- Use NSAIDs with great caution as they may further impair renal function in patients with a nephropathy
- Avoid dexamethasone as it exacerbates insulin resistance

## KEEP IN MIND

- HbA1c has a strong predictive value for complications of diabetes

Diabetes mellitus type 2

## SUGGESTED READING

- Pollard BJ, Kitchen, G. Handbook of Clinical Anaesthesia. Fourth Edition. CRC Press. 2018. 978-1-4987-6289-2.
- Pontes JPJ, Mendes FF, Vasconcelos MM, Batista NR. Avaliação e manejo perioperatório de pacientes com diabetes melito. Um desafio para o anestesiologista [Evaluation and perioperative management of patients with diabetes mellitus. A challenge for the anesthesiologist]. Braz J Anesthesiol. 2018;68(1):75-86.
- Cornelius BW. Patients With Type 2 Diabetes: Anesthetic Management in the Ambulatory Setting: Part 2: Pharmacology and Guidelines for Perioperative Management. Anesth Prog. 2017;64(1):39-44.
- Stubbs, D.J., Levy, N., Dhatariya, K., 2017. Diabetes medication pharmacology. BJA Education 17, 198-207.
- Nicholson G, Hall GM. 2011. Diabetes and adult surgical inpatients. Continuing Education in Anaesthesia Critical CAre & Pain. 11;6:234-238.
- Robertshaw HJ, Hall GM. Diabetes mellitus: anaesthetic management [published correction appears in Anaesthesia. 2007 Jan;62(1):100]. Anaesthesia. 2006;61(12):1187-1190.
- McAnulty GR, Robertshaw HJ, Hall GM. Anaesthetic management of patients with diabetes mellitus. Br J Anaesth. 2000;85(1):80-90.

# EUGLYCEMIC DIABETIC KETOACIDOSIS

## LEARNING OBJECTIVES

- Definition of euglycemic diabetic ketoacidosis (EDKA)
- Management of EDKA

## DEFINITION AND MECHANISM

- Diabetic ketoacidosis (DKA) is defined as metabolic acidosis with hyperglycemia and increased ketone bodies in the blood and urine, with hyperglycemia is the hallmark for the diagnosis of DKA
- However, in a subset of patients, the serum glucose levels are within the normal limits; this is defined as euglycemic diabetic ketoacidosis (EDKA)
- This rare condition is a diagnostic challenge as euglycemia masks the underlying diabetic ketoacidosis
- Occurs in both type 1 and type 2 diabetes mellitus and can be life-threatening
- EDKA is secondary to a carbohydrate deficit resulting in generalized decreased serum insulin and excess hormones such as glucagon, epinephrine, and cortisol
- The increased glucagon/insulin ratio leads to increased lipolysis, increased free fatty acids, and ketoacidosis
- The resulting anion gap metabolic acidosis triggers respiratory compensation and a sensation of dyspnea, as well as nausea, anorexia, and vomiting
- The resulting volume depletion further exacerbates elevations in glucagon, cortisol, and epinephrine, worsening lipolysis and ketogenesis
- Additionally, decreased hepatic gluconeogenesis or increased glucosuria contribute to EDKA

## SIGNS AND SYMPTOMS

- Metabolic acidosis (pH < 7.3, serum bicarbonate < 18 mEq/L)
- Ketonemia or ketonuria
- Normal blood glucose levels < 250 mg/dL
- Malaise
- Dyspnea
- Nausea
- Vomiting
- Confusion
- Excessive thirst/urination
- Kussmaul respiration (deep, rapid)

## ETIOLOGY

- Starvation resulting in ketosis while maintaining normoglycemia
  □ Anorexia
  □ Gastroparesis
  □ Fasting
  □ Use of a ketogenic diet
  □ Alcohol use
  □ Persistent vomiting
- Pregnancy
- Pancreatitis
- Glycogen storage disorders
- Surgery
- Infection
- Cocaine toxicity
- Cirrhosis
- Insulin pump use
- Dehydration
- Sodium-glucose cotransporter 2 (SGLT2) inhibitors:
  □ SGLT2 inhibition in the proximal renal tubules promotes glycosuria
  □ Resulting in diminished insulin production and elevated plasma glucagon concentrations

## COMPLICATIONS

- Dehydration
- Vomiting
- Hypoglycemia
- Hypovolemic shock
- Respiratory failure
- Cerebral edema
- Coma
- Seizures
- Infection
- Thrombosis
- Myocardial infarction

Euglycemic diabetic ketoacidosis

# DIAGNOSIS

- Blood or urine ketone testing
- Laboratory evaluation:
  - Electrolytes
  - Glucose
  - Calcium
  - Magnesium
  - Creatinine
  - Blood urea nitrogen (BUN)
  - Serum and urine ketones
  - Beta-hydroxybutyric acid
  - Arterial or venous blood gas analysis
  - Lactic acid
  - Chest X-ray
  - ECG
  - Serum osmolality
  - Alcohol

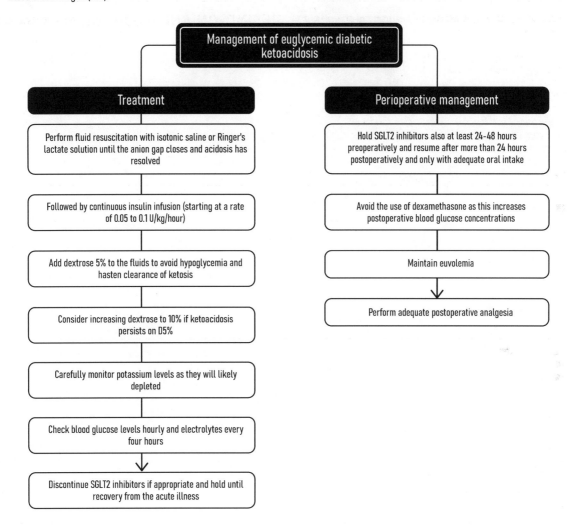

**Management of euglycemic diabetic ketoacidosis**

**Treatment**

- Perform fluid resuscitation with isotonic saline or Ringer's lactate solution until the anion gap closes and acidosis has resolved
- Followed by continuous insulin infusion (starting at a rate of 0.05 to 0.1 U/kg/hour)
- Add dextrose 5% to the fluids to avoid hypoglycemia and hasten clearance of ketosis
- Consider increasing dextrose to 10% if ketoacidosis persists on D5%
- Carefully monitor potassium levels as they will likely depleted
- Check blood glucose levels hourly and electrolytes every four hours
- Discontinue SGLT2 inhibitors if appropriate and hold until recovery from the acute illness

**Perioperative management**

- Hold SGLT2 inhibitors also at least 24-48 hours preoperatively and resume after more than 24 hours postoperatively and only with adequate oral intake
- Avoid the use of dexamethasone as this increases postoperative blood glucose concentrations
- Maintain euvolemia
- Perform adequate postoperative analgesia

## SUGGESTED READING

- Nasa P, Chaudhary S, Shrivastava PK, Singh A. Euglycemic diabetic ketoacidosis: A missed diagnosis. World J Diabetes. 2021;12(5):514-523.
- Thiruvenkatarajan, V., Meyer, E.J., Nanjappa, N., Van Wijk, R.M., Jesudason, D., 2019. Perioperative diabetic ketoacidosis associated with sodium-glucose co-transporter-2 inhibitors: a systematic review. British Journal of Anaesthesia 123, 27–36.
- Rawla, P., Vellipuram, A.R., Bandaru, S.S., Pradeep Raj, J., 2017. Euglycemic diabetic ketoacidosis: a diagnostic and therapeutic dilemma. Endocrinology, Diabetes & Metabolism Case Reports 2017.
- Modi A, Agrawal A, Morgan F. Euglycemic Diabetic Ketoacidosis: A Review. Curr Diabetes Rev. 2017;13(3):315-321.

# HYPERALDOSTERONISM

**84**

## LEARNING OBJECTIVES

- Describe hyperaldosteronism
- Recognize the symptoms and signs of hyperaldosteronism
- Anesthetic management of a patient with hyperaldosteronism

## DEFINITION AND MECHANISM

- Hyperaldosteronism is a condition in which one or both adrenal glands produce too much aldosterone
- Aldosterone regulates blood pressure by controlling the blood levels of potassium and sodium

### Classification

- **Primary hyperaldosteronism (Conn's syndrome):** Overproduction of aldosterone independent from the renin-angiotensin-aldosterone system (RAAS), usually caused by a tumor of the adrenal gland
- **Secondary hyperaldosteronism (hyperreninism):** Overproduction of aldosterone due to overactivity of the RAAS

## SIGNS AND SYMPTOMS

- Hypertension
  - Headache
  - Dizziness
  - Vision changes
  - Difficulty breathing
- Fluid and electrolyte imbalances
  - Hypokalemia
    - Muscle weakness
    - Muscle spasm
    - Tingling and numbness
    - Fatigue
    - Polydipsia
    - Polyuria
  - Hypernatremia
  - Hypomagnesemia
  - Metabolic alkalosis
  - Volume depletion

## COMPLICATIONS

The most common complications are caused by hypertension
- Atrial fibrillation
- Left ventricular hypertrophy
- Heart attack
- Stroke

## PATHOPHYSIOLOGY

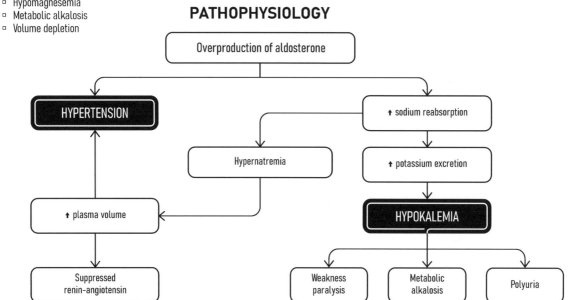

Hyperaldosteronism

# TREATMENT

## Primary hyperaldosteronism

- Surgery to remove the adrenal gland tumor
- Potassium-sparing diuretics that act as aldosterone antagonists (i.e., spironolactone, eplerenone, and amiloride)
- Limit salt intake

## Secondary hyperaldosteronism

- No surgery
- Potassium-sparing diuretics that act as aldosterone antagonists (i.e., spironolactone, eplerenone, and amiloride)
- COX-2 inhibitors
- Limit salt intake

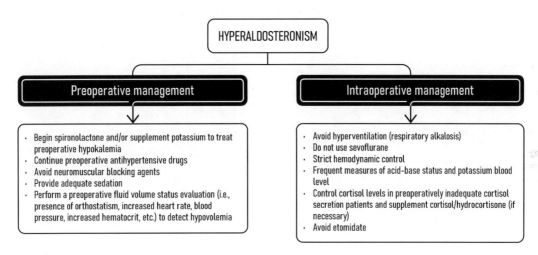

# KEEP IN MIND

- The anesthesiologist must deal with hypertension, hypovolemia, hypokalemia, and cortisol supplementation (depending case by case) in patients with hyperaldosteronism

**SUGGESTED READING**

- Domi R, Sula H, Kaci M, Paparisto S, Bodeci A, Xhemali A. Anesthetic considerations on adrenal gland surgery. J Clin Med Res. 2015;7(1):1-7.
- Jano A, Domi R, Berdica L, et al. Anaesthetic considerations of Conn syndrome: a case presentation and mini-review the anaesthesiologist and Conn syndrome. Clin Med Res 2014;3(5):132-135.
- Davies M, Hardman J. Anaesthesia and adrenocortical disease. Continuing Education in Anaesthesia, Critical Care & Pain. 2005;5(4):122-126.

# HYPERCAPNIA

## LEARNING OBJECTIVES

- Describe the etiology and causes of hypercapnia
- Diagnose hypercapnia
- Manage hypercapnia

## DEFINITION AND MECHANISM

- Hypercapnia is defined as an elevation in the partial pressure of carbon dioxide ($PaCO_2$) above 45 mmHg
- Due to $CO_2$'s role in pH buffering, hypercapnia can lead to acid-base imbalances

## ETIOLOGY

- Hypercapnia is secondary to disease rather than a single etiology
- Hypercapnia is caused by either increased metabolic $CO_2$ production or respiratory failure
- Metabolic processes that increase $CO_2$ production:
  - Fever
  - Thyrotoxicosis
  - Increased catabolism in sepsis or steroid use
  - Overfeeding
  - Metabolic acidosis
  - Exercise
- Respiratory failure: Failure to eliminate $CO_2$ from the pulmonary system, hypoventilation secondary to decreased respiratory rate or decreased tidal volume
  - Causes:
    - Decreased central nervous system respiratory drive
    - Anatomical defects
    - Decreased neuromuscular response
    - Increased dead space within the lung
- Hypercapnia can be acute or chronic, depending on the etiology
  - Acute hypercapnia: $PaCO_2$ > 45 mmHg, $HCO_3$ within normal range (~30 mmHg), resulting decrease in pH < 7.35
  - Chronic hypercapnia: Renal compensation, $PaCO_2$ > 45 mmHg, $HCO_3$ elevated proportionally, less severe pH imbalance

## UNDERLYING PATHOLOGIES

Pathologies that lead to hypercapnia include:
- Acute respiratory distress syndrome
- Asthma exacerbation
- Central or obstructive sleep apnea
- Chronic obstructive pulmonary disease
- Drug overdose
- Exogenous $CO_2$ inhalation
- Head or cervical cord injury
- Myasthenia gravis
- Myxedema
- Obesity-hypoventilation syndrome (Pickwickian syndrome)
- Polyneuropathy
- Poliomyelitis
- Primary muscle disorders
- Porphyria
- Primary alveolar hypoventilation
- Pulmonary edema
- Tetanus

## SIGNS & SYMPTOMS

- Flushed skin
- Lethargy
- Inability to focus
- Mild headache
- Disorientation
- Dizziness
- Dyspnea
- Nausea
- Vomiting
- Fatigue
- Delirium
- Paranoia
- Depression
- Abnormal muscle twitches
- Palpitations
- Hyperventilation
- Hypoventilation
- Seizures
- Anxiety
- Syncope

## DIAGNOSIS

- Signs on physical examination may include:
  - Fever
  - Tachycardia
  - Tachypnea
  - Dyspnea
  - Altered mental status
  - Wheezing on auscultation
  - Rales on auscultation
  - Rhonchi on auscultation
  - Decreased breath sounds
  - Hyper-resonant chest on percussion
  - Increased anterior-posterior diameter of chest
  - Cardiac murmur
  - Signs of hypoxia
  - Hepatosplenomegaly
  - Neurological deficit
  - Confusion
  - Somnolence
  - Muscular weakness
  - Peripheral edema
  - Asterixis
  - Papilledema
  - Superficial vein dilation
- Diagnostic testing:
  - Complete blood count to determine anemia presence
  - Complete metabolic panel (sodium, potassium, chloride, $HCO_3$)
  - Thyroid stimulating hormone to determine underlying hypo- or hyperthyroidism
  - Arterial or venous blood gas (pH status, serum $CO_2$, serum $HCO_3$, anion gap)
  - Spirometry (forced expiratory volume over 1 second, forced vital capacity)
  - Chest X-ray
  - Chest CT
  - Echocardiography if cardiopulmonary abnormality is suspected
  - ECG to evaluate central nervous system malfunctions
  - Electromyography to evaluate neuromuscular disorders
  - Polysomnography for suspected central or obstructive sleep apnea

## MANAGEMENT

- Treat the underlying pathology
- Increase ventilation:
  - Bi-level positive airway pressure
  - Ventilation assist
  - Continuous positive airway pressure ventilation
  - Intubation with mechanical ventilation in critically ill patients
- Maintain oxygen saturation at 90% or higher
- Other options for critically ill ventilated patients:
  - Increase minute ventilation
  - Increase end-inspiratory pause prolongation
  - Buffers: sodium bicarbonate, tromethamine
  - Prone position ventilation
  - Airway pressure release ventilation
  - High-frequency oscillation ventilation
  - Extracorporeal membrane oxygenation
  - Low-flow extracorporeal $CO_2$ removal devices

---

### ■ SUGGESTED READING ■

- Rawat D, Modi P, Sharma S. Hypercapnea. [Updated 2022 Jul 25]. In: StatPearls [Internet]. Treasure Island (FL): StatPearls Publishing; 2022 Jan-. Available from: https://www.ncbi.nlm.nih.gov/books/NBK500012/
- Tiruvoipati R, Gupta S, Pilcher D, Bailey M. Management of hypercapnia in critically ill mechanically ventilated patients-A narrative review of literature. J Intensive Care Soc. 2020;21(4):327-333.

# HYPERGLYCEMIA

**86**

## LEARNING OBJECTIVES

- Recognize signs and symptoms of hyperglycemia
- Manage and prevent hyperglycemia

### DEFINITION AND MECHANISM

- An excessive amount of glucose circulates in the plasma, typically above 180-200 mg/dL (or 10-11.1 mmol/L), or fasting blood glucose above 125 mg/dL
- Symptoms of hyperglycemia develop slowly over several days or weeks
- However, symptoms may not become noticeable until even higher values (250-300 mg/dL or 13.9-16.7 mmol/L)
- Due to a low insulin level or if the body can not process insulin properly (insulin resistance)
- Increased rates of morbidity, mortality, and length of hospital stay

## SIGNS AND SYMPTOMS

- High glucose levels in the urine
- Polyphagia
- Polydipsia
- Polyuria
- Increased thirst
- Blurred vision
- Feeling weak or unusually tired
- Fatigue
- Restlessness
- Weight loss or weight gain
- Dry or itchy skin
- Seizures
- Coma

If hyperglycemia is not treated, ketoacidosis occurs:
- Fruity-smelling breath
- Dry mouth
- Abdominal pain
- Nausea and vomiting
- Shortness of breath
- Kussmaul hyperventilation
- Confusion
- Loss of consciousness

## CAUSES

- Type 1 or type 2 diabetes mellitus
- Infection/illness
- Limited physical activity
- Lack of insulin
- Certain medications: corticosteroids, octreotide, beta blockers, epinephrine, thiazide diuretics, statins, protease inhibitors, antipsychotic medications
- Excess cortisol, catecholamines, growth hormone, glucagon

Hyperglycemia may also be seen in:
- Cushing's syndrome
- Pheochromocytoma
- Acromegaly
- Hyperglucagonemia
- Hyperthyroidism

## COMPLICATIONS

- Diabetic ketoacidosis
- Peripheral neuropathy
- Diabetic retinopathy
- Nephropathy
- Gastroparesis
- Heart disease
- Stroke

## DIAGNOSIS

- Fasting glucose tests
- Glucose tolerance tests
- A1c test

# MANAGEMENT

See also diabetes mellitus type 2

## Preoperative management

- Consider:
  - □ Increased rates of infection
  - □ Medical complications including: acute kidney injury, acute coronary syndromes, and acute cerebrovascular events
- Administer longer-acting analogs and the increased or continuous subcutaneous insulin infusion to cover the fasting period

## Perioperative glycemic control

- As long as HBA1c < 8.5%, no extra precautions are warranted, except to perform regular capillary blood glucose (CBG) measurements
- Administer simultaneously glucose with premixed potassium at a fixed rate and an IV insulin infusion titrated according to the CBG ( variable rate IV insulin infusion)
- Treat a CBG > 12.0 mmol/L
- Check capillary ketones to ensure that the patient had not developed DKA

Example of variable rate continuous insulin infusion:

| Blood Glucose mg/dL (mmol/L) | If BG increased from previous measurement | BG decreased from prior measurement by less than 30 mg/dL | BG decreased from prior measurement by greater than 30 mg/dL |
|---|---|---|---|
| > 241 (13.4) | Increase rate by 3U/h | Increase rate by 3U/h | No change in rate |
| 211-240 (11.7-13.4) | Increase rate by 2U/h | Increase rate by 2U/h | No change in rate |
| 181-210 (10-11.7) | Increase rate by 1U/h | Increase rate by 1U/h | No change in rate |
| 141-180 (7.8-10) | No change in rate | No change in rate | No change in rate |
| 110-140 (6.1-7.8) | Increase rate by 1U/h | Decrease rate by ½ U/h | Hold insulin infusion |
| 100-109 (5.5-6.1) | 1. Hold insulin infusion<br>2. Re-check BG hourly<br>3. Restart infusion at ½ the prior infusion rate if BG > 180mg/dL (10mmol/L) | | |
| 71-99 (3.9-5.5) | 1. Hold insulin infusion<br>2. Check BG every 30 minutes until BG > 100mg/dL (5.5mmol/L)<br>3. Resume BG checks every hour<br>4. Restart infusion at ½ the prior infusion rate if BG > 180mg/dL (10mmol/L) | | |
| 70 (3.9) or lower | If BG 50-70 (2.8-3.9mmol/L),<br>1. Give 25mL D50<br>2. Repeat BG checks every 30 minutes until BG > 100mg/dL (5.5mmol/L)<br>If BG < 50mg/dL (2.8mmol/L)<br>1. Give 50mL D50<br>2. Repeat BG every 15 minutes until > 70mg/dL (3.9mmol/L)<br>3. When BG > 70mg/dL, BG checks every 30 minutes until > 100mg/dL (5.5mmol/L). Repeat 50mL D50 dose if BG < 50mg/dL a second time and start D10 infusion<br>4. After BG > 100mg/dL (5.5mmol/L), resume hourly BG check<br>Restart infusion at ½ the prior infusion rate if BG > 180mg/dL (5.5mmol/L) | | |

BG: Blood Glucose, mg: milligrams, dL: deciliter, mmol: millimoles, L: liter, U: Units, h: hour, D50: 50% dextrose solution, D10: 10% dextrose solution, mL: milliliters

1. If BG > 180mg/dL (10mmol/L), start insulin infusion
2. Consider bolus dose [BG – 100/40]
3. Start rate at BG/100 = U/hr
4. Check BG hourly and correct per table

## SUGGESTED READING

- Duggan EW, Carlson K, Umpierrez GE. Perioperative Hyperglycemia Management: an update. Anesthesiology. 2017;126(3):547-560.
- Stubbs, D.J., Levy, N., Dhatariya, K., 2017. The rationale and the strategies to achieve perioperative glycaemic control. BJA Education 17, 185-193.

# HYPERKALEMIA

**87**

## LEARNING OBJECTIVES

- Definition, diagnosis, and management of hyperkalemia

## DEFINITION AND MECHANISM

- Hyperkalemia is an elevated level of potassium (K+) in the blood:
  - Mild: a serum K+ of 5.5 – 5.9 mmol/L
  - Moderate: a serum K+ of 6.0-6.4 mmol/L
  - Severe: a serum K+ ≥ 6.5 mmol/L

## SIGNS AND SYMPTOMS

- Gastro-intestinal
  - Nausea
  - Vomiting
  - Diarrhea
- Neuromuscular
  - Paresthesias
  - Muscle fasciculations
  - Ascending paralysis of the extremities (quadriplegia)
- Cardiac
  - Dyspnea
  - Progressive ECG changes with increasing severity of hyperkalemia
    - Peaked T wave
    - Wide PR interval
    - Wide QRS duration
    - Loss of P wave
    - Sinusoidal wave

| Causes | |
|---|---|
| Renal failure | |
| Medications | Angiotensin-converting enzyme inhibitors (ACE-i) |
| | Angiotensin II receptor blockers (ARB) |
| | Potassium-sparing diuretics |
| | Non-steroidal anti-inflammatory drugs (NSAIDs) |
| | Beta-blockers |
| | Trimethoprim (antibiotic) |
| | Digitalis overdose |
| Tissue breakdown | Rhabdomyolysis |
| | Trauma |
| Endocrine disorders | Diabetes mellitus type 2 |
| | Adrenocortical insufficiency |

# MANAGEMENT

- First, ensure that the lab result is correct and rule out pseudohyperkalemia
- Typical examples of pseudohyperkalemia cases:
  - Poor storage of blood specimens
  - Long transport time from blood draw of the sample to processing in the lab

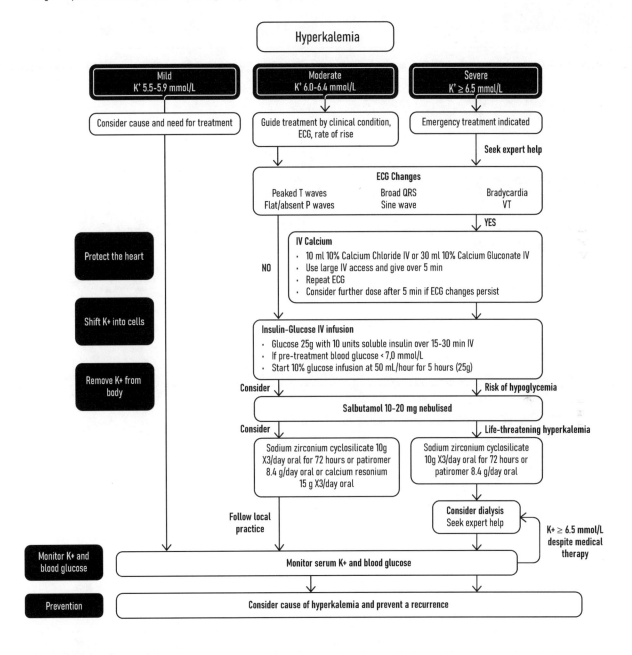

## SUGGESTED READING

- Lott C, Truhlář A, Alfonzo A, et al. European Resuscitation Council Guidelines 2021: Cardiac arrest in special circumstances [published correction appears in Resuscitation. 2021 Oct;167:91-92]. Resuscitation. 2021;161:152-219.
- Palmer BF, Carrero JJ, Clegg DJ, et al. Clinical Management of Hyperkalemia. Mayo Clin Proc. 2021;96(3):744-762.
- Palmer BF, Clegg DJ. Diagnosis and treatment of hyperkalemia. Cleve Clin J Med. 2017;84(12):934-942. doi:10.3949/ccjm.84a.17056

# HYPERNATREMIA

## LEARNING OBJECTIVES

- Definition, diagnosis, and management of hypernatremia

## DEFINITION AND MECHANISM

- Serum sodium > 145 mmol/L
- Severe symptoms usually occur at concentrations > 160 mmol/L

## SIGNS AND SYMPTOMS

| Mild symptoms | Severe symptoms |
|---|---|
| Anorexia | Vomiting |
| Muscle weakness | Seizures |
| Restlessness | Coma |
| Headache | Brain shrinkage, resulting in vascular rupture and intracranial bleeding |
| Confusion | |
| Nausea | |

## CAUSES

- Decreased intake or increased loss of water resulting in a net loss in water
- Increase in sodium intake as a cause is rare

| Causes | |
|---|---|
| Primary hypodipsia | Lack of thirst<br>Usually caused by destruction of the hypothalamic thirst center<br>Due to primary or metastatic tumors, granulomatous disease, vascular disease or trauma |
| Diabetes insipidus | Caused by a defect in the secretion of ADH in the hypothalamus or by a defective response to ADH in the renal tubules<br>Resulting in production of large amounts of urine (polyuria), thereby raising the Na+ |
| Pure hypertonic saline gain | Relatively rare cause of hypernatremia caused by the ingestion of hypertonic solutions |
| Combination of inadequate fluid intake + increased free water loss | The most common cause of hypernatremia in the elderly<br>Pathophysiology: the thirst mechanism weakens and renal function declines with increasing age<br>Frail elderly people, particularly those living alone may also have difficulties obtaining adequate fluid volumes (fever, heat, burns may cause water loss) |
| Hyperglycemia | |
| Hyperaldosteronism | |

# MANAGEMENT

- Estimate volume status and total body water deficit with this formula: $WD1 = 0.6 \times bodymass \times [1 - (140 \div Na+)]$
- Treat the underlying cause and correct the water deficit
  - First choice of fluid: oral free water
  - IV: Use isotonic solutions
  - Isotonic saline is the first fluid of choice and consider hypotonic solution based by vascular bed filling state and severity of hypernatremia
  - Do NOT rapidly correct or overcorrect, this increases the risk for cerebral edema
- A correction rate of 1 mmol/L per hour is considered a safe rate of correction
  - NOTE: This rate is NOT recommended in chronic hypernatremia!
- In patients where hypernatremia is present for a longer period, the sodium level should be corrected at a rate of 0.5 mmol/L per hour, max 8 – 10 mmol/L per 24 hours
- In patients with acute hypernatremia, quick correction of sodium can be perfomed safely with isotonic saline or water without the risk of cerebral edema

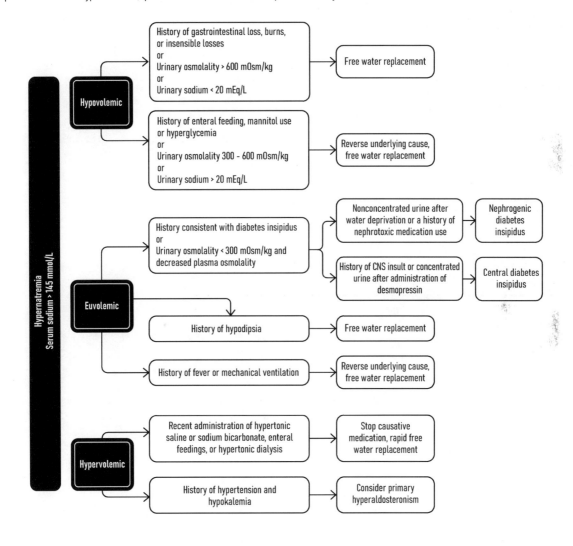

- Braun MM, Barstow CH, Pyzocha NJ. Diagnosis and management of sodium disorders: hyponatremia and hypernatremia. Am Fam Physician. 2015;91(5):299-307.

**89**

# HYPERPARATHYROIDISM

## LEARNING OBJECTIVES

- Describe hyperparathyroidism
- Recognize the symptoms and signs of hypercalcemia, related to hyperparathyroidism
- Anesthetic management of a patient with hyperparathyroidism

## DEFINITION AND MECHANISM

- Hyperparathyroidism (HPT) is a condition in which the parathyroid glands produce too much parathyroid hormone (PTH)
- PTH plays an important role in maintaining normal calcium homeostasis
- The main effector sites responding directly or indirectly to PTH are the intestines, kidneys, and bone
- HPT ultimately results in hypercalcemia

## CLASSIFICATION

- **Primary HPT:** Hyperfunction of the parathyroid glands (i.e., adenoma, carcinoma, or hyperplasia) leading to an overproduction of PTH
- **Secondary HPT:** Appropriate compensatory response of the parathyroid glands to secrete more PTH in response to a condition (i.e., chronic kidney disease, vitamin D deficiency) that produces hypocalcemia
- **Tertiary HPT:** Long-standing secondary HPT starts to behave like primary HPT, usually associated with advanced kidney failure
- **Ectopic HPT:** Secretion of PTH by tissues other than the parathyroid glands

## SIGNS AND SYMPTOMS

The symptoms of HPT are caused by hypercalcemia:

- **Cardiovascular:** Hypertension, shortened QT interval, prolonged PR interval, hypovolemia, conduction blockade
- **Neurological:** Mental status changes, weakness, lethargy
- **Respiratory:** Potential respiratory muscle weakness, poor clearance of secretions
- **Musculoskeletal:** Muscle weakness, osteoporosis, pathological fractures, bone pains
- **Gastrointestinal:** Abdominal pain, peptic ulcer, pancreatitis, nausea/vomiting, increase aspiration risk
- **Renal:** Polyuria, polydipsia, renal stones, renal failure
- **Hematopoietic:** Anemia

## RISK FACTORS

- **Age:** Older adults ( > 60 years)
- **Sex:** Female sex
- **Genetic conditions:** Multiple endocrine neoplasia syndromes (MEN)

# PATHOPHYSIOLOGY

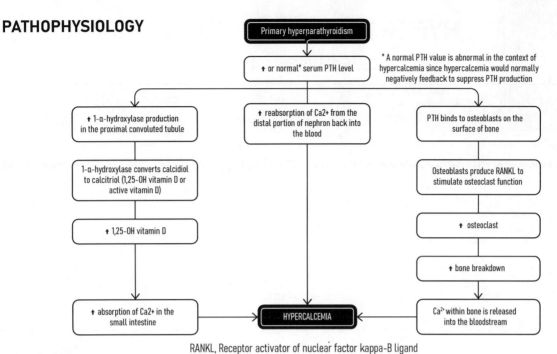

RANKL, Receptor activator of nuclear factor kappa-B ligand

# TREATMENT

- Primary HPT: Parathyroidectomy
- Secondary HPT: Treat underlying cause (i.e., chronic kidney failure, vitamin D deficiency)
- Tertiary HPT: Parathyroidectomy
- Calcimimetics are used in patients with primary HPT unable to undergo parathyroidectomy and for patients with secondary HPT on dialysis

# MANAGEMENT

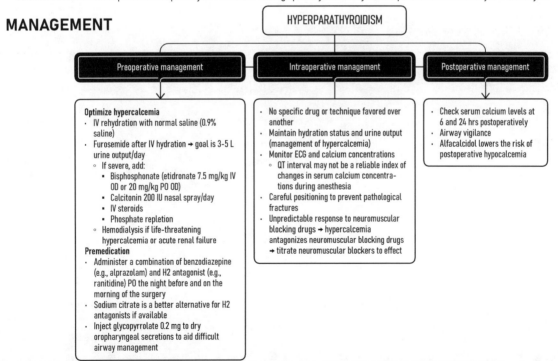

---

## SUGGESTED READING

- Malhotra S, Sodhi V. Anaesthesia for thyroid and parathyroid surgery. Continuing Education in Anaesthesia Critical Care & Pain. 2007;7(2):55-58.

# HYPERTHYROIDISM/THYROID STORM

## LEARNING OBJECTIVES

- Describe the pathophysiology and symptoms of hyperthyroidism
- Diagnose and treat hyperthyroidism
- Manage patients with hyperthyroidism or thyroid storm

## DEFINITION AND MECHANISM

- Hyperthyroidism is a syndrome associated with excess thyroid hormone production
- Can lead to thyroid storm, an acute and life-threatening complication
- Most commonly caused by Graves disease (young population) and toxic multinodular goiter (older population)
- Other causes: Iodine-induced hyperthyroidism (Jod-Basedow phenomenon), thyroid adenomas, de Quervain thyroiditis (subacute thyroiditis), postpartum thyroiditis, factitious thyroiditis (thyrotoxicosis factitia)

## PATHOPHYSIOLOGY

- Graves disease
  - Thyroid-stimulating antibodies mimicking the effects of thyroid-stimulating hormone (TSH)
  - Typical signs: Edema of retro-orbital tissues, pretibial myxedema
- Toxic multinodular goiter
  - Palpable thyroid nodules leading to excess thyroid hormone production
- Thyroid adenoma
  - Solitary palpable nodule causing hyperthyroidism
- Thyroiditis
  - Transient increase in circulating thyroid hormone resulting from mechanical disruption of thyroid follicles
- Iodine-induced hyperthyroidism
  - Typically iatrogenic
  - Due to administration of iodine-containing medications (e.g., contrast media, amiodarone)

## SIGNS & SYMPTOMS

- Weight loss despite increased appetite
- Palpitation
- Nervousness
- Tremors
- Dyspnea
- Fatigability
- Diarrhea
- Increased gastrointestinal motility
- Muscle weakness
- Heat intolerance
- Diaphoresis
- Goiter
- Palpable nodules
- Painful thyroid

## DIAGNOSIS

- Initial test: Serum TSH (decreased)
- Free T3 and T4 (increased)
- ECG when atrial fibrillation is suspected
- Palpitation of the thyroid gland
- 24-hour radioactive iodine (RAIU) uptake to distinguish between etiologies
  - Increased RAIU: Graves disease, toxic multinodular goiter, thyroid adenoma
  - Decreased RAIU: Subacute thyroiditis, painless thyroiditis, iodine-induced hyperthyroidism, factitious hyperthyroidism
- Thyroid receptor antibody measurement as an alternative diagnosis for Graves disease
- Radioisotope thyroid scan

# TREATMENT

- Symptomatic
  - Beta-blockers or calcium channel blockers
- Definitive
  - Radioactive iodine
  - Thionamide
  - Subtotal thyroidectomy
  - Clinical assessment and free T4 monitoring are essential for all treatments

# MANAGEMENT

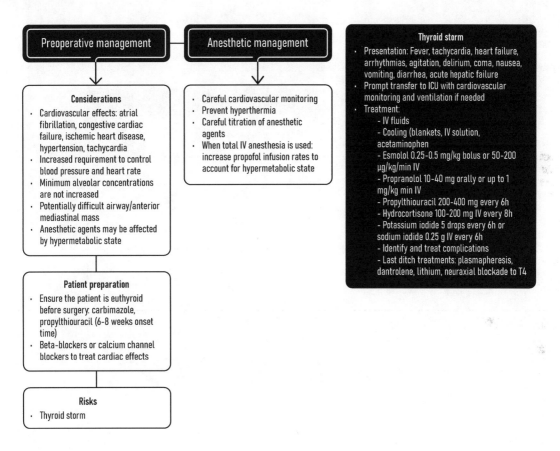

**Preoperative management** → **Anesthetic management**

**Considerations**
- Cardiovascular effects: atrial fibrillation, congestive cardiac failure, ischemic heart disease, hypertension, tachycardia
- Increased requirement to control blood pressure and heart rate
- Minimum alveolar concentrations are not increased
- Potentially difficult airway/anterior mediastinal mass
- Anesthetic agents may be affected by hypermetabolic state

**Patient preparation**
- Ensure the patient is euthyroid before surgery: carbimazole, propylthiouracil (6-8 weeks onset time)
- Beta-blockers or calcium channel blockers to treat cardiac effects

**Risks**
- Thyroid storm

**Anesthetic management considerations**
- Careful cardiovascular monitoring
- Prevent hyperthermia
- Careful titration of anesthetic agents
- When total IV anesthesia is used: increase propofol infusion rates to account for hypermetabolic state

**Thyroid storm**
- Presentation: Fever, tachycardia, heart failure, arrhythmias, agitation, delirium, coma, nausea, vomiting, diarrhea, acute hepatic failure
- Prompt transfer to ICU with cardiovascular monitoring and ventilation if needed
- Treatment:
  - IV fluids
  - Cooling (blankets, IV solution, acetaminophen)
  - Esmolol 0.25-0.5 mg/kg bolus or 50-200 μg/kg/min IV
  - Propranolol 10-40 mg orally or up to 1 mg/kg min IV
  - Propylthiouracil 200-400 mg every 6h
  - Hydrocortisone 100-200 mg IV every 8h
  - Potassium iodide 5 drops every 6h or sodium iodide 0.25 g IV every 6h
  - Identify and treat complications
  - Last ditch treatments: plasmapheresis, dantrolene, lithium, neuraxial blockade to T4

# KEEP IN MIND

- Acute coronary syndrome may be complicated with thyroid dysfunction
- Close monitoring is essential with propylthiouracil administration in pregnant patients as overcorrection can potentially cause fetal hypothyroidism

## SUGGESTED READING

- Carroll R, Matfin G. Endocrine and metabolic emergencies: thyroid storm. Ther Adv Endocrinol Metab. 2010;1(3):139-145.
- Farling PA. Thyroid disease. BJA: British Journal of Anaesthesia. 2000;85(1):15-28.
- Mathew P, Rawla P. Hyperthyroidism. [Updated 2022 Jul 23]. In: StatPearls [Internet]. Treasure Island (FL): StatPearls Publishing; 2022 Jan-. Available from: https://www.ncbi.nlm.nih.gov/books/NBK537053/
- Pokhrel B, Aiman W, Bhusal K. Thyroid Storm. [Updated 2022 Oct 6]. In: StatPearls [Internet]. Treasure Island (FL): StatPearls Publishing; 2022 Jan-. Available from: https://www.ncbi.nlm.nih.gov/books/NBK448095/

# HYPOKALEMIA

## LEARNING OBJECTIVES

- Definition, diagnosis, and management of hypokalemia

**DEFINITION AND MECHANISM**

- Hypokalemia is a reduced level of potassium (K+) in the blood
- Serum potassium < 3.5 mmol/L
- Mild low potassium does not typically cause symptoms
- Life-threatening symptoms usually occur at concentrations < 2.5 mmol/L

| Causes | |
|---|---|
| Gastrointestinal loss | Chronic diarrhea |
| An intracellular shift of K+ | Due to insulin administration or excessive insulin secretion |
| Renal loss | |
| Cushing's syndrome | |
| Primary hyperaldosteronism | |
| Rare syndromes | Bartter syndrome<br>Gitelman syndrome<br>Liddle syndrome<br>Hypokalemic periodic paralysis<br>Hypothermia |
| Hypomagnesemia | |
| Medications | Diuretics (thiazides, loop-, and osmotic diuretics)<br>Laxatives<br>Beta-2-agonists (albuterol, terbutaline)<br>Amphotericin B<br>Antibiotics (carbenicillin and penicillin in high doses)<br>Theophylline |

## SIGNS AND SYMPTOMS

- Gastrointestinal:
  - Nausea
  - Constipation
  - Gastrointestinal paralysis
- Neuromuscular:
  - Paresthesias
  - Muscle cramps
  - Ascending paralysis of the extremities (quadriplegia)
- Respiratory failure

- Cardiac:
  - Heart failure
  - Progressive ECG changes
    - Depressed ST segment
    - Diphasic T wave
    - Prominent U wave

# MANAGEMENT

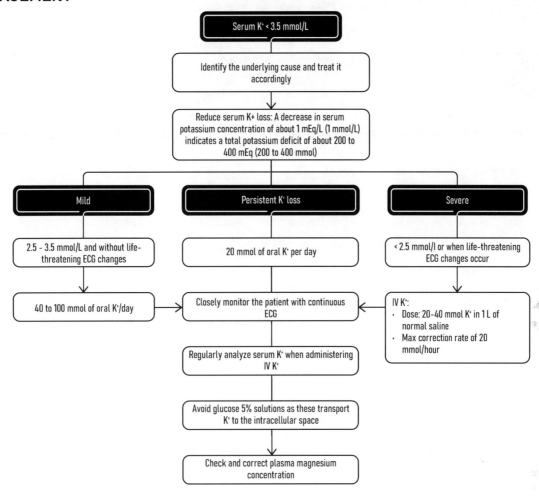

```
                    ┌──────────────────────────┐
                    │   Serum K⁺ < 3.5 mmol/L   │
                    └──────────────────────────┘
                                 │
                    ┌──────────────────────────┐
                    │ Identify the underlying   │
                    │ cause and treat it        │
                    │ accordingly               │
                    └──────────────────────────┘
                                 │
                    ┌──────────────────────────────────┐
                    │ Reduce serum K+ loss: A decrease  │
                    │ in serum potassium concentration  │
                    │ of about 1 mEq/L (1 mmol/L)       │
                    │ indicates a total potassium       │
                    │ deficit of about 200 to 400 mEq   │
                    │ (200 to 400 mmol)                 │
                    └──────────────────────────────────┘
```

**Mild**

2.5 - 3.5 mmol/L and without life-threatening ECG changes

40 to 100 mmol of oral K⁺/day

**Persistent K⁺ loss**

20 mmol of oral K⁺ per day

Closely monitor the patient with continuous ECG

Regularly analyze serum K⁺ when administering IV K⁺

Avoid glucose 5% solutions as these transport K⁺ to the intracellular space

Check and correct plasma magnesium concentration

**Severe**

< 2.5 mmol/l or when life-threatening ECG changes occur

IV K⁺:
- Dose: 20-40 mmol K⁺ in 1 L of normal saline
- Max correction rate of 20 mmol/hour

## SUGGESTED READING

- Kardalas E, Paschou SA, Anagnostis P, Muscogiuri G, Siasos G, Vryonidou A. Hypokalemia: a clinical update. Endocr Connect. 2018;7(4):R135-R146.
- Viera AJ, Wouk N. Potassium Disorders: Hypokalemia and Hyperkalemia. Am Fam Physician. 2015;92(6):487-495.

# HYPONATREMIA

**92**

## LEARNING OBJECTIVES

- Defining, diagnosing, and managing hyponatremia

## DEFINITION AND MECHANISM

- Hyponatremia is defined as:
  - Mild: a serum sodium concentration between 130-135 mmol/L
  - Moderate: a serum sodium concentration between 125-129 mmol/L
  - Severe: A serum sodium concentration < 125 mmol/L
- Hyponatremia is acute if it is documented to exist < 48 hours and chronic if it is documented to exist for at least 48 hours
- If unsure, consider chronic hyponatremia unless there is clinical or anamnestic evidence of the contrary

## SIGNS AND SYMPTOMS

- Moderate symptoms
  - Nausea without vomiting
  - Confusion
  - Headache
- Severe symptoms
- ECG changes
  - Prolonged PR
  - Wide QRS
  - Sinus arrest
  - Vomiting
  - Cardiorespiratory distress
  - Somnolence
  - Seizures
  - Coma

## DIFFERENTIAL DIAGNOSIS

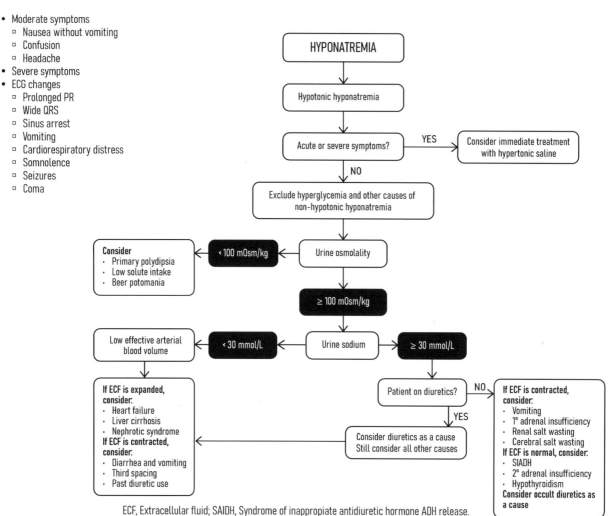

ECF, Extracellular fluid; SAIDH, Syndrome of inappropiate antidiuretic hormone ADH release.

# MANAGEMENT IN ADULTS

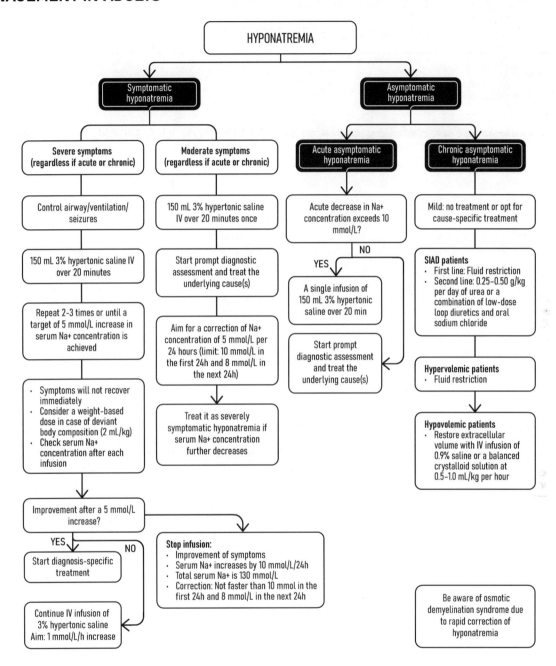

**SUGGESTED READING**

- Hoorn EJ, Zietse R. Diagnosis and Treatment of Hyponatremia: Compilation of the Guidelines. J Am Soc Nephrol. 2017;28(5):1340-1349.
- Spasovski G, Vanholder R, Allolio B, et al. Clinical practice guideline on diagnosis and treatment of hyponatraemia [published correction appears in Nephrol Dial Transplant. 2014 Jun;40(6):924]. Nephrol Dial Transplant. 2014;29 Suppl 2:i1-i39.

# HYPOPARATHYROIDISM

## LEARNING OBJECTIVES

- Describe hypoparathyroidism
- Recognize the symptoms and signs of hypocalcemia, related to hypoparathyroidism
- Anesthetic management of a patient with hypoparathyroidism

## DEFINITION AND MECHANISM

- Hypoparathyroidism is a condition in which the parathyroid glands do not produce enough parathyroid hormone (PTH)
- PTH plays an important role in maintaining normal calcium homeostasis
- The main effector sites responding directly or indirectly to PTH are the intestines, kidneys, and bone
- Hypoparathyroidism ultimately results in hypocalcemia and hyperphosphatemia

### Classification

- **Acquired hypoparathyroidism:** Develops after the removal of, or trauma to, the parathyroid glands due to thyroid surgery (thyroidectomy), parathyroid surgery (parathyroidectomy), or other surgical interventions in the central part of the neck (i.e., chemotherapy or radiation); hypomagnesemia
- **Autoimmune hypoparathyroidism:** The immune system mistakenly attacks the parathyroid glands or PTH
- **Congenital hypoparathyroidism:** Occurs at birth resulting from gene mutations or if someone is born without parathyroid glands (i.e., DiGeorge syndrome)
- **Familial (inherited) hypoparathyroidism:** Genetically passed down from family

## SIGNS AND SYMPTOMS

The symptoms of hypoparathyroidism are caused by hypocalcemia:
- **Acute:** Perioral paresthesia, restlessness, neuromuscular irritability, and stridor
- **Chronic:** Fatigue, muscle cramps, severe spasms (tetany), lethargy, personality changes, and cerebral defects
Neuromuscular signs:
- **Positive Chvostek sign:** Facial contracture elicited by tapping the facial nerve
- **Positive Trousseau sign:** Fingers and wrist contracture elicited by inflation of a blood pressure cuff above the patient's systolic blood pressure for $\geq 3$ minutes

## COMPLICATIONS

- Seizures
- Hypotension
- QT prolongation and arrhythmias
- Congestive heart failure
- Bronchospasm, laryngospasm, and resulting respiratory failure
- Problems with kidney function (e.g., kidney stones and chronic kidney failure) due to treatment with calcium and vitamin D supplements
- Hardening and changes in the shape of the bones, and poor growth
- Delayed mental development in children
- Clouded vision due to cataracts

## RISK FACTORS

- Recent neck surgery, particularly if the thyroid was involved
- Family history
- Certain autoimmune or endocrine conditions (e.g., Addison's disease)

# PATHOPHYSIOLOGY

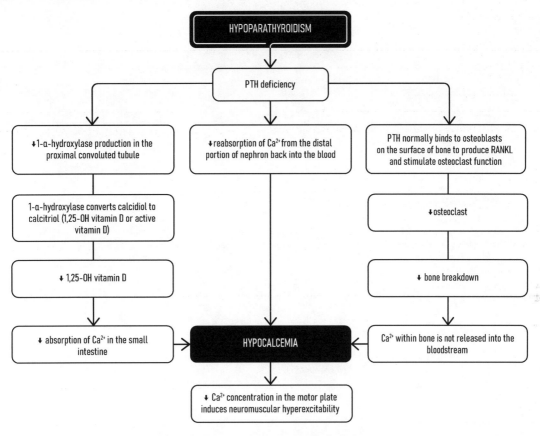

RANKL, Receptor activator of nuclear factor kappa beta.

## TREATMENT

- **Acute hypocalcemia:** IV infusion of calcium (e.g., calcium chloride or calcium gluconate) until the neuromuscular irritability resolves
- **Chronic hypocalcemia:** Oral calcium and vitamin D supplements

# MANAGEMENT

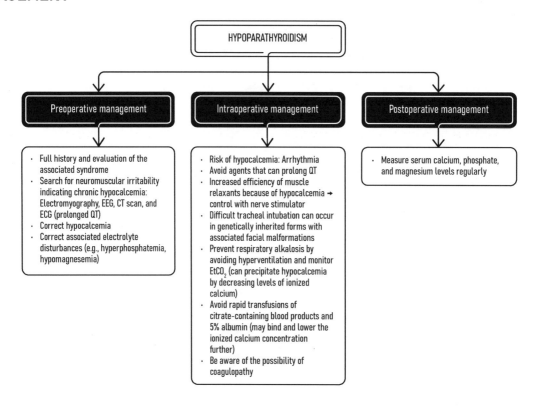

```
                          ┌─────────────────────────┐
                          │    HYPOPARATHYROIDISM    │
                          └─────────────────────────┘
```

**Preoperative management**

- Full history and evaluation of the associated syndrome
- Search for neuromuscular irritability indicating chronic hypocalcemia: Electromyography, EEG, CT scan, and ECG (prolonged QT)
- Correct hypocalcemia
- Correct associated electrolyte disturbances (e.g., hyperphosphatemia, hypomagnesemia)

**Intraoperative management**

- Risk of hypocalcemia: Arrhythmia
- Avoid agents that can prolong QT
- Increased efficiency of muscle relaxants because of hypocalcemia → control with nerve stimulator
- Difficult tracheal intubation can occur in genetically inherited forms with associated facial malformations
- Prevent respiratory alkalosis by avoiding hyperventilation and monitor $EtCO_2$ (can precipitate hypocalcemia by decreasing levels of ionized calcium)
- Avoid rapid transfusions of citrate-containing blood products and 5% albumin (may bind and lower the ionized calcium concentration further)
- Be aware of the possibility of coagulopathy

**Postoperative management**

- Measure serum calcium, phosphate, and magnesium levels regularly

## SUGGESTED READING

- Hypoparathyroidism. In: Bissonnette B, Luginbuehl I, Marciniak B, Dalens BJ. eds. Syndromes: Rapid Recognition and Perioperative Implications. Mgraw Hill; 2006. Accessed March 06, 2023. https://accessanesthesiology.mhmedical.com/content.aspx?bookid=852&sectionid=49517707

Hypoparathyroidism

# HYPOTHYROIDISM

## LEARNING OBJECTIVES

- Describe the etiology and symptoms of hypothyroidism
- Diagnose and treat hypothyroidism
- Manage patients with hypothyroidism presenting for surgery

## DEFINITION AND MECHANISM

- Hypothyroidism results from low levels of thyroid hormone
- Autoimmune thyroid disease and lack of dietary iodine are the most common causes
- Can range from asymptomatic to myxedema coma
- Can be treated with exogenous thyroid hormone

## ETIOLOGY

- Primary hypothyroidism: The thyroid gland does not produce adequate amounts of thyroid hormone
  - Iodine deficiency
  - Autoimmune (Hashimoto thyroiditis)
  - Medications (amiodarone, thalidomide, oral tyrosine kinase inhibitors, stavudine, interferon, bexarotene, perchlorate, rifampin, ethionamide, phenobarbital, phenytoin, carbamazepine, interleukin-2, lithium)
  - Thyroid radioactive iodine therapy
  - Thyroid surgery
  - Radiotherapy to head or neck area
  - Subacute granulomatous thyroiditis
  - Postpartum thyroiditis
- Secondary hypothyroidism: Thyroid gland is normal, pathology is related to pituitary gland or hypothalamus
  - Neoplastic, infiltrative, inflammatory, genetic, or iatrogenic disorders of the pituitary or hypothalamus
  - Sheehan syndrome
  - Thyrotropin-releasing hormone (TRH) resistance
  - TRH deficiency
  - Lymphocytic hypophysitis
  - Radiation therapy to the brain
  - Medications such as dopamine, prednisone, or opioids

## RISK FACTORS

- Women > 60 years of age
- Pregnancy
- History of head and neck irradiation
- Autoimmune disorders
- Type I diabetes mellitus
- Positive thyroid peroxidase antibodies
- Family history of hypothyroidism

# SIGNS & SYMPTOMS

- Cold intolerance
- Puffiness
- Decreased sweating
- Dry skin
- Hair loss
- Constipation
- Fatigue
- Muscle cramps
- Sleep disturbance
- Menstrual cycle abnormalities
- Weight gain
- Galactorrhea
- Depression
- Anxiety
- Psychosis
- Cognitive impairments
- Carpal tunnel syndrome
- Sleep apnea
- Hyponatremia
- Hypercholesterolemia
- Congestive heart failure
- Prolonged QT interval
- Fullness of throat
- Painless thyroid enlargement
- Episodic neck pain/sore throat
- Pallor and jaundice
- Dull facial expressions
- Macroglossia
- Bradycardia
- Pericardial effusion
- Prolonged ankle reflex relaxation time

# DIAGNOSIS

- Serum thyroid stimulating hormone (TSH) level to test for primary hypothyroidism
- Serum-free T4 level to test for secondary hypothyroidism
- Serum Cortisol levels
- Serum anti-thyroid antibodies to test for autoimmune thyroid disease
- Other laboratory tests may reveal hyperlipidemia, elevated serum creatine kinase (CK), elevated hepatic enzymes, anemia, blood urea nitrogen, creatinine, and uric acid levels

# DIFFERENTIAL DIAGNOSIS

- Euthyroid sick syndrome
- Goiter
- Myxedema coma
- Anemia
- Riedel thyroiditis
- Subacute thyroiditis
- Thyroid lymphoma
- Iodine deficiency
- Addison disease
- Chronic fatigue syndrome
- Depression
- Dysmenorrhea
- Erectile dysfunction
- Familial hypercholesterolemia
- Infertility

# TREATMENT

- Main treatment: levothyroxine monotherapy 1.6 µg/kg per day
- Lower the dose in elderly and atrial fibrillation patients
- IV levothyroxine in patients who cannot take it orally (half of the oral dose)
- Treat adrenal insufficiency first

Hypothyroidism

# MANAGEMENT

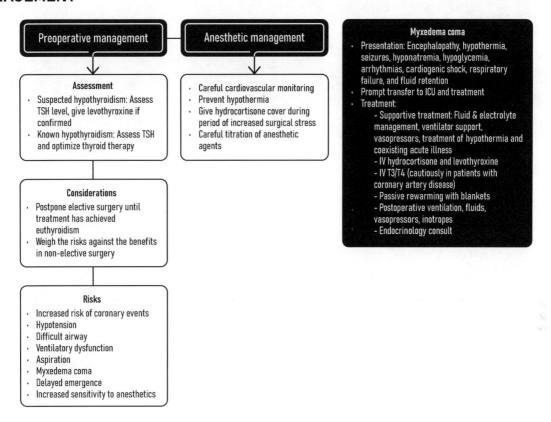

**Preoperative management** — **Anesthetic management**

**Assessment**
- Suspected hypothyroidism: Assess TSH level, give levothyroxine if confirmed
- Known hypothyroidism: Assess TSH and optimize thyroid therapy

**Anesthetic management**
- Careful cardiovascular monitoring
- Prevent hypothermia
- Give hydrocortisone cover during period of increased surgical stress
- Careful titration of anesthetic agents

**Considerations**
- Postpone elective surgery until treatment has achieved euthyroidism
- Weigh the risks against the benefits in non-elective surgery

**Risks**
- Increased risk of coronary events
- Hypotension
- Difficult airway
- Ventilatory dysfunction
- Aspiration
- Myxedema coma
- Delayed emergence
- Increased sensitivity to anesthetics

**Myxedema coma**
- Presentation: Encephalopathy, hypothermia, seizures, hyponatremia, hypoglycemia, arrhythmias, cardiogenic shock, respiratory failure, and fluid retention
- Prompt transfer to ICU and treatment
- Treatment:
    - Supportive treatment: Fluid & electrolyte management, ventilator support, vasopressors, treatment of hypothermia and coexisting acute illness
    - IV hydrocortisone and levothyroxine
    - IV T3/T4 (cautiously in patients with coronary artery disease)
    - Passive rewarming with blankets
    - Postoperative ventilation, fluids, vasopressors, inotropes
    - Endocrinology consult

TSH, thyroid stimulating hormone; T3, triiodothyronine; T4, thyroxine

## SUGGESTED READING

- Farling PA. Thyroid disease. BJA: British Journal of Anaesthesia. 2000;85(1):15-28.
- Palace MR. Perioperative Management of Thyroid Dysfunction. Health Serv Insights. 2017;10:1178632916689677. Published 2017 Feb 20.
- Patil N, Rehman A, Jialal I. Hypothyroidism. [Updated 2022 Aug 8]. In: StatPearls [Internet]. Treasure Island (FL): StatPearls Publishing; 2022 Jan-. Available from: https://www.ncbi.nlm.nih.gov/books/NBK519536/

# MALNUTRITION

## LEARNING OBJECTIVES

- Define malnutrition
- Describe how malnutrition affects different body systems
- Anesthetic management of the malnourished patient

## DEFINITION AND MECHANISM

- Malnutrition or nutritional deficiency occurs when there is a negative balance between nutritional supply and demand
  - Reduced supply states are caused by mechanical obstruction, poor absorption, and psychogenic eating disorders (e.g., anorexia nervosa)
  - Increased demand occurs in hypermetabolic states (e.g., sepsis, trauma, and cancer)
- It is a deficiency, excess, or imbalance of energy, protein, and other nutrients, which adversely affects the body's tissues and form
- Malnutrition occurs in approximately half of the surgical patients, resulting in an increased incidence of postoperative complications
- The main symptoms are unintentional weight loss ($\geq$ 5-10% over 3-6 months) and a low body weight (BMI < 18.5 kg/m2)

**Note:** Malnutrition involves both undernutrition and overnutrition, however, this article will only discuss undernutrition, for overnutrition the reader is referred to the obesity considerations

## SIGNS AND SYMPTOMS

Body systems affected by malnutrition

| System | Features |
|---|---|
| Central nervous system | Impaired mental ability<br>Mental depression<br>Depressed cognitive function<br>Fatigue and generalized weakness |
| Musculoskeletal | Reduced muscle mass and strength<br>Histologically confirmed myopathy in severe anorexia nervosa patients<br>Reduced bone mass, osteopenia, and osteoporosis with secondary fractures<br>Impaired thermoregulation<br>Impaired wound healing |
| Cardiovascular | Reduction in cardiac output<br>Hypotension and bradycardia<br>Increased risk of arrhythmia due to vitamin and electrolyte disturbance<br>Mitral valve prolapse<br>Loss of cardiac muscle mass with associated reduced left ventricular function and ejection fraction<br>Increased vagal tone<br>Peripheral vasoconstriction<br>Sinus arrest and wandering atrial pacemakers<br>ECG changes: Prolonged QTc, ST depression and T-wave inversion |
| Respiratory | Reduced respiratory muscle strength and function<br>Spontaneous pneumothorax<br>Pneumomediastinum from persistent vomiting<br>Decreased respiratory compliance (due to decreased elasticity of lung tissues) |
| Renal | Reduced glomerular filtration rate<br>Total body water proportionally higher<br>Proteinuria<br>High urea due to dehydration |

| System | Features |
|---|---|
| Gastrointestinal | Decreased enteral feeding leading to gut atrophy, bacterial translocation, and impaired immune function<br>Esophagitis and Mallory-Weiss tear from purging<br>Gastric dilatation<br>Paradoxical decrease in gastric emptying time |
| Micronutrient disturbances | Vitamin A insufficiency - blindness (xerophthalmia due to corneal ulceration is the leading cause of childhood blindness), immunosuppression<br>Reduced iron, ferritin, and iron deficiency anemia<br>Low folic acid and zinc levels |
| Electrolyte disturbances | Hypokalemia (due to repeated purging and vomiting)<br>Hypocalcemia (prolonged nondepolarizing muscle relaxation action)<br>Hypoglycemia and hypoglycemic coma<br>Metabolic alkalosis (more likely in patients who purge)<br>Increased cortisol and corticotrophin-releasing hormone levels with blunted response<br>Starvation ketosis/ketoacidosis |
| Hematological | Leucopenia<br>Often normal immune function until 50% drop in normal expected body weight<br>Elevated liver transaminases<br>Anemia<br>Pancytopenia |
| Pharmacological | Delayed or reduced absorption of drugs<br>Hypoalbuminemia increases free fraction of drugs, decreased protein binding occurs<br>Pseudocholinesterase deficiency in severe malnutrition (severe albumin < 2 g/dL) → prolonged neuromuscular blockade with succinylcholine and mivacurium<br>Lower total body mass means reduced drug doses required and lowered thresholds for toxicity<br>Neostigmine, edrophinium, and catecholamines can cause life-threatening arrhythmias |

## RISK FACTORS

- Lack of breastfeeding
- Anorexia nervosa
- Bulimia nervosa
- Bariatric surgery
- Gastroenteritis
- Pneumonia
- Malaria
- Measles
- HIV/AIDS
- Hyperemesis
- Abnormal nutrient loss due to diarrhea or chronic small bowel illnesses (e.g., Crohn's disease, untreated celiac disease)
- Poverty
- Homelessness
- Social isolation

## TREATMENT

- Improve nutrition
- Supplementation
- Ready-to-use therapeutic foods
- Treat underlying cause

# MANAGEMENT

```
                         ┌─────────────────────────────┐
                         │        MALNUTRITION         │
                         └─────────────────────────────┘
```

**Preoperative assessment**

**Nutritional assessment**
- Quantify overall daily calorie intake
- Balanced diet or lacking in crucial micronutrients?
- **Moderate malnutrition:** 15% loss of ideal body weight
- **Severe malnutrition:** 30% loss of ideal body weight

**Clinical assessment**
- Assess each organ system for symptoms and signs of dysfunction
- Optimize nutrition preoperatively
- General inspection: Evidence of fat and muscle loss, quality of skin, hair, and fingernails
- Reduced pulmonary function: Complaints of shortness of breath on minimal exertion
- Heart failure: Peripheral edema, orthopnea
- Recent history of multiple infections
- Presence of a feeding tube

**Investigations**
- **Routine blood:** Full blood count, creatinine and electrolytes, liver function tests, calcium, phosphate, magnesium, glucose, transferrin, and albumin
- **Urinalysis:** Proteinuria and ketonuria
- **ECG:** Cardiovascular complications or electrolyte imbalance
- **Echocardiogram:** Reduced myocardial contractility
- **Pulmonary function tests:** FVC 50 mL/kg in the absence of obvious lung disease, reduced maximal ventilatory volume

**Preoperative optimization**

- Discuss preoperative nutrition with surgeons and dieticians
- Delay surgery where possible to allow for nutritional assessment and implementation of a feeding plan
- Adequate hydration and correction of electrolyte abnormalities for emergency cases
- Correct dietary problems before major surgery in elective cases with albumin < 34 g/dL or lymphocyte count < 1400
- Use total parenteral nutrition (TPN) in case of intestinal failure
  ○ Examine patients on TPN for potential complications (e.g., improper central line placement, line infection, fluid overload, and metabolic disturbances [hyperglycemia, hypercarbia, hypokalemia, hypomagnesemia, hypophosphatemia])
  ○ Do not suddenly stop TPN → risk of rebound hypoglycemia
    - Continue TPN at the same rate, controlling hyperglycemia perioperatively as in the diabetic patient
    - Wean to half the maintenance rate over 12 hours preoperatively
    - Replace with 10% glucose infused at the same rate (in unstable patients)
- Enteral route in other cases
- Start feeding (enteral or parenteral) 7-10 days preoperatively for the maximum nutritional benefit
- Take appropriate precautions to prevent and monitor for refeeding syndrome
- Identify and correct any existing infections
- Blood transfusion for anemia and correction of clotting abnormalities

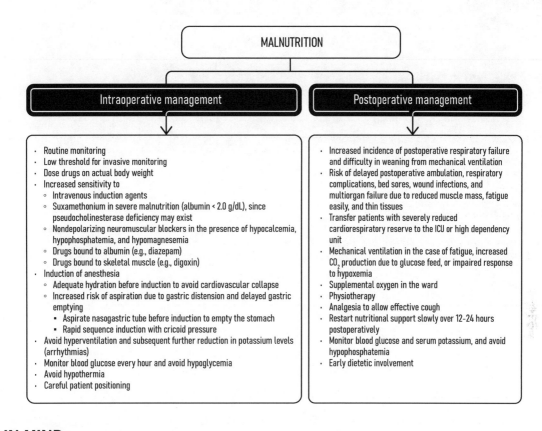

```
                    ┌─────────────────────────┐
                    │       MALNUTRITION       │
                    └─────────────────────────┘
                   ┌───────────────┴───────────────┐
        ┌──────────────────────┐      ┌──────────────────────┐
        │ Intraoperative       │      │ Postoperative        │
        │ management           │      │ management           │
        └──────────────────────┘      └──────────────────────┘
```

**Intraoperative management**

- Routine monitoring
- Low threshold for invasive monitoring
- Dose drugs on actual body weight
- Increased sensitivity to
  - Intravenous induction agents
  - Suxamethonium in severe malnutrition (albumin < 2.0 g/dL), since pseudocholinesterase deficiency may exist
  - Nondepolarizing neuromuscular blockers in the presence of hypocalcemia, hypophosphatemia, and hypomagnesemia
  - Drugs bound to albumin (e.g., diazepam)
  - Drugs bound to skeletal muscle (e.g., digoxin)
- Induction of anesthesia
  - Adequate hydration before induction to avoid cardiovascular collapse
  - Increased risk of aspiration due to gastric distension and delayed gastric emptying
    - Aspirate nasogastric tube before induction to empty the stomach
    - Rapid sequence induction with cricoid pressure
- Avoid hyperventilation and subsequent further reduction in potassium levels (arrhythmias)
- Monitor blood glucose every hour and avoid hypoglycemia
- Avoid hypothermia
- Careful patient positioning

**Postoperative management**

- Increased incidence of postoperative respiratory failure and difficulty in weaning from mechanical ventilation
- Risk of delayed postoperative ambulation, respiratory complications, bed sores, wound infections, and multiorgan failure due to reduced muscle mass, fatigue easily, and thin tissues
- Transfer patients with severely reduced cardiorespiratory reserve to the ICU or high dependency unit
- Mechanical ventilation in the case of fatigue, increased $CO_2$ production due to glucose feed, or impaired response to hypoxemia
- Supplemental oxygen in the ward
- Physiotherapy
- Analgesia to allow effective cough
- Restart nutritional support slowly over 12-24 hours postoperatively
- Monitor blood glucose and serum potassium, and avoid hypophosphatemia
- Early dietetic involvement

## KEEP IN MIND

- Malnutrition affects all systems, organs, and cells
- Treat all malnourished patients as if they have a full stomach (increased aspiration risk)
- Careful adjustment of drug dosing and understanding of the pharmacokinetics specific to the malnourished patient is vital

## SUGGESTED READING

- Edwards S. Anaesthetising the malnourished patient. Update in Anaesthesia. 2016;31:31-37.
- Pollard BJ, Kitchen G. Handbook of Clinical Anaesthesia. 4th ed. Taylor & Francis group; 2018. Chapter 4 Gastrointestinal tract, Jackson MJ.

# METABOLIC ACIDOSIS

## LEARNING OBJECTIVES

- Describe the physiology, causes, and effects of metabolic acidosis
- Diagnose metabolic acidosis
- Manage metabolic acidosis

## DEFINITION AND MECHANISM

- Metabolic acidosis is a disturbance in the homeostasis of plasma acidity
- Any process that increases the serum hydrogen ion concentration is a distinct acidosis
- A patient can have multiple acidoses contributing to the decrease of serum pH
- Adicosis can be either respiratory (changes in $CO_2$) or metabolic (changes in bicarbonate)
- Metabolic acidosis is characterized by an increase in serum hydrogen ion concentration resulting in serum bicarbonate ($HCO_3$) < 24 mEq/L
- May be associated with organ failure, especially respiratory and cardiovascular
- Can be acute or chronic

## ETIOLOGY

- Classification of metabolic acidosis is based on the presence or absence of an anion gap (concentration of unmeasured serum anions)
- Sodium, the main plasma cation, is balanced by the sum of the anions bicarbonate and chloride in addition to the unmeasured anions (e.g., lactate, acetoacetate), which represent the anion gap
- Anion gap metabolic acidosis is often caused by anaerobic metabolism and lactic acid accumulation
- Non-gap metabolic acidosis is primarily caused by the loss of bicarbonate (e.g., diarrhea, renal tubular acidosis)

## CAUSES

| Anion gap metabolic acidosis | Non-gap metabolic acidosis associated with normal or high serum K+ | Non-gap metabolic acidosis associated with low serum K+ |
|---|---|---|
| Acute kidney injury | Administration of HCl or precursors | Diarrhea |
| Chronic kidney disease | Administration of cationic amino acids | Intestinal, pancreatic, or biliary fistula |
| Diabetic ketoacidosis | Chronic kidney disease | Proximal renal tubular acidosis |
| Alcoholic ketoacidosis | Adrenal insufficiency (primary or secondary) | Distal renal tubular acidosis |
| Lactic acidosis | Hyporeninemic hypoaldosteronism | Ureterosigmoidostomy |
| Salicylate intoxication | Hyperkalemic distal renal tubular acidosis | Ureteroileostomy |
| Toxic alcohol intoxication (methanol, ethylene glycol, diethylene glycol, propylene glycol) | Pseudoaldosteronism type I | Diabetic ketoacidosis |
| Pyroglutamic acidosis | Pseudoaldosteronism type II (Gordon's syndrome) | Toluene intoxication |
| Fasting ketoacidosis | Drugs (spironolactone, prostaglandin inhibitors, triamterene, amiloride, trimethoprim, pentamidine, ciclosporin) | Lactic acidosis |
| Toluene intoxication | | |

| Anion gap metabolic acidosis | Non-gap metabolic acidosis associated with normal or high serum K+ | Non-gap metabolic acidosis associated with low serum K+ |
|---|---|---|
| Acute kidney injury | Administration of HCl or precursors | Diarrhea |
| Chronic kidney disease | Administration of cationic amino acids | Intestinal, pancreatic, or biliary fistula |
| Toluene intoxication | | |

## ADVERSE EFFECTS

| Acute metabolic acidosis | Chronic metabolic acidosis |
|---|---|
| Impaired leukocyte function | Generation or exacerbation of bone disease |
| Predisposition to ventricular arrhythmias | Growth retardation (in children) |
| Arterial vasodilation and hypotension | Impaired glucose tolerance |
| Resistance to action of infused catecholamines | Acceleration of progression of kidney disease |
| Resistance to action of insulin | Increased muscle wasting |
| Suppression of lymphocyte function | Reduced albumin synthesis |
| Impaired cellular energy production | Enhanced production of β2-microglobulin |
| Stimulation of apoptosis | |
| Changes in mental status | |
| Stimulation of interleukin production | |
| Alteration in oxygen binding to hemoglobin | |
| Venoconstriction | |
| Decreased cardiac contractility and cardiac output | |

## DIAGNOSIS

- History: Identify potential causes (vomiting, diarrhea, medications, possible overdoses, chronic conditions such as diabetes mellitus)
- Physical examination: dry mucus membranes in diabetic ketoacidosis, compensatory hyperventilation
- Lab tests;
  - Blood pH < 7.35
  - $pCO_2$:
    - > 40-45: respiratory acidosis
    - < 40: metabolic acidosis

Metabolic acidosis

- Anion gap
  - Anion gap = Na+ – (Cl- + $HCO_3$-)
  - Normal anion gap = 12
  - Anion gap > 12: Anion gap metabolic acidosis
- Respiratory compensation
  - Winter's formula: Expected $CO_2$ = ($HCO_3$- x 1.5) + 8 +/- 2
  - If $pCO_2$ is within the predicted range, there is no additional respiratory disturbance
  - If $pCO_2$ is greater than expected, there is an additional respiratory acidosis
  - If $pCO_2$ is less than expected, there is an additional respiratory alkalosis
- Additional metabolic disturbances
  - If anion gap is present, determine delta gap
  - Delta gap = Delta anion gap – Delta $HCO_3$- = (anion gap – 12) – (24 – $HCO_3$-)
  - Delta gap < -6: Non anion gap metabolic acidosis
  - Delta gap > 6: underlying metabolic alkalosis
  - Delta gap between -6 and 6: only anion gap metabolic acidosis

# MANAGEMENT

- Address the cause of acidosis
- Fluid resuscitation and electrolyte imbalance correction for sepsis and diabetic ketoacidosis
- Antidotes for poisoning, dialysis, antibiotics, bicarbonate administration

### LACTIC ACIDOSIS

- Lactic acid may increase dramatically in anaerobic conditions
- Beta-adrenergic receptor activation (due to stress or catecholamine infusions) increases lactic acid
- Lactic acidosis occurs when the production of lactic acid is greater than its hepatic clearance
- A lactic acid level of 2 mmol/L is clinically significant, 5 mmol/L is considered severe
- Initial management: Fluid resuscitation
- Consider base administration if serum pH < 7.1 in patients with suspected cardiovascular compromise

### KETOACIDOSIS

- Ketosis is seen in malnutrition, bowel disease, and alcoholism
- Ketoacidosis occurs when the production of ketones exceeds their hepatic clearance
- Management: Fluid resuscitation including glucose and insulin therapy
- Consider base administration if serum pH < 7.1, there is evidence of cardiovascular compromise, and insulin and fluids fail to rapidly improve acidemia

### RENAL ACIDOSIS

- Metabolic acidosis associated with acute kidney failure is multifactorial
- The presence of metabolic acidosis in the setting of oliguria can indicate uremia, fluid overload and abdominal compartment syndrome
- Conservative approach involving fluid restriction and diuretic therapy
- If the patient develops clinically significan hyperkalemia, cardiovascular instability, fluid overload, or arunia, renal replacement therapy is indicated
- Sodium bicarbonate therapy can be used to provide cardiovascular stability as a bridg to hemodiafiltration

### GENERAL MANAGEMENT

- If sodium bicarbonate is given, administer slowly as an isotonic solution, with the initial dose limited to ≤ 1–2 mEq/kg
- Consider increasing alveolar ventilation temporarily while monitoring for possible barotrauma
- Carefully monitor acid-base status
- In patients with $CO_2$ retention and adequate renal function, consider administration of Tromethamine
- In patients with hyperchloremic acidosis, administer base if serum pH < 7.1

## SUGGESTED READING

- Burger MK, Schaller DJ. Metabolic Acidosis. [Updated 2022 Jul 19]. In: StatPearls [Internet]. Treasure Island (FL): StatPearls Publishing; 2022 Jan-. Available from: https://www.ncbi.nlm.nih.gov/books/NBK482146/
- Fleisher, Lee A., and Stanley H. Rosenbaum. Complications in Anesthesia. Elsevier, 2018.
- Kraut, J., Madias, N. Metabolic acidosis: pathophysiology, diagnosis and management. Nat Rev Nephrol 6, 274–285 (2010).

Metabolic acidosis

# METABOLIC ALKALOSIS

## LEARNING OBJECTIVES

- Describe the pathophysiology of metabolic alkalosis
- Diagnose metabolic alkalosis
- Manage metabolic alkalosis

## DEFINITION AND MECHANISM

- Metabolic alkalosis is defined as an increase in serum pH to > 7.45
- Mostly due to a primary increase in serum bicarbonate ($HCO_3$-)
- Associated with a compensatory increase in $CO_2$ arterial pressure ($PaCO_2$)
- Usually accompanied by hypokalemia and hypochloremia
- Common acid-base disorder in critically ill patients

## PATHOPHYSIOLOGY

- Intracellular shift of hydrogen ions
  - E.g., hypokalemia
  - Decrease in serum hydrogen ions results in a relative increase in bicarbonate
- Renal loss of hydrogen ions
  - Pathologies that increase the levels of mineralocorticoids or the effect of aldosterone lead to hypernatremia, hypokalemia, and hydrogen loss
  - Loop and thiazide diuretics can induce secondary hyperaldosteronism
  - Genetic defects leading to decreased expression of ion transporters in the loop of Henle (Bartter disease, Gitelman disease)
- Retention/addition of bicarbonate
  - Overdose of exogenous sodium bicarbonate
  - Compensatory mechanism for hypercarbia: hypoventilation and $CO_2$ retention result in renal compensation over time by retaining bicarbonate (post-hypercapnia syndrome)
- Contraction alkalosis
  - Occurs when a large volume of sodium-rich, bicarbonate low fluid is lost
  - Diuretic use, cystic fibrosis, congenital chloride diarrhea
  - Net concentration of bicarbonate increases
- Evaluation of etiology: Urinary chloride
  - Chloride responsive (urine chloride < 10 mEq/L): Gastrointestinal hydrogen loss, congenital chloride diarrhea syndrome, contraction alkalosis, diuretic therapy, post-hypercapnia syndrome, cystic fibrosis, exogenous alkalotic agent use, villous adenoma, high volume ileostomy output
  - Chloride resistant (urine chloride > 20 mEq/L): Retention of bicarbonate, intracellular shift of hydrogen, hyperaldosteronism, Bartter syndrome, Gitelman syndrome, Cushing's syndrome, exogenous mineralocorticoids, congenital adrenal hyperplasia, licorice, Liddle syndrome
- Adverse effects
  - Decreased myocardial contractility
  - Arrhythmias
  - Decreased cerebral blood flow
  - Delirium
  - Increased neuromuscular excitability
  - Impaired peripheral oxygen unloading
  - Compensatory increase in arterial $pCO_2$
  - Net effect resulting in hypoxia

## DIAGNOSIS

- Elevated serum $HCO_3$- and $pCO_2$
- Determine respiratory compensation
  - $PaCO_2$ (mmHg) = $40 + 0.6 \times (HCO_3- - 24 \text{ mmol/L})$

# MANAGEMENT

- Alkalosis is rarely life-threatening in itself
- Prolonged alkalosis can however be associated with dyselectrolytemias and associated adverse effects

### CHLORIDE-RESPONSIVE ALKALOSIS

- Give isotonic saline and replete potassium with potassium chloride orally, intravenously or both
- Replace magnesium in patients with hypomagnesemia
- Discontinue diuretics if possible, otherwise reduce the dose
- Add a potassium sparing diuretic (spironolactone, eplerenone, amiloride, or triamterene) in patients where discontinuation of diuretics is not possible

### GENERAL MANAGEMENT

- Address the underlying etiology
- Treat vomiting and investigate the cause
- Proton pump inhibitors or H2 blockers may be helpful in patients with ongoing gastric fluid losses
- Identify exogenous sources of alkali
- Instruct patients to avoid licorice or licorice-containing tobacco products

### CHLORIDE-RESISTANT ALKALOSIS

- Replace potassium with potassium chloride orally, intravenously or both
- Main focus of treatment: Underlying etiology
- Bilateral adrenal hyperplasia: Aldosterone blockers (spironolactone or eplerenone)
- Hyperaldosteronism: Low-sodium diet
- Advanced chronic kidney disease: Peritoneal dialysis or hemodialysis, continuous renal replacement therapy
- Bartter syndrome: Potassium repletion, potassium-sparing diuretics, non-steroidal anti-inflammatory drugs
- Gitelman syndrome: Magnesium repletion, potassium repletion, potassium-sparing diuretics, non-steroidal anti-inflammatory drugs

## SUGGESTED READING

- Brinkman JE, Sharma S. Physiology, Metabolic Alkalosis. [Updated 2022 Jul 18]. In: StatPearls [Internet]. Treasure Island (FL): StatPearls Publishing; 2022 Jan-. Available from: https://www.ncbi.nlm.nih.gov/books/NBK482291/
- Tinawi M. Pathophysiology, Evaluation, and Management of Metabolic Alkalosis. Cureus. 2021;13(1):e12841. Published 2021 Jan 21.

# MULTIPLE ENDOCRINE NEOPLASIA SYNDROMES

## 98

## LEARNING OBJECTIVES

- Define multiple endocrine neoplasia syndromes
- Describe the differences between MEN type 1 and MEN type 2
- Anesthetic management of patients with multiple endocrine neoplasia syndromes

## DEFINITION AND MECHANISM

- Multiple endocrine neoplasia (MEN) syndromes are characterized by hyperplasia of or a tumor in specific endocrine system glands and tissues
- Caused by a genetic mutation, autosomal dominant inheritance

### Classification

MEN type 1
- Genetic condition in which multiple tumors affect different aspects of the endocrine system
- **Most common affected areas:** Parathyroid glands, gastroenteropancreatic tract, and anterior pituitary gland
- **Less common types of tumors:** Neuroendocrine tumors of the thymus and bronchi, adrenocortical tumors, lipomas, visceral leiomyomas, truncal and facial collagenomas, facial angiofibromas, breast cancer, meningioma, ependymomas
- Most tumors are benign
- Tumors are due to the inactivation of the MEN 1 oncosuppressor gene located on chromosome 11q13

MEN type 2
- Genetic polyglandular cancer syndrome
- All patients develop medullary thyroid carcinoma and have an increased risk of developing other tumors affecting other endocrine glands
- Patients with MEN type 2 also develop one or both of the following conditions
- Pheochromocytoma
- Hyperparathyroidism
- Tumors result from oncogenic point mutations of the c-Ret proto-oncogene located on chromosome 10cen-10q11.2

## SIGNS AND SYMPTOMS

- Symptoms vary depending on which glands are affected by the hyperplasia or tumor
- Hyperplasia or tumors cause the affected glands to produce and release more hormones than normal
- Symptoms vary from person to person

## MEN type 1

| Tumor/condition | Incidence | Associated hormone | Symptoms |
|---|---|---|---|
| Hyperparathyroidism | 90% | Parathyroid hormone | Related to hypercalcemia<br>Mild: Joint pain, muscle weakness, fatigue, depression, trouble concentrating, loss of appetite<br>Severe: Nausea and vomiting, confusion and forgetfulness, increased thirst and frequent urination, constipation, bone pain |
| Gastrinomas | 40% | Gastrin | Abdominal pain, diarrhea, gastroesophageal reflux (acid reflux), peptic ulcers |
| Insulinomas | 10% | Insulin | Related to hypoglycemia<br>Confusion, shakiness, sweating, hunger, anxiety, heart palpitations, temporary vision changes |
| Prolactinomas | 25% | Prolactin | Women: Changes in menstruation unrelated to menopause (i.e., irregular menstruation or amenorrhea), infertility, milky discharge from the nipples when not pregnant or breastfeeding (galactorrhea), decreased libido<br>Men: Decreased libido, erectile dysfunction, infertility<br>Large tumor: Nausea and vomiting, vision changes (i.e., double vision or decreased peripheral vision) |

## MEN type 2

| Tumor/condition | Incidence | Associated hormone | Symptoms |
|---|---|---|---|
| Medullary thyroid carcinoma | 100% | Calcitonin | Lump and pain in front of the neck, voice changes (e.g., hoarseness), coughing, trouble swallowing, dyspnea |
| Pheochromocytomas | 50% | Epinephrine and norepinephrine | Hypertension, headache, excessive sweating, tachycardia, arrhythmia, feeling shaky |
| Hyperparathyroidism | 20% | Parathyroid hormone | Related to hypercalcemia<br>Mild: Joint pain, muscle weakness, fatigue, depression, trouble concentrating, loss of appetite<br>Severe: Nausea and vomiting, confusion and forgetfulness, increased thirst and frequent urination, constipation, bone pain |

# DIAGNOSIS

| | MEN Type 1 | MEN Type 2 |
|---|---|---|
| Diagnosis | At least two of the three endocrine tumors associated with the condition<br>One of the associated tumors and a family history | Medullary thyroid carcinoma and pheochromocytoma and/or parathyroid enlargement (hyperplasia) or tumor (adenoma) |
| Tests | Blood tests to detect elevated levels of certain hormones<br>- Hyperparathyroidism: Parathyroid hormone + hypercalcemia<br>- Gastrinomas: Gastrin<br>- Insulinomas: Insulin<br>- Prolactinomas: Prolactine<br>CT and MRI scans<br>Genetic testing of MEN 1 gene | Blood tests to detect elevated levels of certain hormones<br>- Medullary thyroid carcinoma: Calcitonin<br>- Pheochromocytoma: Catecholamines<br>- Hyperparathyroidism: Parathyroid hormone + hypercalcemia<br>CT and MRI scans<br>Genetic testing of RET gene |

Multiple endocrine neoplasia syndromes

# TREATMENT

Dependent on what endocrine glands and organs are affected, treatment may include
- Medications (e.g., bisphosphonates, calcitonin) to treat symptoms and counteract the side effects of excess hormones
- Surgery to remove tumors or entire affected glands (e.g., thyroidectomy, parathyroidectomy)
- Replacement hormones if an endocrine gland is surgically removed
- Cancer treatment (e.g., chemotherapy and radiation) in case of metastasis

# MANAGEMENT

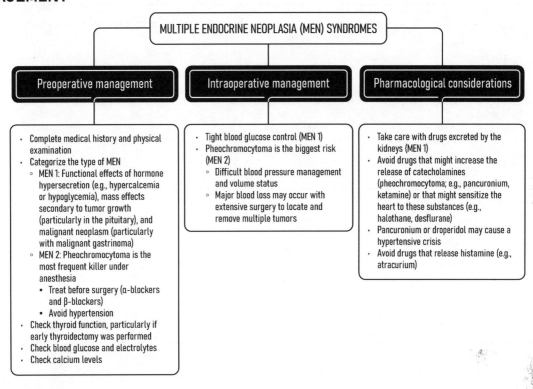

## *Anesthetic challenges per tumor*
- Parathyroid tumors: Hypercalcemia
  - Maintain hydration and urinary output
  - Main risk: Potential for cardiac dysrhythmias
  - Unpredictable responses to muscle relaxants
  - Careful positioning due to the possible presence of osteoporosis and the potential for pathologic fractures
- Gastrinomas
  - Correct hypovolemia and electrolyte imbalance (hypokalemia and metabolic alkalosis)
  - Large gastric fluid volumes from gastric hypersecretion → vulnerable to aspiration during anesthetic induction
  - Gastroesophageal reflux is common → rapid sequence induction with maintenance of cricoid pressure
- Insulinomas: Hypoglycemia
  - Maintain normal blood glucose concentrations to prevent cerebral damage
    - Place an intra-arterial catheter to measure glucose levels regularly
    - Administer IV glucose
  - Anesthetic technique should focus on agents that decrease the cerebral metabolic rate for oxygen (avoid ketamine)
  - Maintain normocarbia during controlled ventilation
- Patients might be obese → pay attention to the airway and address respiratory and cardiac issues
- Prolactinoma
  - No specific anesthetic considerations

- Medullary thyroid carcinoma
  - Enlarged thyroid causing airway compromise
  - Intraoperative damage to the recurrent laryngeal nerve → may cause hoarseness, stridor, and complete airway obstruction upon extubation of the trachea or in the PACU
  - Airway may also become compromised by hematoma formation compressing the trachea
- Pheochromocytoma: Hypertension
  - Prevent hypertension and tachycardia → smooth anesthesia induction and endotracheal intubation
  - Avoid catecholamine release induced by anesthetic or surgical maneuvers
  - Correct hypovolemia and electrolyte imbalances

See also hyperparathyroidism considerations
See also pheochromocytoma considerations

## KEEP IN MIND

- The anesthetic course may range from routine with no special requirements to severe and life-threatening depending on the tumor
- Some syndromes demand specific management techniques, but a carefully and thoughtfully administered anesthetic is the key to a successful outcome in patients with MEN

## SUGGESTED READING

- Grant F. Anesthetic considerations in the multiple endocrine neoplasia syndromes. Curr Opin Anaesthesiol. 2005;18(3):345-352.
- Multiple Endocrine Neoplasia (MEN). In: Bissonnette B, Luginbuehl I, Marciniak B, Dalens BJ. eds. Syndromes: Rapid Recognition and Perioperative Implications. Mgraw Hill; 2006. Accessed March 07, 2023. https://accessanesthesiology.mhmedical.com/content.aspx?bookid=852&sectionid=49517985

# OBESITY

## LEARNING OBJECTIVES

- Understand the impact of obesity and related health conditions upon the provision of anesthesia
- Identify the high-risk obese patient
- Plan safe and individualized perioperative care determined by comorbidities and the extent of surgery

## DEFINITION AND MECHANISM

- Obesity is an excessive fat accumulation that presents a risk to health, defined by the WHO as having a body mass index (BMI) over 30 kg/m2
- Obesity is a leading preventable cause of death worldwide
- The prevalence of obesity has tripled over the past 40 years, and there are more than 650 million obese adults worldwide

## RISK FACTORS

- Family inheritance and influences
- Lifestyle choices: Unhealthy diet, liquid calories, inactivity, sedentary lifestyle
- Certain diseases: Prader-Willi syndrome, Cushing syndrome, hypothyroidism, growth hormone deficiency, eating disorders (i.e., binge eating disorder, night eating syndrome)
- Certain medications: Antidepressants, insulin, sulfonylureas, thiazolidinediones, atypical antipsychotics, steroids, β-blockers, anticonvulsants (i.e., phenytoin and valproate), pizotifen, some forms of hormonal contraception
- Socioeconomic issues
- Aging
- Other factors: Pregnancy, quitting smoking, lack of sleep, stress, microbiome

## COMPLICATIONS

- Hypertension
- Cardiovascular diseases and stroke
- Type 2 diabetes mellitus
- Metabolic syndrome
- Increased risk of cancer of the uterus, cervix, endometrium, ovary, breast, colon, rectum, esophagus, liver, gallbladder, pancreas, kidney, and prostate
- Digestive problems
- Obstructive sleep apnea (OSA)
- Obesity hypoventilation syndrome (OHS)
- Osteoarthritis
- Depression

## TREATMENT

- **Goal:** Reach and stay at a healthy weight → improve overall health and lower the risk of developing complications related to obesity
- **Initial treatment:** Modest weight loss (5-10% of total weight)
- Changes in eating habits and increased physical activity

### Dietary changes

- Reduce calories
- Eat healthier
- Restrict certain foods (e.g., high carbohydrates, full-fat foods)
- Choose satiating foods with high fiber content
- Meal replacements (e.g., low-calorie shakes or meal bars)

### Exercise and activity

- Exercise: 150 minutes/week of moderate-intensity physical activity
- Keep moving

### Behavior changes

- Counseling
- Support groups

### Weight-loss medication

- Used along with diet, exercise, and behavior changes
- Bupropion-naltrexone
- Liraglutide
- Orlistat
- Phentermine-topiramate

### Endoscopic procedures for weight loss

- Endoscopic sleeve gastroplasty
- Intragastric balloon for weight loss

### Bariatric surgery

- Limits the amount of food the patient can comfortably eat or decreases the absorption of food and calories
- May result in nutritional and vitamin deficiencies
- Reserved for individuals with a BMI > 40 kg/m² or BMI > 35 kg/m² with weight-related comorbidities
- Adjustable gastric banding
- Gastric bypass surgery
- Sleeve gastrectomy

## MANAGEMENT

### Preoperative assessment and risk prediction

- Most important to identify
  - Central or peripheral distribution of fat
  - Central obesity is more risky
  - Presence of metabolic syndrome
  - Peripheral oxygen saturation < 95% breathing air
- Optimize associated health conditions before scheduling surgery (see table)

| Conditions | Suggestive features | Perioperative actions |
|---|---|---|
| **Respiratory** | | |
| Sleep-disordered breathing (OSA, OHS) | Shortness of breath<br>$SpO_2$ < 95% breathing air<br>Stop-BANG ≥ 5<br>OHS-BMI > 30, hypercapnia when awake, raised $HCO_3$, hypoxia, exclusion other causes of hypoventilation | ABG initially<br>Spirometry<br>Cardiopulmonary excercise testing (CPET) if abnormalities found in above tests<br>Airway planning, 4x ↑ risk of difficult intubation and difficult mask ventilation<br>Refer for further investigation and treatment<br>Commence CPAP before surgery and continue after surgery<br>BiPAP sometimes necessary for improvement in symptoms (especially OHS)<br>Plan for postoperative HDU/ICU admission if symptoms not improved by time of surgery |
| Asthma | Dyspnea<br>Wheezing | Asthmatic symptoms common but reversibility with β2-agonists not always found - cause is partly chronic pro-inflammatory state from excess adipose tissue and fat within/around chest/abdomen causing small airway collapse<br>Weight loss: Symptoms from asthma and fat-related wheeze will improve |

| Conditions | Suggestive features | Perioperative actions |
|---|---|---|
| **Cardiovascular** | | |
| Hypertension<br>Left ventricular hypertrophy<br>Left ventricular failure<br>Conduction abnormalities<br>Cardiomyopathy | Clinical signs of heart failure<br>History of cardiac syncope<br>Increased SBP<br>Reduced exercise capacity | Preoperative ECG<br>ECHO if structural or functional disease suspected<br>Referral to cardiologist<br>Medical management and optimization before surgery |
| Right heart failure | Pulmonary hypertension resulting from sleep-disordered breathing<br>Polycythemia | |
| Reduced functional capacity | Difficult to assess in obese patients<br>Ability to achieve 4 metabolic equivalents indicates fitness and low risk patient | Assess ability to walk on a flat level surface<br>Assess climbing stairs<br>CPET |
| **Metabolic** | | |
| Diabetes mellitus | Deranged serum glucose, HbA1C, or associated complications | Optimize glucose control with referral to endocrinologist<br>Avoid delaying surgery based on HbA1C concentrations only |
| Liver involvement (NASH/NAFLD) | Evidence of cirrhosis, deranged liver function tests | Liver-shrinking diet (< 1000 calories/day) can reverse the disease processes somewhat |
| Metabolic syndrome | Central obesity, hypertension, impaired glucose handing or diabetes, increased triglycerides, decreased HDL cholesterol | Actively seek components of metabolic syndrome ($\geq 3$ required for diagnosis) |

## *Organization and equipment*

Preparation and positioning
- Ensure availability of theatre gowns of appropriate size
- Assess deep vein thrombosis risk and use prophylaxis measures
- Maintain patient's dignity and safety
- Use gel pads to protect pressure points

Monitoring and ventilation
- Use non-invasive blood pressure cuffs of the correct size
- Anesthetic ventilators should be able to deliver high driving pressures and PEEP
- Potential for incomplete neuromuscular block antagonism requires routine neuromuscular monitoring

Ultrasound
- Facilitate successful regional blocks and aid with difficult venous access

## Induction of anesthesia

Patient position
- Ramped position (head-up tilt) until the ear tragus and sternal notch are aligned horizontally
- Position offers advantages
  - Increased comfort for the patient
  - Maintain functional residual capacity
  - Reduce dyspnea
  - Facilitate bag-mask ventilation
  - Improve laryngoscopy

Airway
- Tracheal intubation is the recommended technique for airway management
- Obesity is associated with a higher risk of developing airway problems under anesthesia
- Routine airway assessment to determine potential difficult laryngoscopy or ventilation
  - Mallampati score 3 (predicts difficult facemask ventilation and intubation)
  - Neck circumference > 42 cm (predicts difficult intubation)
  - BMI > 50 kg/m2 (independent predictor of difficult intubation and facemask ventilation)
  - Symptoms of gastroesophageal reflux disease
- Obese patients have increased oxygen consumption and $CO_2$ production due to increased total body tissue mass and increased work of breathing → can lead to hypercapnia and hypoxemia when ventilation is impaired
- Delay onset of hypoxemia by
  - Preoxygenation of the lungs
  - Induction of anesthesia in the semi-upright position with application of CPAP or high-flow nasal oxygen
  - Avoid prolonged apnea
- Excess adipose tissue reduces chest wall compliance, which reduces functional residual capacity (FRC) to closing capacity, leading to atelectasis

Routine rapid sequence intubation (RSI)
- Obesity is associated with an increased incidence of known risk factors for aspiration (e.g., hiatus hernia, diabetes with autonomic neuropathy causing delayed gastric emptying)
- RSI is not routinely required in the absence of risk factors for aspiration
- Failed intubation after induction of anesthesia requires antagonism of neuromuscular block

Awareness
- Reduce awareness shortly after induction of anesthesia by
  - Ensuring adequate dosing of IV anesthetic agents
  - Prompt delivery of maintenance anesthetic agent
  - Further IV bolus(es) of the anesthetic agent before airway manipulation or protracted airway maneuvers

## Maintenance of anesthesia

- TIVA with propofol offers advantages over volatile anesthetics
  - Reduced incidence of laryngospasm
  - Reliable clearance of hypnotic agents
  - Reduced postoperative nausea and vomiting
  - Maintained anesthesia during protracted airway manipulation
- To minimize the risk of accidental awareness, the use of processed EEG-based depth of anesthesia monitoring, continuous clinical observation, and interpretation of vital signs should guide titration of drug infusion targets and rates
- Volatile anesthetics with a rapid offset of action (i.e., desflurane and sevoflurane) limit absorption into adipose tissue, reduce the risk of resedation, deteriorate respiration function, and may obstruct the airway at emergence

Ventilation
- Obesity is an independent risk factor for developing postoperative pulmonary complications
- Use lung protective volumes (6-8 mL/kg), plateau pressures < 30 cm $H_2O$, and titration of PEEP guided by the patient's respiratory and cardiovascular state
- Position the patient in the 20° reverse Trendelenburg position with 45° hip flexion for laparoscopy for upper abdominal surgery to reduce airway pressures
- Position the patient in the flat Trendelenburg position for lower abdominal surgery to reduce airway pressures

## Postoperative care

- Place the patient in a 30-45° head up position in the recovery room
- CPAP may enhance recovery of normal respiratory function if started in the early postoperative period
- Use multimodal and opioid-free analgesia; if required monitor $SpO_2$ continuously and consider a higher level of care
- Early mobilization with regular reviews
- Discharge criteria
  - Unsupported stable vital signs with minimal inspired oxygen requirement
  - No evidence of hypoventilation
  - Free from apneas without stimulation
  - Patient must be able to use a CPAP device if required
- Consider critical care admission for all patients with significant comorbidities (e.g., diabetes mellitus, chronic respiratory disease)

## Day-case surgery

| | Patient-specific factors | Anesthetic factors | Surgical factors |
|---|---|---|---|
| Appropriate for day-case surgery | Any BMI<br>Good functional capacity<br>OSA/OHS effectively treated with CPAP/Non-invasive ventilation (NIV)<br>Able to continue venous thromboembolism (VTE) prophylaxis at home if required | Adequate time on list to anesthetize<br>Regional anesthesia possible<br>Experienced anesthesiologist, OR, and day-case ward team required | Adequate time on operating list to perform surgery, taking into account expected time to discharge<br>Appropriate equipment for surgery and postoperative care available |
| Inappropriate for day-case surgery | Poor functional capacity<br>Unstable hypertension, ischemic heart disease, congestive heart failure<br>Unstable respiratory disease (low $SpO_2$, OSA/OHS untreated or no symptomatic improvement after treatment)<br>Previous VTE<br>Metabolic syndrome | Likely to require long-acting potent opioids | |

## Implications of previous bariatric surgery

- **Sleeve gastrectomy:** Routinely intubate these patients as there is a risk of reflux of gastric contents, regardless of presence of symptoms
- **Roux-en-Y gastric bypass; one anastomosis gastric bypass:** May affect bioavailability of oral medications due to shortening of the small bowel and loss of surface area (e.g., postoperative analgesia absorption)
- **Adjustable gastric banding**
  - High risk of aspiration despite prolonged fasting times
  - RSI with antacid premedication should be routine
  - Avoid nasogastric tubes unless acute abdomen or bowel obstruction (risk of displacing band or perforation of proximal stomach)
  - The band should not be deflated (risk infection to system, band erosion in stomach or damage to the band)

# KEEP IN MIND

- Obesity only increases perioperative risk significantly when BMI is $\geq 40$ kg/m2, or when associated with significant comorbidities
- Day-case surgery is usually appropriate if BMI is < 50 kg/m2 and comorbidities are optimized
- OSA and OHS are common high-risk conditions that influence the management of anesthesia
- RSI should not be routine in the absence of specific indications
- Previous bariatric surgery has important implications for subsequent anesthesia

# SUGGESTED READING

- Dority J, Hassan ZU, Chau D. Anesthetic implications of obesity in the surgical patient. Clin Colon Rectal Surg. 2011;24(4):222-228.
- Seyni-Boureima R, Zhang Z, Antoine MM, Antoine-Frank CD. A review on the anesthetic management of obese patients undergoing surgery. BMC Anesthesiol. 2022; 22(98).
- Wynn-Hebden A, Bouch DC. Anaesthesia for the obese patient. BJA Education. 2020;20(11):388-395.

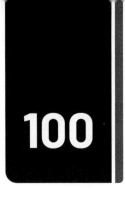

# PANHYPOPITUITARISM

## LEARNING OBJECTIVES

- Definition of panhypopituitarism
- Management of panhypopituitarism

## DEFINITION AND MECHANISM

- A rare condition in which there's a deficiency in **all of the hormones produced** by the pituitary gland
- The anterior lobe of the pituitary gland produces:
  - Adrenocorticotropic hormone (ACTH or corticotropin)
  - Follicle-stimulating hormone (FSH)
  - Growth hormone (GH)
  - Luteinizing hormone (LH)
  - Prolactin (PRL)
  - Thyroid stimulation hormone (TSH)
- The posterior lobe of the pituitary gland produces:
  - Antidiuretic hormone (ADH)/vasopressin
  - Oxytocin
- Can affect anyone at any age
- It can be life-threatening, especially if significant deficiencies of ACTH are present, and affects 4 people per 100,000 people
- Panhypopituitarism is a type of hypopituitarism
  - A deficiency or lack in one or multiple of the hormones produced by the pituitary gland
- Patients with hormonal deficiencies present with the following:
  - ACTH deficiency – adrenal insufficiency
  - TSH deficiency – hypothyroidism
  - Gonadotropin deficiency – hypogonadism
  - GH deficiency – difficult to thrive and short stature in children, adults are usually asymptomatic; however, they may feel fatigued and weak
  - ADH deficiency – diabetes insipidus presenting with polydipsia and polyuria

## SIGNS AND SYMPTOMS

- Symptoms depend on which hormone is deficient
  - Growth problems (in children)
  - Obesity
  - Hair loss
  - Bradycardia
  - Hypoglycemia
  - Hypotension
  - Fatigue
  - Nausea or dizziness
  - Depression and/or anxiety
  - Frequent infections
  - Sensitivity to cold
  - Unusually dry skin
  - Unexplained weight loss or weight gain
  - Dyslipidemia
  - Tachycardia
  - Excessive thirst and urination
  - Female and male infertility
- Additional symptoms specific to infants, children, or adolescents
  - Prolonged jaundice in newborns
  - Micropenis
  - Slowed growth
  - Delayed puberty

# CAUSES

| Pituitary-related | Hypothalamus-related |
|---|---|
| Pituitary adenoma | Traumatic brain injury |
| Infection | Brain surgery |
| Injury | Tumors such as craniopharyngiomas |
| Pituitary gland surgery | Secondary metastasis |
| Radiation therapy | Pressure from hydrocephalus |
| Pituitary apoplexy | Stroke |
| Congenital (related to midline craniofacial defects) | Tuberculous meningitis |
| Kallman syndrome | |
| Idiopathic | |

# COMPLICATIONS

- Adrenal crisis (acute cortisol insufficiency) which is characterized by the following symptoms:
  - Fever
  - Weakness
  - Confusion
  - Hypotension
  - Tachycardia
  - Vomiting
  - Diarrhea
  - Hypoglycemia
- Secondary diseases:
  - Obesity
  - Increased cholesterol
  - Metabolic syndrome
  - Estradiol deficiency potentially leads to osteoporosis

# DIAGNOSIS

- MRI
- CT
- Hormone level tests:
  - Blood tests
  - ACTH-stimulation test
  - Growth hormone stimulation test
  - Insulin tolerance test
  - Modern combined test

# TREATMENT

- Hormone replacement therapy
- Pituitary surgery
- Radiation therapy
- Corticosteroids

# MANAGEMENT

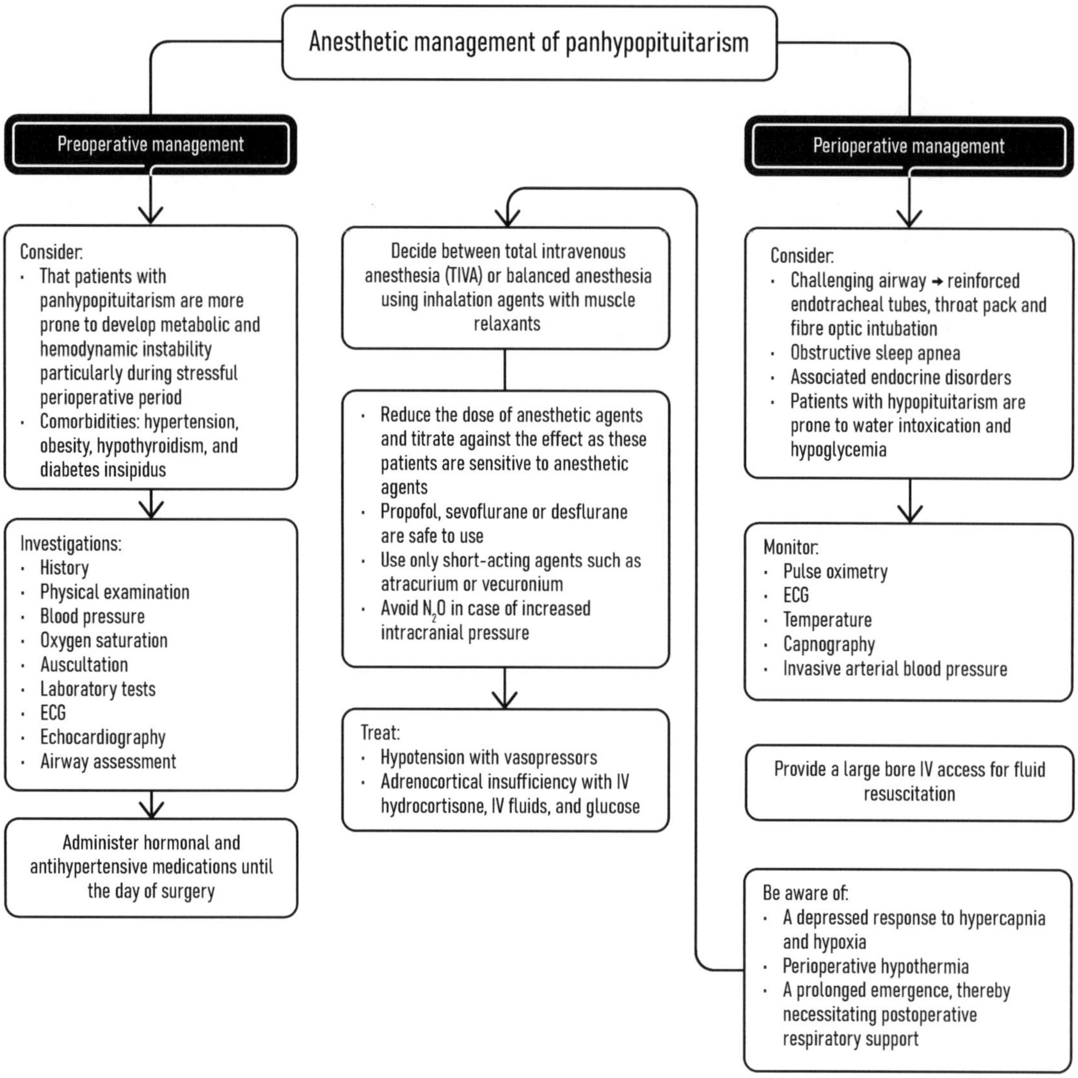

Anesthetic management of panhypopituitarism

## Preoperative management

Consider:
- That patients with panhypopituitarism are more prone to develop metabolic and hemodynamic instability particularly during stressful perioperative period
- Comorbidities: hypertension, obesity, hypothyroidism, and diabetes insipidus

Investigations:
- History
- Physical examination
- Blood pressure
- Oxygen saturation
- Auscultation
- Laboratory tests
- ECG
- Echocardiography
- Airway assessment

Administer hormonal and antihypertensive medications until the day of surgery

Decide between total intravenous anesthesia (TIVA) or balanced anesthesia using inhalation agents with muscle relaxants

- Reduce the dose of anesthetic agents and titrate against the effect as these patients are sensitive to anesthetic agents
- Propofol, sevoflurane or desflurane are safe to use
- Use only short-acting agents such as atracurium or vecuronium
- Avoid $N_2O$ in case of increased intracranial pressure

Treat:
- Hypotension with vasopressors
- Adrenocortical insufficiency with IV hydrocortisone, IV fluids, and glucose

## Perioperative management

Consider:
- Challenging airway → reinforced endotracheal tubes, throat pack and fibre optic intubation
- Obstructive sleep apnea
- Associated endocrine disorders
- Patients with hypopituitarism are prone to water intoxication and hypoglycemia

Monitor:
- Pulse oximetry
- ECG
- Temperature
- Capnography
- Invasive arterial blood pressure

Provide a large bore IV access for fluid resuscitation

Be aware of:
- A depressed response to hypercapnia and hypoxia
- Perioperative hypothermia
- A prolonged emergence, thereby necessitating postoperative respiratory support

Panhypopituitarism

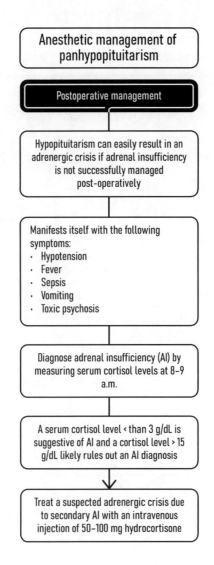

**Anesthetic management of panhypopituitarism**

**Postoperative management**

Hypopituitarism can easily result in an adrenergic crisis if adrenal insufficiency is not successfully managed post-operatively

Manifests itself with the following symptoms:
· Hypotension
· Fever
· Sepsis
· Vomiting
· Toxic psychosis

Diagnose adrenal insufficiency (AI) by measuring serum cortisol levels at 8–9 a.m.

A serum cortisol level < than 3 g/dL is suggestive of AI and a cortisol level > 15 g/dL likely rules out an AI diagnosis

Treat a suspected adrenergic crisis due to secondary AI with an intravenous injection of 50–100 mg hydrocortisone

**SUGGESTED READING**

• Malhotra, Surender & Jangra, Kiran & Saini, Vikas. (2013). Pituitary Surgery and Anesthetic Management: An Update. World Journal of Endocrine Surgery. 5. 1-5. 10.5005/jp-journals-10002-1114.
• Menon R, Murphy PG, Lidnley AM. 2011. Anaesthesia and pituitary disease. Continuing Education in Anaesthesia Critical Care & Pain. 11;4:133-137.
• Raut MS, Kar S, Maheshwari A, Shivnani G, Dubey S. Perioperative management in a patient with panhypopituitarism – evidence based approach: a case report. Eur Heart J Case Rep. 2019;3(3):ytz145. Published 2019 Sep 18.

# PARATHYROIDECTOMY

**101**

## LEARNING OBJECTIVES

- Define parathyroidectomy
- Describe the complications that are associated with parathyroidectomy
- Management of a patient undergoing a parathyroidectomy

## DEFINITION AND MECHANISM

- Parathyroidectomy is the surgical removal of one or more of the four parathyroid glands
- The surgery is performed to remove an adenoma or hyperplasia of the parathyroid glands and treat excessive parathyroid hormone (PTH) production (i.e., hyperparathyroidism) and associated hypercalcemia

## INDICATIONS

- **Primary hyperparathyroidism:** Hyperfunction of the parathyroid glands (i.e., adenoma, carcinoma, or hyperplasia) leading to an overproduction of PTH
- **Secondary hyperparathyroidism:** Appropriate compensatory response of the parathyroid glands to secrete more PTH in response to a condition (i.e., chronic kidney disease, vitamin D deficiency) that produces hypocalcemia
- **Tertiary hyperparathyroidism:** Long-standing secondary hyperparathyroidism starts to behave like primary hyperparathyroidism, usually associated with advanced kidney failure
- **Ectopic hyperparathyroidism:** Secretion of PTH by tissues other than the parathyroid glands

## PATIENT CHARACTERISTICS

- Skeletal muscle weakness, myopathy
- Nephrolithiasis, polyuria, polydipsia, renal failure
- Anemia
- Peptic ulcer disease, vomiting, pancreatitis
- Hypertension, prolonged PR interval, short QT interval
- Generalized osteopenia, bone pain, pathological fractures
- A decline in mental function, personality changes, lethargy, mood disturbances

## COMPLICATIONS

- Hypoparathyroidism and associated hypocalcemia
- Recurrent laryngeal nerve damage
- Hematoma
- Infection
- Edema of the glottis and pharynx

# MANANGEMENT

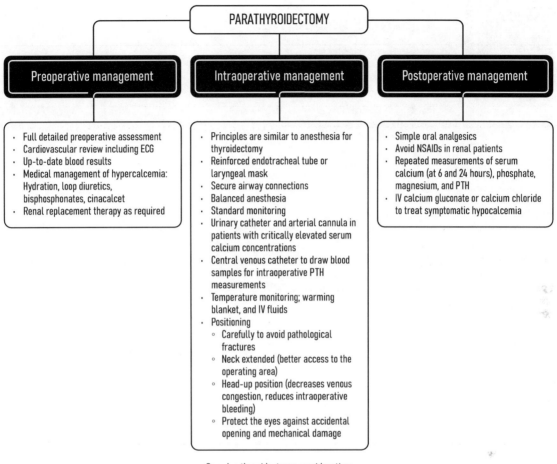

**PARATHYROIDECTOMY**

**Preoperative management**

- Full detailed preoperative assessment
- Cardiovascular review including ECG
- Up-to-date blood results
- Medical management of hypercalcemia: Hydration, loop diuretics, bisphosphonates, cinacalcet
- Renal replacement therapy as required

**Intraoperative management**

- Principles are similar to anesthesia for thyroidectomy
- Reinforced endotracheal tube or laryngeal mask
- Secure airway connections
- Balanced anesthesia
- Standard monitoring
- Urinary catheter and arterial cannula in patients with critically elevated serum calcium concentrations
- Central venous catheter to draw blood samples for intraoperative PTH measurements
- Temperature monitoring; warming blanket, and IV fluids
- Positioning
  - Carefully to avoid pathological fractures
  - Neck extended (better access to the operating area)
  - Head-up position (decreases venous congestion, reduces intraoperative bleeding)
  - Protect the eyes against accidental opening and mechanical damage

See also thyroidectomy considerations

**Postoperative management**

- Simple oral analgesics
- Avoid NSAIDs in renal patients
- Repeated measurements of serum calcium (at 6 and 24 hours), phosphate, magnesium, and PTH
- IV calcium gluconate or calcium chloride to treat symptomatic hypocalcemia

## SUGGESTED READING

- Malhotra S, Sodhi V. Anaesthesia for thyroid and parathyroid surgery. Continuing Education in Anaesthesia Critical Care & Pain. 2007;7(2):55-58.
- Pollard BJ, Kitchen G. Handbook of Clinical Anaesthesia. 4th ed. Taylor & Francis group; 2018. Chapter 20 Head and neck surgery, Macnab R and Bexon K.

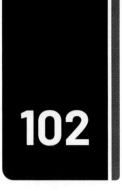

# PHEOCHROMOCYTOMA

## LEARNING OBJECTIVES

- Describe pheochromocytoma
- Recognize the symptoms and signs of pheochromocytoma
- Anesthetic management of a patient with a pheochromocytoma

## DEFINITION AND MECHANISM

- Pheochromocytomas are neuroendocrine tumors arising from chromaffin cells in the adrenal medulla
- Pheochromocytomas synthesize and secrete catecholamines (i.e., dopamine, norepinephrine, and epinephrine)
- The clinical presentation depends on the profile of the catecholamine secretion
  - **Norepinephrine:** Hypertension
  - **Epinephrine:** Tachycardia and tachydysrhythmias
- Neuroendocrine chromaffin tumors arising outside of the adrenal medulla are called paragangliomas

## SIGNS AND SYMPTOMS

- Hypertension
- Headache
- Heavy sweating
- Tachycardia
- Tachydysrhythmias
- Tremors
- Pallor
- Shortness of breath
- Panic attack-type symptoms
- Hyperglycemia
- Intravascular volume depletion (hypovolemia)
- Abdominal pain

Less common symptoms
- Anxiety
- Weight loss
- Blurred vision
- Constipation

## TREATMENT

- **Primary treatment:** Surgery to remove the tumor

## RISK FACTORS

- Family history of pheochromocytoma
- Family history of related genetic disorders
  - Multiple endocrine neoplasia, type 2 (MEN 2)
  - Von Hippel-Lindau disease
  - Neurofibromatosis 1
  - Hereditary paraganglioma syndromes

## COMPLICATIONS

Hypertension can damage other organs, particularly the cardiovascular system, brain, and kidneys. This damage may result in the following critical conditions:
- Cardiovascular disease
- Stroke
- Kidney failure
- Problems with the nerves of the eye

# MANAGEMENT

```
                        ┌─────────────────────────┐
                        │     PHEOCHROMOCYTOMA     │
                        └─────────────────────────┘
```

| Preoperative management | Intraoperative management | Postoperative management |
|---|---|---|

**Preoperative management**

- Control arterial pressure and correct hypovolemia
  - **α-blockers:** Phenoxybenzamine and doxazosin
- Control heart rate and arrhythmia
  - Selective β1-antagonists (i.e., atenolol or metoprolol) are preferred and must be started after complete α-blockade
- Assess and optimize myocardial function
  - ECG to diagnose ventricular hypertrophy, tachyarrhythmias, or myocardial ischemia
  - Echocardiography
- Correct glucose and electrolyte disturbances
- Invasive blood pressure monitoring and central venous access

**Intraoperative management**

- Avoid drug-induced catecholamine release → avoid drugs that increase sympathetic tone (e.g., ketamine, morphine, pethidine, ephedrine, pancuronium, atracurium, droperidol, metoclopramide, and desflurane)
- Avoid catecholamine release induced by anesthetic or surgical maneuvers → control hypertension
- Anti-hypertensive agents
  - Use short-acting agents only
  - **Sodium nitroprusside:** 50 mg in 250 mL normal saline (200 mcg/mL), run at 25-200 mcg/min or 0.3-3 mcg/kg/min, prepare syringe of 100 mcg/mL for bolusing
  - **Esmolol:** 10 mg/mL, run at 50-250 mcg/kg/min
  - **Phentolamine:** Administer 1-2 mg boluses, may increase to 5 mg/dose
  - **Magnesium sulphate:** 4-6 g at induction over 30 min, then 1-2 g/hr
- Smooth anesthesia induction and tracheal intubation to avoid hypertension and tachycardia
- Correct volume depletion by infusion of crystalloids or colloids

**Postoperative management**

- Invasive arterial pressure monitoring for at least 24 hrs after surgery
- Focused on metabolic changes (i.e., hyperglycemia and decreased cortisol level), pain treatment, and residual postoperative hypertension
  - Regular blood glucose monitoring and appropriate titration of dextrose infusions in case of hypoglycemia
  - Administer steroids if hypoadrenalism occurs → wean the IV hydrocortisone dose to 25 mg twice daily before converting to oral prednisolone in the first postoperative 72 hrs
  - Use vasopressors if hypotension occurs
    - Norepinephrine: 4 mg in 250 mL normal saline (16 mcg/mL), run at 1-20 mcg/min, bolus 20-30 mcg/dose
    - Vasopressin: Run at 0.01-0.04 U/min and boluses 4 U/dose for hypotension refractory to norepinephrine

# SUGGESTED READING

- Connor D, Boumphrey S. Perioperative care of phaeochromocytoma. BJA Education. 2016;16(5):153-158.
- Domi R, Sula H. Pheochromocytoma, the Challenge to Anesthesiologists. Journal Of Endocrinology And Metabolism. 2011;1(3):97-100.

# PERIOPERATIVE STEROIDS

## LEARNING OBJECTIVES

- Recognize the signs and symptoms of a perioperative adrenal crisis
- Be able to treat a perioperative adrenal crisis
- Anesthetic management of a patient on chronic steroid therapy

## DEFINITION AND MECHANISM

- Chronic steroid therapy is used in the treatment of many common conditions (e.g., inflammatory bowel disease, rheumatologic disease, asthma, chronic obstructive pulmonary disease, and immunosuppression for transplant recipients)
- Patients on chronic steroid therapy may develop secondary adrenal insufficiency
  - Patients on chronic steroids may experience hypothalamic-pituitary-adrenal (HPA) axis suppression
  - Result in low corticotropin-releasing hormone (CRH) and adrenocorticotropic hormone (ACTH) levels, leading to atrophy of the adrenal zona fasciculata and a decrease in cortisol production = secondary adrenal insufficiency
  - The renin-angiotensin-aldosterone system remains intact
  - No mineralocorticoid deficiency
  - Inadequate cortisol levels may predispose to vasodilation and hypotension
- Secondary adrenal insufficiency can manifest as an adrenal crisis in the perioperative period

### HPA axis

- Acute physiologic or psychologic stress activates the HPA axis
- Hypothalamus produces CRH
- CRH stimulates the production of ACTH in the anterior pituitary
- ACTH signals cortisol production in the adrenal glands
- Cortisol production is self-regulated via negative feedback loops, leading to decreased production of CRH and ACTH

Roles of cortisol

- Stimulate gluconeogenesis
- Catecholamine production
- Activation of anti-stress and anti-inflammatory pathways
- Maintain cardiac output and contractility via modulation of β-receptor synthesis and function
- Enhance vascular tone via an increased sensitivity to catecholamines

## SIGNS AND SYMPTOMS

Signs and symptoms of an adrenal crisis in the awake patient may include:

- Altered mental status
- Abdominal pain
- Nausea and vomiting
- Weakness
- Hypotension

These signs and symptoms are largely absent in the anesthetized patient and nonspecific in the postoperative patient ➔ severe, persistent hypotension that is poorly responsive to fluid and vasopressor therapy

## TREATMENT

Perioperative adrenal crisis can be life-threatening and requires prompt recognition and treatment

- Stress-dose steroids
- Supportive care with fluids and vasopressors

# MANAGEMENT

## *Risk stratification*

**1. Patients who have been diagnosed with secondary adrenal insufficiency**
- Demonstrated by short-acting ACTH test
- Require perioperative stress-dose steroids with dosing based on surgical stress risk

**2. Patients at high risk of HPA axis suppression**
- Patients treated with a glucocorticoid in doses equivalent to > 20 mg/day of prednisone for > 3 weeks or who have clinical features of Cushing syndrome
- Perioperative stress-dose steroids with dosing based on surgical stress

**3. Patient at low risk of HPA axis suppression**
- Patients treated with any dose of glucocorticoid for < 3 weeks, morning doses of prednisone ≤ 5 mg/day, or prednisone 10 mg/day every other day
- Perioperative stress-dose steroids are not required unless these patients exhibit signs of HPA axis suppression

**4. Patients at intermediate risk of HPA axis suppression**
- Patients on chronic steroid therapy who do not fall into one of the above categories (> 5 mg/day but < 20 mg/day)
- Refer patients for preoperative testing to determine HPA axis integrity
- Decide whether or not to administer stress-dose steroids based on the patient's perioperative condition (e.g., hemodynamic status) and surgical risk

## *Dosing*
- **Moderate risk surgery:** Hydrocortisone 50 mg IV q8h x 3 doses
- **High-risk surgery:** Hydrocortisone 100 mg IV q8h x 3 doses

# KEEP IN MIND

- Patients on chronic steroids are at risk for an adrenal crisis during periods of stress due to their attenuated ability to mount a cortisol response
- The patient's risk for an adrenal crisis must be weighed against the risks of unnecessary steroid supplementation

## SUGGESTED READING

- Liu MM, Reidy AB, Saatee S, Collard CD. Perioperative Steroid Management: Approaches Based on Current Evidence. Anesthesiology. 2017;127:166-172.

# PORPHYRIA

**104**

## LEARNING OBJECTIVES

- Describe porphyria
- Recognize the symptoms and signs of porphyria
- Anesthetic management of a patient with porphyria

## DEFINITION AND MECHANISM

- Porphyrias are a heterogeneous group of inherited genetic disorders of heme biosynthesis
- The heme biosynthetic pathway is most active in the liver and bone marrow
- The porphyrins are cyclic structures formed by the linkage of four pyrrole rings through methene (–CH=) bridges
- The porphyrin ring can, via the nitrogen atom of the pyrrole subunits, form complexes with many metals, giving metalloporphyrins
- Of the metalloporphyrins, the most biologically important are those containing iron (to form haem) and magnesium (to form chlorophyll)
- In human physiology, haem is the most important of the porphyrins
- In its biologically active form, haem is bound to various proteins to form haemoproteins, which include haemoglobin, myoglobin and all of the cytochromes (including the P450 series) together with numerous other compounds involved in oxidation and hydroxylation reactions
- Acute attacks of porphyria are most commonly precipitated by events that decrease haem concentrations, thus increasing the activity of ALA synthetase and stimulating the production of porphyrinogens
- Acute exacerbations may be precipitated by a number of factors, including physiological hormonal fluctuations (such as those occurring with menstruation), fasting, dehydration, stress and infection

### *Classification*

- **Acute porphyrias:** Potential to develop acute neurovisceral crises
  - Acute intermittent porphyria (AIP)
  - Variegate porphyria (VP)
  - Hereditary coproporphyria (HCP)
  - 5-aminolaevulinic acid (ALA) dehydrase deficiency: (also called plumboporphyria)
    - Triggers for an acute crisis
    - Fasting
    - Dehydration
    - Infection
    - Drugs: (barbiturates, steroids)
    - Endogenous hormones
    - Stress
    - Smoking
    - Alcohol
- **Non-acute:** Do not deteriorate into acute crises, less relevant for anesthesiologists
  - Porphyria cutanea tarda
  - Congenital erythropoietic porphyria
  - Erythropoietic protoporphyria

# SIGNS AND SYMPTOMS

## *Presentation of an acute crisis*

- Almost all patients have severe abdominal pain, usually associated with tachycardia
- Symptoms and signs of acute crises vary greatly and can mimic other conditions

| Symptoms & signs | Features | May be misdiagnosed as |
|---|---|---|
| Abdominal pain | Recurrent, severe, poorly localized<br>Associated nausea and vomiting<br>Absence of fever or leucocytosis | Another cause of acute abdomen<br>Endometriosis/pelvic inflammatory disease<br>Irritable bowel syndrome<br>Opiate addiction |
| Cardiovascular signs | Tachycardia<br>Tachyarrhythmia<br>Hypertension | |
| Weakness | Proximal > distal<br>Upper limbs > lower<br>Up to 20% develop respiratory failure<br>May progress to bulbar paresis in severe cases | Guillain-Barré syndrome<br>Poliomyelitis<br>Acute lead poisoning<br>Vasculitis |
| Psychiatric features | Mood disturbance<br>Confusion<br>Psychosis | Anxiety disorder<br>Somatization disorder<br>Acute psychosis<br>Acute confusional state |
| Pain and sensory disturbance | Back, thigh, or extremity pain<br>Sensory neuropathy over the trunk | Chronic fatigue syndrome<br>Fibromyalgia<br>Chronic pain syndromes |
| Seizures | CNS manifestation of porphyria<br>Secondary to hyponatremia | Epilepsy |
| Other autonomic features | Constipation<br>Gastoparesis<br>Postural hypotension | |
| Cutaneous lesions | Only in VP and HCP<br>Vesicular rash<br>Photosensitivity | Porphyria cutanea tarda<br>Bullous skin disease |
| Hyponatremia and other electrolyte disturbance | Low serum sodium<br>Low serum magnesium | Other disorders of sodium and water balance |

# RISK FACTORS

- Women are 4 to 5 times more likely to develop crises in their early thirties

# PATHOPHYSIOLOGY

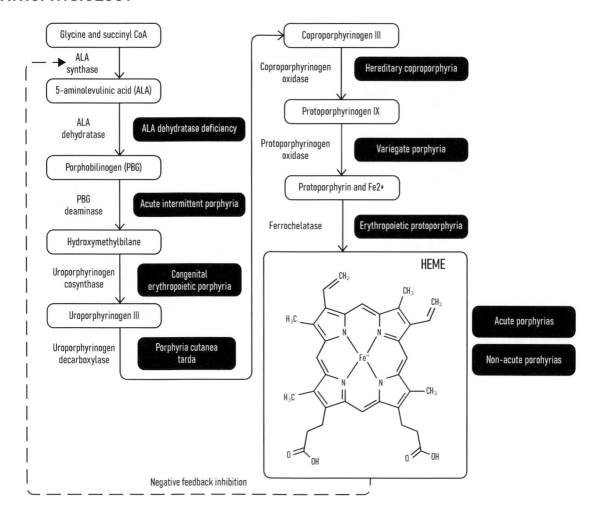

# TREATMENT

Once an acute crisis has been diagnosed, management consists of the following:

- Remove or treat potential triggering factors and avoid a catabolic state
- Administration of IV heme arginate 3 mg/kg daily for 4 days
- Supportive measures
  - May require large doses of morphine to control pain
  - Antiemetics prochlorperazine and ondansetron are safe
  - Control tachycardia and hypertension with β-blockers
  - Avoid seizures via correcting hyponatremia and treating with gabapentin, vigabatrin, or levetiracetam
  - Sedation with propofol and alfentanil is safe

# MANAGEMENT

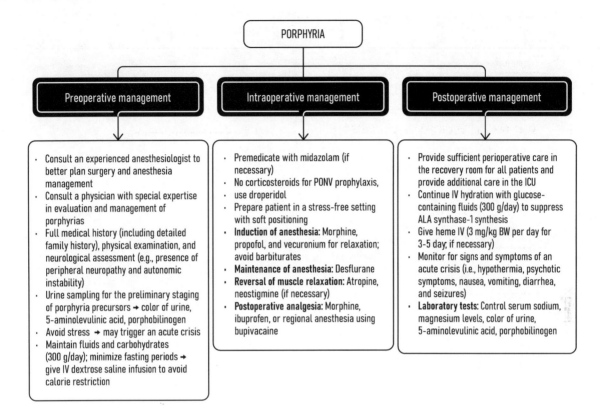

**PORPHYRIA**

**Preoperative management**

- Consult an experienced anesthesiologist to better plan surgery and anesthesia management
- Consult a physician with special expertise in evaluation and management of porphyrias
- Full medical history (including detailed family history), physical examination, and neurological assessment (e.g., presence of peripheral neuropathy and autonomic instability)
- Urine sampling for the preliminary staging of porphyria precursors → color of urine, 5-aminolevulinic acid, porphobilinogen
- Avoid stress → may trigger an acute crisis
- Maintain fluids and carbohydrates (300 g/day); minimize fasting periods → give IV dextrose saline infusion to avoid calorie restriction

**Intraoperative management**

- Premedicate with midazolam (if necessary)
- No corticosteroids for PONV prophylaxis, use droperidol
- Prepare patient in a stress-free setting with soft positioning
- **Induction of anesthesia:** Morphine, propofol, and vecuronium for relaxation; avoid barbiturates
- **Maintenance of anesthesia:** Desflurane
- **Reversal of muscle relaxation:** Atropine, neostigmine (if necessary)
- **Postoperative analgesia:** Morphine, ibuprofen, or regional anesthesia using bupivacaine

**Postoperative management**

- Provide sufficient perioperative care in the recovery room for all patients and provide additional care in the ICU
- Continue IV hydration with glucose-containing fluids (300 g/day) to suppress ALA synthase-1 synthesis
- Give heme IV (3 mg/kg BW per day for 3-5 day; if necessary)
- Monitor for signs and symptoms of an acute crisis (i.e., hypothermia, psychotic symptoms, nausea, vomiting, diarrhea, and seizures)
- **Laboratory tests:** Control serum sodium, magnesium levels, color of urine, 5-aminolevulinic acid, porphobilinogen

*Commonly used drugs and their safety profile*

| Drug | Safe | Unsafe | Undetermined |
|---|---|---|---|
| IV anesthetic agents | Propofol | Thiopentone, ketamine | Etomidate |
| Inhalational anesthetic agents | Isoflurane, desflurane, nitrous oxide | Sevoflurane | |
| Local anesthetics | Bupivacaine, prilocaine, lidocaine | | Levobupivacaine, ropivacaine |
| Neuromuscular blocking agents and removal | Succinylcholine, all non-depolarizing muscle relaxants, neostigmine | | |
| Analgesics | Fentanyl, alfentanil, remifentanil, morphine, hydromorphone, meperidine, tramadol, ibuprofen, aspirin | Oxycodone, diclofenac | Etomidate |
| Sedative premedication | Lorazepam, phenothiazines (chlorpromazine), temazepam | | |
| Antibiotics | Gentamicin, co-amoxiclav, penicillins, vancomycin, piperacillin tazobactam, meropenem | Rifampicin, erythromycin | |
| Cardiovascular drugs | Adrenaline, noradrenaline, milrinone, atropine, glycopyrrolate, β-blockers, phenylephrine, magnesium, angiotensin 2 inhibitors, fibrinolytic drugs | Ephedrine | Vasopressin, metaraminol |
| Miscellaneous | Synthetic oxytocin, carboprost, tranexamic acid, aprotinin | | Dexamethasone, hydrocortisone |

## KEEP IN MIND

- Anesthesiologists should be aware of the perioperative factors that may trigger or worsen an acute crisis in porphyria

## SUGGESTED READING

- Findley H, Philips A, Cole D, Nair A. Porphyrias: implications for anaesthesia, critical care, and pain medicine. Continuing Education in Anaesthesia Critical Care & Pain. 2012;12(3):128-133.

# SIADH

## LEARNING OBJECTIVES

- Describe SIADH
- Recognize the symptoms and signs of SIADH
- Anesthetic management of a patient with SIADH

## DEFINITION AND MECHANISM

- Syndrome of inappropriate antidiuretic hormone secretion (SIADH) is characterized by excessive release of antidiuretic hormone (ADH) or vasopressin from the posterior pituitary gland or an abnormal non-pituitary source
- Overproduction of ADH leads to water retention, urinary sodium loss, and hyponatremia, resulting in volume expansion promoting urine flow rate, and thus limiting further water retention

## SIGNS AND SYMPTOMS

Hyponatremia is mainly responsible for the symptoms associated with SIADH
- **Mild to moderate:** Headache, lethargy, slowness, poor concentration, depressed mood, lack of attention, impaired memory, nausea, restlessness, instability of gait and falls, muscle cramps, tremor
- **Advanced:** Confusion, disorientation, somnolence, vomiting, hallucinations, acute psychosis, limb weakness, dysarthria
- **Serious:** Seizures, hemiplegia, severe somnolence, respiratory insufficiency, coma, death if untreated

## CAUSES

- Conditions dysregulating ADH secretion in the central nervous system (e.g., meningitis, encephalitis, subarachnoid hemorrhage, subdural hematoma, hydrocephalus, Guillain-Barré syndrome, acute porphyria, multiple system atrophy, multiple sclerosis)
- Tumors secreting ADH
- Various lung diseases (e.g., pneumonia, lung abscess, asthma, cystic fibrosis)
- Drugs increasing ADH secretion
- Inherited mutations
- Transient causes (e.g., general anesthesia)

## PATHOPHYSIOLOGY

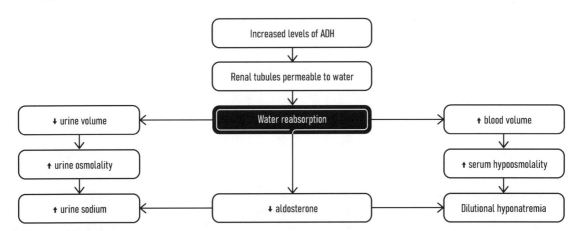

# TREATMENT

- Restore fluid and electrolyte balance
  - Water restriction
  - PO or IV administration of hypertonic saline
- Medications
  - Reduce fluid retention: Loop diuretics (i.e., furosemide)
  - ADH antagonists (i.e., demeclocycline, tolvaptan, conivaptan)
- Eliminate underlying cause
- Caution with rapid correction of serum sodium concentration → may cause central pontine myelinolysis

# MANAGEMENT

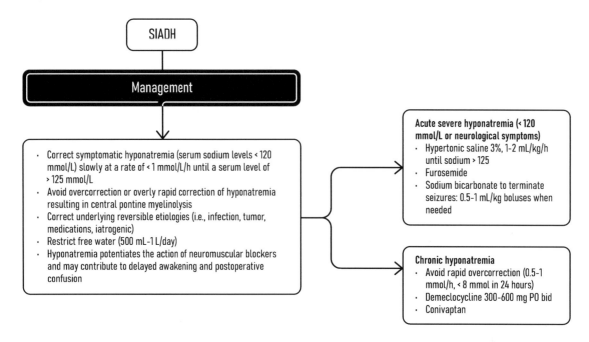

**SIADH**

**Management**

- Correct symptomatic hyponatremia (serum sodium levels < 120 mmol/L) slowly at a rate of < 1 mmol/L/h until a serum level of > 125 mmol/L
- Avoid overcorrection or overly rapid correction of hyponatremia resulting in central pontine myelinolysis
- Correct underlying reversible etiologies (i.e., infection, tumor, medications, iatrogenic)
- Restrict free water (500 mL-1 L/day)
- Hyponatremia potentiates the action of neuromuscular blockers and may contribute to delayed awakening and postoperative confusion

**Acute severe hyponatremia (< 120 mmol/L or neurological symptoms)**
- Hypertonic saline 3%, 1-2 mL/kg/h until sodium > 125
- Furosemide
- Sodium bicarbonate to terminate seizures: 0.5-1 mL/kg boluses when needed

**Chronic hyponatremia**
- Avoid rapid overcorrection (0.5-1 mmol/h, < 8 mmol in 24 hours)
- Demeclocycline 300-600 mg PO bid
- Conivaptan

## SUGGESTED READING

- Gross P. Clinical management of SIADH. Therapeutic advances in endocrinology and metabolism. 2012;3(2):61-73.
- SIADH. In: Bissonnette B, Luginbuehl I, Marciniak B, Dalens BJ. eds. Syndromes: Rapid Recognition and Perioperative Implications. Mgraw Hill; 2006. Accessed January 20, 2023.

# THYROIDECTOMY

## LEARNING OBJECTIVES

- Define and classify the different types of thyroidectomy
- Describe the complications that are associated with thyroidectomy
- Management of a patient undergoing a thyroidectomy

## DEFINITION AND MECHANISM

- Thyroidectomy is the surgical removal of all or part of the thyroid gland
- The surgery is performed to treat thyroid disorders including thyroid cancer, a noncancerous enlargement of the thyroid (goiter), and overactive thyroid (hyperthyroidism)
- A skin crease incision is made approximately 4 cm above the sternum
- The recurrent laryngeal nerves and parathyroid glands should be preserved

### Classification

- **Total thyroidectomy:** The entire thyroid gland is removed
- **Near-total thyroidectomy:** Both lobes of the thyroid are removed except for a small amount of thyroid tissue (on one or both sides) in the vicinity of the recurrent laryngeal nerve entry point and the superior parathyroid gland
- **Partial thyroidectomies**
  - **Hemithyroidectomy or unilateral thyroid lobectomy:** One lobe of the thyroid is removed
  - **Isthmusectomy:** The band of tissue (thyroid isthmus) connecting the two lobes of the thyroid is removed
  - **Open thyroid biopsy:** The thyroid nodule is removed directly (rarely performed)

## INDICATIONS

Thyrotoxicosis
- 2% of females, 0.02% of males
- Graves disease (hyperthyroidism) in younger women is the most common cause (up to 80%)
- Multinodular goiter (older patients)
- Toxic solitary nodule
- Other causes: Thyroiditis, pregnancy, drug-induced (amiodarone)

Thyroid malignancy
- Papillary (80%)
  - 30-40 years old
  - 95% 10-year survival rate
- Follicular (10%)
  - May be hormone producing
  - Older population
  - 85% 10-year survival rate
- Medullary (8%)
  - Older patients
  - May be associated with multiple endocrine neoplasias
  - May produce calcitonin
  - 65% 10-year survival rate
- Anaplastic (1%)
  - Mean survival 6 months from diagnosis

## PATIENT CHARACTERISTICS

- Up to 5% of the population has a goiter
- Most patients are female
- Approximately 10% of thyroid nodules will be malignant

## COMPLICATIONS

- Hypothyroidism → need for lifelong thyroid hormone replacement
- Recurrent laryngeal nerve palsy
  - Unilateral damage: Temporary or permanent hoarseness
  - Bilateral damage: Airway obstruction and acute respiratory distress → emergency tracheostomy may be required
- Damage to the parathyroid glands → temporary or permanent hypoparathyroidism and hypocalcemia
- Anesthetic complications
- Infection
- Hemorrhage/hematoma which may compress the airway → acute respiratory distress
- Stich granuloma
- Chyle leak

# MANAGEMENT

## *Preoperative assessment*

Detailed history and examination
- Airway
  - Marked tracheal deviation
  - Stridor or respiratory distress, especially when supine
  - Assess vocal cords movement to recognize preexisting laryngeal nerve palsy
- Cardiovascular system
  - Hyperthyroidism can cause tachycardia, atrial fibrillation, or heart failure
  - Large goiters may obstruct venous drainage, and superior vena cava obstruction can occur with retrosternal spread
- Eyes
  - Protect the eyes from intraoperative drying or trauma in case of lid retraction and exophthalmos
- Other conditions
  - May be part of multiple endocrine neoplasia syndromes, and conditions such as diabetes mellitus, hyperparathyroidism, and pheochromocytoma must be considered

## *Drug treatment in hyperthyroidism*

Patients should be clinically and biochemically euthyroid before surgery
- **Carbimazole:** Inhibits iodination of tyrosyl residues in thyroglobulin
- **Propylthiouracil:** Same as carbimazole but also reduces peripheral deiodination of T4 to T3
- **β-blockers:** Control cardiovascular effects; propranolol also decreases the extrathyroidal conversion of T4 to T3
- **Iodine:** Give potassium iodine for 7-10 days preoperatively

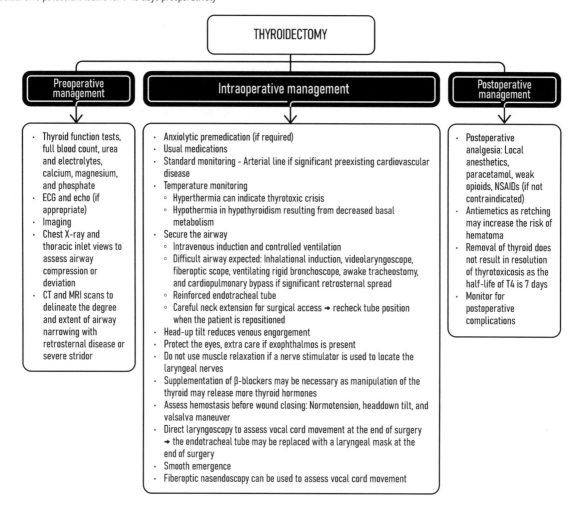

THYROIDECTOMY

**Preoperative management**
- Thyroid function tests, full blood count, urea and electrolytes, calcium, magnesium, and phosphate
- ECG and echo (if appropriate)
- Imaging
- Chest X-ray and thoracic inlet views to assess airway compression or deviation
- CT and MRI scans to delineate the degree and extent of airway narrowing with retrosternal disease or severe stridor

**Intraoperative management**
- Anxiolytic premedication (if required)
- Usual medications
- Standard monitoring - Arterial line if significant preexisting cardiovascular disease
- Temperature monitoring
  - Hyperthermia can indicate thyrotoxic crisis
  - Hypothermia in hypothyroidism resulting from decreased basal metabolism
- Secure the airway
  - Intravenous induction and controlled ventilation
  - Difficult airway expected: Inhalational induction, videolaryngoscope, fiberoptic scope, ventilating rigid bronchoscope, awake tracheostomy, and cardiopulmonary bypass if significant retrosternal spread
  - Reinforced endotracheal tube
  - Careful neck extension for surgical access → recheck tube position when the patient is repositioned
- Head-up tilt reduces venous engorgement
- Protect the eyes, extra care if exophthalmos is present
- Do not use muscle relaxation if a nerve stimulator is used to locate the laryngeal nerves
- Supplementation of β-blockers may be necessary as manipulation of the thyroid may release more thyroid hormones
- Assess hemostasis before wound closing: Normotension, headdown tilt, and valsalva maneuver
- Direct laryngoscopy to assess vocal cord movement at the end of surgery → the endotracheal tube may be replaced with a laryngeal mask at the end of surgery
- Smooth emergence
- Fiberoptic nasendoscopy can be used to assess vocal cord movement

**Postoperative management**
- Postoperative analgesia: Local anesthetics, paracetamol, weak opioids, NSAIDs (if not contraindicated)
- Antiemetics as retching may increase the risk of hematoma
- Removal of thyroid does not result in resolution of thyrotoxicosis as the half-life of T4 is 7 days
- Monitor for postoperative complications

Thyroidectomy

```
┌─────────────────────────────────────────────────┐
│   THYROIDECTOMY: MANAGEMENT OF POSTOPERATIVE      │
│                 COMPLICATIONS                      │
└─────────────────────────────────────────────────┘
```

**Complications**

**Rare complications**

- Hypocalcemia
  - Check serum calcium to ensure normal parathyroid function
  - Tetany or low serum calcium requires calcium supplementation (PO or IV)
- Recurrent laryngeal nerve palsy
  - Temporary 3-4%, permanent < 1%
  - Cause the affected vocal cord to lie in adduction → hoarse voice, poor cough, dyspnea, and stridor
  - Bilateral palsies can result in complete airway obstruction, requiring urgent reintubation
- Hematoma
  - Early detection of signs of postoperative hemorrhage
  - Incidence 0-2%, usually early within 4 hours
  - Can be life-threatening
  - Neck hematoma and surgical tracheal retraction may cause laryngeal edema
  - Immediate removal of wound clips and sutures will decompress the neck and trachea before urgent evacuation and hemostasis

- Tracheomalacia following resection of long-standing large compressive retrosternal thyroid masses
- Pneumothorax following extensive and difficult retrosternal resection
- Thyroid storm (rare due to use of antithyroid medication)
  - Signs: Hyperpyrexia, tachycardia, hypertension, arrhythmias, vomiting, diarrhea, and altered mental state
  - May mimic malignant hyperpyrexia intraoperatively, may also occur postoperatively
  - Treatment includes
    - Supplemental oxygen
    - Temperature monitoring, antipyretics, and active cooling
    - IV fluids
    - β-blockers: Propranolol inhibits peripheral conversion T4 to T3; Esmolol for acute management (short-acting, β1-selective)
    - Antithyroid drugs: Carbimazole or propylthiouracil orally or via a nasogastric tube
    - Dexamethasone
    - Magnesium if hypertension and/or arrhythmia
    - Dantrolene

## SUGGESTED READING

- Pollard BJ, Kitchen G. Handbook of Clinical Anaesthesia. 4th ed. Taylor & Francis group; 2018. Chapter 20 Head and neck surgery, Macnab R and Bexon K.

# HEMATOLOGY

# ACUTE LEUKEMIA

## LEARNING OBJECTIVES

- Definition, symptoms, and perioperative management of acute leukemia

## DEFINITION AND MECHANISM

- Defined as the proliferation of immature white blood cells that comprise more than 20% of the cells of the bone marrow or peripheral blood
- Characterized by a rapid increase in the number of immature blood cells
- The bone marrow is unable to produce healthy blood cells resulting in low hemoglobin and low platelets
- Immediate treatment is required because of the rapid progression and accumulation of the malignant cells
- Two types according to the type of blood cell affected:
  - Acute lymphoblastic leukemia (ALL)
  - Acute myelogenous leukemia (AML)

## SIGNS AND SYMPTOMS

| Acute lymphoblastic leukemia (ALL) | Acute myelogenous leukemia (AML) |
| --- | --- |
| Pale skin | Skin looking pale or "washed out" |
| Feeling tired and breathless | Tiredness |
| Repeated infections over a short time | Breathlessness |
| Unusual and frequent bleeding, such as bleeding gums or nosebleeds | Losing weight without trying |
| High temperature | Frequent infections |
| Night sweats | High temperature/fever |
| Bone and joint pain | Night sweats |
| Easily bruised skin | Unusual and frequent bleeding, such as bleeding gums or nosebleeds |
| Swollen lymph nodes | Easily bruised skin |
| Abdominal pain – caused by a swollen liver or spleen | Flat red or purple spots on the skin |
| Unintentional weight loss | Bone and joint pain |
| A purple skin rash (purpura) | A feeling of fullness or discomfort in the abdomen |
| | Swollen glands in your neck, armpit, or groin |

## RISK FACTORS

- Radiation exposure
- Benzene and smoking
- Chemotherapy
- Blood disorders: myelodysplasia, myelofibrosis, polycythemia
- Genetic disorders: Down syndrome, Fanconi's anemia

Acute leukemia

# MANAGEMENT

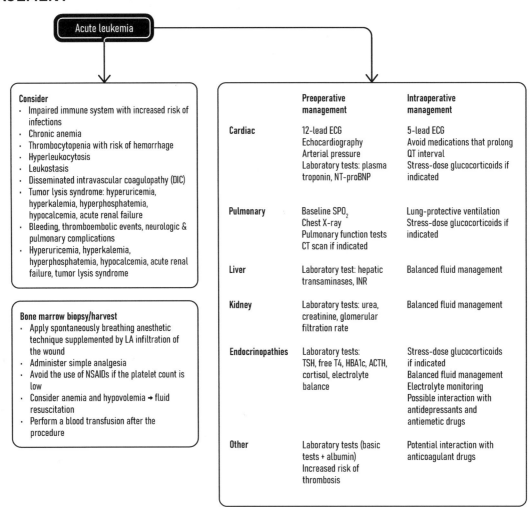

**Acute leukemia**

**Consider**
- Impaired immune system with increased risk of infections
- Chronic anemia
- Thrombocytopenia with risk of hemorrhage
- Hyperleukocytosis
- Leukostasis
- Disseminated intravascular coagulopathy (DIC)
- Tumor lysis syndrome: hyperuricemia, hyperkalemia, hyperphosphatemia, hypocalcemia, acute renal failure
- Bleeding, thromboembolic events, neurologic & pulmonary complications
- Hyperuricemia, hyperkalemia, hyperphosphatemia, hypocalcemia, acute renal failure, tumor lysis syndrome

**Bone marrow biopsy/harvest**
- Apply spontaneously breathing anesthetic technique supplemented by LA infiltration of the wound
- Administer simple analgesia
- Avoid the use of NSAIDs if the platelet count is low
- Consider anemia and hypovolemia → fluid resuscitation
- Perform a blood transfusion after the procedure

|  | Preoperative management | Intraoperative management |
|---|---|---|
| **Cardiac** | 12-lead ECG<br>Echocardiography<br>Arterial pressure<br>Laboratory tests: plasma troponin, NT-proBNP | 5-lead ECG<br>Avoid medications that prolong QT interval<br>Stress-dose glucocorticoids if indicated |
| **Pulmonary** | Baseline $SPO_2$<br>Chest X-ray<br>Pulmonary function tests<br>CT scan if indicated | Lung-protective ventilation<br>Stress-dose glucocorticoids if indicated |
| **Liver** | Laboratory test: hepatic transaminases, INR | Balanced fluid management |
| **Kidney** | Laboratory tests: urea, creatinine, glomerular filtration rate | Balanced fluid management |
| **Endocrinopathies** | Laboratory tests: TSH, free T4, HBA1c, ACTH, cortisol, electrolyte balance | Stress-dose glucocorticoids if indicated<br>Balanced fluid management<br>Electrolyte monitoring<br>Possible interaction with antidepressants and antiemetic drugs |
| **Other** | Laboratory tests (basic tests + albumin)<br>Increased risk of thrombosis | Potential interaction with anticoagulant drugs |

DIC, disseminated intravascular coagulopathy; LA, local anesthetic; NT-proBNP, N-terminal prohormone of brain natriuretic peptide; TSH, thyroid stimulating hormone; HBA1c, glycated hemoglobin; ACTH, adrenocorticotropic hormone; T4, thyroxine.

## SUGGESTED READING

- Allan N, Siller C, Breen A. Anaesthetic implications of chemotherapy, Continuing Education in Anaesthesia Critical Care & Pain, Volume 12, Issue 2, April 2012, Pages 52–56.
- Groenewold MD, Olthof CG, Bosch DJ. Anaesthesia after neoadjuvant chemotherapy, immunotherapy or radiotherapy. BJA Educ. 2022;22(1):12-19.
- Louise Oduro-Dominah L, Brennan LH, Anaesthetic management of the child with haematological malignancy, Continuing Education in Anaesthesia Critical Care & Pain, Volume 13, Issue 5, October 2013, Pages 158-164.

# ANTIPHOSPHOLIPID ANTIBODY SYNDROME

## LEARNING OBJECTIVES

- Describe antiphospholipid antibody syndrome (APS)
- Signs and symptoms and management of APS

## DEFINITION AND MECHANISM

- Antiphospholipid syndrome (APS) or Hughes syndrome is a disorder of immune system that creates antibodies that attack tissues in the body by mistake
- These antibodies can cause blood clots to form in arteries and veins, leading to a heart attack, stroke, and other conditions
- Can result miscarriage and stillbirth during pregnancy
- Primary APS: The sole manifestation of an autoimmune process
- Secondary APS: In association with another disease such as systemic lupus erythematosus
- Antiphospholipid syndrome is more common in women than in men
- Causes are not completely understood and include environmental or genetic factors or an existing autoimmune disorder
- In very rare cases, blood clots can suddenly form throughout the body, resulting in multiple organ failures → catastrophic antiphospholipid syndrome (CAPS), or Asherson syndrome
  - CAPS requires immediate emergency treatment with high-dose anticoagulants

| Signs and symptoms | | |
|---|---|---|
| Vascular thrombosis | Arterial thrombosis | Stroke<br>Transient ischemic attack<br>Myocardial infarction<br>Venous thrombosis |
| | Venous thromboembolism | Venous thromboembolism<br>Pulmonary embolism<br>Small vessel thrombosis |
| Obstetric morbidity | ≥ 1 unexplained fetal death at or beyond week 10 of gestation<br>≥ 1 premature birth due to severe pre-eclampsia, eclampsia, or consequences of placental insufficiency<br>≥ 3 unexplained consecutive spontaneous abortions before week 10 of gestation | |
| Cardiac manifestations | Valvular heart disease<br>Cardiomyopathies | |
| Neurological manifestations | Cognitive dysfunction<br>Headache or migraine<br>Multiple sclerosis<br>Transverse myelopathy<br>Epilepsy | |

## Signs and symptoms

| | |
|---|---|
| Dermatologic manifestations | Livedo reticularis<br>Skin ulceration<br>Pseudo-vasculitic lesion<br>Distal gangrene<br>Superficial phlebitis<br>Malignant atrophic papulosis-like lesion<br>Subungual splinter hemorrhage |
| Renal manifestations | Thrombotic microangiopathy<br>Chronic vascular damage |
| Hematologic manifestations | Thrombocytopenia<br>Hemolytic anemia |

## RISK FACTORS

- Pregnancy
- Immobility
- Surgery
- Smoking
- Oral contraceptives or estrogen therapy for menopause
- High cholesterol and triglyceride levels
- Systemic autoimmune diseases such as lupus

## COMPLICATIONS

- Kidney failure
- Stroke
- Cardiovascular problems
- Pulmonary embolism
- Pregnancy complications
  - Miscarriages
  - Stillbirths
  - Premature delivery
  - Slow fetal growth
  - Preeclampsia

## TREATMENT

- Primary thromboprophylaxis for APS carriers with no prior history of vascular thrombosis and/or obstetric events
  - Low-dose aspirin (75-100 mg/day)
  - Lifestyle changes: smoking cessation, weight loss, control of hypertension and hyperlipidemia
  - A prophylactic dose of low-molecular-weight heparin (LMWH) in high-risk situations such as surgery, prolonged immobilization, and the puerperium
- Secondary thromboprophylaxis for the prevention of recurrence after thrombotic and/or obstetric events in patients with a prior history
  - Previous venous thrombosis:
    - Anticoagulation: target INR of 2.0-3.0
  - Previous arterial thrombosis:
    - High-intensity anticoagulation: target INR of 3.0-4.0 or a target INR of 2.0-3.0 combined with low-dose aspirin
- CAPS
  - Combination therapy with glucocorticoid, heparin, and plasmapheresis or IV immunoglobulin, rituximab, cyclophosphamide, or eculizumab
- Pregnant women
  - Combination therapy:
    - Low-dose aspirin and unfractionated heparin or LMWH
  - Withdraw oral anticoagulants as soon as pregnancy is confirmed to prevent teratogenicity
  - Patients without a history of thrombosis:
    - Low-dose aspirin and a prophylactic dose of unfractionated heparin or LMWH are used for primary prevention
  - Patients with a history of thrombotic events:
    - Low-dose aspirin and a prophylactic dose of unfractionated heparin or LMWH are used for secondary prevention
  - After delivery:
    - Administer a prophylactic dose of LMWH for at least 6 weeks after delivery
    - Start warfarin as soon as possible after bleeding is controlled
    - Patients with APS who have not received any thromboprophylaxis before delivery and do not carry any risk factors for thrombosis, require LMWH for only 7 days following delivery

Antiphospholipid antibody syndrome

# MANAGEMENT

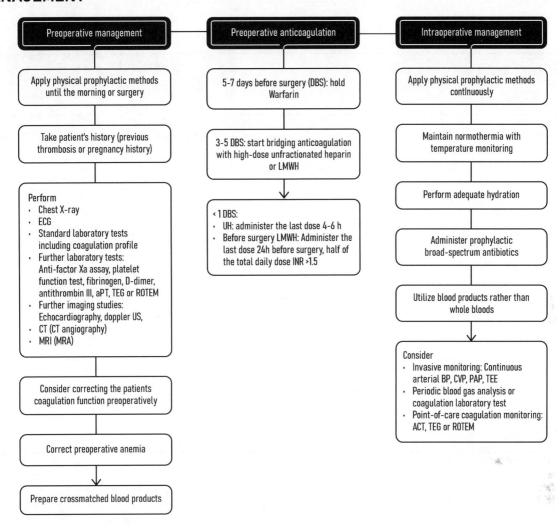

DBS, days before surgery; UH, unfractionated heparin; LMWH, low molecular weight heparin; INR, international normalized ratio; ECG, electrocardiogram; aPTT, activated partial thromboplastin time; TEG, thromboelastography; ROTEM, rotational thromboelastometry; US, ultrasound; CT, computed tomography; MRI, magnetic resonance imaging; MRA, magnetic resonance angiography; BP, blood pressure; CVP, central venous pressure; PAP, pulmonary artery pressure; TEE, transesophageal echocardiography; ACT, activated clotting time

Antiphospholipid antibody syndrome

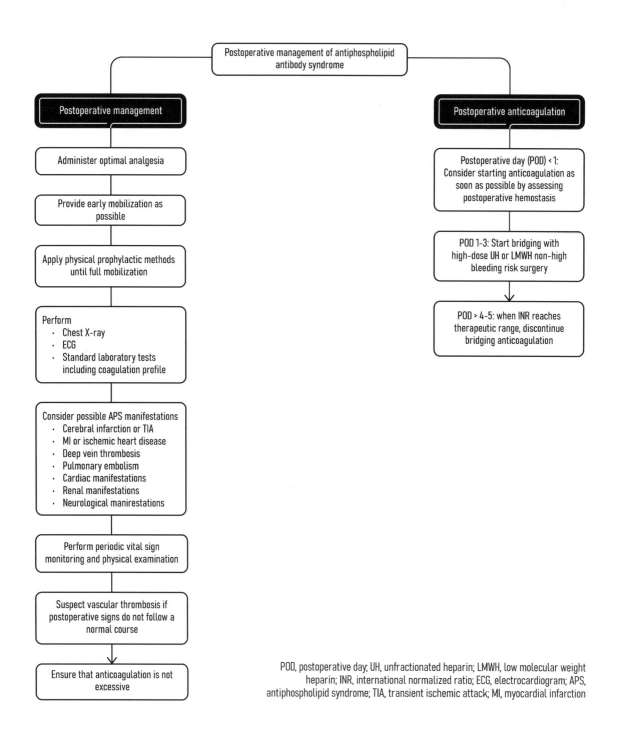

**Postoperative management of antiphospholipid antibody syndrome**

**Postoperative management**

- Administer optimal analgesia
- Provide early mobilization as possible
- Apply physical prophylactic methods until full mobilization
- Perform
  - Chest X-ray
  - ECG
  - Standard laboratory tests including coagulation profile
- Consider possible APS manifestations
  - Cerebral infarction or TIA
  - MI or ischemic heart disease
  - Deep vein thrombosis
  - Pulmonary embolism
  - Cardiac manifestations
  - Renal manifestations
  - Neurological manirestations
- Perform periodic vital sign monitoring and physical examination
- Suspect vascular thrombosis if postoperative signs do not follow a normal course
- Ensure that anticoagulation is not excessive

**Postoperative anticoagulation**

- Postoperative day (POD) < 1: Consider starting anticoagulation as soon as possible by assessing postoperative hemostasis
- POD 1-3: Start bridging with high-dose UH or LMWH non-high bleeding risk surgery
- POD > 4-5: when INR reaches therapeutic range, discontinue bridging anticoagulation

POD, postoperative day; UH, unfractionated heparin; LMWH, low molecular weight heparin; INR, international normalized ratio; ECG, electrocardiogram; APS, antiphospholipid syndrome; TIA, transient ischemic attack; MI, myocardial infarction

## SUGGESTED READING

- Kim JW, Kim TW, Ryu KH, Park SG, Jeong CY, Park DH. Anaesthetic considerations for patients with antiphospholipid syndrome undergoing non-cardiac surgery. J Int Med Res. 2020;48(1):300060519896889.

# COAGULOPATHY

## LEARNING OBJECTIVES

- Definition of coagulopathy
- Management of coagulopathy

## DEFINITION AND MECHANISM

- Coagulopathy is a condition in which the blood's ability to coagulate (form clots) is impaired
- Leading to a tendency toward prolonged or excessive bleeding and occurring spontaneously or following an injury
- Caused by:
  □ Genetic conditions such as hemophilia and Von Willebrand disease
  □ Acquired factors: anticoagulant medications (warfarin), the continued use of antibiotics, liver disease, or disseminated intravascular coagulation (DIC)
- Activation of coagulation will lead to consumption of clotting factors, particularly factor V and fibrinogen, leading to a consumptive coagulopathy

## SIGNS AND SYMPTOMS

- Easy bruising
- Hemarthrosis (bleeding into a joint cavity)
- Hemorrhage after childbirth
- Hemothorax
- Very heavy menstrual flow
- Loss of blood through the nose
- Anal bleeding
- Livedo reticularis
- Thrombocytopenia
- Gingival bleeding

- Rheumatism
- Bloody gums
- Joint pain and swelling
- Blood in the urine
- Double vision
- Severe head or neck pain
- Repeated vomiting
- Difficulty walking
- Convulsions or seizures

## MANAGEMENT

- Obtain a blood sample for a full coagulation screen
- Perform near-patient testing such as rotational thromboelastometry (ROTEM) or thromboelastography (TEG)
- Consider permissive hypotension in patients with moderate bleeding
- Perform massive volume resuscitation in a patient with severe hypovolemic shock
- Limit crystalloid and colloid infusions as this leads to acidosis, hypothermia and coagulopathy
- Transfuse red blood cells → hemoglobin target is between 7-9 dL/L
- Administer fresh frozen plasma, platelets, cryoprecipitate, and concentrated red cells, depending on clotting results and blood loss
- Correct hyperfibrinolysis with tranexamic acid
- Avoid volatile anesthetics as they lead to vasodilation
- Administer multimodal analgesia (opioids, NMDA glutamate receptor antagonists)
- Regional anesthesia is not indicated as it takes too much time and could mask compartment syndrome
- Avoid hypothermia as this worsens coagulopathy
  □ With passive rewarming, active external rewarming, and active internal rewarming
  □ Hypothermia impairs thrombin generation
  □ Hypothermia contributes to platelet dysfunction
- Consider complications associated with plasma administration such as transfusion-related acute lung injury (TRALI), sepsis, and ABO incompatibility

Coagulopathy

# TRAUMA-INDUCED COAGULOPATHY

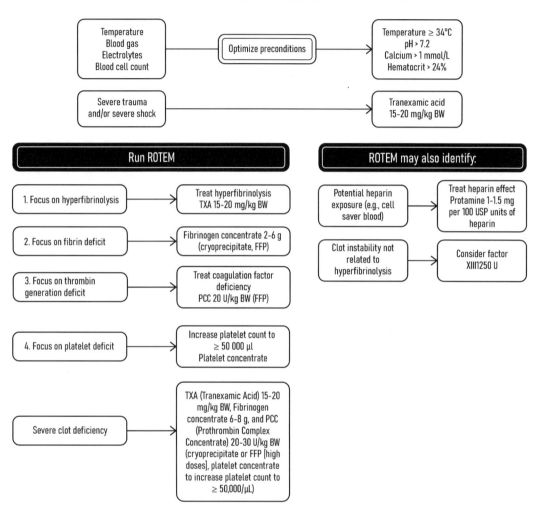

ROTEM, rotational thromboelastometry; TXA, tranexamic acid; BW, body weight; FFP, fresh frozen plasma; PCC, prothrombin complex concentrate

## SUGGESTED READING

- Daniel Bolliger, Klaus Görlinger, Kenichi A. Tanaka, David S. Warner; Pathophysiology and Treatment of Coagulopathy in Massive Hemorrhage and Hemodilution. Anesthesiology 2010; 113:1205-1219.
- Gaunt, C., Woolley, T., 2014. Management of haemorrhage in major trauma. Continuing Education in Anaesthesia Critical Care & Pain 14, 251-255.
- Hofer S, Schlimp CJ, Casu S, Grouzi E. Management of Coagulopathy in Bleeding Patients. J Clin Med. 2021;11(1):1.
- Pollard BJ, Kitchen, G. Handbook of Clinical Anaesthesia. Fourth Edition. CRC Press. 2018. 978-1-4987-6289-2.
- Simmons J, Powel M. 2016. Acute traumatic coagulopathy: pathophysiology and resuscitation. BJA: British journal of anaesthesia. 17;3:31-43.

# DISSEMINATED INTRAVASCULAR COAGULATION (DIC)

## LEARNING OBJECTIVES

- Recognize Disseminated Intravascular Coagulation (DIC)
- Management of DIC

## DEFINITION AND MECHANISM

- Disseminated intravascular coagulation is a life-threatening disease characterized by systemic activation of blood coagulation
- Resulting in the generation and deposition of fibrin
- Leading to microvascular thrombi in various organs and contributing to multiple organ dysfunction syndrome (MODS)
- Consumption of clotting factors and platelets in DIC can result in life-threatening hemorrhage
- A patient with DIC can present with a simultaneously occurring thrombotic and bleeding problem, obviously complicating the proper treatment
- DIC affects approximately 10% of critically ill patients, including those with sepsis, cancer, or pancreatitis, as well as patients recovering from traumatic injuries such as burns or serious pregnancy and delivery complications

## SIGNS AND SYMPTOMS

- Bleeding at wound sites or from the nose, gums, or mouth
- Blood in the stool or urine
- Bruising
- Chest pain
- Pain, redness, warmth, and swelling of the leg
- Confusion, memory loss, or change of behavior
- Difficulty breathing
- Fever

## COMPLICATIONS

- Acute respiratory distress syndrome (ARDS)
- Bleeding in the gastrointestinal tract
- Heart attack
- Shock
- Stroke
- Venous thromboembolism

| Causes | |
| --- | --- |
| Sepsis | |
| Major damage to organs or tissues | Cirrhosis<br>Pancreatitis<br>Severe injury<br>Burns<br>Major surgery |
| Severe immune reactions | Failed blood transfusion<br>Organ transplant rejection<br>Toxin: snake venom |
| Serious pregnancy-related problems | Separation of the placenta from the uterus before delivery<br>Amniotic fluid in the bloodstream<br>Serious bleeding during or after delivery |
| Cancer | |
| Covid-19 | |

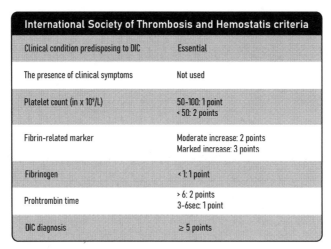

| International Society of Thrombosis and Hemostatis criteria | |
|---|---|
| Clinical condition predisposing to DIC | Essential |
| The presence of clinical symptoms | Not used |
| Platelet count (in x 10⁹/L) | 50-100: 1 point<br>< 50: 2 points |
| Fibrin-related marker | Moderate increase: 2 points<br>Marked increase: 3 points |
| Fibrinogen | < 1: 1 point |
| Prohtrombin time | > 6: 2 points<br>3-6sec: 1 point |
| DIC diagnosis | ≥ 5 points |

# MANAGEMENT

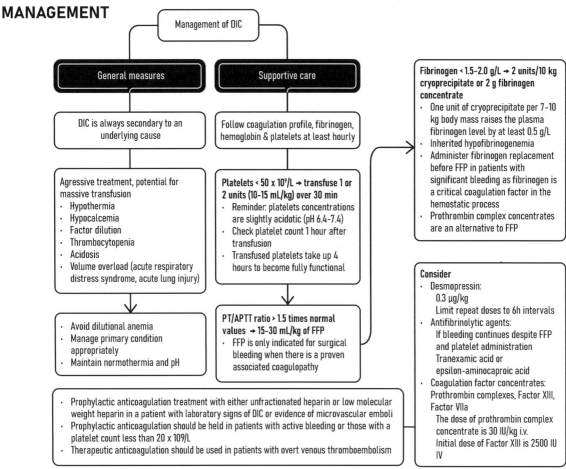

**Management of DIC**

**General measures**

DIC is always secondary to an underlying cause

Agressive treatment, potential for massive transfusion
- Hypothermia
- Hypocalcemia
- Factor dilution
- Thrombocytopenia
- Acidosis
- Volume overload (acute respiratory distress syndrome, acute lung injury)

- Avoid dilutional anemia
- Manage primary condition appropriately
- Maintain normothermia and pH

**Supportive care**

Follow coagulation profile, fibrinogen, hemoglobin & platelets at least hourly

**Platelets < 50 x 10⁹/L → transfuse 1 or 2 units (10-15 mL/kg) over 30 min**
- Reminder: platelets concentrations are slightly acidotic (pH 6.4-7.4)
- Check platelet count 1 hour after transfusion
- Transfused platelets take up 4 hours to become fully functional

**PT/APTT ratio > 1.5 times normal values → 15-30 mL/kg of FFP**
- FFP is only indicated for surgical bleeding when there is a proven associated coagulopathy

**Fibrinogen < 1.5-2.0 g/L → 2 units/10 kg cryoprecipitate or 2 g fibrinogen concentrate**
- One unit of cryoprecipitate per 7-10 kg body mass raises the plasma fibrinogen level by at least 0.5 g/L
- Inherited hypofibrinogenemia
- Administer fibrinogen replacement before FFP in patients with significant bleeding as fibrinogen is a critical coagulation factor in the hemostatic process
- Prothrombin complex concentrates are an alternative to FFP

**Consider**
- Desmopressin:
  0.3 µg/kg
  Limit repeat doses to 6h intervals
- Antifibrinolytic agents:
  If bleeding continues despite FFP and platelet administration
  Tranexamic acid or epsilon-aminocaproic acid
- Coagulation factor concentrates:
  Prothrombin complexes, Factor XIII, Factor VIIa
  The dose of prothrombin complex concentrate is 30 IU/kg i.v.
  Initial dose of Factor XIII is 2500 IU IV

- Prophylactic anticoagulation treatment with either unfractionated heparin or low molecular weight heparin in a patient with laboratory signs of DIC or evidence of microvascular emboli
- Prophylactic anticoagulation should be held in patients with active bleeding or those with a platelet count less than 20 x 10⁹/L
- Therapeutic anticoagulation should be used in patients with overt venous thromboembolism

PT, prothrombin time; aPTT, activated partial thromboplastin time; FFP, fresh frozen plasma; DIC, disseminated intravascular coagulation; pH, potential of hydrogen; IV, intravenous

# SUGGESTED READING

- Adelborg K, Larsen JB, Hvas AM. Disseminated intravascular coagulation: Epidemiology, biomarkers, and management. Br J Haematol. 2021;192(5):803-18.
- Ridley, S., Taylor, B., Gunning, K., 2007. Medical management of bleeding in critically ill patients. Continuing Education in Anaesthesia Critical Care & Pain 7, 116-121.
- Thachil J. Disseminated Intravascular Coagulation: A Practical Approach. Anesthesiology. 2016;125(1):230-236.

# FACTOR V LEIDEN

## LEARNING OBJECTIVES

- Description and management of Factor V Leiden

## DEFINITION AND MECHANISM

- Factor V Leiden is an autosomal dominant inherited mutation of the F5 gene that controls the production of factor V, one of the clotting factors in the blood
- Resulting in resistance to activated protein C thereby leading to thrombosis
- It is the most common inherited blood clotting disorder
- Factor V Leiden increases the chance of developing a deep vein thrombosis or pulmonary embolism
- However, most people with factor V Leiden never develop abnormal blood clots

## SIGNS AND SYMPTOMS

- The factor V Leiden mutation does not itself cause any symptoms and the first indication is the development of a blood clot
- Deep vein thrombosis
  - Pain
  - Swelling
  - Redness
  - Warmth
  - Tenderness
  - Abdominal pain
  - A severe, sudden headache and/or seizures
- Pulmonary embolism
  - Sudden shortness of breath
  - Chest pain when breathing in
  - A cough that produces bloody or blood-streaked sputum
  - Wheezing
  - Tachycardia
  - Feeling light-headed or fainting

## RISK FACTORS

- Immobility
- Intake of estrogen-based therapies
- Surgeries or injuries
- Non-O blood type

## DIAGNOSIS

- Activated protein C blood test
- Genetic testing

# MANAGEMENT

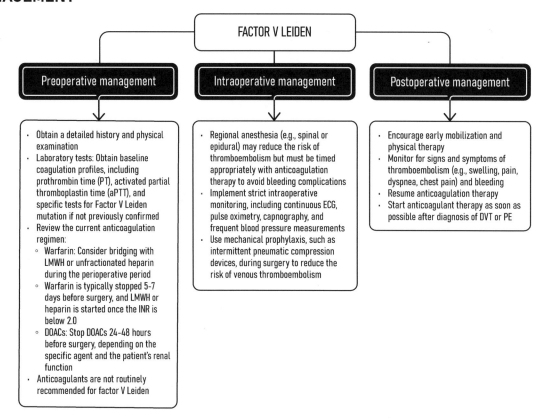

**FACTOR V LEIDEN**

**Preoperative management**

- Obtain a detailed history and physical examination
- Laboratory tests: Obtain baseline coagulation profiles, including prothrombin time (PT), activated partial thromboplastin time (aPTT), and specific tests for Factor V Leiden mutation if not previously confirmed
- Review the current anticoagulation regimen:
  - Warfarin: Consider bridging with LMWH or unfractionated heparin during the perioperative period
  - Warfarin is typically stopped 5-7 days before surgery, and LMWH or heparin is started once the INR is below 2.0
  - DOACs: Stop DOACs 24-48 hours before surgery, depending on the specific agent and the patient's renal function
- Anticoagulants are not routinely recommended for factor V Leiden

**Intraoperative management**

- Regional anesthesia (e.g., spinal or epidural) may reduce the risk of thromboembolism but must be timed appropriately with anticoagulation therapy to avoid bleeding complications
- Implement strict intraoperative monitoring, including continuous ECG, pulse oximetry, capnography, and frequent blood pressure measurements
- Use mechanical prophylaxis, such as intermittent pneumatic compression devices, during surgery to reduce the risk of venous thromboembolism

**Postoperative management**

- Encourage early mobilization and physical therapy
- Monitor for signs and symptoms of thromboembolism (e.g., swelling, pain, dyspnea, chest pain) and bleeding
- Resume anticoagulation therapy
- Start anticoagulant therapy as soon as possible after diagnosis of DVT or PE

## SUGGESTED READING

- Shah UJ, Madan Narayanan M, J Graham Smith JH. 2015. Anaesthetic considerations in patients with inherited disorders of coagulation. Continuing Education in Anaesthesia Critical Care & Pain. 15;1 26-31.

# G6PD DEFICIENCY

## LEARNING OBJECTIVES

- Describe glucose-6-phosphate dehydrogenase or G6PD deficiency
- Management of G6PD deficiency

## DEFINITION AND MECHANISM

- G6PD deficiency is the most common inherited metabolic disorder of red blood cells (RBCs)
- A genetic X-linked recessive disorder characterized by a lack of G6PD in the blood
- Caused by mutations in the G6DP gene
- GD6P protects red blood cells from reactive oxygen species
- Can cause hemolytic anemia as RBCs are vulnerable to hemolysis
- 400 million people are globally affected and males are affected more often than females
  □ Particularly common in certain parts of Africa, Asia, the Mediterranean area, and the Middle East
- Affected persons must avoid dietary triggers such as fava beans
- A spectrum of disease: chronic hemolysis, intermittent hemolysis, hemolysis only with triggers, no hemolysis

## SIGNS AND SYMPTOMS

Most individuals with G6PD deficiency are asymptomatic
- Pale skin
- Jaundice
- Dark-colored urine
- Fever
- Weakness
- Dizziness
- Confusion
- Trouble with physical activity
- Enlarged spleen and liver
- Increased heart rate
- Heart murmur

## TRIGGERS

- Foods: fava beans
- Medicines: aspirin, quinine, and other antimalarials derived from quinine
- Mothballs (naphthalene)
- Bacterial and viral infections

## DIAGNOSIS

- Complete blood count and reticulocyte count: Heinz bodies can be seen in red blood cells
- Liver enzymes: to exclude other causes of jaundice
- Lactate dehydrogenase: elevated in hemolysis
- Haptoglobin: decreased in hemolysis
- A direct antiglobulin test (Coombs' test): should be negative as hemolysis in G6DP is not immune-mediated

# MANAGEMENT

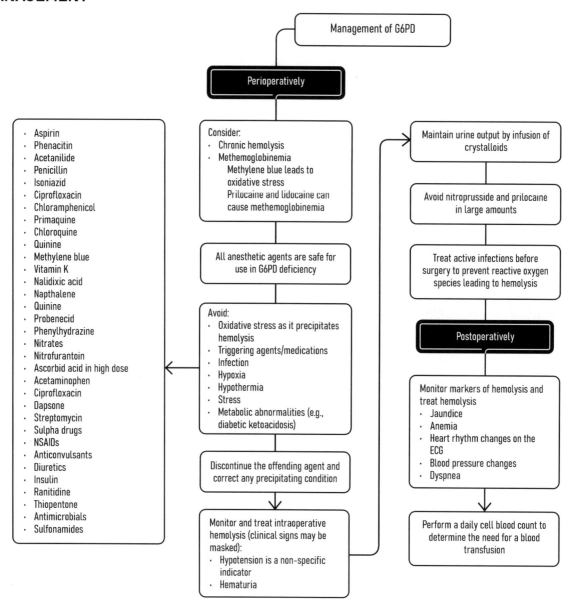

Management of G6PD

**Perioperatively**

- Aspirin
- Phenacitin
- Acetanilide
- Penicillin
- Isoniazid
- Ciprofloxacin
- Chloramphenicol
- Primaquine
- Chloroquine
- Quinine
- Methylene blue
- Vitamin K
- Nalidixic acid
- Napthalene
- Quinine
- Probenecid
- Phenylhydrazine
- Nitrates
- Nitrofurantoin
- Ascorbid acid in high dose
- Acetaminophen
- Ciprofloxacin
- Dapsone
- Streptomycin
- Sulpha drugs
- NSAIDs
- Anticonvulsants
- Diuretics
- Insulin
- Ranitidine
- Thiopentone
- Antimicrobials
- Sulfonamides

Consider:
- Chronic hemolysis
- Methemoglobinemia
  Methylene blue leads to oxidative stress
  Prilocaine and lidocaine can cause methemoglobinemia

All anesthetic agents are safe for use in G6PD deficiency

Avoid:
- Oxidative stress as it precipitates hemolysis
- Triggering agents/medications
- Infection
- Hypoxia
- Hypothermia
- Stress
- Metabolic abnormalities (e.g., diabetic ketoacidosis)

Discontinue the offending agent and correct any precipitating condition

Monitor and treat intraoperative hemolysis (clinical signs may be masked):
- Hypotension is a non-specific indicator
- Hematuria

Maintain urine output by infusion of crystalloids

Avoid nitroprusside and prilocaine in large amounts

Treat active infections before surgery to prevent reactive oxygen species leading to hemolysis

**Postoperatively**

Monitor markers of hemolysis and treat hemolysis
- Jaundice
- Anemia
- Heart rhythm changes on the ECG
- Blood pressure changes
- Dyspnea

Perform a daily cell blood count to determine the need for a blood transfusion

---

## SUGGESTED READING

- Cicvarić, A., Glavaš Tahtler, J., Vukoja Vukušić, T., Bekavac, I., Kvolik, S., 2022. Management of Anesthesia and Perioperative Procedures in a Child with Glucose-6-Phosphate Dehydrogenase Deficiency. Journal of Clinical Medicine 11, 6476.
- Goi T, Shionoya Y, Sunada K, Nakamura K. General Anesthesia in a Glucose-6-Phosphate Dehydrogenase Deficiency Child: A Case Report. Anesth Prog. 2019;66(2):94-96.
- Pollard BJ, Kitchen, G. Handbook of Clinical Anaesthesia. Fourth Edition. CRC Press. 2018. 978-1-4987-6289-2.
- Valiaveedan S, Mahajan C, Rath GP, Bindra A, Marda MK. Anaesthetic management in patients with glucose-6-phosphate dehydrogenase deficiency undergoing neurosurgical procedures. Indian J Anaesth. 2011;55(1):68-70.

# HEMOPHILIA

## LEARNING OBJECTIVES

- Definition and types of hemophilia
- Management of hemophilia

## DEFINITION AND MECHANISM

- Inherited bleeding disorder in which the blood does not clot properly
- Resulting in a longer bleeding time: ↑ PTT, normal INR
- Spontaneous bleeding as well as bleeding following injuries or surgery
- The severity depends on the amount of clotting factors in the blood
- Three types of hemophilia:
  - Hemophilia A (Classic hemophilia): Caused by a lack or decrease of clotting factor VIII
  - Hemophilia B (Christmas Disease): Caused by a lack or decrease of clotting factor IX
  - Hemophilia C (Rosenthal syndrome): Factor 11 deficiency, extremely rare, autosomal recessive transmission
  - Hemophilia A is 4 times as common as hemophilia B
  - A normal value of coagulation factor is 0.5-1.5 IU/ml or 50-150%

| Hemophilia | Mild | Moderate | Severe |
|---|---|---|---|
| % activity of factors | 5-40 | 1-5 | <1 |
| Factor levels (IU/mL) | 0.05-0.40 | 0.01-0.05 | <0.01 |

## SIGNS AND SYMPTOMS

- Unexplained and excessive bleeding from cuts or injuries, or after surgery or dental work
- Many large or deep bruises
- Unusual bleeding after vaccinations
- Pain, swelling, or tightness in the joints
- Blood in the urine or stool
- Nosebleeds without a known cause
- Unexplained irritability in infants

## CAUSES

- Congenital:
  - Caused by an X-linked genetic mutation
  - Occurs in 1/5000 male births
- Acquired hemophilia:
  - Pregnancy
  - Autoimmune disorders
  - Cancer
  - Multiple sclerosis
  - Drug reactions

## COMPLICATIONS

- Deep internal bleeding
- Bleeding into the throat or neck
- Damage to joints
- Infection: hepatitis C
- Adverse reaction to clotting factor treatment

# MANAGEMENT

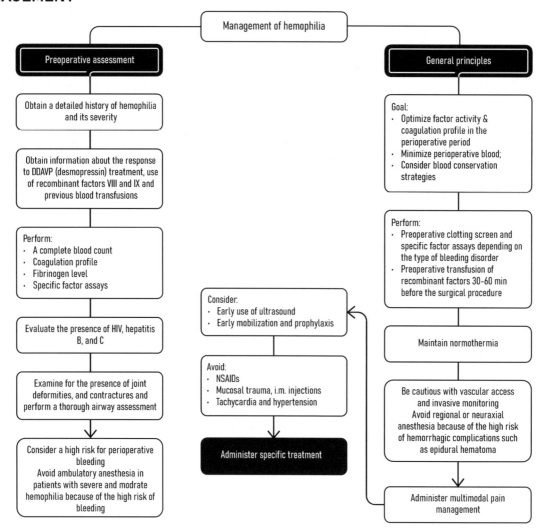

**Management of hemophilia**

## Preoperative assessment

Obtain a detailed history of hemophilia and its severity

Obtain information about the response to DDAVP (desmopressin) treatment, use of recombinant factors VIII and IX and previous blood transfusions

Perform:
- A complete blood count
- Coagulation profile
- Fibrinogen level
- Specific factor assays

Evaluate the presence of HIV, hepatitis B, and C

Examine for the presence of joint deformities, and contractures and perform a thorough airway assessment

Consider a high risk for perioperative bleeding
Avoid ambulatory anesthesia in patients with severe and modrate hemophilia because of the high risk of bleeding

Consider:
- Early use of ultrasound
- Early mobilization and prophylaxis

Avoid:
- NSAIDs
- Mucosal trauma, i.m. injections
- Tachycardia and hypertension

**Administer specific treatment**

## General principles

Goal:
- Optimize factor activity & coagulation profile in the perioperative period
- Minimize perioperative blood;
- Consider blood conservation strategies

Perform:
- Preoperative clotting screen and specific factor assays depending on the type of bleeding disorder
- Preoperative transfusion of recombinant factors 30-60 min before the surgical procedure

Maintain normothermia

Be cautious with vascular access and invasive monitoring
Avoid regional or neuraxial anesthesia because of the high risk of hemorrhagic complications such as epidural hematoma

Administer multimodal pain management

# SPECIFIC TREATMENT

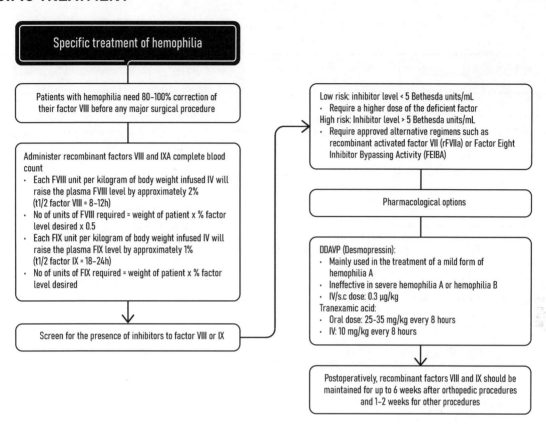

**Specific treatment of hemophilia**

Patients with hemophilia need 80-100% correction of their factor VIII before any major surgical procedure

Administer recombinant factors VIII and IXA complete blood count
- Each FVIII unit per kilogram of body weight infused IV will raise the plasma FVIII level by approximately 2% (t1/2 factor VIII = 8-12h)
- No of units of FVIII required = weight of patient x % factor level desired x 0.5
- Each FIX unit per kilogram of body weight infused IV will raise the plasma FIX level by approximately 1% (t1/2 factor IX = 18-24h)
- No of units of FIX required = weight of patient x % factor level desired

Screen for the presence of inhibitors to factor VIII or IX

Low risk: inhibitor level < 5 Bethesda units/mL
- Require a higher dose of the deficient factor

High risk: Inhibitor level > 5 Bethesda units/mL
- Require approved alternative regimens such as recombinant activated factor VII (rFVIIa) or Factor Eight Inhibitor Bypassing Activity (FEIBA)

Pharmacological options

DDAVP (Desmopressin):
- Mainly used in the treatment of a mild form of hemophilia A
- Ineffective in severe hemophilia A or hemophilia B
- IV/s.c dose: 0.3 µg/kg

Tranexamic acid:
- Oral dose: 25-35 mg/kg every 8 hours
- IV: 10 mg/kg every 8 hours

Postoperatively, recombinant factors VIII and IX should be maintained for up to 6 weeks after orthopedic procedures and 1-2 weeks for other procedures

## SUGGESTED READING

- Shah UJ, Madan Narayanan M, J Graham Smith JH. Anaesthetic considerations in patients with inherited disorders of coagulation, Continuing Education in Anaesthesia Critical Care & Pain, Volume 15, Issue 1, February 2015, Pages 26-31.

# HEPARIN-INDUCED THROMBOCYTOPENIA (HIT)

**114**

## LEARNING OBJECTIVES

- Description and types of heparin-induced thrombocytopenia (HIT)
- Management of HIT

## DEFINITION AND MECHANISM

- Heparin-induced thrombocytopenia (HIT) is a potentially life-threatening complication of heparin therapy leading to the formation of new blood cloths rather than preventing new blood clots
- HIT occurs in approximately 5% of patients taking heparin for > 4 days and is more common in women
- Administration of heparin can lead to the formation of an immune complex between heparin and a specific blood factor (PF4) released by platelets
- This complex triggers the immune system to form antibodies that bind to the heparin-PF4 complex leading to the clotting of platelets
- The clotting platelets release more PF4, causing a chain reaction
- Immune-mediated HIT usually occurs between 5-14 days after first starting heparin therapy with typically a decrease of platelets by > 30%
  - Platelets rarely drop < 20%
- Mortality is 10-20%

## TWO TYPES OF HIT

| HIT I (nonimmune) | HIT II (immune-mediated) |
|---|---|
| Occurs 1-4 days after initiation of therapy | Occurs 5-14 days after initial therapy |
| Mild thrombocytopenia despite continued use of heparin | Thrombocytopenia is usually severe |
| Usually resolves spontaneously | Occurs with any dose of heparin by any route |
| Occurs primarily with a high dose of intravenous heparin | May cause serious thromboembolic complications |
| Usually no clinical sequelae | Heparin must be discontinued |
| Treatment is not required | Occurs less frequently, however, is dangerous |
| Occurs most frequently | |

## SIGNS AND SYMPTOMS

- Low levels of platelets may be a sign of HIT when taking heparin
- About 50% of patients with HIT develop deep vein thrombosis or pulmonary embolism and symptoms include:
  - Pain, swelling, redness, or tenderness in the arm or leg
  - Sudden sharp pain in the chest
  - Hypertension
  - Feeling faint, dizzy, or light-headed
  - Tachycardia
  - Coughing and wheezing
  - Feeling out of breath
  - Excessive sweating
  - Fever and chills

# RISK FACTORS

- Gender
- Taking certain low-molecular-weight heparin (LMWH) instead of unfractionated heparin (UFH)
- Taking heparin after surgery

# COMPLICATIONS

- New venous or arterial thrombotic event
- Treatment-related bleeding
- Limb amputation
- Venous gangrene

# 4TS PROBABILITY SCALE

This scale can be used to estimate the probability of a patient having HIT
- High: 6-8 points
- Intermediate: 4-5 points
- Low: 0-3 points

| Thrombocytopenia | Timing of onset of decrease in platelet count (or other sequelae of HIT) | Thrombosis or other sequelae | Other causes of decrease in platelet count |
|---|---|---|---|
| 0 points if <30% decrease in the platelet count, or if the nadir is < 10×109 /L | 0 points if onset is within four days of first time heparin use (no recent heparin) | 0 points if there is no thrombosis or other finding | 0 points if there is another definite cause |
| 1 point if 30-50% decrease in platelet count, or if the nadir is 10-19×109 /L | 1 point if onset is >10 days after starting heparin or if timing is unclear, or if < 1 day after starting heparin with recent heparin use (past 31-100 days) | 1 point if there is progressive or recurrent thrombosis, erythematous skin lesions at injections sites, or suspected thrombosis (not proved) | 1 point if there is another possible cause |
| 2 points if > 50% decrease in platelet count to a platelet count nadir of ≥ 20×109 /L | 2 points if onset is 5-10 days after starting heparin, or <1 day if there has been recent heparin use (within past 30 days) | 2 point if there is progressive or recurrent thrombosis, erythematous skin lesions at injections sites, or suspected thrombosis (not proved) | 2 points if none evident |

# DIAGNOSIS

- Normal platelet count before the commencement of heparin
- Thrombocytopenia is defined as a drop in platelet count by 30% or more if the count falls below 100 x 10^9/L or a drop of > 50% from the patient's baseline platelet count
- The onset of thrombocytopenia typically occurs 5-10 days after initiation of heparin treatment, but can also occur earlier with previous heparin exposure (within 100 days)
- Acute thrombotic event
- The exclusion of other causes of thrombocytopenia
- The resolution of thrombocytopenia after cessation of heparin
- IT antibody seroconversion

# PREVENTION

- Avoid heparin where possible
- Use low molecular weight heparin instead of unfractionated heparin where possible
- Monitor platelet counts daily in high-risk patients

# MANAGEMENT

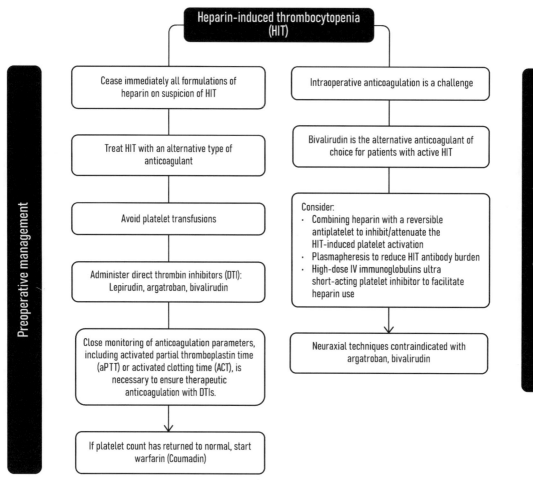

**Heparin-induced thrombocytopenia (HIT)**

## Preoperative management

- Cease immediately all formulations of heparin on suspicion of HIT
- Treat HIT with an alternative type of anticoagulant
- Avoid platelet transfusions
- Administer direct thrombin inhibitors (DTI): Lepirudin, argatroban, bivalirudin
- Close monitoring of anticoagulation parameters, including activated partial thromboplastin time (aPTT) or activated clotting time (ACT), is necessary to ensure therapeutic anticoagulation with DTIs.
- If platelet count has returned to normal, start warfarin (Coumadin)

## Perioperative management

- Intraoperative anticoagulation is a challenge
- Bivalirudin is the alternative anticoagulant of choice for patients with active HIT
- Consider:
  - Combining heparin with a reversible antiplatelet to inhibit/attenuate the HIT-induced platelet activation
  - Plasmapheresis to reduce HIT antibody burden
  - High-dose IV immunoglobulins ultra short-acting platelet inhibitor to facilitate heparin use
- Neuraxial techniques contraindicated with argatroban, bivalirudin

## SUGGESTED READING

- Ahmed I, Majeed A, Powell R. Heparin induced thrombocytopenia: diagnosis and management update. Postgrad Med J. 2007;83(983):575-582.
- Andreas Koster, Michael Nagler, Gabor Erdoes, Jerrold H. Levy; Heparin-induced Thrombocytopenia: Perioperative Diagnosis and Management. Anesthesiology 2022; 136:336-344
- Baroletti, S.A., Goldhaber, S.Z., 2006. Heparin-Induced Thrombocytopenia. Circulation 114, e355-e356.
- Linkins LA. Heparin induced thrombocytopenia. BMJ. 2015;350:g7566. Published 2015 Jan 8.

# IDIOPATHIC THROMBOCYTOPENIC PURPURA (ITP)

## LEARNING OBJECTIVES

- Definition of idiopathic thrombocytopenia purpura (ITP)
- Treatment and perioperative management of ITP

## DEFINITION AND MECHANISM

- Idiopathic thrombocytopenic purpura (ITP) is an autoimmune disease characterized by a low platelet count, purpura, and hemorrhagic episodes
- Resulting in easy or excessive bruising and bleeding due to unusually low levels of platelets
- The immune system produces antibodies against platelets
  - Most often against platelet membrane glycoproteins IIB-IIIa or Ib-IX
- Normal platelet count is between 150.000 and 450.000, the platelet count is less than 10.000 with ITP
- Pregnant women with ITP have an increased incidence of fetal loss, a low fetal birth rate, and a higher incidence of premature births
- Two types:
  - Acute thrombocytopenic purpura
    - Affects young children between 2-6 years, often following a viral infection
    - Starts suddenly and symptoms usually disappear in less than 6 months, often within a few weeks
    - Most common form and resolves spontaneously
  - Chronic thrombocytopenic purpura
    - Onset can happen at any age
    - Symptoms can last a minimum of 6 months to several years or a lifetime
    - More common in adults and in females
    - Requires continual follow-up care

## SIGNS AND SYMPTOMS

- Easy or excessive bruising
- Petechiae
- Bleeding from the gums or nose
- Blood in urine or stools
- Unusually heavy menstrual flow

## CAUSES

- Medication (the medication absorbs the platelet cell membrane)
- Infection: the virus that causes chickenpox, hepatitis C, and AIDS
- Pregnancy
- Immune disorders: Rheumatoid arthritis, lupus
- Cancer: Low-grade lymphomas and leukemia
- The cause is sometimes unknown

## COMPLICATIONS

- Subarachnoid or intracerebral hemorrhage
- Lower gastrointestinal bleeding

## DIAGNOSIS

- Complete blood count
- Low platelet count, usually < $40×10^9$/L for over three months
- Bleeding time
- Blood and urine tests to detect a possible infection
- Antiplatelet antibody test
- Bone marrow examination shows an increased number of megakaryocytes

# MANAGEMENT

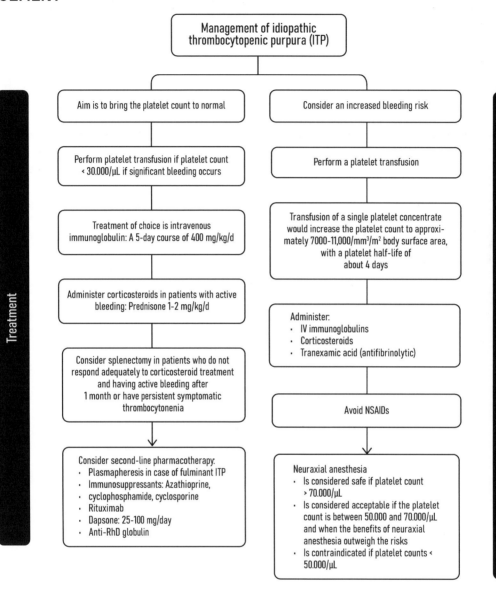

**Management of idiopathic thrombocytopenic purpura (ITP)**

## Treatment

Aim is to bring the platelet count to normal

Perform platelet transfusion if platelet count < 30.000/μL if significant bleeding occurs

Treatment of choice is intravenous immunoglobulin: A 5-day course of 400 mg/kg/d

Administer corticosteroids in patients with active bleeding: Prednisone 1-2 mg/kg/d

Consider splenectomy in patients who do not respond adequately to corticosteroid treatment and having active bleeding after 1 month or have persistent symptomatic thrombocytonenia

Consider second-line pharmacotherapy:
- Plasmapheresis in case of fulminant ITP
- Immunosuppressants: Azathioprine, cyclophosphamide, cyclosporine
- Rituximab
- Dapsone: 25-100 mg/day
- Anti-RhD globulin

## Preoperative management

Consider an increased bleeding risk

Perform a platelet transfusion

Transfusion of a single platelet concentrate would increase the platelet count to approximately 7000-11,000/mm³/m² body surface area, with a platelet half-life of about 4 days

Administer:
- IV immunoglobulins
- Corticosteroids
- Tranexamic acid (antifibrinolytic)

Avoid NSAIDs

Neuraxial anesthesia
- Is considered safe if platelet count > 70.000/μL
- Is considered acceptable if the platelet count is between 50.000 and 70.000/μL and when the benefits of neuraxial anesthesia outweigh the risks
- Is contraindicated if platelet counts < 50.000/μL

## SUGGESTED READING

- Guidelines for the investigation and management of idiopathic thrombocytopenic purpura in adults, children and in pregnancy. 2003. British Journal of Haematology 120, 574–596.
- Ramalingam, G., Jones, N., Besser, M., 2016. Platelets for anaesthetists—part 1: physiology and pathology. BJA Education 16, 134–139.
- Toyomasu Y, Shimabukuro R, Moriyama H, et al. Successful perioperative management of a patient with idiopathic thrombocytopenic purpura undergoing emergent appendectomy: Report of a case. Int J Surg Case Rep. 2013;4(10):898-900.
- Warrier R, Chauhan A. Management of immune thrombocytopenic purpura: an update. Ochsner J. 2012;12(3):221-227.

# JEHOVAH'S WITNESS PATIENTS

## LEARNING OBJECTIVES

- Understand the beliefs of Jehovah's Witness patients
- Perioperative management of Jehovah's Witness patients

## DEFINITION AND MECHANISM

- Jehovah's witnesses believe that the Bible prohibits Christians from accepting blood component transfusions, even when necessary to prevent morbidity/mortality as they believe that the removed blood is 'unclean' and should be disposed off
- That means that their beliefs prevent them from accepting transfusion of whole blood or its primary components and not accepting blood transfusions and not donating or storing their own blood for transfusion
- It is illegal to administer a blood transfusion to a Jehovah's Witness who has expressly forbidden it
- Preoperative planning, preparation, and an experienced team are essential for a successful outcome
- Blood-free major surgery in the Jehovah's Witness patient presents a challenge to the anesthetic and surgical team
- In case of emergency or life-threatening circumstances:
  - If Jehovah's Witness status is unknown/unsure, administer blood if required, unless documentary evidence such as an advance directive is available
  - If Jehovah's Witness is competent to refuse a transfusion - provide standard treatment except for a blood transfusion, even if it may lead to the patient's death

| Acceptability of blood products and transfusion-related procedures | |
|---|---|
| Unacceptable | Whole blood |
| | Packed red cells |
| | Plasma |
| | Autologous pre-donation |
| Acceptable | Cardiopulmonary bypass |
| | Renal dialysis |
| | Acute hypervolemic hemodilution |
| | Recombinant erythropoietin |
| | Recombinant factor VIIa |
| May be acceptable | Platelets |
| | Clotting factors |
| | Albumin |
| | Immunoglobulins |
| | Epidural blood patch |
| | Cell saver |

# MANAGEMENT

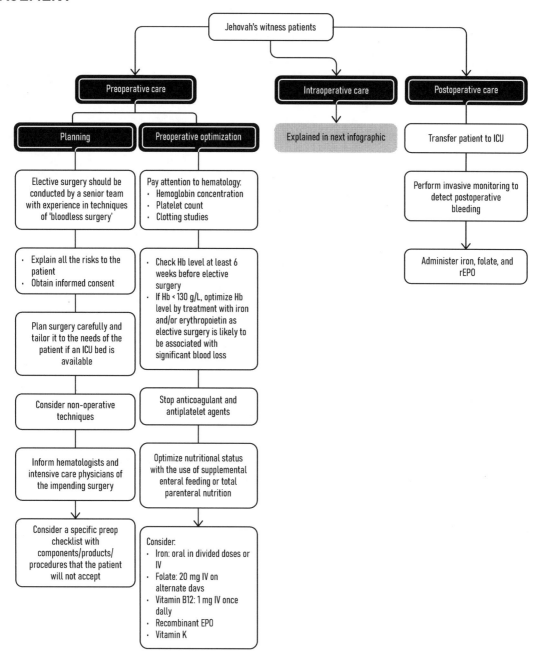

**Jehovah's witness patients**

**Preoperative care** → **Intraoperative care** → **Postoperative care**

**Preoperative care**

**Planning** / **Preoperative optimization**

**Planning:**

Elective surgery should be conducted by a senior team with experience in techniques of 'bloodless surgery'

- Explain all the risks to the patient
- Obtain informed consent

Plan surgery carefully and tailor it to the needs of the patient if an ICU bed is available

Consider non-operative techniques

Inform hematologists and intensive care physicians of the impending surgery

Consider a specific preop checklist with components/products/procedures that the patient will not accept

**Preoperative optimization:**

Pay attention to hematology:
- Hemoglobin concentration
- Platelet count
- Clotting studies

- Check Hb level at least 6 weeks before elective surgery
- If Hb < 130 g/L, optimize Hb level by treatment with iron and/or erythropoietin as elective surgery is likely to be associated with significant blood loss

Stop anticoagulant and antiplatelet agents

Optimize nutritional status with the use of supplemental enteral feeding or total parenteral nutrition

Consider:
- Iron: oral in divided doses or IV
- Folate: 20 mg IV on alternate davs
- Vitamin B12: 1 mg IV once dally
- Recombinant EPO
- Vitamin K

**Intraoperative care:**

Explained in next infographic

**Postoperative care:**

Transfer patient to ICU

Perform invasive monitoring to detect postoperative bleeding

Administer iron, folate, and rEPO

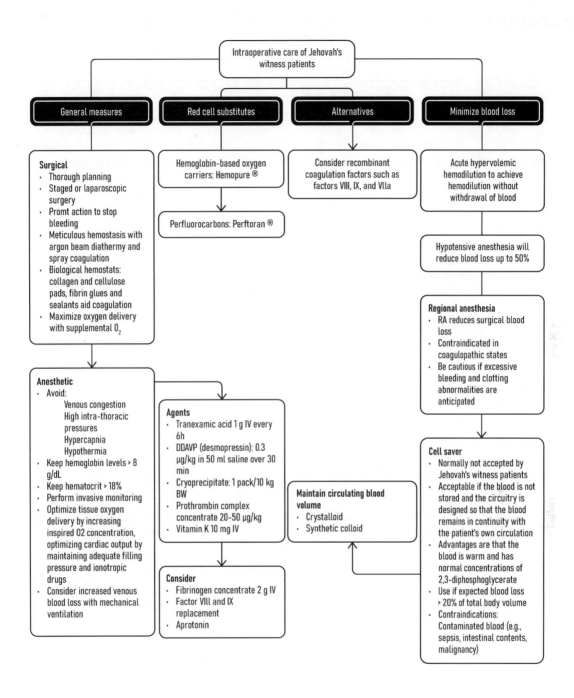

Intraoperative care of Jehovah's witness patients

**General measures**

**Surgical**
- Thorough planning
- Staged or laparoscopic surgery
- Promt action to stop bleeding
- Meticulous hemostasis with argon beam diathermy and spray coagulation
- Biological hemostats: collagen and cellulose pads, fibrin glues and sealants aid coagulation
- Maximize oxygen delivery with supplemental $O_2$

**Anesthetic**
- Avoid:
  Venous congestion
  High intra-thoracic pressures
  Hypercapnia
  Hypothermia
- Keep hemoglobin levels > 8 g/dL
- Keep hematocrit > 18%
- Perform invasive monitoring
- Optimize tissue oxygen delivery by increasing inspired O2 concentration, optimizing cardiac output by maintaining adequate filling pressure and ionotropic drugs
- Consider increased venous blood loss with mechanical ventilation

**Red cell substitutes**

Hemoglobin-based oxygen carriers: Hemopure ®

Perfluorocarbons: Perftoran ®

**Agents**
- Tranexamic acid 1 g IV every 6h
- DDAVP (desmopressin): 0.3 µg/kg in 50 ml saline over 30 min
- Cryoprecipitate: 1 pack/10 kg BW
- Prothrombin complex concentrate 20-50 µg/kg
- Vitamin K 10 mg IV

**Consider**
- Fibrinogen concentrate 2 g IV
- Factor VlII and IX replacement
- Aprotonin

**Alternatives**

Consider recombinant coagulation factors such as factors VIII, IX, and VIIa

**Maintain circulating blood volume**
- Crystalloid
- Synthetic colloid

**Minimize blood loss**

Acute hypervolemic hemodilution to achieve hemodilution without withdrawal of blood

Hypotensive anesthesia will reduce blood loss up to 50%

**Regional anesthesia**
- RA reduces surgical blood loss
- Contraindicated in coagulopathic states
- Be cautious if excessive bleeding and clotting abnormalities are anticipated

**Cell saver**
- Normally not accepted by Jehovah's witness patients
- Acceptable if the blood is not stored and the circuitry is designed so that the blood remains in continuity with the patient's own circulation
- Advantages are that the blood is warm and has normal concentrations of 2,3-diphosphoglycerate
- Use if expected blood loss > 20% of total body volume
- Contraindications: Contaminated blood (e.g., sepsis, intestinal contents, malignancy)

## SUGGESTED READING

- Lawson, T., Ralph, C., 2015. Perioperative Jehovah's Witnesses: a review. British Journal of Anaesthesia 115, 676–687.
- Klein AA, Bailey CR, Charlton A, et al. Association of Anaesthetists: anaesthesia and peri-operative care for Jehovah's Witnesses and patients who refuse blood. Anaesthesia. 2019;74(1):74–82.
- Milligan LC, Bellamy MC. Anaesthesia and critical care of Jehovah's Witnesses. Continuing Education in Anaesthesia Critical Care & Pain. 2004/ 4;(2); 35–39.

# PERIOPERATIVE ANEMIA

## LEARNING OBJECTIVES

- Optimize blood hemoglobin levels to avoid or minimize transfusion necessity during surgery

## DEFINITION AND MECHANISM

- Anemia is a condition in which the number of red blood cells or the hemoglobin concentration within them is lower than normal
- Normal blood hemoglobin levels range from:
  - 13 - 17.2 g/dL in men
  - 12 - 15.1 g/dL in women
- A Hb trigger treshold of 7-8 mg/dL for blood transfusion is widely accepted
- Blood transfusion is not an optimal treatment for preoperative anemia
- Preoperative anemia is associated with increased risk of blood transfusion, in-hospital complications, delayed hospital discharge and poor recovery
- Preoperative anemia - common, 25%-75% of patients. Higher prevalence in elderly
- Post-operative anemia - 90% of patients following major surgery

## SIGNS AND SYMPTOMS

- Fatigue
- Shortness of breath
- Pallor
- Resting tachycardia

Note that these symptoms are unreliable as people with long-existing anemia might be asymptomatic

## CAUSES AND CLASSIFICATION

- Anemia is classified depending on the size of the RBCs

|  | Microcytic (MCV < 80 fL) | Normocytic | Macrocytic (MCV > 100 fL) |
|---|---|---|---|
| Causes | Iron deficiency<br>Thalassemia<br>Anemia of inflammation<br>Sideroblastic anemia | Acute bleeding<br>Renal disease<br>Acute inflammation | Vitamin B12 deficiency<br>Folate deficiency<br>Myelodysplastic syndrome<br>Chemotherapy<br>Aplastic anemia<br>Liver and renal disease<br>Hypothyroidism<br>Reticulocytosis |

MCV, Mean corpuscular volume.

# MANAGEMENT

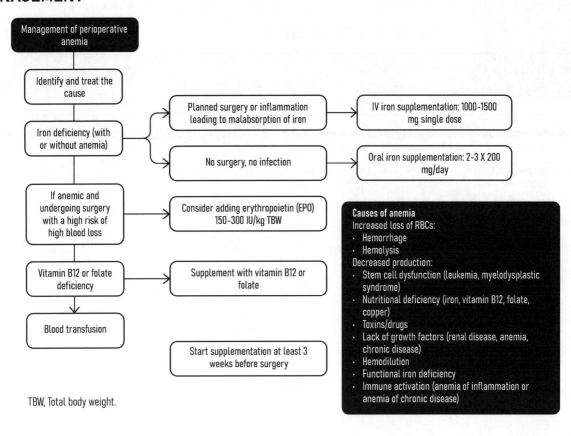

TBW, Total body weight.

━━━━━ **SUGGESTED READING** ━━━━━

- Cascio MJ, DeLoughery TG. Anemia: Evaluation and Diagnostic Tests. Med Clin North Am. 2017;101(2):263-284.
- Chernecky CC et al. Laboratory Tests and Diagnostic Procedures. 6th ed. Philadelphia, PA: Elsevier; 2013:621-623.
- Hare GMT, Mazer CD. Anemia: Perioperative Risk and Treatment Opportunity. Anesthesiology. 2021;135(3):520-530.

# POLYCYTHEMIA (ERYTHROCYTOSIS)

## LEARNING OBJECTIVES

- Define polycythemia
- Describe the classification of polycythemia
- Anesthetic management of a patient with polycythemia

## DEFINITION AND MECHANISM

- Polycythemia or erythrocytosis is an increase in red blood cell mass, and is associated with an increase in hemoglobin concentration (Hb) and hematocrit (Hct)
- The condition increases blood viscosity and can reduce cerebral blood flow

## CLASSIFICATION

- Absolute polycythemia (increased red cell mass)
  - Primary (polycythemia vera; PV)
  - Secondary
  - Idiopathic
- Apparent polycythemia (normal red cell mass)
  - Reduced plasma volume

### Primary polycythemia (polycythemia vera; PV)

- PV is characterized by the clonal proliferation of myeloid cells and is a chronic progressive myeloproliferative disease
- > 95% of patients have a genetic mutation of JAK2 → stimulates overproduction of erythrocytes, platelets, and granulocytes
- JAK2 mutation is not specific for PV, also found in patients with primary thrombocytosis and primary myelofibrosis
- Clinical manifestations result from thrombotic episodes secondary to increased blood viscosity
- Production of immature platelets with variable function and acquired von Willebrand's disease (vWD) are thought to be behind the bleeding tendency
- The criteria for a diagnosis of PV include an elevated hematocrit, normal arterial oxygenation, normal erythropoietin levels, and splenomegaly not attributable to another cause
- Associated laboratory findings:
  - Thrombocytosis
  - Leukocytosis
  - Elevated lactate dehydrogenase
  - A steep increase in viscosity above 55% is thrombogenic
- Clinical features
  - Hypertension (46%)
  - Splenomegaly (36%)
  - Pruritus (36%)
  - Erythromelalgia (29%)
  - Arterial thrombosis (16%)
  - Venous thrombosis (7%)
  - Hemorrhage (4%)
  - Facial plethora
  - Hepatomegaly
  - Gout
  - Peripheral vascular occlusion

### Secondary polycythemia

- Increased red cell mass is due to increased erythropoietin (EPO) production
- Compensatory mechanism in response to chronic tissue hypoxia or inappropriate production of EPO by the kidneys
- Causes include:
  - Chronic obstructive pulmonary disease (COPD)
  - Obstructive sleep apnea (OSA)
  - Cyanotic heart disease
  - High altitude
  - Renal artery stenosis
  - Renal tumors
  - Transplanted kidneys

### Idiopathic polycythemia

- Increased red cell mass without an identifiable cause
- Patients are more commonly male and > 50% present with vascular occlusive complications

### Apparent polycythemia

- Reduced plasma volume results in an increased Hct and Hb on laboratory tests, but the red cell mass is normal
- Associated with the following clinical conditions:
  - Obesity
  - Hypertension
  - Smoking
  - Excessive alcohol intake
  - Diuretic use

## SIGNS AND SYMPTOMS

- Fatigue
- Headaches
- Dizziness
- Episodic blurred vision
- Red skin (particularly on the face, hands, and feet)
- Peripheral tingling, or burning and itching
- Hypertension
- Mucosal cyanosis
- Bruising
- Petechiae
- Unusual bleeding, nosebleeds
- Enlarged spleen or liver

## DIAGNOSIS

| Measurement | Male | Female |
|---|---|---|
| Hemoglobin (g/L) | > 185 | > 165 |
| Hematocrit | > 0.52 | > 0.48 |

## COMPLICATIONS

- Pulmonary embolism
- Deep vein thrombosis
- Increased risk of heart attack and stroke
- Perioperative complications:
  - Most common cause of hypoxia
  - Greater risk of perioperative thrombosis
  - Increased risk of bleeding diathesis

Polycythemia (erythrocytosis)

# TREATMENT

| Classification | Treatment |
|---|---|
| Primary polycythemia | Reduce the risk of thrombosis, hemorrhage, and transformation to acute leukemia or myelofibrosis<br>Phlebotomy or venesection (Hct < 0.45) and aspirin<br>Consider hydroxyurea or interferon alpha (myelosupressive therapy) if the above treatments fail |
| Secondary polycythemia | Phlebotomy and management of the underlying condition (if possible) |
| Idiopathic polycythemia | Phlebotomy, cytoreductive therapy is contraindicated |
| Apparent polycythemia | Lifestyle modification and phlebotomy (if required) |

# MANAGEMENT

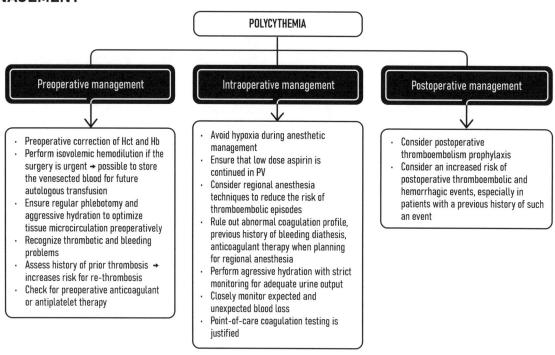

**POLYCYTHEMIA**

**Preoperative management**

- Preoperative correction of Hct and Hb
- Perform isovolemic hemodilution if the surgery is urgent → possible to store the venesected blood for future autologous transfusion
- Ensure regular phlebotomy and aggressive hydration to optimize tissue microcirculation preoperatively
- Recognize thrombotic and bleeding problems
- Assess history of prior thrombosis → increases risk for re-thrombosis
- Check for preoperative anticoagulant or antiplatelet therapy

**Intraoperative management**

- Avoid hypoxia during anesthetic management
- Ensure that low dose aspirin is continued in PV
- Consider regional anesthesia techniques to reduce the risk of thromboembolic episodes
- Rule out abnormal coagulation profile, previous history of bleeding diathesis, anticoagulant therapy when planning for regional anesthesia
- Perform agressive hydration with strict monitoring for adequate urine output
- Closely monitor expected and unexpected blood loss
- Point-of-care coagulation testing is justified

**Postoperative management**

- Consider postoperative thromboembolism prophylaxis
- Consider an increased risk of postoperative thromboembolic and hemorrhagic events, especially in patients with a previous history of such an event

## SUGGESTED READING

- Pollard BJ, Kitchen G. Handbook of Clinical Anaesthesia. 4th ed. Taylor & Francis group; 2018. Chapter 7 The blood, Duncan A.
- Zhao, J., Huang, L., Matson, D., Li, N., & Liu, H. (2021). Perioperative management of polycythemia. In Essentials of Blood Product Management in Anesthesia Practice (pp. 405-409). Springer International Publishing. https://doi.org/10.1007/978-3-030-59295-0_42

# SICKLE CELL DISEASE

## LEARNING OBJECTIVES

- Signs and symptoms and management of sickle cell disease

## DEFINITION AND MECHANISM

- Sickle cell disease is a group of inherited hemoglobinopathies
- The most common type is known as sickle cell anemia or homozygous sickle cell disease (HbSS), other types include the double heterozygote conditions sickle C (HbSC) and sickle thalassemia (HbSThal)
- The average life expectancy is 40 to 60 years
- The dominant hemoglobin (Hb) is replaced by the unstable hemoglobin S resulting in the deformation of the red cell membrane into the characteristic sickle shape
- These sickle cells become rigid and aggregate, thereby occluding small blood vessels and leading to tissue infarction
- Hemolysis occurs due to the damaged cell membrane leading to an inflammatory response
- The major features of sickle cell disease are chronic hemolytic anemia and the occurrence of painful vaso-occlusive crises in which multiple episodes of tissue infarction occur
- Crises can be provoked by temperature changes, stress, dehydration, and high altitude

## SIGNS AND SYMPTOMS

- Symptoms of sickle cell anemia usually appear around 6 months of age
- Vary from person to person and may change over time
- Anemia
- Episodes of pain (acute painful crises)
- Swelling of hands and feet
- Frequent infections
- Delayed growth or puberty
- Vision problems

## MANAGEMENT

- Avoid precipitants of sickle cell crisis
  - Hypoxia
  - Vascular stasis
  - Hypothermia
  - Hypovolemia/hypotension
  - Acidosis

## COMPLICATIONS

### Acute sickle-related complications

- Acute painful crises
- Hyposplenism
- Adenotonsillar hypertrophy
- Priapism
- Acute splenic sequestration crisis
- Aplastic crisis
- Acute chest syndrome
- Neurological (stroke, intracranial hemorrhage)

### Chronic sickle-related complications

- **Renal**
  - Hyposthenuria
  - Proteinuria
  - Renal insufficiency
- **Cardiorespiratory**
  - Obstructive sleep apnea
  - Chronic lung disease
  - Congestive cardiac failure
  - Pulmonary hypertension
- **Orthopedic**
  - Avascular necrosis of the femoral head
  - Osteomyelitis
- **Surgical/urological**
  - Cholelithiasis
  - Erectile dysfunction
- **Ophthalmological**
  - Retinopathy
- **Dermatological**
  - Leg ulcers
- **Infection-related**
  - Gram-negative sepsis
  - Urinary tract infection
  - Biliary sepsis
  - Non-typhi salmonella infection
- **Transfusion/treatment-related**
  - Acquired red cell antibodies
  - Iron overload
  - Neutropenia (hydroxycarbamide treatment)
  - Hyperhemolysis

## SICKLE CELL DISEASE

### Preoperative management

Screen patients from susceptible populations for hemoglobin S with a quick solubility test

Identify and evaluate for wider systemic manifestations and complications

Identify the frequency, pattern, and severity of recent sickle crises + presence of organ damage

Note that sickle cell crises may mimic acute surgical conditions such as an acute abdomen

Assess the patient for signs of fever, dehydration, and vaso-occlusion

Preoperative investigations
- Chest X-ray
- ECG: may be required for adults with symptoms suggestive of pulmonary hypertension ($SpO_2$ < 94%, reduced exercise capacity)
- Full blood count
- Urea
- Electrolytes
- Liver function test
- Oxygen saturation
- Arterial blood gas
- Pulmonary function tests
- Venous access assessment as access may be difficult

Schedule early on the list to avoid prolonged starving

Blood transfusions are usually unnecessary for patients undergoing minor surgery

Avoid elective surgery if patient is febrile or having painful crisis

Major surgery. Red blood cell transfusion to increase the Hb concentration to 10 g/dL

### Intraoperative management

Avoid factors that promote sickling: e.g., stress or infections: dehydration, hypoxia, acidosis, hypothermia, and pain

GA or RA but avoid the use of epinephrine with LA solutions

Regional/central neuraxal blocks
Advantages:
- Fewer sickle cell complications
- Postoperative analgesia
- Improved peripheral blood flow
Risks
- Hypotension
- Hypoperfusion, treat early with vasopressors and intravenous fluids
- Priapism may be missed - counsel/examine regularly

GA:
- ECG
- Perform preoxygenation
- Avoid hypotension
- Controlled ventilation
- Replace fluid losses
- Monitor central venous pressure
- Avoid venous stasis

Maintain:
- Adequate oxygenation
- Hydration
- Normothermia
- Normal acid-base balance
- Aseptic precautions
- Urine output

Consider thromboembolism prophylaxis

Avoid limb tourniquets or apply them as distally as possible

### Postoperative management

Transfer patient to ICU
- Avoid factors that promote sickling
- Extend monitoring
- Supplement oxygen
- Optimize fluid balance
- Perform chest physiotherapy
- Be cautious for complications of sickle cell disease

Pain management
- Note that opioids may cause respiratory depression with acidosis and hypoxia
- Some patients have developed opioids tolerance
- Distinguish painful sickle crises from surgical pain

Acute chest syndrome is an acute pain crisis
- Presents as pleuritic chest pain, fever, hypoxemia, and lung infiltrates on the chest X-ray
- Requires urgent oxygen therapy and exchange transfusion

Analgesia:
- Consider opioid tolerance and thus higher doses
- Multimodal analgesia: acetaminophen, NSAIDs, local anesthetics, RA, PCA, oral or IV administration
- Avoid NSAIDs if there is evidence of renal dysfunction

Consider:
- Early mobilization
- Physiotherapy
- Incentive spirometry after moderate to major surgery
- Thromboprophylaxis
- Antibiotic prophylaxis as per surgical procedure

| Genotype | Baseline Hb (g/L) | Suggested preoperative transfusion |
|---|---|---|
| All genotypes | - | Exchange transfusion aiming for Hb of 100 g/L |
| HbSS/HbSβ⁰ | < 90 g/L | Top-up transfusion aiming for Hb of 100 g/L |
| HbSS/HbSβ⁰ | ≥ 90 g/L | Partial exchange transfusion aiming for Hb of 100 g/L |
| HbSC | - | Top-up transfusion or partial exchange transfusion aiming for Hb of 100 g/L |

## SUGGESTED READING

- Pollard BJ, Kitchen, G. Handbook of Clinical Anaesthesia. Fourth Edition. CRC Press. 2018. 978-1-4987-6289-2.
- Walker, I., Trompeter, S., Howard, J., Williams, A., Bell, R., Bingham, R., Bankes, M., Vercueil, A., Dalay, S., Whitaker, D. and Elton, C. (2021), Guideline on the peri-operative management of patients with sickle cell disease. Anaesthesia, 76: 805-817. https://doi.org/10.1111/anae.15349
- Wilson, M., Forsyth, P., Whiteside, J.. Haemoglobinopathy and sickle cell disease. Continuing Education in Anaesthesia Critical Care & Pain. 2010. 10, 24-28.

Sickle cell disease

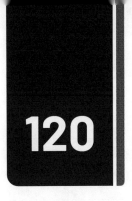

# THALASSEMIA

## LEARNING OBJECTIVES

- Difference between α- and β thalassemia
- Recognize thalassemia
- Management of thalassemia

## DEFINITION AND MECHANISM

- Thalassemia is an inherited group of hematological disorders
- The synthesis of alpha or beta globin chains is deficient in thalassemia, and is characterized by a decreased hemoglobin production
- The majority of hemoglobin is HbA in normal adults, which has two α and two β chains, i.e., $\alpha 2\beta 2$
- More frequently found in the Mediterranean, Central Africa, China, and South East Asian regions

### α thalassemia

- $\alpha^0$ thalassemia results from the elimination of α1 and α2 genes and/or regulatory sequences
- α' thalassemia minor results from a single gene deletion or point mutation that prevents normal α chain production
    □ The resulting anemia is mild and of little anesthetic significance
- Hemoglobin H disease is caused by the interaction of α0 and α+ determinants (loss of three genes)
    □ The clinical picture is of chronic hemolytic anemia with Hb levels of 8–10 g/dL
    □ Stimulates erythropoietin production and results in excess production of large amounts of β-chains
- "α thalassemia major" occurs when all four alpha globin genes are nonfunctioning
    □ Is almost uniformly fatal in-utero without intervention

### β thalassemia

- Is an autosomal recessive defect of the beta-globin chains of the hemoglobin A molecule
- The clinical presentation typically manifests at approximately 4 to 6 months of age
- A defect in one beta globin allele will result in beta thalassemia minor
    □ An effective carrier state as individuals are usually asymptomatic or present with anemia
    □ Hemoglobin levels 2–3 g/dL below the normal range for their age
- A defect in both alleles results in β thalassemia major (Cooley anemia)
    □ Results in profound anemia requiring lifelong blood transfusions

| Signs and symptoms | |
|---|---|
| Intravascular hemolysis: | Perioperative anemia<br>Jaundice, gallstones<br>Splenic sequestration causes anemia and other hematological effects<br>Free iron causes a vascular endothelial inflammatory response and its consequences, e.g., leading to systemic and pulmonary hypertension (PH), cerebral ischemia, platelet activation, hypercoagulability |
| Extramedullary erythropoiesis: | Frontoparietal bossing, prominent maxilla and zygomatic arch (characteristic 'rodent' or 'chipmunk' face), compression of neural structures in bony canal including the spinal cord, bony deformities e.g., thoracic cage, spinal column, optic neuropathy, conductive hearing loss<br>Defects in bone mineralisation, osteopenia, osteomalacia and microfractures due to expansion of the marrow cavity |
| Systemic effects of anemia: | High output cardiac failure, decreased oxygen delivery leading to poor growth |
| Multiple transfusions: | Hypervolemia, coagulation defects, immunosuppression, iron overload |
| Iron overload: | Cardiomyopathy, cardiac hypertrophy, myocarditis, pericarditis<br>Liver failure and cirrhosis<br>Renal tubular dysfunction, loss of concentrating renal function, and increased excretion of calcium, magnesium, and phosphate<br>Endocrinopathy (diabetes, hypothyroidism, hypoparathyroidism, adrenal insufficiency)<br>Immunosuppression: Increased risk of infection<br>Lung fibrosis, interstitial edema<br>Risk of venous thromboembolic events (B-thalassemia intermedia), while arterial (major type) |

Thalassemia

# DIAGNOSIS

- Complete blood count
- Hemoglobin electrophoresis
- DNA-testing
- Metzer index, not a definitive test but in can suggest the possibility of thalassemia

# MANAGEMENT

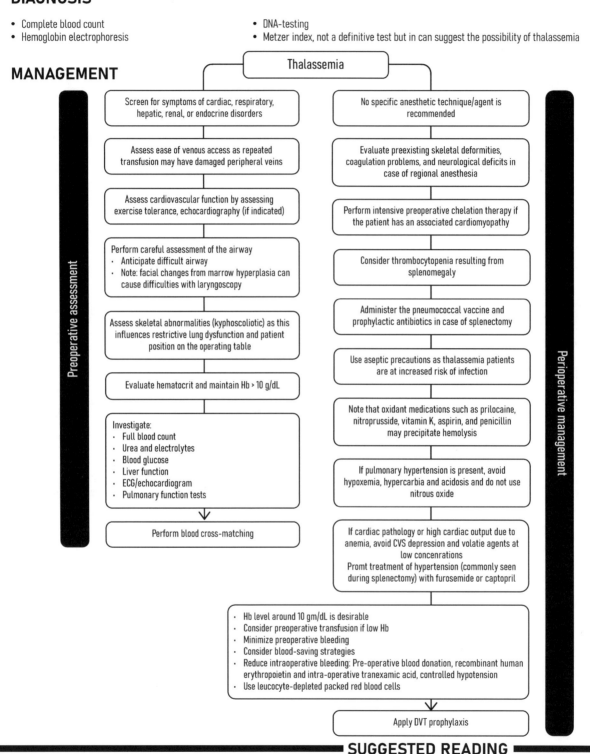

**Thalassemia**

**Preoperative assessment**

- Screen for symptoms of cardiac, respiratory, hepatic, renal, or endocrine disorders
- Assess ease of venous access as repeated transfusion may have damaged peripheral veins
- Assess cardiovascular function by assessing exercise tolerance, echocardiography (if indicated)
- Perform careful assessment of the airway
  - Anticipate difficult airway
  - Note: facial changes from marrow hyperplasia can cause difficulties with laryngoscopy
- Assess skeletal abnormalities (kyphoscoliotic) as this influences restrictive lung dysfunction and patient position on the operating table
- Evaluate hematocrit and maintain Hb > 10 g/dL
- Investigate:
  - Full blood count
  - Urea and electrolytes
  - Blood glucose
  - Liver function
  - ECG/echocardiogram
  - Pulmonary function tests
- Perform blood cross-matching

**Perioperative management**

- No specific anesthetic technique/agent is recommended
- Evaluate preexisting skeletal deformities, coagulation problems, and neurological deficits in case of regional anesthesia
- Perform intensive preoperative chelation therapy if the patient has an associated cardiomyopathy
- Consider thrombocytopenia resulting from splenomegaly
- Administer the pneumococcal vaccine and prophylactic antibiotics in case of splenectomy
- Use aseptic precautions as thalassemia patients are at increased risk of infection
- Note that oxidant medications such as prilocaine, nitroprusside, vitamin K, aspirin, and penicillin may precipitate hemolysis
- If pulmonary hypertension is present, avoid hypoxemia, hypercarbia and acidosis and do not use nitrous oxide
- If cardiac pathology or high cardiac output due to anemia, avoid CVS depression and volatie agents at low concenrations
- Promt treatment of hypertension (commonly seen during splenectomy) with furosemide or captopril

- Hb level around 10 gm/dL is desirable
- Consider preoperative transfusion if low Hb
- Minimize preoperative bleeding
- Consider blood-saving strategies
- Reduce intraoperative bleeding: Pre-operative blood donation, recombinant human erythropoietin and intra-operative tranexamic acid, controlled hypotension
- Use leucocyte-depleted packed red blood cells

- Apply DVT prophylaxis

# SUGGESTED READING

- Pollard BJ, Kitchen, G. Handbook of Clinical Anaesthesia. Fourth Edition. CRC Press. 2018. 978-1-4987-6289-2.
- Thomas, C., Lumb, A.B., 2012. Physiology of haemoglobin. Continuing Education in Anaesthesia Critical Care & Pain 12, 251-256.
- Wilson, M., Forsyth, P., Whiteside, J., 2010. Haemoglobinopathy and sickle cell disease. Continuing Education in Anaesthesia Critical Care & Pain 10, 24-28.

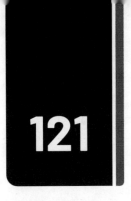

# TUMOR LYSIS SYNDROME

## 121

## LEARNING OBJECTIVES

- Describe tumor lysis syndrome (TLS)
- Management of TLS

## DEFINITION AND MECHANISM

- Tumor lysis syndrome (TLS) is a condition that occurs when a large number of cancer cells die within a short period, releasing their contents into the blood
- Occurs most commonly after the treatment of lymphomas and leukemias and in particular when treating non-Hodgkin lymphoma, acute myeloid leukemia, and acute lymphoblastic leukemia
- TLS can occur spontaneously (before cancer treatment) but is more common within a week of starting treatment
- Not limited to patients receiving traditional chemotherapy, can also occur in patients receiving steroids, hormonal therapy, targeted therapy, or radiation therapy
- Characterized by hyperkalemia, hyperphosphatemia, hypocalcemia, hyperuricemia, and higher-than-normal levels of blood urea nitrogen (BUN)
- TLS is analogous to rhabdomyolysis

## SIGNS AND SYMPTOMS

- Nausea with or without vomiting
- Lack of appetite and fatigue
- Dark urine, reduced urine output, or flank pain
- Numbness, seizures, or hallucinations
- Muscle cramps and spasms
- Heart palpitations
- Hyperkalemia and secondary arrhythmias
- Hyperphosphatemia and prolonged QT interval
- Hypocalcemia and risk of seizures
- Hyperuricemia and acute renal failure
- Hyperuricosuria

## COMPLICATIONS

- Acute uric acid nephropathy
- Acute kidney failure
- Seizures
- Cardiac arrhythmias

## DIAGNOSIS

- Large tumor burden
- Hyperuricemia > 15 mg/dL
- Hyperphosphatemia > 8 mg/d
- Urine analysis: Uric acid crystals or amorphous urates
- Detection of hypersecretion of uric acid with a high urine uric acid/creatinine ratio > 1.0

| Risk factors | |
|---|---|
| Tumor characteristics | High cell turnover rate<br>Rapid growth rate<br>High tumor bulk |
| Type of cancer | Burkitt's lymphoma<br>Other Non-Hodgkin lymphomas<br>Acute lymphoblastic leukemia<br>Acute myeloid leukemia |
| Patient characteristics | Baseline serum creatine<br>Kidney failure<br>Dehydration |
| Chemotherapy characteristics | Chemo-sensitive tumors, such as lymphomas<br>Use of steroids |
| Spontaneous tumor lysis syndrome | Triggered without any treatment |

# MANAGEMENT

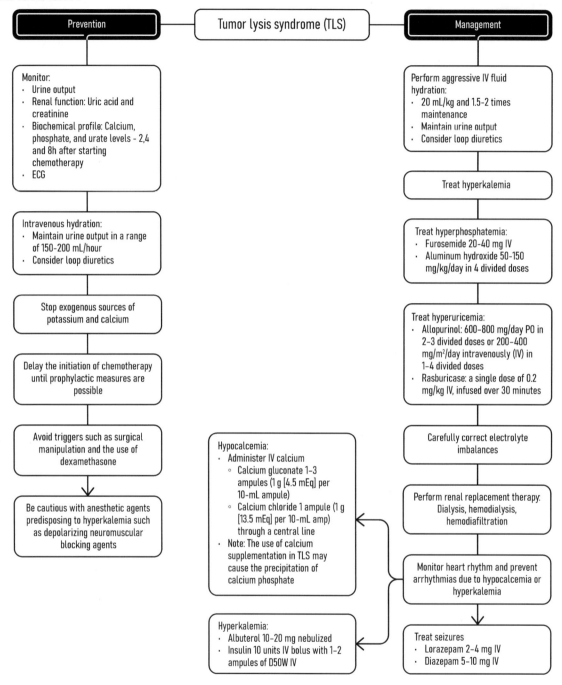

```
                          ┌──────────────────────────┐
                          │ Tumor lysis syndrome (TLS)│
                          └──────────────────────────┘
         ┌──────────────┐                            ┌──────────────┐
         │  Prevention  │                            │  Management  │
         └──────────────┘                            └──────────────┘
```

**Prevention**

Monitor:
· Urine output
· Renal function: Uric acid and creatinine
· Biochemical profile: Calcium, phosphate, and urate levels - 2,4 and 8h after starting chemotherapy
· ECG

Intravenous hydration:
· Maintain urine output in a range of 150-200 mL/hour
· Consider loop diuretics

Stop exogenous sources of potassium and calcium

Delay the initiation of chemotherapy until prophylactic measures are possible

Avoid triggers such as surgical manipulation and the use of dexamethasone

Be cautious with anesthetic agents predisposing to hyperkalemia such as depolarizing neuromuscular blocking agents

**Management**

Perform aggressive IV fluid hydration:
· 20 mL/kg and 1.5-2 times maintenance
· Maintain urine output
· Consider loop diuretics

Treat hyperkalemia

Treat hyperphosphatemia:
· Furosemide 20-40 mg IV
· Aluminum hydroxide 50-150 mg/kg/day in 4 divided doses

Treat hyperuricemia:
· Allopurinol: 600-800 mg/day PO in 2-3 divided doses or 200-400 mg/m²/day intravenously (IV) in 1-4 divided doses
· Rasburicase: a single dose of 0.2 mg/kg IV, infused over 30 minutes

Carefully correct electrolyte imbalances

Perform renal replacement therapy: Dialysis, hemodialysis, hemodiafiltration

Monitor heart rhythm and prevent arrhythmias due to hypocalcemia or hyperkalemia

Treat seizures
· Lorazepam 2-4 mg IV
· Diazepam 5-10 mg IV

Hypocalcemia:
· Administer IV calcium
  ○ Calcium gluconate 1-3 ampules (1 g [4.5 mEq] per 10-mL ampule)
  ○ Calcium chloride 1 ampule (1 g [13.5 mEq] per 10-mL amp) through a central line
· Note: The use of calcium supplementation in TLS may cause the precipitation of calcium phosphate

Hyperkalemia:
· Albuterol 10-20 mg nebulized
· Insulin 10 units IV bolus with 1-2 ampules of D50W IV

---

# SUGGESTED READING

- Behl D, Hendrickson AW, Moynihan TJ. Oncologic emergencies. Crit Care Clin. 2010;26(1):181-205.
- Beed M, Levitt M, Bokhari SW. Intensive care management of patients with haematological malignancy. Continuing Education in Anaesthesia Critical Care & Pain. 2010.10;(6);167-171.
- Gupta, A., Moore, J.A., 2018. Tumor Lysis Syndrome. JAMA Oncology 4, 895.
- Oduro-Dominah L, Brennan LJ. Anaesthetic management of the child with haematological malignancy. Continuing Education in Anaesthesia Critical Care & Pain. 2013. 13;(5);158-164.
- Puri I, Sharma D, Gunturu KS, Ahmed AA. Diagnosis and management of tumor lysis syndrome. J Community Hosp Intern Med Perspect. 2020;10(3):269-272.

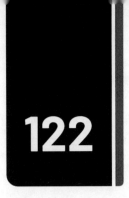

# VON WILLEBRAND'S DISEASE (VWD)

## LEARNING OBJECTIVES

- Definition and types of Von Willebrand's Disease (VWD)
- Treatment of VWD
- Anesthetic management of VWD

## DEFINITION AND MECHANISM

- Von Willebrand Disease is the most common inherited bleeding disorder with a prevalence of approximately 1% in the population
- Due to a qualitative or quantitative defect of the von Willebrand factor (vWF)
- Three types (mild, moderate, severe):
  - Type 1 is a quantitative defect
  - Type 2 is a qualitative defect
  - Type 3 is a very rare but severe form characterized by a mutant inhibitor protein against the vWF (vWF inhibitor)
    - It demonstrates autosomal dominant (e.g., type 1, 2B) & - recessive (e.g., types 2M, 2N, 3) inheritance, with marked phenotypic variations
- It may be discovered at any age and in either sex

## SIGNS AND SYMPTOMS

- Easy bruising
- Recurrent nose bleeds
- Prolonged postoperative or posttraumatic bleeding
- Bleeding gums

## COMPLICATIONS

- Anemia
- Swelling
- Pain
- Menorrhagia or in extreme cases even chronic joint bleeding

### Acquired von Willebrand Syndrome

- Is extremely rare but has been documented in clonal hematological, cardiovascular (aortic valve stenosis with higher sheer stresses in the vessels), immunological (hypothyroidism), and other lymphoproliferative auto-immune diseases
- A vWF-inhibitor protein or the adhesion of vWF with malignant cells can occur
- It has a marked reduced vWF activity interfering with the production and/or the stability of vWF
- Leading to the production of autoantibodies to endogenous vWF which can result in decreased functional high molecular weight vWF multimers
- Acquired vWS responds well to vWF-concentrates administration but the effects can be mitigated by these inhibitor proteins since they affect the half-life time of the administered vWF

### von Willebrand factor

- vWF is a ligand between platelets and subendothelial cells
- vWF stabilizes circulating factor VIII hereby preventing its degradation
- The levels of vWF and FVIII are on average lower in humans with type O blood and are increased in inflammatory conditions and during pregnancy
- Bleeding time and platelet function analysis will be prolonged in relation to the severity of the abnormality
- APTT can be prolonged in relation to the remaining quantity of FVIII

## DIAGNOSIS

- Laboratory testing: VWF-antigen, VWF-activity, and FVIII
- Familial history

## TYPES

Determination of the exact type is of utmost importance for the therapeutical approach

| Type 1 | Type 2 | Type 3 |
|---|---|---|
| ~ 85% with vWD have this form. Decreased quantities of vWF in several degrees. Characterized by a mild bleeding tendency but has increased risks perioperatively. Responds well to desmopressin infusion | ~ 5% with vWD have this form. Subtypes 2A, 2B, 2M, and 2N are described. Types 2A and 2B differ in the platelet binding capacity but the amount of high molecular weight multimers circulating in the plasma is decreased in both. Type 2A presents with a decreased platelet binding. Type 2B presents with an increased platelet agglutination with a concomitant increased risk of thrombosis. Type 2B is marked by accompanying thrombocytopenia due to a higher clearance of platelets. Subtype 2M has a decreased platelet binding with normal quantities of HMW multimers. Subtype 2N is characterized by a flawed ability to stabilize circulating FVIII and results in a factor VIII deficiency | A complete defect in vWF synthesis. Plasma factor VIII is decreased despite normal synthesis due to the lack of stabilization by the total absence of vWF |

## MAJOR BLEEDING RISKS

- Need to be considered when FVIII < 30IU/dL & Thrombocytopenia < 50000/mm³

## TREATMENT

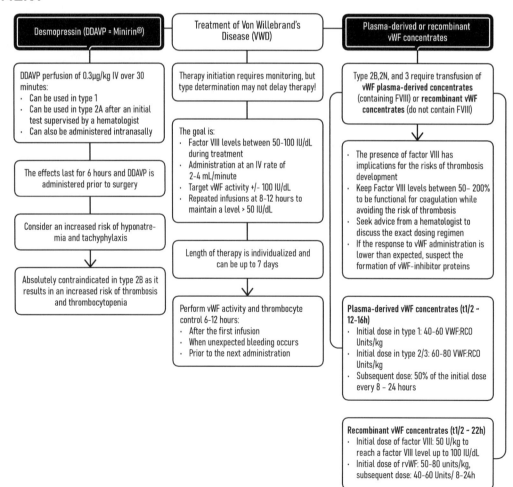

Von Willebrand's Disease (VWD)

# MANAGEMENT

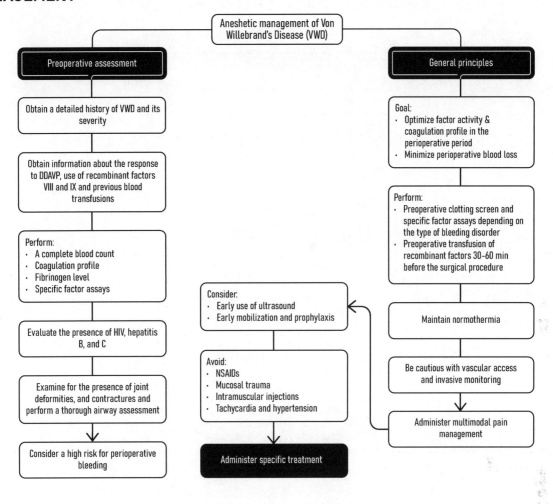

Aneshetic management of Von Willebrand's Disease (VWD)

**Preoperative assessment**

Obtain a detailed history of VWD and its severity

Obtain information about the response to DDAVP, use of recombinant factors VIII and IX and previous blood transfusions

Perform:
- A complete blood count
- Coagulation profile
- Fibrinogen level
- Specific factor assays

Evaluate the presence of HIV, hepatitis B, and C

Examine for the presence of joint deformities, and contractures and perform a thorough airway assessment

Consider a high risk for perioperative bleeding

Consider:
- Early use of ultrasound
- Early mobilization and prophylaxis

Avoid:
- NSAIDs
- Mucosal trauma
- Intramuscular injections
- Tachycardia and hypertension

Administer specific treatment

**General principles**

Goal:
- Optimize factor activity & coagulation profile in the perioperative period
- Minimize perioperative blood loss

Perform:
- Preoperative clotting screen and specific factor assays depending on the type of bleeding disorder
- Preoperative transfusion of recombinant factors 30-60 min before the surgical procedure

Maintain normothermia

Be cautious with vascular access and invasive monitoring

Administer multimodal pain management

# SPECIFIC TREATMENT DURING ANESTHESIA

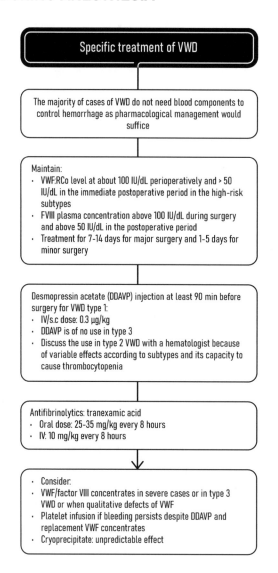

**Specific treatment of VWD**

The majority of cases of VWD do not need blood components to control hemorrhage as pharmacological management would suffice

Maintain:
- VWF:RCo level at about 100 IU/dL perioperatively and > 50 IU/dL in the immediate postoperative period in the high-risk subtypes
- FVIII plasma concentration above 100 IU/dL during surgery and above 50 IU/dL in the postoperative period
- Treatment for 7-14 days for major surgery and 1-5 days for minor surgery

Desmopressin acetate (DDAVP) injection at least 90 min before surgery for VWD type 1:
- IV/s.c dose: 0.3 µg/kg
- DDAVP is of no use in type 3
- Discuss the use in type 2 VWD with a hematologist because of variable effects according to subtypes and its capacity to cause thrombocytopenia

Antifibrinolytics: tranexamic acid
- Oral dose: 25-35 mg/kg every 8 hours
- IV: 10 mg/kg every 8 hours

- Consider:
- VWF/factor VIII concentrates in severe cases or in type 3 VWD or when qualitative defects of VWF
- Platelet infusion if bleeding persists despite DDAVP and replacement VWF concentrates
- Cryoprecipitate: unpredictable effect

---

## SUGGESTED READING

- Shah UJ, Madan Narayanan M, J Graham Smith JH. Anaesthetic considerations in patients with inherited disorders of coagulation. Continuing Education in Anaesthesia Critical Care & Pain, Volume 15, Issue 1, February 2015, Pages 26–31.
- Training in anaesthesia: the essential curriculum; Oxford Specialty Training, Chapter 15 pp392-393; ISBN: 978-0-19-922726-6
- Uptodate: von Willebrand disease (vWD):Treatment of major bleeding and major surgery, Paula James, MD, FRCPC, literature review current Nov 2022, last updated Sep 12, 2022.

# HEPATIC DISEASES

# END STAGE LIVER DISEASE (ESLD)

## LEARNING OBJECTIVES

- Recognize end-stage liver disease (ESLD)
- Management of ESLD

## DEFINITION AND MECHANISM

- Chronic liver failure progresses over months to years
- Often the result of cirrhosis of the liver
- ESLD is the final stage of acute and chronic liver failure accompanied by ascites, variceal bleeding, hepatic encephalopathy, or renal impairment
- Patients with severe symptoms of cirrhosis may benefit from a liver transplant

## SIGNS AND SYMPTOMS

- Weakness
- Fatigue
- Loss of appetite
- Nausea
- Vomiting
- Weight loss
- Abdominal pain and bloating
- Itching
Decompensated cirrhosis
- Bleeding varices
- Ascites
- Encephalopathy
- Jaundice

## COMPLICATIONS

- Edema and ascites
- Bruising and bleeding
- Portal hypertension
- Esophageal varices and gastropathy
- Splenomegaly
- Jaundice
- Gallstones
- Sensitivity to medications
- Hepatic encephalopathy
- Insulin resistance and type 2 diabetes mellitus
- Liver cancer

# MANAGEMENT

Management of ESLD

**Preperative care**

**Consider**
· Aspiration risk
· Friable/edematous tissues
· Altered drug pharmacology:
  ↑ volume of distribution, ↓ hepatic clearance, ↓ protein binding
· Altered fluid physiology: total body water excess (ascites) with intravascular volume depletion en low albumin state
· GA reduces hepatic arterial blood flow and predisposes to ischemic injury
· Spinal or epidural anesthesia reduces MAP
· Chronic alcohol use may increase anesthetic requirements

**Multiorgan dysfunction**
· CNS: encephalopathy
· Cardiovascular: hyperdynamic circulation (↑ cardiac output, ↓ SVR), cardiomyopathy, portopulmonary hypertension
· Pulmonary: hypoxemia (intrapulmonary AV shunting, V/Q mismatch); restrictive lung physiology (ascites & pleural effusions)
· GU: hepatorenal syndrome/renal failure
· GI: U/LGIB from varices & AVM's
· Hematology: Coagulopathy (↓ platelets, ↓ clotting factors, ↑ fibrinolysis) & immunodeficiency
· Endocrine: Hypoglycemia, hyponatremia, lactic acidosis

**The following agents are safe to use**
· Volatile anesthetics isoflurane, sevoflurane and desflurane
· Desflurane is the ideal volatile agent (preserves hepatic blood flow and CO)
· Remifentanil
· Etomidate
· Propofol (cirrhosis does not affect the elimination half-life)
· Atracurium and cisatracurium (these neuromuscular blocking agents are not hepatically excreted)

**Avoid**
· Morphine, fentanyl, and alfentanil (reduced elimination)
· Vecuronium (prolongs the duration of action of the neuromuscular blockade and the time to recovery)

**Periopeartive care**

· Perform invasive monitoring
· Pay attention to intravascular volume status, coagulation function, liver blood flow, renal function, encephalopathy, and prevention of sepsis
· Avoid sedative premedication
· Large bore IV access is mandatory
· Consider draining ascites to optimize respiratory mechanics
· Anticipate fluid shifts & major blood loss
· Appropriate use of hepatically-metabolized drugs

Consult the next infographic for extended perioperative management

Perform meticulous monitoring as surgical traction on the liver augments the reduction in hepatic blood ↓ causes a rise in TAP

Reduce the IV thionental dose

GA, General anesthesia; MAP, Mean arterial pressure; CNS, Central nervous system; SVR, Systemic vascular resistance; AV, Atrioventricular; V/Q, Ventilation/perfusion; GU, Genitourinary; GI, Gastrointestinal; U/LGIB, Upper/Lower gastrointestinal bleeding; AVM, Arteriovenous malformation; CO, Cardiac output; TAP, Transaminase activity parameters.

## Management of ESLD

| Clinical areas to be addressed in bold | Perioperative management |
|---|---|
| Nutrition and metabolism | Diet with high carbohydrate, high lipid content, and low in amino acid<br>Protein intake of 1.0 to 1.5 g/kg daily<br>Monitoring for hypoglycemia and hyperglycemia<br>Vitamin B1 in alcoholics |
| Portal hypertension and ascites | Salt and water restriction<br>Diuretics<br>Ascitic fluid analysis<br>SBP treatment and prophylaxis<br>Large-volume paracentesis for uncontrolled ascites with albumin<br>TIPS for refractory ascites |
| Renal | Fluid and electrolyte balance<br>Avoid nephrotoxic drugs including contrast agents<br>Combination of albumin and terlipressin or octreotide with midodrine in HRS |
| Cerebral | Use of lactulose, metronidazole, and neomycin<br>Rifaximin and branched-chain amino acids<br>Treat infections, avoid diuretics, and constipation<br>Correct electrolyte abnormalities |
| Pulmonary | Optimize pulmonary functions<br>Incentive spirometry<br>Intravenous prostacyclin in selective cases |
| Cardiac | Optimization of fluid status<br>ACC and AHA guidelines for noncardiac surgery<br>β-blockers in perioperative period |
| Electrolytes and Metabolism | Monitor and correct hyponatremia and hypokalemia<br>Blood sugar monitoring |
| Hematology | Maintain HB > 10 g/dL and < 50 000<br>INR correction with intravenous vitamin K, FFP, and cryoprecipitate<br>May need DDAVP, recombinant factor VIIa, aprotinin, and tranexamic acid<br>Prophylactic platelets transfusion for platelets < 50 000 |

*Perioperative care*

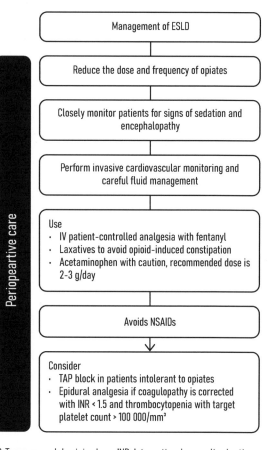

TAP, Transverse abdominis plane; INR, International normalised ratio.

SBP, Spontaneous bacterial peritonitis; TIPS, Transjugular intrahepatic portosystemic shunt; HRS, Hepatorenal syndrome; ACC, American College of Cardiology; AHA, American Heart Association; HB, Hemoglobin; INR, International normalised ratio; FFP, Fresh frozen plasma; DDAVP, Desmopressin acetate.

## KEEP IN MIND

- Patients with end-stage liver disease can also develop kidney failure
- This is often reversible with a liver transplant but some patients may need a combined liver and kidney transplant

## SUGGESTED READING

- Abbas N, Makker J, Abbas H, Balar B. Perioperative Care of Patients With Liver Cirrhosis: A Review. Health Serv Insights. 2017;10:1178632917691270. Published 2017 Feb 24.
- Rakesh Vaja, BSc MBChB FRCA, Larry McNicol, MBBS (Hons) FRCA FANZCA, Imogen Sisley, MBChB MRCP FRCA, Anaesthesia for patients with liver disease, Continuing Education in Anaesthesia Critical Care & Pain, Volume 10, Issue 1, February 2010, Pages 15-19

# JAUNDICED PATIENT

## LEARNING OBJECTIVES

- Outline the signs and symptoms of jaundice
- Describe the causes of jaundice and their classification
- Anesthetic management of a jaundiced patient

## DEFINITION AND MECHANISM

- Jaundice, or icterus, is a yellowish discoloration of the skin and sclera due to high bilirubin levels
- Jaundice in adults indicates the presence of underlying diseases involving abnormal heme metabolism, liver dysfunction, or biliary tract obstruction
- Surgery should be avoided in these patients, only emergency procedures

## SIGNS AND SYMPTOMS

- Hyperbilirubinemia (serum bilirubin $\geq$ 3 mg/dL)
- Yellowish discoloration of the skin, mucous membranes, and sclera
- Itchiness (pruritus)
- Pale fatty stool (steatorrhea)
- Dark urine (bilirubinuria)
- Abdominal pain
- Fatigue
- Weight loss
- Vomiting
- Fever

## COMPLICATIONS

- Hyperbilirubinemia-induced neurological damage → kernicterus (especially in newborns)
- Coagulopathy
  - Vitamin K-dependent coagulation factors (II, VII, IX, and X) are reduced, resulting in a prolonged prothrombin time
  - Hepatocellular coagulopathy is often refractory to vitamin K administration
  - Disseminated intravascular coagulation (DIC) is associated with secondary biliary tract infection
- Altered drug handling
  - Drugs excreted via the biliary system have prolonged elimination half-life in cholestasis
  - Atracurium is the drug of choice for muscular relaxation
- Acute oliguric renal failure (17%)
- Stress ulceration with gastrointestinal hemorrhage (16%)
- Reduced wound healing

# CAUSES

| Category | Definition | Causes |
|---|---|---|
| Prehepatic/hemolytic | Pathology occurs prior to liver metabolism, due to increased breakdown of erythrocytes → increased rate of erythrocyte hemolysis → increased unconjugated serum bilirubin → increased deposition of unconjugated bilirubin into mucosal tissue | Sickle-cell anemia<br>Spherocytosis<br>Thalassemia<br>Pyruvate kinase deficiency<br>Glucose-6-phosphate dehydrogenase deficiency<br>Microangiopathic hemolytic anemia<br>Hemolytic-uremic syndrome<br>Severe malaria |
| Hepatic/hepatocellular | Pathology is due to damage of parenchymal liver cells → abnormal liver metabolism of bilirubin | Acute hepatitis<br>Chronic hepatitis<br>Hepatotoxicity<br>Cirrhosis<br>Drug-induced hepatitis<br>Alcoholic liver disease<br>Gilbert syndrome<br>Crigler-Najjar syndrome<br>Leptospirosis |
| Posthepatic/cholestatic (obstructive jaundice) | Pathology occurs after bilirubin conjugation in the liver, due to obstruction of the biliary tract and/or decreased bilirubin excretion | Choledocholithiasis (common bile duct gallstones)<br>Cancer of the pacreas<br>Biliary tract strictures<br>Biliary atresia<br>Primary biliary cholangitis<br>Cholestasis of pregnancy<br>Acute pancreatitis<br>Chronic pancreatitis<br>Pancreatic pseudocysts<br>Mirizzi syndrome<br>Parasites |

## RISK FACTORS

- Male gender
- White ethnicities
- Active smoking

## TREATMENT

- Based on the underlying cause

Jaundiced patient

# MANAGEMENT

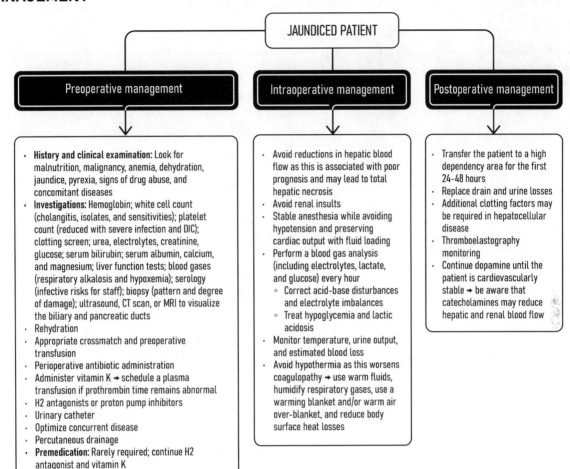

**JAUNDICED PATIENT**

**Preoperative management**

- **History and clinical examination:** Look for malnutrition, malignancy, anemia, dehydration, jaundice, pyrexia, signs of drug abuse, and concomitant diseases
- **Investigations:** Hemoglobin; white cell count (cholangitis, isolates, and sensitivities); platelet count (reduced with severe infection and DIC); clotting screen; urea, electrolytes, creatinine, glucose; serum bilirubin; serum albumin, calcium, and magnesium; liver function tests; blood gases (respiratory alkalosis and hypoxemia); serology (infective risks for staff); biopsy (pattern and degree of damage); ultrasound, CT scan, or MRI to visualize the biliary and pancreatic ducts
- Rehydration
- Appropriate crossmatch and preoperative transfusion
- Perioperative antibiotic administration
- Administer vitamin K → schedule a plasma transfusion if prothrombin time remains abnormal
- H2 antagonists or proton pump inhibitors
- Urinary catheter
- Optimize concurrent disease
- Percutaneous drainage
- **Premedication:** Rarely required; continue H2 antagonist and vitamin K

**Intraoperative management**

- Avoid reductions in hepatic blood flow as this is associated with poor prognosis and may lead to total hepatic necrosis
- Avoid renal insults
- Stable anesthesia while avoiding hypotension and preserving cardiac output with fluid loading
- Perform a blood gas analysis (including electrolytes, lactate, and glucose) every hour
  - Correct acid-base disturbances and electrolyte imbalances
  - Treat hypoglycemia and lactic acidosis
- Monitor temperature, urine output, and estimated blood loss
- Avoid hypothermia as this worsens coagulopathy → use warm fluids, humidify respiratory gases, use a warming blanket and/or warm air over-blanket, and reduce body surface heat losses

**Postoperative management**

- Transfer the patient to a high dependency area for the first 24-48 hours
- Replace drain and urine losses
- Additional clotting factors may be required in hepatocellular disease
- Thromboelastography monitoring
- Continue dopamine until the patient is cardiovascularly stable → be aware that catecholamines may reduce hepatic and renal blood flow

## SUGGESTED READING

- Pollard BJ, Kitchen G. Handbook of Clinical Anaesthesia. 4th ed. Taylor & Francis group; 2018. Chapter 4 Gastrointestinal tract, Jackson MJ.
- Wang L, Yu W. Obstructive jaundice and perioperative management. Acta Anaesthesiol Taiwan. 2014;52(1):22-29.

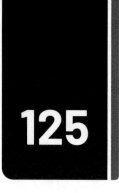

# LIVER RESECTION

## LEARNING OBJECTIVES

- Definition and types of liver resections
- Anesthetic management of liver resection

## DEFINITION AND MECHANISM

- Hepatectomy or liver resection is a surgical operation to remove part or all of the liver
- Up to two-thirds can be removed as long as the rest of the liver is healthy
- The liver can regenerate functionally active tissue after resection by hyperplasia of the remnant tissue
- Liver is highly vascular and receives 25% of cardiac output, 80% is supplied by the portal vein and 20% by the hepatic artery
- Liver resection is the treatment of choice for colorectal hepatic metastases without evidence of more distant disease spread
- Also used in the management of benign and malignant primary hepato-biliary tumors, donation for transplantation, or hepatic trauma
- The most common liver cancers treated by partial hepatectomy include:
  - Hepatocellular carcinoma
  - Cholangiocarcinoma
  - Metastatic colorectal cancer
- Other benign lesions include:
  - Gallstones in the intrahepatic ducts
  - Adenoma
  - Liver cystadenoma or a cyst

## COMPLICATIONS

- Infection
- Bleeding
- Bile leakage
- Pleural effusion
- Ascites
- Deep vein thrombosis
- Kidney failure
- Liver failure

| Types of liver resections | |
| --- | --- |
| Major liver resection | Right or left hepatectomy or lobectomy removes the right or left lobe |
| Minor liver resection | Segmental or wedge resection removes a segment or a part of a segment with a tumor with a margin around it<br>Another minor liver resection is the left lateral sectionectomy, which removes the lateral part (section) of the left lobe |
| Multiple liver resections | Multiple tumors may be resected at the same time |
| Two-stage liver resection | If it is too dangerous to remove all the tumors at once |

## MANAGEMENT

- Consider:
  - The potential for massive blood loss
  - Risk of postoperative liver dysfunction and coagulopathy
  - Altered drug metabolism
  - Temporary occlusion of blood supply during liver resection (surgical technique to minimize bleeding) → ↓ cardiac output (CO) up to 10%, ↑ left ventricle (LV) afterload by 20-30%
  - Surgical manipulation may cause transient inferior vena cava (IVC) compression and a decrease in venous return

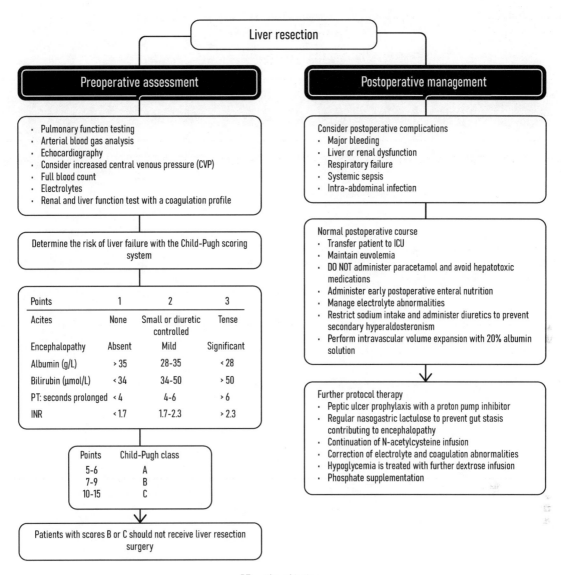

```
                              ┌─────────────────────┐
                              │   Liver resection   │
                              └─────────────────────┘
```

**Preoperative assessment**

- Pulmonary function testing
- Arterial blood gas analysis
- Echocardiography
- Consider increased central venous pressure (CVP)
- Full blood count
- Electrolytes
- Renal and liver function test with a coagulation profile

Determine the risk of liver failure with the Child-Pugh scoring system

| Points | 1 | 2 | 3 |
|---|---|---|---|
| Acites | None | Small or diuretic controlled | Tense |
| Encephalopathy | Absent | Mild | Significant |
| Albumin (g/L) | > 35 | 28-35 | < 28 |
| Bilirubin (µmol/L) | < 34 | 34-50 | > 50 |
| PT: seconds prolonged | < 4 | 4-6 | > 6 |
| INR | < 1.7 | 1.7-2.3 | > 2.3 |

| Points | Child-Pugh class |
|---|---|
| 5-6 | A |
| 7-9 | B |
| 10-15 | C |

Patients with scores B or C should not receive liver resection surgery

**Postoperative management**

Consider postoperative complications
- Major bleeding
- Liver or renal dysfunction
- Respiratory failure
- Systemic sepsis
- Intra-abdominal infection

Normal postoperative course
- Transfer patient to ICU
- Maintain euvolemia
- DO NOT administer paracetamol and avoid hepatotoxic medications
- Administer early postoperative enteral nutrition
- Manage electrolyte abnormalities
- Restrict sodium intake and administer diuretics to prevent secondary hyperaldosteronism
- Perform intravascular volume expansion with 20% albumin solution

Further protocol therapy
- Peptic ulcer prophylaxis with a proton pump inhibitor
- Regular nasogastric lactulose to prevent gut stasis contributing to encephalopathy
- Continuation of N-acetylcysteine infusion
- Correction of electrolyte and coagulation abnormalities
- Hypoglycemia is treated with further dextrose infusion
- Phosphate supplementation

PT, prothrombin time.

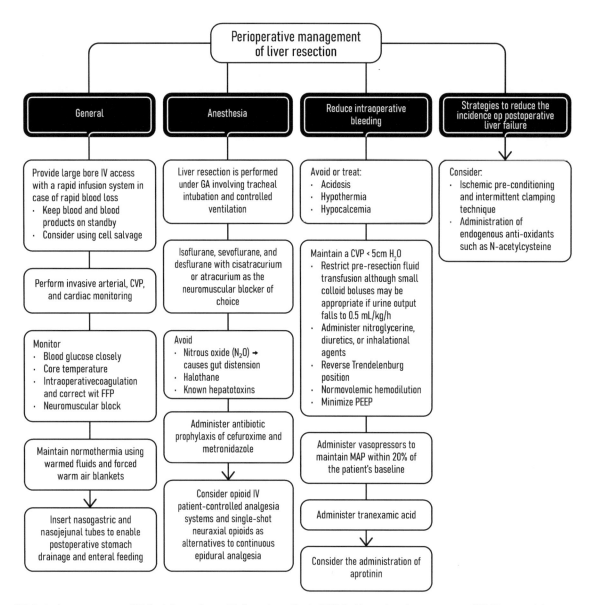

**Perioperative management of liver resection**

**General**

Provide large bore IV access with a rapid infusion system in case of rapid blood loss
- Keep blood and blood products on standby
- Consider using cell salvage

Perform invasive arterial, CVP, and cardiac monitoring

Monitor
- Blood glucose closely
- Core temperature
- Intraoperativecoagulation and correct wit FFP
- Neuromuscular block

Maintain normothermia using warmed fluids and forced warm air blankets

Insert nasogastric and nasojejunal tubes to enable postoperative stomach drainage and enteral feeding

**Anesthesia**

Liver resection is performed under GA involving tracheal intubation and controlled ventilation

Isoflurane, sevoflurane, and desflurane with cisatracurium or atracurium as the neuromuscular blocker of choice

Avoid
- Nitrous oxide ($N_2O$) → causes gut distension
- Halothane
- Known hepatotoxins

Administer antibiotic prophylaxis of cefuroxime and metronidazole

Consider opioid IV patient-controlled analgesia systems and single-shot neuraxial opioids as alternatives to continuous epidural analgesia

**Reduce intraoperative bleeding**

Avoid or treat:
- Acidosis
- Hypothermia
- Hypocalcemia

Maintain a CVP < 5cm $H_2O$
- Restrict pre-resection fluid transfusion although small colloid boluses may be appropriate if urine output falls to 0.5 mL/kg/h
- Administer nitroglycerine, diuretics, or inhalational agents
- Reverse Trendelenburg position
- Normovolemic hemodilution
- Minimize PEEP

Administer vasopressors to maintain MAP within 20% of the patient's baseline

Administer tranexamic acid

Consider the administration of aprotinin

**Strategies to reduce the incidence op postoperative liver failure**

Consider:
- Ischemic pre-conditioning and intermittent clamping technique
- Administration of endogenous anti-oxidants such as N-acetylcysteine

CVP, Central venous pressure, FFP, Fresh frozen plasma, GA, General anesthesia; PEEP, Positive end-expiratory pressure; MAP, Mean arterial pressure.

## SUGGESTED READING

- Harto A, Mills G. 2009. Anaesthesia for hepatic resection surgery. Continuing Education in Anaesthesia Critical Care & Pain9;1:1-5.
- Page AJ, Kooby DA. Perioperative management of hepatic resection. J Gastrointest Oncol. 2012;3(1):19-27.
- Pollard BJ, Kitchen, G. Handbook of Clinical Anaesthesia. Fourth Edition. CRC Press. 2018. 978-1-4987-6289-2.

# PATIENT WITH A LIVER TRANSPLANT

**126**

## LEARNING OBJECTIVES

- Define orthotopic liver transplantation
- Understand the considerations of patients with a previous liver transplant
- Manage patients with a liver transplant liver undergoing nontransplant surgery

## DEFINITION AND MECHANISM

- Liver transplantation is a treatment option for end-stage living disease (ESLD) and acute liver failure
- Orthotopic liver transplantation is the most common technique and involves the substitution of a diseased native liver with a normal liver (or part of one) taken from a deceased or living donor in the same anatomic position as the original liver
- Recipients may present for nontransplant surgery later in life

## CONSIDERATIONS

- The majority of recipients are 30-60 years old and in good health
- Cardiopulmonary effects of ESLD reverse shortly after transplantation
- Most patients have normal liver function unless there is rejection, sepsis, or recurrence of the original disease
- High incidence of hypertension after liver transplantation
- Immunosuppression increases susceptibility to infection and other common side effects
  - **Corticosteroids:** Hypertension, hypokalemia, hyperglycemia, adrenal suppression
  - **Tacrolimus:** Hypertension, renal dysfunction, electrolyte abnormalities, hyperglycemia
  - **Cyclosporine:** Nephrotoxicity and hyperkalemia, hepatotoxicity, neurotoxicity, hypertension
  - **Azathioprine:** Bone marrow suppression

## KEEP IN MIND

- Increasing numbers of patients have a successful liver transplant and may require nontransplant surgery later in life
- Careful preoperative assessment is essential, especially for liver and kidney function
- The goal of perioperative management is to avoid any factors that might compromise hepatic and renal function and to minimize the infection risk with antibiotic prophylaxis and careful aseptic techniques

Patient with a liver transplant

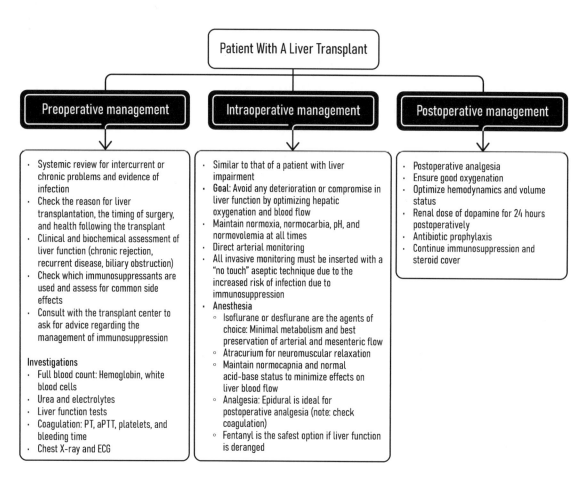

## Patient With A Liver Transplant

### Preoperative management

- Systemic review for intercurrent or chronic problems and evidence of infection
- Check the reason for liver transplantation, the timing of surgery, and health following the transplant
- Clinical and biochemical assessment of liver function (chronic rejection, recurrent disease, biliary obstruction)
- Check which immunosuppressants are used and assess for common side effects
- Consult with the transplant center to ask for advice regarding the management of immunosuppression

**Investigations**
- Full blood count: Hemoglobin, white blood cells
- Urea and electrolytes
- Liver function tests
- Coagulation: PT, aPTT, platelets, and bleeding time
- Chest X-ray and ECG

### Intraoperative management

- Similar to that of a patient with liver impairment
- **Goal:** Avoid any deterioration or compromise in liver function by optimizing hepatic oxygenation and blood flow
- Maintain normoxia, normocarbia, pH, and normovolemia at all times
- Direct arterial monitoring
- All invasive monitoring must be inserted with a "no touch" aseptic technique due to the increased risk of infection due to immunosuppression
- Anesthesia
  - Isoflurane or desflurane are the agents of choice: Minimal metabolism and best preservation of arterial and mesenteric flow
  - Atracurium for neuromuscular relaxation
  - Maintain normocapnia and normal acid-base status to minimize effects on liver blood flow
  - Analgesia: Epidural is ideal for postoperative analgesia (note: check coagulation)
  - Fentanyl is the safest option if liver function is deranged

### Postoperative management

- Postoperative analgesia
- Ensure good oxygenation
- Optimize hemodynamics and volume status
- Renal dose of dopamine for 24 hours postoperatively
- Antibiotic prophylaxis
- Continue immunosuppression and steroid cover

PT, Prothrombin time; aPTT, Activated partial thromboplastin time.

## SUGGESTED READING

- Pollard BJ, Kitchen G. Handbook of Clinical Anaesthesia. 4th ed. Taylor & Francis group; 2018. Chapter 4 Gastrointestinal tract, Jackson MJ.

# MISCELLANEOUS

# AWARENESS DURING ANESTHESIA

## LEARNING OBJECTIVES

- Describe the implications and risk factors of awareness during anesthesia
- Prevent awareness during anesthesia
- Diagnose and manage patients who experienced awareness during anesthesia

## DEFINITION AND MECHANISM

- Rare but severe complication of anesthetic care
- Also referred to as "accidental awareness during general anesthesia" (AAGA)
- Mostly occurs during induction and emergence
- Can range from only auditory or tactile awareness to being fully awake with paralysis and pain
- Traumatic experience with possibly severe long-term effects (post-traumatic stress disorder)

## RISK FACTORS

- Neuromuscular blocking
- Female gender
- Pregnancy
- Cardiothoracic patients
- Obesity
- Total intravenous anesthesia

- Trauma & emergency surgery
- Ketamine, etomidate, and thiopental use
- Difficult intubation
- History of AAGA
- Chronic drug use
- Lack of monitoring

## PSYCHOLOGICAL ASSESSMENT AND DIAGNOSIS

- Acute stress disorder (ASD): Occurs shortly after traumatic event (3 days to 1 month)
    - Diagnosis: at least 9 of the following symptoms:
        - Recurring, uncontrollable, and intrusive distressing memories of the event
        - Recurring nightmares of the event
        - Flashbacks of the event
        - Intense psychological or physical distress when reminded of the event
        - Persistent inability to experience positive emotions
        - Altered sense of reality
        - Memory loss for an important part of the traumatic event
        - Efforts to avoid distressing memories, thoughts, or feelings associated with the event
        - Efforts to avoid external reminders associated with the event
        - Disturbed sleep
        - Irritability or angry outbursts
        - Hypervigilance
        - Concentration difficulties
        - Exaggerated startle response
- Post-traumatic stress disorder (PTSD): Diagnosed when symptoms persist for more than 1 month after the traumatic event

## PREVENTION

- Check equipment and medications
- Depth of anesthesia monitoring (Electroencephalography (EEG) is superior to bispectral index monitoring (BIS))
- Avoid or minimize the use of neuromuscular blocking agents
- Monitor neuromuscular block if neuromuscular blocking is necessary
- Use target-controlled infusion for total IV anesthesia

## MANAGEMENT

Management is based on treating psychological symptoms:
- Early face-to-face postoperative meeting with the patient and consultation with a psychiatrist or psychologist
- Psychological interventions (e.g., cognitive behavioral therapy)
- Antidepressants
- Benzodiazepines for acute anxiety (beware of potential abuse)
- Antipsychotics may be helpful in some patients

**SUGGESTED READING**

- Kim MC, Fricchione GL, Akeju O. Accidental awareness under general anaesthesia: Incidence, risk factors, and psychological management. BJA Education. 2021;21(4):154-61.
- Mashour GA, Avidan MS. Intraoperative awareness: controversies and non-controversies. Br J Anaesth. 2015;115 Suppl 1:i20-i26.
- Mashour GA, Orser BA, Avidan MS, Warner DS. Intraoperative Awareness: From Neurobiology to Clinical Practice. Anesthesiology. 2011;114(5):1218-33.
- Tasbihgou SR, Vogels MF, Absalom AR. Accidental awareness during general anaesthesia - a narrative review. Anaesthesia. 2018;73(1):112-22.

# BARIATRIC SURGERY

## LEARNING OBJECTIVES

- Define and classify the different types of bariatric surgery
- Describe the complications that are associated with bariatric surgery
- Anesthetic management of a patient undergoing bariatric surgery

## DEFINITION AND MECHANISM

- Bariatric or weight loss surgery limits the amount of food a patient can comfortably eat or decreases the absorption of food and calories or a combination of both mechanisms
- It is used as a later treatment option for obesity and helps to improve obesity-related conditions:

  - Hypertension
  - Hyperglycemia
  - Diabetes mellitus type 2
  - Hypercholesterolemia
  - Cardiovascular disease and stroke

  - Kidney disease
  - Obstructive sleep apnea
  - Osteoarthritis
  - Non-alcohol-related fatty liver disease

### Classification

**A. Restrictive procedures: that limit gastric volume**
1. Adjustable gastric banding (Placement of an inflatable silicone band around the top portion of the stomach)
2. Sleeve gastrectomy. The stomach is reduced to 15% of its original size via surgical removal of a large portion of the stomach along the greater curvature

**B. Malabsortive procedures: that limit food absorption by bypassing the small bowel; now they are less commonly performed due to significant nutritional complications**
1. Biliopancreatic diversion with or without doudenal switch: By removing the pylorus, and dividing the ileum. The distal ileum is anastomosed to the stomach and the proximal ileum is anastomosed with the output from the liver, pancreas, and duodenum
2. Gastric bypass (e.g., Roux-en-Y, one anastomosis gastric bypass): The stomach is divided into a small upper pouch and a much larger lower "remnant" pouch, and the small intestine is rearranged to connect to both

## WORKING MECHANISM

Each procedure exerts its effects through at least one of the three mechanisms
→ procedures often affect several of these mechanisms:
- **Restricting:** Restricting food intake (e.g., gastric sleeve)
  - Reduce the size of the stomach that is available to hold a meal
  - Filling the stomach faster enables the individual to feel more full after a smaller meal
- **Blocking:** Decreasing nutrient absorption (e.g., Roux-en-Y gastric bypass)
  - Reduce the amount of intestine that the food passes through
  - Reduces the ability of the intestines to absorb nutrients from the food
- **Mixed:** Affecting cell signaling pathways
  - Alter hormones responsible for hunger (e.g., ghrelin) and satiety (e.g., leptin)

## PATIENT CHARACTERISTICS

- Morbid obesity and high BMI
- Adults, and a selected group of young adults
- Males and females equally affected
- Increased incidence of
  - Diabetes mellitus
  - Cardiovascular disease
  - Respiratory disease
  - Sleep apnea syndrome

## COMPLICATIONS

- Early (intraop and early postop):
  - Bleeding
  - Surgical emphysema and $CO_2$ embolism
  - Blood Clots (Deep Vein Thrombosis and Pulmonary embolism)
  - Infection; surgical site infection and pneumonia
  - Anastomotic leak and peritonitis
  - Bowel obstruction
  - Vomiting

**356**

- Late complications:
  - Pancreatitis
  - excess skin folds
  - Malabsorption and malnutrition
  - GERD and Bile reflux
  - Gallstones with or without Cholecystitis
  - Renal stones
  - Small bowel obstruction
  - Hernias
  - Recurrent hypoglycemia
  - Dumping syndrome
  - Ulcers
  - Metabolic bone disease (e.g., osteopenia and secondary hyperparathyroidism)

## MANAGEMENT

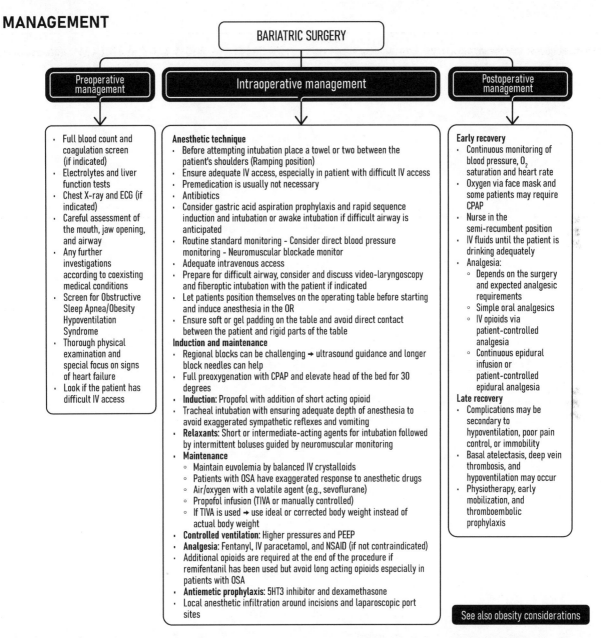

**BARIATRIC SURGERY**

**Preoperative management**

- Full blood count and coagulation screen (if indicated)
- Electrolytes and liver function tests
- Chest X-ray and ECG (if indicated)
- Careful assessment of the mouth, jaw opening, and airway
- Any further investigations according to coexisting medical conditions
- Screen for Obstructive Sleep Apnea/Obesity Hypoventilation Syndrome
- Thorough physical examination and special focus on signs of heart failure
- Look if the patient has difficult IV access

**Intraoperative management**

**Anesthetic technique**
- Before attempting intubation place a towel or two between the patient's shoulders (Ramping position)
- Ensure adequate IV access, especially in patient with difficult IV access
- Premedication is usually not necessary
- Antibiotics
- Consider gastric acid aspiration prophylaxis and rapid sequence induction and intubation or awake intubation if difficult airway is anticipated
- Routine standard monitoring - Consider direct blood pressure monitoring - Neuromuscular blockade monitor
- Adequate intravenous access
- Prepare for difficult airway, consider and discuss video-laryngoscopy and fiberoptic intubation with the patient if indicated
- Let patients position themselves on the operating table before starting and induce anesthesia in the OR
- Ensure soft or gel padding on the table and avoid direct contact between the patient and rigid parts of the table

**Induction and maintenance**
- Regional blocks can be challenging → ultrasound guidance and longer block needles can help
- Full preoxygenation with CPAP and elevate head of the bed for 30 degrees
- **Induction:** Propofol with addition of short acting opioid
- Tracheal intubation with ensuring adequate depth of anesthesia to avoid exaggerated sympathetic reflexes and vomiting
- **Relaxants:** Short or intermediate-acting agents for intubation followed by intermittent boluses guided by neuromuscular monitoring
- **Maintenance**
  - Maintain euvolemia by balanced IV crystalloids
  - Patients with OSA have exaggerated response to anesthetic drugs
  - Air/oxygen with a volatile agent (e.g., sevoflurane)
  - Propofol infusion (TIVA or manually controlled)
  - If TIVA is used → use ideal or corrected body weight instead of actual body weight
- **Controlled ventilation:** Higher pressures and PEEP
- **Analgesia:** Fentanyl, IV paracetamol, and NSAID (if not contraindicated)
- Additional opioids are required at the end of the procedure if remifentanil has been used but avoid long acting opioids especially in patients with OSA
- **Antiemetic prophylaxis:** 5HT3 inhibitor and dexamethasone
- Local anesthetic infiltration around incisions and laparoscopic port sites

**Postoperative management**

**Early recovery**
- Continuous monitoring of blood pressure, O$_2$ saturation and heart rate
- Oxygen via face mask and some patients may require CPAP
- Nurse in the semi-recumbent position
- IV fluids until the patient is drinking adequately
- Analgesia:
  - Depends on the surgery and expected analgesic requirements
  - Simple oral analgesics
  - IV opioids via patient-controlled analgesia
  - Continuous epidural infusion or patient-controlled epidural analgesia

**Late recovery**
- Complications may be secondary to hypoventilation, poor pain control, or immobility
- Basal atelectasis, deep vein thrombosis, and hypoventilation may occur
- Physiotherapy, early mobilization, and thromboembolic prophylaxis

See also obesity considerations

## SUGGESTED READING

- Pollard BJ, Kitchen G. Handbook of Clinical Anaesthesia. 4th ed. Taylor & Francis group; 2018. Chapter 10 Abdominal surgery.
- Reeve K, Kennedy N. Anaesthesia for bariatric surgery. BJA Education. 2022;22(6):231-237. doi:10.1016/j.bjae.2021.12.007
- Soleimanpour H, Safari S, Sanaie S, Nazari M, Alavian SM. Anesthetic Considerations in Patients Undergoing Bariatric Surgery: A Review Article. Anesth Pain Med. 2017 Jul 11;7(4):e57568.

# BEACH CHAIR POSITION

## LEARNING OBJECTIVES

- Describe the advantages and risks of the beach chair position
- Manage patients presenting for surgery in the beach chair position

## DEFINITION AND MECHANISM

- Patients are often positioned in the beach chair or sitting position for shoulder surgery, posterior fossa craniotomy, and post-c-spine surgery

## ADVANTAGES

- Improved surgical access
- Decreased brachial traction injury
- Ease of setup and conversion to an open approach
- Decreased risk of bleeding

## MANAGEMENT

Management of patients presenting for surgery in the beach chair position comprises minimizing the risk of complications, mainly by maintaining cerebral perfusion

## RISKS

- Hypotension
- Decrease in cerebral perfusion
- Venous air embolism
- Paradoxical air embolism
- Excessive neck flexion
- Bradycardia or cardiac arrest
- Macroglossia
- Upper airway obstruction
- Pneumocephalus
- Subdural hematoma
- Quadriplegia
- Stroke

---

**AVOID HYPERVENTILATION**

- Avoid excessive PEEP which compromises venous return
- Hypocapnia causes cerebral vasoconstriction and decreased blood flow
- Beware: Hypercapnia may decrease blood flow to the ischemic brain by vasodilating the vasculature in the normal brain

---

**ANESTHETIC MODALITY**

- Regional anesthesia
  - Better sympathetic response to sitting upright: Increase in systemic vascular resistance maintains blood pressure
  - Better postoperative analgesia
  - Shorter operating theater time
  - Avoidance of potential airway, respiratory, and cardiovascular complications of general anesthesia
- Inhalational anesthesia in favor of total IV anesthesia

---

**AVOID PNEUMOCEPHALUS**

- Discontinue nitrous oxide and keep on 100% $O_2$ 20-30 min before completion of the procedure

---

**AVOID QUADRIPLEGIA**

- Avoid neck hyperflexion by keeping at least two fingerbreadths distance between chin and neck
- Avoid hip flexion > 90 degrees in order to minimize stretch on lower extremity nerves
- Slightly flex the knees to avoid stretching of the sciatic nerve
- Arms should be supported to avoid nerve plexus stretching

---

**MAINTAIN BLOOD PRESSURE**

- Support mean arterial pressure above the lower limit of cerebral autoregulation
- Vasopressors (e.g., ephedrine or phynelephrine infusion)
- IV fluids
- Ensure adequate hydration and avoid hypovolemia
- Compression stockings
- Consider invasive blood pressure monitoring, and place the transducer at the level of carotid bifurcation
- If unable to treat hypotension, lay patient supine

---

**AVOID VENOUS AIR EMBOLISM**

- Preoperative "bubble test" in awake patient using transesophageal or transthoracic echocardiography
- Precordial transthoracic Doppler for early detection
- Air embolism causes increase in dead space
- Large air embolus causes acute right ventricular failure.
- Small air embolus causes reflex bronchoconstriction and pulmonary edema.
- 20-30% of adults have patent foramen ovale. in that case air embolus may cause MI or stroke (Paradoxical embolism)

Air embolism is avoided by:

- Flooding the surgical field with saline
- Immediate ligation of open veins and venous sinuses

## SUGGESTED READING

- Hewson DW, Oldman M, Bedforth NM. Regional anaesthesia for shoulder surgery. BJA Education. 2019;19(4):98-104.
- Murphy GS, Greenberg SB, Szokol JW. Safety of Beach Chair Position Shoulder Surgery: A Review of the Current Literature. Anesth Analg. 2019;129(1):101-118.
- Rozet I, Vavilala MS. Risks and benefits of patient positioning during neurosurgical care. Anesthesiol Clin. 2007;25(3):631-x.

# BLEOMYCIN EXPOSURE

## LEARNING OBJECTIVES

- Describe the effects and underlying mechanisms of bleomycin therapy
- Diagnose bleomycin pulmonary toxicity
- Manage patients who have received bleomycin therapy

## DEFINITION AND MECHANISM

- Bleomycin is an antitumor antibiotic often used systemically to treat germ cell tumors and Hodgkin's disease and is used locally by installation if pleural cavity to treat malignant effusions
- Side-effect: Potential for subacute pulmonary damage that can progress to life-threatening pulmonary fibrosis
- Pulmonary toxicity occurs in 6-10% of patients
- "Bleomycin lung" is associated with cumulative dosing greater than 400 U and occurs rarely with a total dose of 150 U and is potentiated by thoracic radiation and by hyperoxia
- Exposure to high-inspired concentration oxygen therapy, even for short periods, can cause rapidly progressive pulmonary toxicity in patients previously treated with bleomycin
- Lung injury typically develops within 6 months after the start of bleomycin treatment
- Pulmonary function studies show decreased CO diffusing capacity and restrictive ventilatory changes
- The potential for high-inspired fractions of oxygen to provoke pulmonary toxicity remains a life-long risk in these patients
- Symptoms of bleomycin-induced pulmonary toxicity include pneumonitis, dry cough, breathlessness, pleuritic chest pain, and fever

## PATHOPHYSIOLOGY

- Bleomycin oxidatively damages DNA by binding to metal ions such as iron, resulting in reactive oxygen species formation
- Is inactivated by bleomycin hydrolase
- Low concentrations of bleomycin hydrolase in skin and lung tissues contribute to the sensitivity to bleomycin of these tissues
- Contributing factors to bleomycin pulmonary toxicity:
  □ Inflammatory cell infiltration into pulmonary endothelial cells
  □ Fibrotic changes with elevated collagen content
  □ Increased expression of fibrogenic mediators (TGF-beta, connective tissue growth factor, PDGF-C) in endothelial cells
  □ Decrease in thapsigargin-induced prostaglandin I2 and nitric oxide (vasodilators) in endothelial pneumocytes

## RISK FACTORS FOR PULMONARY TOXICITY

- Advanced age
- Renal insufficiency
- Increased cumulative drug dose
- Severity of underlying malignancy
- Concomitant high $FiO_2$ therapy
- Concomitant radiation therapy
- Other chemotherapeutic agents
- Smoking

## DIAGNOSIS

| Diagnosis | |
|---|---|
| Physical examination | Dyspnea<br>Pulmonary crackles<br>Hypoxemia |
| Radiology | Linear interstitial shadowing, which can look similar to Kerly B lines seen in pulmonary edema<br>Confluent airspace shadowing, which may be diagnosed as infection if the diagnosis of bleomycin lung injury is not considered<br>Pneumothorax and pneumomediastinum are recognized complications in severe bleomycin lung injury |
| Pulmonary function studies | Decreased CO diffusing capacity<br>Restrictive ventilatory changes |

# MANAGEMENT

- Minimize peak airway pressure and judicious use of PEEP during mechanical ventilation
- Avoid oxygen therapy when possible and use least possible $FiO_2$
- Avoid clinical procedures (and leisure activities) involving a high $FiO_2$
- If a patient is hypoxic, $O_2$ therapy should be minimized to least possible $FiO_2$ to maintain $O_2$ saturation of 88–92%
- High oxygen concentrations should be used with extreme caution for immediate life-saving indications only (to maintain $O_2$ saturation of 88–92%)
- Minimize IV fluids to avoid volume overload and pulmonary edema

## SUGGESTED READING

- Allan N, Siller C, Breen A. Anaesthetic implications of chemotherapy. Continuing Education in Anaesthesia Critical Care & Pain. 2012;12(2):52-6.
- Brandt JP, Gerriets V. Bleomycin. [Updated 2022 Aug 29]. In: StatPearls [Internet]. Treasure Island (FL): StatPearls Publishing; 2022 Jan-. Available from: https://www.ncbi.nlm.nih.gov/books/NBK555895/
- Della Latta V, Cecchettini A, Del Ry S, Morales MA. Bleomycin in the setting of lung fibrosis induction: From biological mechanisms to counteractions. Pharmacological Research. 2015;97:122-30.
- Groenewold MD, Olthof CG, Bosch DJ. Anaesthesia after neoadjuvant chemotherapy, immunotherapy or radiotherapy. BJA Educ. 2022;22(1):12-19.

Bleomycin exposure

# CANNABIS USE

## LEARNING OBJECTIVES

- Describe the mechanisms and clinical effects of cannabis
- Manage patients who consumed cannabis preoperatively
- Manage patients who present with cannabis withdrawal syndrome postoperatively

## DEFINITION AND MECHANISM

- According to the United Nations, approximately 284 million individuals used cannabis in 2020
- This number is expected to grow as many countries are starting to legalize cannabis use
- The number of patients who use cannabis perioperatively will consequently rise

## MECHANISMS

Overview:
- Cannabinoids are divided into three categories:
- Endocannabinoids: naturally produced ligands of CB1 and CB2 receptors in our bodies
- Synthetic cannabinoids: recreational/illicit used (e.g. K2) and FDA-approved medicinal (e.g. nabilone) compounds
- Phytocannabinoids: plant-derived

There are more than 100 cannabinoid compounds
- Most potent of them are THC (most psychoactive) and CBD
- Tetrahydrocannabinol (THC) and cannabidiol (CBD) are the most studied cannabinoid constituents of cannabis
- THC is a cannabinoid receptor type 1 and type 2 partial agonist
- CBD is a negative allosteric modulator of the cannabinoid receptor
- Clinical effects of cannabis vary with the quantity and chronicity of its use

## CLINICAL EFFECTS

|  | Acute | Chronic |
|---|---|---|
| Cardiovascular | Tachycardia<br>Vasodilation<br>Orthostasis | Atheromatous disease |
| Pulmonary | Bronchodilation<br>Hyperreactivity<br>Airway edema | Chronic bronchitis<br>Emphysema |
| Central nervous system | Anxiolysis<br>Anxiety<br>Paranoia/psychosis<br>Euphoria<br>Dizziness<br>Headache<br>Memory dysfunction<br>Analgesia | Similar to acute effects but tolerance develops, requiring higher doses for similar effects |
| Gastrointestinal | Antinausea<br>Increased appetite<br>Abdominal pain | Hyperemesis |
| Endocrine | / | Gynecomastia<br>Anovulation<br>Galactorrhea |

## WITHDRAWAL SYNDROME

- Withdrawal symptoms can develop within a day of cessation for high-dose chronic users and may take weeks to resolve fully:

### Signs & symptoms

- Irritability/anger
- Anxiety/depressed mood
- Insomnia
- Altered dreams
- Anorexia
- Abdominal cramping
- Headaches
- Tremors
- Fevers/chills

### Onset

< 1 day for high-dose, chronic users

### Duration

Up to several weeks

### Treatment

Symptomatic therapy, synthetic THC

# CANNABIS USE: PREOPERATIVE MANAGEMENT

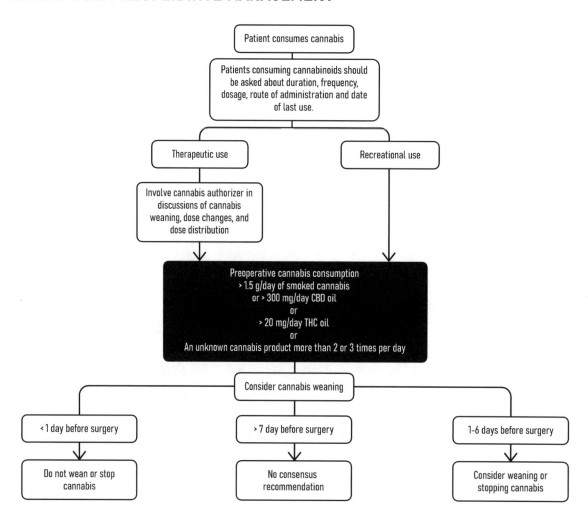

Patient consumes cannabis

Patients consuming cannabinoids should be asked about duration, frequency, dosage, route of administration and date of last use.

Therapeutic use

Recreational use

Involve cannabis authorizer in discussions of cannabis weaning, dose changes, and dose distribution

Preoperative cannabis consumption
> 1.5 g/day of smoked cannabis
or > 300 mg/day CBD oil
or
> 20 mg/day THC oil
or
An unknown cannabis product more than 2 or 3 times per day

Consider cannabis weaning

< 1 day before surgery

> 7 day before surgery

1-6 days before surgery

Do not wean or stop cannabis

No consensus recommendation

Consider weaning or stopping cannabis

# CANNABIS USE: INTRAOPERATIVE AND POSTOPERATIVE MANAGEMENT

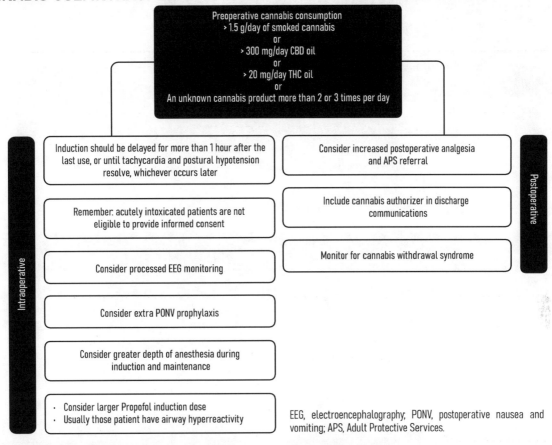

**Preoperative cannabis consumption**
> 1.5 g/day of smoked cannabis
or
> 300 mg/day CBD oil
or
> 20 mg/day THC oil
or
An unknown cannabis product more than 2 or 3 times per day

**Intraoperative**

- Induction should be delayed for more than 1 hour after the last use, or until tachycardia and postural hypotension resolve, whichever occurs later
- Remember: acutely intoxicated patients are not eligible to provide informed consent
- Consider processed EEG monitoring
- Consider extra PONV prophylaxis
- Consider greater depth of anesthesia during induction and maintenance
- · Consider larger Propofol induction dose
  · Usually those patient have airway hyperreactivity

**Postoperative**

- Consider increased postoperative analgesia and APS referral
- Include cannabis authorizer in discharge communications
- Monitor for cannabis withdrawal syndrome

EEG, electroencephalography; PONV, postoperative nausea and vomiting; APS, Adult Protective Services.

## CANNABIS WITHDRAWAL SYNDROME (CWS) MANAGEMENT

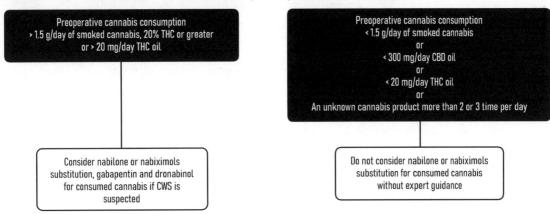

**Preoperative cannabis consumption**
> 1.5 g/day of smoked cannabis, 20% THC or greater
or > 20 mg/day THC oil

Consider nabilone or nabiximols substitution, gabapentin and dronabinol for consumed cannabis if CWS is suspected

**Preoperative cannabis consumption**
< 1.5 g/day of smoked cannabis
or
< 300 mg/day CBD oil
or
< 20 mg/day THC oil
or
An unknown cannabis product more than 2 or 3 time per day

Do not consider nabilone or nabiximols substitution for consumed cannabis without expert guidance

## ━━ SUGGESTED READING ━━

- Alexander JC, Joshi GP. A review of the anesthetic implications of marijuana use. Proc (Bayl Univ Med Cent). 2019;32(3):364-371. Published 2019 May 21.
- Ladha KS, McLaren-Blades A, Goel A, Buys MJ, Farquhar-Smith P, Haroutounian S, et al. Perioperative Pain and Addiction Interdisciplinary Network (PAIN): consensus recommendations for perioperative management of cannabis and cannabinoid-based medicine users by a modified Delphi process. British Journal of Anaesthesia. 2021;126(1):304-18.
- UNODC World Drug Report 2022 highlights trends on cannabis post-legalization, environmental impacts of illicit drugs, and drug use among women and Youth. United Nations: Office on Drugs and Crime. https://www.unodc.org/unodc/en/press/releases/2022/June/unodc-world-drug-report-2022-highlights-trends-on-cannabis-post-legalization-environmental-impacts-of-illicit-drugs-and-drug-use-among-women-and-youth.html. Published June 27, 2022. Accessed February 3, 2023.

**132**

# CORNEAL ABRASION

## LEARNING OBJECTIVES

- Describe the causes and risk factors for corneal abrasion
- Prevent corneal abrasion
- Manage corneal abrasion occurrence

## DEFINITION AND MECHANISM

- Corneal abrasion is the most common ophthalmologic complication in patients undergoing general anesthesia for nonocular surgery
- Can result in eye pain or soreness in response to bright light
- May develop into inflammation or ulcers by infection of bacteria or fungi on the scar
- Postoperative pain can be more severe than pain from the operative site

| Causes | |
|---|---|
| Mechanical injury | Direct contact with drapes, masks, or other equipment/items<br>Inadvertent pressure on the eyeball<br>Loss of pain perception and inhibition of protective corneal reflexes further increase risk |
| Chemical injury | Spillage of antimicrobial solutions into the eyes during skin preparation<br>Contact with cleaning solutions retained on the anesthetic mask<br>Ocular hypersensitivity to inhaled anesthetic agents (e.g., halothane)<br>Antiseptic solutions containing detergents or alcohol |
| Exposure keratopathy | Sedatives and neuromuscular blocking agents inhibit active contraction of the orbicularis oculi muscle, resulting in incomplete eyelid closure, corneal exposure, and dryness<br>Correlated with the duration of corneal exposure |
| Reduced tear production | General anesthesia suppresses the autonomic nerve supply to the lacrimal gland<br>Specific drugs (e.g., beta-blockers, hydrochlorothiazide) inhibit tear production<br>Ocular hypoperfusion secondary to deliberate hypotension<br>Anesthetic gases delivered via face mask add to corneal dehydration<br>General anesthesia inhibits the blink reflex and redistribution of tears over the ocular surface<br>Bell's phenomenon (upward rotation of the eyeball to protect the cornea during sleep) is absent during anesthesia |

## RISK FACTORS

- General anesthesia
- Lower ASA status
- History of dry eyes
- Advanced age
- Proptosis or exorbitism
- History of corneal trauma
- Longer procedures
- Preoperative anemia
- Prone, lateral or Trendelenburg position
- Procedures near head/neck
- Intraoperative hypotension
- Cardiovascular surgery

## SIGNS AND SYMPTOMS

- Blurry vision
- Tearing
- Redness
- Photophobia
- Foreign body sensation in the eye

## PREVENTION

- Eyelid taping and cushioned covering of the eyeballs immediately after induction (preferred method)
- Ocular lubricants (fat-based ointments are retained longer than aqueous solutions but pose a higher risk of complications)
- Hydrogel dressings
- Bio-occlusive dressings
- Continuous perioperative eye monitoring

## MANAGEMENT

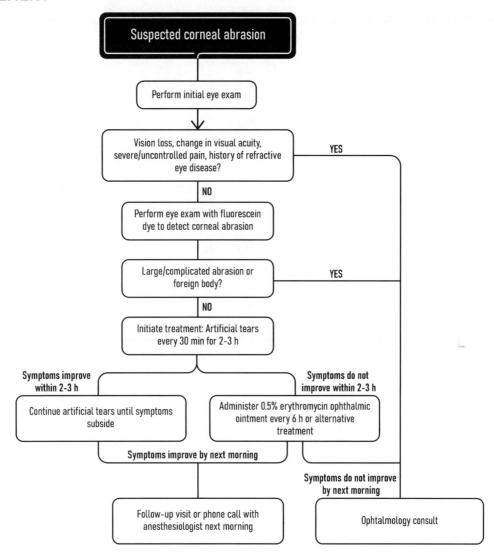

**SUGGESTED READING**

- Grixti A, Sadri M, Watts MT. Corneal protection during general anesthesia for nonocular surgery. Ocul Surf. 2013;11(2):109-118.
- Hewson DW, Hardman JG. Physical injuries during anaesthesia. BJA Educ. 2018;18(10):310-316.
- Lichter JR, Marr LB, Schilling DE, et al. A Department-of-Anesthesiology-based management protocol for perioperative corneal abrasions. Clin Ophthalmol. 2015;9:1689-1695. Published 2015 Sep 11
- Malafa MM, Coleman JE, Bowman RW, Rohrich RJ. Perioperative Corneal Abrasion: Updated Guidelines for Prevention and Management. Plast Reconstr Surg. 2016 May;137(5):790e-798e.

# EXTRAVASATION OF NMBDs

## LEARNING OBJECTIVES

- Risk factors and effects of extravasation of NMBDs
- Management of extravasation of NMBDs

## DEFINITION AND MECHANISM

- Neuromuscular blocking drugs (NMBDs) are widely used in anesthesia, including depolarizing (e.g., succinylcholine) and non-depolarizing (e.g., rocuronium, vecuronium, pancuronium, cisatracurium, atracurium) types
- NMBDs facilitate airway management, improve surgical conditions, and ensure immobility during critical points in an operation
- NMBDs are typically given intravenously, but accidental extravasation can occur if the IV catheter is mispositioned
- Up to 39% of cannulas become dislocated after 72h
- Depending on the drug, leakage into surrounding tissue can cause local irritation or tissue necrosis
- The injected drug may be absorbed into the circulation and cause systemic effect
- When to suspect
- Sudden increase in infusion pressure
- Lack of iv drug effect (infusion and boluses)
- Sudden increasing pain at site of extravasation in awake patients

## RISK FACTORS

- Small or fragile veins
- Advanced age
- Obesity
- Multiple venipunctures
- High injection pressure
- Poor cannula fixation
- Disseminated skin diseases
- Patient movement during cannula placement
- Thrombophlebitis
- Neonates
- Impaired neurocognition or communication

## KEEP IN MIND

- The adductor pollicis muscle is optimal for quantitative neuromuscular monitoring

## MANAGEMENT

> **Key challenges**
> - No established guidelines for managment of extravasation of NMBDs
> - Extravasation results in unpredictable neuromusucular blocks whit slower onset and prologed duration

```
Suspected extravasation of NMBDs
          ↓
Do not remove the old line and do not
           flush the line
          ↓
Secure new IV cannula
          ↓
Monitor TOF count/ratio  ←──────┐
          ↓                      │ NO
Stable or increaseing? ─────────┘
          ↓ YES
TOF ratio > 0.9?
   YES ↓        ↓ NO
Extubation    Reversal or maintain sedation until
              spontaneuos recovery
   ↓
Monitor in PACU ( 4-5h)
```

- Monitor for signs of compartment with large extravasation
- If necrosis, ulceration or compartment syndrome occur consult surgery immediately
- Consider washout procedure
- Cold compress the area to limit drug distribution into the circulation
- Caution if the extravasate contained mixed drug infusion, especially vasoactive drugs
- Limb elevation

NMBDs, neuromuscular blocking drugs; TOF, train-of-four; PACU, post-anesthesia care unit.

## SUGGESTED READING

- Nietvelt F, Van Herreweghe I, Godschalx V, Soetens F. Extravascular injection of neuromuscular blocking drugs: A systematic review of current evidence and management. European Journal of Anaesthesiology | EJA. 2024;41(5)
- Thilen SR, Weigel WA, Todd MM, et al. 2023 American Society of Anesthesiologists Practice Guidelines for Monitoring and Antagonism of Neuromuscular Blockade: A Report by the American Society of Anesthesiologists Task Force on Neuromuscular Blockade. Anesthesiology. 2023;138(1):13-41.

# FLUID AND ELECTROLYTE BALANCE

## LEARNING OBJECTIVES

- Describe the fluid compartments and the distribution of fluid and electrolytes
- Manage the fluid and electrolyte balance in surgical patients

## DEFINITION AND MECHANISM

- Body water content varies with age and gender
- Approximately two-thirds of total body water (TBW) is intracellular fluid (ICF) and one-third is extracellular fluid (ECF)
- ECF is further divided into interstitial fluid (ISF) and plasma

|  | TBW (% body weight) | ICF (% body weight) | ECF (% body weight) |
|---|---|---|---|
| Neonate | 75% | 40% | 35% |
| Infant | 70% | 40% | 30% |
| Adult male | 60% | 40% | 20% |
| Adult female | 55% | 35% | 20% |
| Elderly female | 45% | 30% | 15% |

## TBW AND ELECTROLYTE DISTRIBUTION

- Example of TBW and electrolyte distribution in a healthy 70-kg man:

|  | ICF | Interstitial fluid | Plasma |
|---|---|---|---|
| Water (L) | 28 | 11 | 3 |
| $Na^+$ (mmol/L) | 10 | 140 | 140 |
| $K^+$ (mmol/L) | 150 | 4 | 4 |
| $Ca^{2+}$ (mmol/L) | / | 2.5 | 2.5 |
| $Mg^{2+}$ (mmol/L) | 26 | 1.5 | 1.5 |
| $Cl^-$ | / | 114 | 114 |
| $HCO_3^-$ | 10 | 25 | 25 |
| $HPO_4^{2-}$ | 38 | 1 | 1 |
| $SO_4^{2-}$ | / | 0.5 | 0.5 |
| $Prot^-$ | 74 | 2 | 16 |

# REDISTRIBUTION OF INFUSED FLUIDS

- The redistribution of infused fluids depends on their composition relative to that of each compartment:

| | ICF (%) | Interstitial fluid (%) | Plasma (%) |
|---|---|---|---|
| Saline (0.9%) | 0 | 79 | 21 |
| Dextrose (5%) | 67 | 26 | 7 |

# HOMEOSTASIS MAINTENANCE

- Homeostasis maintenance requirements for surgical patients:
  - Water: 25-30 mL/kg/day for adults (use ideal body weight for obese patients)
  - Sodium: 1 mmol/kg/day, can be administered by:
    - 2500 mL of 4% dextrose/0.18% saline over 24 hours
    - 2000 mL of 5% dextrose and 500 mL of 0.9% saline over 24 hours
- Potassium: 1 mmol/kg/day

# MANAGEMENT

### PERIOPERATIVE FLUID MANAGEMENT: PREOPERATIVE ASSESSMENT

- Fluid status depends on the surgical indication, history of the patient and whether the surgery is elective or urgent
- Determine fluid and electrolyte balance by repeated clinical assessment throughout the perioperative period
- Include an estimate of total balance and intravascular volume

**Total balance**

- Note the duration of preoperative fasting
- Review the patient's ability to maintain fluid balance during illness
- Consider normal variations in fluid balance at extremes of age
- Identify increased losses (pyrexia, diarrhea, vomiting, hemorrhage)
- Acute abdomen may result in large volumes of fluid sequestered in the abdominal compartment
- Monitor body weight
- Review charts to identify urine output and losses via nasogastric tubes
- Analyze fluid prescription charts to identify the volume and type of fluid administered
- Blood tests for additional information (urea, creatinine, hematocrit, plasma levels of sodium and potassium)

**Intravascular volume**

- Arterial catheters (arterial pressure and pulse pressure variation)
- Transesophageal Doppler (stroke volume, flow time corrected)
- Devices utilizing pulse contour analysis to derive hemodynamic parameters (stroke volume, flow time corrected)
- Echocardiography (e.g., inferior vena cava diameter and collapsibility, left ventricular end-diastolic area)
- Pulmonary artery catheters (cardiac output, central and pulmonary capillary wedge pressures)
- Central venous pressure does not correlate with volume status

Fluid and electrolyte balance

# PERIOPERATIVE FLUID THERAPY

- Patients should commence surgery with a normal and stable fluid and electrolyte balance
- Healthy patients presenting for minor elective surgery generally do not need perioperative fluid replacement unless unable to drink normally in the early postoperative period

### Prevention and replacement of preoperative deficits

- Encourage patient to maintain their oral intake of clear fluids until 2 hours prior to induction of anesthesia
- Correct a deficit in maintenance with the equivalent of 1.25 mL/kg/h of balanced crystalloid in proportion to the oral intake of the patient
- Emergency patients may have a significantly reduced intake over several days, this can be exacerbated by repeated periods of fasting while awaiting surgery
- Possible abnormal losses and redistribution: Bowel preparation, sequestration, vomiting and diarrhea, enterocutaneous fistula, stoma, wounds, hemorrhage
- Significant hypovolemia may occur with inflammatory conditions (e.g., sepsis, peritonitis, pancreatitis)
- Replacement is based on an estimate of the composition and volume of loss (losses from the gut are particularly important)
- Monitor serum biochemistry
- Severe hypovolemia with signs of shock: Give isotonic crystalloid 10 mL/kg as bolus, the reassess and give additional fluid acording to the response

### Blood loss

- Blood transfusion to maintain hemoglobin level
- Guided by clinical assessment of the patient, the pattern of bleeding and measures of hemoglobin and hematocrit

### Intraoperative management

- Goal: Maintain ideal tissue perfusion while avoiding fluid compartments getting overloaded
- Maintenance fluid: Balanced crystalloid or dextrose (4%) with saline (0.18%) at 1.25 mL/kg/h
- Administer additional fluids based on continuous clinical assessment and the physiological goals of the patient
- Monitor heart rate, tissue perfusion, and urine output (not less than 0.5 mL/kg/h)
- Goal-directed hemodynamic therapy can be beneficial in high-risk patients: Vascular filling guided by measures of stroke volume and cardiac output, continuous flow measurement. Boluses (250 mL) of crystalloid or colloid to maximize stroke volume early and maintain optimal tissue perfusion. Maintain oxygen delivery above baseline

### Postoperative requirements

- Potassium is not required for the first 24-48 h in most patients
- Avoid IV fluids if possible
- Tailor postoperative fluids to the specific patient
- Starting point: 25-30 mL/kg/day of 4% dextrose with 0.18% saline, estimate and replace other fluid and electrolyte losses

## SUGGESTED READING

- Pollard BJ, Kitchen, G. Handbook of Clinical Anaesthesia. Fourth Edition. CRC Press. 2018. 978-1-4987-6289-2.
- Rassam SS, Counsell DJ. Perioperative electrolyte and fluid balance. Continuing Education in Anaesthesia Critical Care & Pain. 2005;5(5):157-60.

# GASTROESOPHAGEAL REFLUX DISEASE

## LEARNING OBJECTIVES

- Define gastrointestinal reflux disease
- Describe the signs and symptoms of gastrointestinal reflux disease
- Anesthetic management of a patient with gastrointestinal reflux disease

## DEFINITION AND MECHANISM

- Gastroesophageal reflux disease (GERD) occurs when gastric content repeatedly and regularly flows back into the distal esophagus, this regurgitation (acid reflux) can irritate the lining of the esophagus
- Caused by frequent acid reflux or reflux of nonacidic content from the stomach due to inadequate closure of the lower esophageal sphincter (LES)

## SIGNS AND SYMPTOMS

Classic symptoms
- Heartburn (burning sensation in the chest), especially after eating, might be worse at night or while lying down
- Regurgitation (acid reflux)
- Taste of acid
- Upper abdominal or non-cardiac chest pain
- Globus
- Swallowing difficulties (dysphagia) and painful swallowing (odynophagia)
- Bad breath
- Bloating and belching

Extraesophageal symptoms
- Chronic cough
- Sore throat
- Dental corrosion
- Sinusitis
- Bronchitis
- Pulmonary fibrosis
- Recurrent aspiration pneumonia
- Hoarseness
- Hiccups
- Laryngitis
- Hypersalivation (water brash)
- New or worsening asthma

## COMPLICATIONS

- Reflux esophagitis: Inflammation of the esophageal epithelium which can cause ulcer formation
- Esophageal stricture: Persistent narrowing of the esophagus caused by reflux-induced inflammation
- Barrett's esophagus (precancerous changes to the esophagus): Intestinal metaplasia (changes of the epithelial cells from squamous to intestinal columnar epithelium) of the distal esophagus
- Esophageal carcinoma

# RISK FACTORS

- Obesity
- Hiatal or diaphragmatic hernia
- Pregnancy
- Connective tissue disorders (e.g., scleroderma)
- Delayed stomach emptying
- Family history of GERD

Factors that exacerbate acid reflux:
- Smoking
- Eating large meals or eating late at night
- Eating certain foods (e.g., fatty or fried foods)
- Drinking certain beverages (e.g., alcohol, coffee)
- Taking certain medications (e.g., aspirin, benzodiazepines, calcium channel blockers, tricyclic antidepressants, NSAIDs, and certain asthma medicines)

# TREATMENT

- Lifestyle changes
  - Avoid chocolate, mint, high-fat food, coffee, and alcohol
  - Weight loss in overweight and obese patients
  - Avoid bedtime snacks or lying down immediately after meals
  - Avoid smoking
- Medications: Antacids, H2 receptor blockers, proton pump inhibitors (PPIs), prokinetics
- Surgery: Nissen fundoplication (the gastric fundus (upper part) of the stomach is wrapped around the lower end of the esophagus and stitched in place, reinforcing the closing function of the LES)

# MANAGEMENT

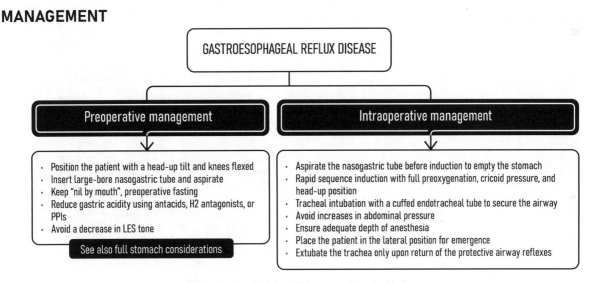

PPI, proton pump inhibitor; LES, lower esophageal sphincter.

# KEEP IN MIND

- Patients with GERD are at an increased risk of pulmonary aspiration during anesthesia
- Factors that increase the risk of aspiration include the urgency of surgery, airway problems, inadequate depth of anesthesia, use of the lithotomy position, gastrointestinal problems, depressed consciousness, increased severity of illness, and obesity
- The main anesthetic goal in patients with GERD is to minimize regurgitation and aspiration of gastric contents
- Avoid drugs that decrease LES tone (e.g., opioids, anticholinergics, tricyclics, dopamine, and beta-agonists)

## SUGGESTED READING

- Fass, R., Boeckxstaens, G.E., El-Serag, H. et al. Gastro-oesophageal reflux disease. Nat Rev Dis Primers 7, 55 (2021).
- Jolliffe DM. Practical gastric physiology. Continuing Education in Anaesthesia Critical Care & Pain. 2009;9(6):173-177.
- Maret-Ouda J, Markar SR, Lagergren J. Gastroesophageal Reflux Disease: A Review. JAMA. 2020;324(24):2536-2547.

# GERIATRIC PATIENTS

## LEARNING OBJECTIVES

- Describe the physiological changes associated with aging
- Manage geriatric patients presenting for surgery

## DEFINITION AND MECHANISM

- Geriatric patients often present with conditions requiring surgery
- Age increases perioperative risks associated with anesthesia
- Geriatric patients have a greater risk of perioperative morbidity and mortality

## PHYSIOLOGICAL CHANGES ASSOCIATED WITH AGING

**Cardiovascular**
- Limited tachycardic response to hypotension: Preload dependent
- Less sensitive baroreceptor reflexes: Limited response to decreased cardiac contractility and hypovolemia
- Rigid arteries: Increased systemic vascular resistance and decreased compliance, wider pulse pressure and labile blood pressures
- Higher prevalence of coronary artery disease, left ventricular hypertrophy, aortic valve calcification, arrhythmias (most commonly atrial fibrillation)
- Commonly reliant on pacemakers or implanted defibrillators
- Chronic anticoagulant use is common

**Neurologic**
- Lower anesthetic doses required for both volatile and IV anesthetics
- Increased prevalence of memory loss, cognitive decline, delirium, depression, dementia
- Increased risk of postoperative delirium and cognitive decline

**Pulmonary**
- Decreased inspiratory capacity
- Ventilation-perfusion mismatch
- Decreased functional residual capacity, increased closing capacity: earlier closure of small airways, diffuse atelectasis, shunting
- Limited central responses to hypoxia and hypercarbia
- Weaker pharyngeal muscles and less effective upper airway reflexes and coughing
- Commonly colonized with gram-negative bacteria

**Renal**
- Decreased glomerular filtration rate
- Increased risk of acute kidney injury secondary to nephrotoxic agents

**Endocrine & metabolism**
- Malnutrition is common
- Decreased heat production, insulation and thermoregulation
- Type 2 diabetes mellitus is common

## COMMON SURGERIES IN THE ELDERLY

- Cataract surgery
- Trans-urethral resection of the prostate
- Hip fracture surgery
- Knee arthroplasty
- Cholecystectomy
- Pacemaker implantation
- Colorectal excision
- Breast excision

# MANAGEMENT

**Preoperative assessment**
- Screen for cognitive impairment using a brief cognitive screening tool (e.g., Minicog, Mini-Mental State Examination)
- Assess capacity for medical decision-making
- Assess frailty
- Routine blood tests
- Additional tests based on comorbidities

**Induction agents**
- Lower dose and slower administration

**Inhalational agents**
- Reduce minimum alveolar concentration by 20-40%
- Use sevoflurane in favor of desflurane
- More easily lost airway can cause problems

**Neuromuscular blocking**
- Time of onset and duration of action are prolonged
- Reduce the dose
- Agents that do not rely on hepatic metabolism and clearance are safer

**Cardiovascular**
- Increased incidence of hypotension on induction
- Administer vasopressors (ephedrine, metaraminol, phenylephrine)
- Administer fluids (limit to 8 mL/kg)

**Respiratory**
- Leave false teeth in situ to prevent difficult airway maintenance
- Be vigilant of airway obstruction

**Fluid management**
- Urinary catheter for monitoring of fluid status
- Avoid hypovolemia and overhydration

**Temperature**
- Maintain normothermia using reflective drapes, warmed IV fluids, warm air systems or warming mattresses

**Practical considerations**
- Carefully protect pressure points
- Avoid excessive joint manipulation
- Venous access may be difficult or easily lost
- Adhesive tapes will damage fragile skin

## SUGGESTED READING

- Staheli B, Rondeau B. Anesthetic Considerations In The Geriatric Population. [Updated 2022 Jun 5]. In: StatPearls [Internet]. Treasure Island (FL): StatPearls Publishing; 2022 Jan-. Available from: https://www.ncbi.nlm.nih.gov/books/NBK572137/
- Murray D, Dodds C. Perioperative care of the elderly. Continuing Education in Anaesthesia Critical Care & Pain. 2004;4(6):193-6.

# INFLAMMATORY BOWEL DISEASE

## LEARNING OBJECTIVES

- Define inflammatory bowel disease
- Describe the differences between Crohn's disease and ulcerative colitis
- Anesthetic management of patients with inflammatory bowel disease

## DEFINITION AND MECHANISM

- Inflammatory bowel disease (IBD) is a term for two conditions (Crohn's disease and ulcerative colitis) that are characterized by chronic inflammation of the gastrointestinal (GI) tract
- Prolonged inflammation results in damage to the GI tract
- Caused by an interaction of environmental and genetic factors leading to immune responses and inflammation in the intestine → autoimmune disease

| IBD | Crohn's disease | Ulcerative colitis |
|---|---|---|
| Affected location | Can affect any part of the GI tract (from mouth to anus), most often affects the portion of the small intestine before the large intestine (i.e., ileocecal region) | Restricted to the large intestine (colon) and rectum |
| Damaged areas | Damaged areas appear in patches that are next to areas of healthy tissue | Damaged areas are continuous (not patchy), usually starting at the rectum and spreading further into the colon |
| Inflammation | Inflammation may reach through the multiple layers of the walls of the GI tract → transmural inflammation leading to abscesses or granulomatous disease | Inflammation is present only in the innermost layer of the lining of the colon (i.e., mucosa) → loss of colonic mucosa |

## SIGNS AND SYMPTOMS

- Persistent diarrhea
- Fatigue
- Abdominal pain and cramping

- Rectal bleeding, bloody stools
- Reduced appetite
- Unintended weight loss

## COMPLICATIONS

**Both conditions**
- Anemia (due to prolonged GI bleeding, often iron and/or vitamin B12 deficiency)
- Colorectal cancer
- Skin, eye, and joint inflammation (e.g., iritis/uveitis, ankylosing spondylitis)
- Medication side effects (e.g., infections, corticosteroids are associated with a risk of osteoporosis and hypertension)
- Primary sclerosing cholangitis
- Blood clots (i.e., venous thromboembolism [VTE])
- Severe dehydration

**Crohn's disease**
- Bowel obstruction
- Malnutrition
- (Perianal) fistulas, may form an abscess
- Anal fissure

**Ulcerative colitis**
- Toxic megacolon
- Perforated colon

## RISK FACTORS

- Age
  - Most patients are diagnosed before 30 years of age
  - Some patients do not develop the disease until their 50-60s
- White ethnicity

- Family history
- Smoking
- NSAIDs (e.g., ibuprofen, naproxen sodium, diclofenac sodium)

## DIAGNOSIS

Combination of endoscopy (for Crohn's disease) or colonoscopy (for ulcerative colitis) and imaging studies
- Contrast radiography
- MRI
- CT
- Stool samples
- Blood tests

## TREATMENT

- Antidiarrheal medications (i.e., psyllium powder, methylcellulose, loperamide)
- Anti-inflammatory drugs (i.e., glucocorticoids, 5-aminosalicylic acids)
- Immunosuppressants (i.e., cyclosporine, azathioprine, mercaptopurine, methotrexate)
- Antibiotics (i.e., ciprofloxacin, metronidazole)
- Biologics (i.e., TNF-α inhibitor infliximab)
- Nutritional support
- Surgery to remove damaged parts of the GI tract

## MANAGEMENT

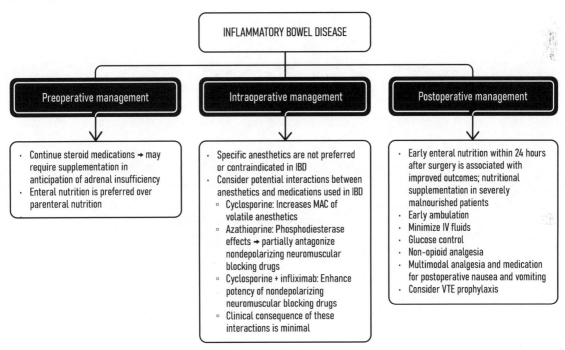

MAC, mean alveolar concentration; VTE, venous thromboembolism.

*IBD medication management during the perioperative period*

| Drug | Recommendation |
|---|---|
| Glucocorticoids | Continue; administer stress dose (see next table) |
| 5-aminosalicylic acid | Discontinue on day of surgery and resume 3 days after surgery if normal renal function |
| Azathioprine, 6-mercaptopurine | Discontinue on day of surgery and resume 3 days after surgery if normal renal function |
| Methotrexate | Continue unless previous poor wound healing or postoperative infections |
| Cyclosporine | Continue but carefully monitor for infectious complications |
| Infliximab | Continue without interruption |

*Glucocorticoid management during the perioperative period*

| Axis suppression | Minor surgical stress | Moderate surgical stress | Major surgical stress |
|---|---|---|---|
| **No:** Prednisone < 5 mg/d Glucocorticoids < 3 weeks Negative corticotropin test | Daily dose No supplementation | Daily dose No supplementation | Daily dose No supplementation |
| **Documented or suspected:** Prednisone > 10 mg/d for > 3 weeks Positive corticotropin test | Daily dose No supplementation | Hydrocortisone 50 mg IV (induction) 25 mg IV every 8 hours for 24-48 hours | Hydrocortisone 100 mg IV (induction) 50 mg IV every 8 hours for 24 hours 25 mg IV every 8 hours from 24-48 hours |
| **Unknown:** Prednisone 5-10 mg ≥ 3 weeks | Daily dose No supplementation | Positive corticotropin test: Hydrocortisone 50 mg IV (induction) 25 mg IV every 8 hours for 24-48 hours | Hydrocortisone 100 mg IV (induction) 50 mg IV every 8 hours for 24 hours 25 mg IV every 8 hours from 24-48 hours |

See also perioperative steroids considerations

**SUGGESTED READING**

- Nickerson TP, Merchea A. Perioperative Considerations in Crohn Disease and Ulcerative Colitis. Clin Colon Rectal Surg. 2016;29(2):80-84.
- Kumar A, Auron M, Aneja A, Mohr F, Jain A, Shen B. Inflammatory bowel disease: perioperative pharmacological considerations. Mayo Clin Proc. 2011;86(8):748-757.

# 138

# LAPAROSCOPIC SURGERY

## LEARNING OBJECTIVES

- Anesthetic management of laparoscopic surgery

---

## DEFINITION AND MECHANISM

- A minimally invasive surgical technique to explore the abdominal and pelvic cavities
- 2–4 small incisions (usually 0.5–1.5 cm) are made to insert surgical instruments and a laparoscope with a camera at the end
- The laparoscope aids in diagnosis or therapeutic interventions

## RISKS AND BENEFITS OF LAPAROSCOPIC SURGERY

| Benefits | Risks |
|---|---|
| Reduced wound infection | Visceral and vascular damage |
| Faster recovery | Complications associated with extremes of positioning |
| Reduced morbidity | Acute kidney injury (AKI) |
| Reduced pain | Cardiocerebral vascular insufficiency |
| Cosmetic benefits | Pulmonary atelectasis |
| | Venous air embolism (VAE) |
| | Well leg compartment syndrome |
| | Pneumoperitoneum challenges |

## LIST OF SURGERIES PERFORMED LAPAROSCOPICALLY

- Cyst, fibroid, stone, and polyp removals
- Small tumor removals
- Biopsies
- Tubal ligation and reversal
- Ectopic pregnancy removal
- Endometriosis surgery
- Urethral and vaginal reconstruction surgery
- Orchiopexy (testicle correction surgery)
- Rectopexy (rectal prolapse repair)
- Hernia repair surgery
- Esophageal anti-reflux surgery (fundoplication)
- Gastric bypass surgery
- Cholecystectomy (gallbladder removal) for gallstones
- Appendectomy (appendix removal) for appendicitis
- Colectomy (bowel resection surgery)
- Abdominoperineal resection (rectum removal)
- Cystectomy (bladder removal)
- Prostatectomy (prostate removal)
- Adrenalectomy (adrenal gland removal)
- Nephrectomy (kidney removal)
- Splenectomy (spleen removal)
- Radical nephroureterectomy (for transitional cell cancer)
- Whipple procedure (pancreaticoduodenectomy) for pancreatic cancer
- Gastrectomy (stomach removal)
- Liver resection
- Hysterectomy

## COMPLICATIONS

- Occult hemorrhage – may not be visible due to small surgical field
- Vascular or solid organ injury
- Gas embolism
- Subcutaneous emphysema
- Capnothorax: suspect of unexplained increase in airway pressure, hypoxemia, & hypercapnia
- Capnomediastinum & capnopericardium
- Complications related to positioning

# MANAGEMENT

Perioperative management of laparoscopic surgery

**General**
- Goal: IAP ≤ 15 mmHg
- IV access: at least one catheter
- Fluid management: balanced crystalloid solution 3-5 mL/kg/hour

**Monitoring**
- Capnography
- Pulse oximetry
- Peak and plateau airway pressures
- Delivered tidal volumes
- Dynamic flow-volume loops
- Blood pressure
- ECG
- Temperature
- Consider arterial monitoring

**Airway**
- Minimize bag and mask ventilation before intubation to avoid gastric distention
- Place a cuffed oral tracheal tube
- Maintain $ETCO_2$ around 35 mmHg
- Adminster neuromuscular relaxation
- Apply positive pressure ventilation to protect against gastric acid aspiration and allow optimal control of $CO_2$
- Insert a nasogastric tube to deflate the stomach

**Analgesia**
- Administer opioid analgesia
- Consider opiate-sparing techniques such as subdural, epidural, or TAP block
- Consider wound infiltration with local anesthetic
- Intraperitoneal levobupivacaine reduces postoperative pain and opiate requirements

**Ventilation**
- Maintain lung-protective ventilation
- If this ventilation is unavailable:
  - $FiO_2$: 0.5
  - Tidal volumes: 6-8 mL/kg/body weight
  - PEEP: 5-10 $cmH_2O$ use PEEP with caution as it can reduce the cardiac ouput especially in the presene of pneumoperitoneum
  - Respiratory rate: 8 breaths/min (consider higher respiratory rate (12 to 15), to achieve the $EtCO_2$ goal with less tidal volumes, = less airway pressure)
- Pressure-controlled ventilation is probably better than volume-controlled ventilation in the morbidly obese patient during laparoscopy
  - $ETCO_2$: 35-40 mmHg
  - $SaO_2$ > 90%

**Anesthesia**
The ideal anesthetic maintains:
- Stable cardiovascular and respiratory functions
- Provides rapid postoperative recovery
- Leads to minimal postoperative nausea and vomiting
- Provides good postoperative pain relief for early mobility
- GA with controlled ventilation is the most acceptable technique:
  - Propofol
  - Etomidate
  - Sevoflurane or desflurane
  - Remifentanil
  - Rocuronium, reversal at the end of the surgery with sugmmadex

**Postoperative pain management**
- Administer supplemental oxygen
- Acetaminophen
- NSAIDs
- COX2-specific inhibitors
- Dexamethasone Infiltration of incision with LA at the time of wound closure
- Weak opioids (tramadol) or strong opioids (hydrocodone or oxycodone)
- Abdominal wall blocks (e.g.: TAP block)

**Antiemetics**
- Dexamethasone 4-8 mg IV after induction
- Ondansetron: 4 mg at the end of the procedure
- Deflate the stomach
- Avoid known emetogenic agents (opiates)

IAP, intra-abdominal pressure.

## SUGGESTED READING

- Bajwa SJ, Kulshrestha A. Anaesthesia for laparoscopic surgery: General vs regional anesthesia. J Minim Access Surg. 2016;12(1):4-9.
- Hayden P, Sarah Cowman S. Continuing Education in Anaesthesia Critical Care & Pain, Volume 11, Issue 5, October 2011, Pages 177-180.
- Jo YY, Kwak HJ. What is the proper ventilation strategy during laparoscopic surgery?. Korean J Anesthesiol. 2017;70(6):596-600.

Laparoscopic surgery

# METHEMOGLOBINEMIA

**139**

## LEARNING OBJECTIVES

- Describe the definition and underlying mechanisms of methemoglobinemia
- Diagnose methemoglobinemia
- Manage patients with methemoglobinemia

## DEFINITION AND MECHANISM

- Methemoglobin is the form of the hemoglobin molecule where the iron moiety is oxidized ($Fe3^+$)
- It is formed in the presence of an oxidizing substrate and does not carry oxygen
- It shifts the oxygen-hemoglobin dissociation curve to the left, hindering the unloading of oxygen to the tissues
- These effects are proportional to the concentration of methemoglobin and reversible
- Normal methemoglobin levels: 1-2 %
- Methemoglobinemia refers to an abnormally high concentration of methemoglobin and results in functional anemia
- Methemoglobinemia can be a life-threatening condition

## ETIOLOGY

- Congenital (rare)
  - Autosomal recessive defects in cytochrome b5 reductase (CYB5R)
    - Congenital methemoglobinemia type I: CYB5R defect only in erythrocytes
    - Congenital methemoglobinemia type II: CYB5R defect in all cells
  - Autosomal dominant mutations in hemoglobin M (hemoglobin M disease)
- Acquired
  - Exposure to oxidizing agents leading to methemoglobin production that exceeds the body's reduction capacity
  - Oxidizing agents:
    - Direct
      - Benzocaine
      - Prilocaine
      - Lidocaine
      - Tetracaine
    - Indirect
      - Nitrates, nitrites
    - Metabolic activation
      - Aniline
      - Dapsone

## PATHOPHYSIOLOGY

- Reduction of methemoglobin by cytochrome b5 reductase:

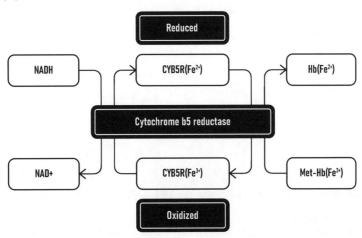

- Hemoglobin M disease:
  - Mutation in globin protein allows for stabilization of iron in the ferric state ($Fe^{3+}$)
  - Most patients have methemoglobin levels between 15-30% and remain asymptomatic
- Congenital methemoglobinemia: Defect in CYB5R function raising methemoglobin levels
- Acquired methemoglobinemia: CYB5R is overwhelmed by oxidative stress resulting in raised methemoglobin levels

## DIAGNOSIS

- Pulse oximetry measurements of oxygen saturation ($SpO_2$): Refractory hypoxemia
- Refractory hypoxemia is usually not detected using blood gas analysis using the partial oxygen pressure ($SaO_2$)
- Saturation gap: Difference between depressed $SpO_2$ measurement and falsely normal $SaO_2$ calculation
- A saturation gap > 5% indicates the presence of abnormal forms of hemoglobin

## MANAGEMENT

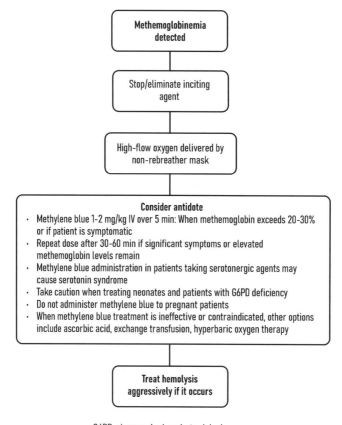

G6PD, glucose-6-phosphate dehydrogenase.

## SUGGESTED READING

- Guay J. Methemoglobinemia related to local anesthetics: a summary of 242 episodes. Anesth Analg. 2009;108(3):837-845.
- Ludlow JT, Wilkerson RG, Nappe TM. Methemoglobinemia. [Updated 2022 Aug 29]. In: StatPearls [Internet]. Treasure Island (FL): StatPearls Publishing; 2022 Jan-. Available from: https://www.ncbi.nlm.nih.gov/books/NBK537317/

# NON-OPERATING ROOM ANESTHESIA (NORA)

## LEARNING OBJECTIVES

- Consider the limitations and challenges of non-operating room anesthesia
- Describe the anesthetic considerations for specific non-operating room anesthesia procedures

## DEFINITION AND MECHANISM

- Non-operating room anesthesia (NORA) refers to all anesthetic procedures performed outside of the operating room
- NORA is a growing field in healthcare
- Unfamiliarity with the environment can be a challenge

## CONSIDERATIONS

- Limitations of the room
- Equipment may be lacking
- Unfamiliar environment
- Staff may be unfamiliar with anesthetic procedures
- Exposure to radiation

- NORA sites have a greater proportion of ASA status III-V patients
- Anesthetic procedures, monitoring, and analgesia should be held to the same standards as in the operating room
- Potential for ad hoc requests, scheduling inconsistencies, poor communication, and less patience

## COMMON NORA PROCEDURES

### ENDOSCOPY

- E.g., esophagogastroduodenoscopy, endoscopic retrograde cholangiopancreatography
- Presence of the endoscope and its placement can cause external compression and lead to upper airway obstruction
- May require patient to be in the prone/semi-prone position
- Topical lidocaine or benzocaine can be applied to the pharynx
- Propofol and midazolam are commonly used

### INTERVENTIONAL RADIOLOGY

- Mostly performed under general anesthesia
- Many procedures can be done under light to moderate sedation and peripheral nerve blocks
- E.g., phrenic nerve block for CT-guided pulmonary biopsies, paravertebral block for biliary drainage

### INTERVENTIONAL CARDIOLOGY

- E.g., percutaneous coronary intervention, percutaneous transcatheter aortic valve replacement, transcatheter mitral valve repair
- Monitor for hemodynamic changes
- Have external defibrillator pads readily available
- Sedation can reduce length of stay compared to general anesthesia

### INTERVENTIONAL PULMONOLOGY

- E.g., endobronchial ultrasound, transbronchial needle aspiration, balloon bronchoplasty, airway stents, bronchoalveolar lavages
- Assess for risk factors for unstable cervical spine
- Topical and/or nebulized lidocaine
- Sedation or general anesthesia may be required depending on the procedure

### MAGNETIC RESONANCE IMAGING

- Use MRI compatible pumps or extension tubing to run infusions from outside the MRI zone
- When an emergency takes place, remove patient from MRI zone to zone 3
- Typically minimal sedation
- Sedation or general anesthesia in patients who are claustrophobic, phonophobic, or unable to remain motionless
- When general anesthesia is required, perform induction and airway management outside of the MRI zone

### IVF

- Retrieval of oocytes can be performed under paracervical, epidural, spinal, and general anesthesia, as well as IV sedation

## SUGGESTED READING

- Chung M, Vazquez R. Non-Operating Room Anesthesia. In: Gropper MA, editor. Miller's Anesthesia, Ninth Edition, 2020. Elsevier, Philadelphia. p. 2284-2312.
- Wong T, Georgiadis PL, Urman RD, Tsai MH. Non-Operating Room Anesthesia: Patient Selection and Special Considerations. Local Reg Anesth. 2020;13:1-9. Published 2020 Jan 8. doi:10.2147/LRA.S181458

# PERIOPERATIVE HYPOTHERMIA

## LEARNING OBJECTIVES

- Describe the causes, risk factors, and consequences of perioperative hypothermia
- Prevent and manage perioperative hypothermia

## DEFINITION AND MECHANISM

- Perioperative hypothermia is defined as a core body temperature < 36.0°C
- Common consequence of anesthesia
- Inability of the body to respond effectively to the multiple causes of heat loss during surgery and anesthesia

## CAUSES

3 phases:

1. Redistribution: Vasodilatation leads to warm blood reaching the peripheries and cool blood from the peripheries entering the core circulation, causing a rapid decline in temperature
2. Heat loss exceeds heat produced from metabolism as the metabolic rate is reduced by 15-40% during general anesthesia, causing a linear decline in temperature
   Sources of heat loss:
   - Radiation
   - Convection
   - Evaporation
   - Conduction
3. Plateau phase: Heat loss is balanced by heat produced metabolically, mostly due to maximal vasoconstriction

## RISK FACTORS

- ASA grade 2-5 (higher grade, greater risk)
- Preoperative temperature < 36.0°C
- Combined general and regional anesthesia
- Major or intermediate surgery
- At risk of cardiovascular complications
- Low BMI
- Diabetic neuropathy
- Paraplegia
- Severe hypothyroidism

## CONSEQUENCES

- Increased risk of surgical site infection
- Decrease in drug metabolism
- Increased bleeding and transfusion requirements
- Increased risk of cardiac events
- Shivering
- Delayed discharge from the post-anesthesia care unit

# MANAGEMENT

```
              INTRAOPERATIVE HYPOTHERMIA
                PREVENTION & MANAGEMENT
```

| Preoperative | Intraoperative | Postoperative |
| --- | --- | --- |

**Preoperative**
- Identify high-risk patients
- Measure core temperature
- Do not transfer patient to operating room unless their core temperature is > 36°C
- Encourage patients to walk to operating room when possible (increase metabolic heat production)
- Start active warming before surgery in hypothermic or high-risk patients

**Intraoperative**
- Do not start induction until core temperature is > 36°C unless clinically urgent
- Use active warming for all high-risk patients with a total anesthesia time of > 30 min
- Keep ambient temperature > 21°C while the patient is exposed
- Use warm IV fluids
- Humidify respiratory gases
- Measure patient's temperature at least every 30 min and titrate active warming to effect

**Postoperative**
- Measure core temperature with the observations in post-anesthesia care unit and then every 15 min
- Keep patients comfortably warm with a duvet and blankets for 24 h after surgery
- Keep patient in post-anesthesia care unit until core temperature > 36°C

**Active warming techniques**
- Forced air
- Resistive heating
- Circulating water garment devices

## SUGGESTED READING

- Rauch S, Miller C, Bräuer A, Wallner B, Bock M, Paal P. Perioperative Hypothermia-A Narrative Review. Int J Environ Res Public Health. 2021;18(16):8749. Published 2021 Aug 19.
- Riley C, Andrzejowski J. Inadvertent perioperative hypothermia. BJA Educ. 2018;18(8):227-233.

# PERIOPERATIVE MALNUTRITION

**142**

## LEARNING OBJECTIVES

- Consequences of perioperative malnutrition
- Recommendations to avoid perioperative malnutrition

## DEFINITION AND MECHANISM

- Malnutrition in the perioperative period is associated with increased morbidity, mortality, length-of-stay, and healthcare costs
- Is often a direct result of an underlying disease process
- The importance of perioperative nutrition optimization continues to be poorly appreciated
- The prevalence of preoperative malnutrition is up to 65% in patients undergoing surgery for cancer or gastrointestinal disease
- However, perioperative malnutrition has proven to be challenging to define, diagnose, and treat
- Patients are at risk of cancer cachexia, muscle protein depletion, poor wound healing, and systemic inflammation
- Appropriate perioperative nutritional therapy improves perioperative outcomes in gastrointestinal/oncologic surgery specifically
- Preventive, rather than 'reactive' boosting of nutritional stores and general metabolic reserve can protect against the catabolic stress response of surgery
- Nutritional optimization should start as early as feasible in the perioperative process
- Enhanced recovery after surgery (ERAS) pathways recommend the use of clear fluid carbohydrate drinks in the immediate preoperative period to decrease the incidence of insulin resistance and postoperative hyperglycemia
- Wishmeyer et al. 2018 on behalf of the American Society for Enhanced Recovery and Perioperative Quality Initiative 2 (POQI-2) pointed out the importance of nutritional screening and therapy within a surgically enhanced recovery pathway

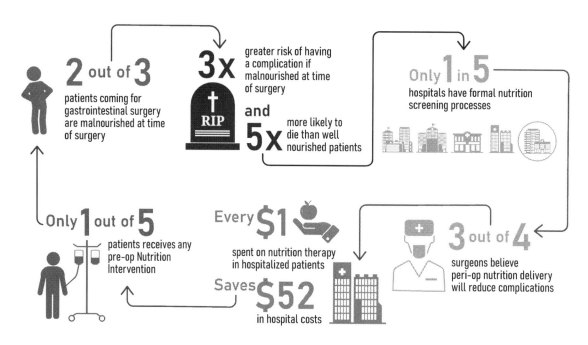

Summary of current challenges and known benefits of perioperative nutrition interventions. Figure adapted from Wischmeyer et al. 2018.

# PERIOPERATIVE NUTRITION SCREENING SCORE (PONS)

• To determine high-risk nutritional groups requiring referral to nutritionists for initiation or oral nutritional supplementation

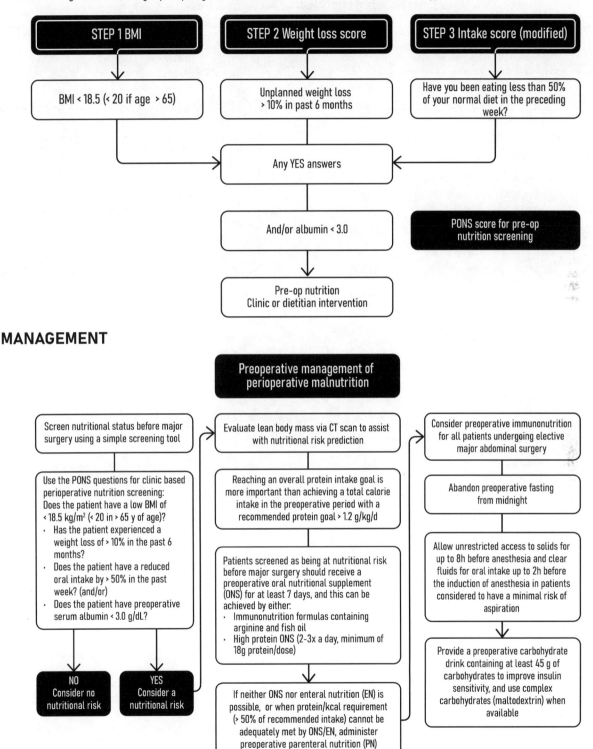

## MANAGEMENT

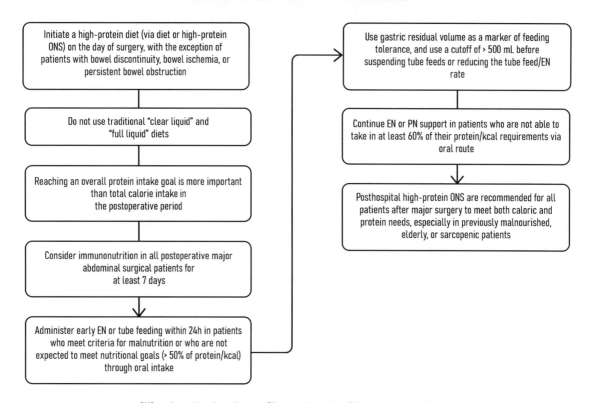

**Postoperative management of perioperative malnutrition**

Initiate a high-protein diet (via diet or high-protein ONS) on the day of surgery, with the exception of patients with bowel discontinuity, bowel ischemia, or persistent bowel obstruction

Do not use traditional "clear liquid" and "full liquid" diets

Reaching an overall protein intake goal is more important than total calorie intake in the postoperative period

Consider immunonutrition in all postoperative major abdominal surgical patients for at least 7 days

Administer early EN or tube feeding within 24h in patients who meet criteria for malnutrition or who are not expected to meet nutritional goals (> 50% of protein/kcal) through oral intake

Use gastric residual volume as a marker of feeding tolerance, and use a cutoff of > 500 mL before suspending tube feeds or reducing the tube feed/EN rate

Continue EN or PN support in patients who are not able to take in at least 60% of their protein/kcal requirements via oral route

Posthospital high-protein ONS are recommended for all patients after major surgery to meet both caloric and protein needs, especially in previously malnourished, elderly, or sarcopenic patients

ONS, oral nutritional supplement; EN, enteral nutrition; PN, parenteral nutrition.

## SUGGESTED READING

- Matthews, L.S., Wootton, S.A., Davies, S.J., Levett, D.Z.H., 2021. Screening, assessment and management of perioperative malnutrition: a survey of UK practice. Perioperative Medicine 10.
- Schonborn, J.L., Anderson, H., 2019. Perioperative medicine: a changing model of care. BJA Education 19, 27–33.
- Williams, D.G.A., Molinger, J., Wischmeyer, P.E., 2019. The malnourished surgery patient. Current Opinion in Anaesthesiology 32, 405–411.
- Wischmeyer, P.E., Carli, F., Evans, D.C., Guilbert, S., Kozar, R., Pryor, A., Thiele, R.H., Everett, S., Grocott, M., Gan, T.J., Shaw, A.D., Thacker, J.K.M., Miller, T.E., Hedrick, T.L., Mcevoy, M.D., Mythen, M.G., Bergamaschi, R., Gupta, R., Holubar, S.D., Senagore, A.J., Abola, R.E., Bennett-Guerrero, E., Kent, M.L., Feldman, L.S., Fiore, J.F., 2018. American Society for Enhanced Recovery and Perioperative Quality Initiative Joint Consensus Statement on Nutrition Screening and Therapy Within a Surgical Enhanced Recovery Pathway. Anesthesia & Analgesia 126, 1883–1895.

# PERIOPERATIVE STROKE

## LEARNING OBJECTIVES

- Describe the definition and risk factors of perioperative stroke
- Diagnose perioperative stroke
- Manage perioperative stroke

## DEFINITION AND MECHANISM

- Perioperative stroke is a devastating complication of surgery
- Defined as an ischemic or hemorrhagic brain infarction that occurs during surgery or within 30 days of surgery
- Overt stroke: Acute brain infarct with clinical manifestation lasting longer than 24 hours
- Covert stroke: Infarct that is not immediately recognized, often detected later through imaging or other diagnostic methods
- Incidence 0.1-1.9%
- Higher morbidity and mortality rates compared to stroke unrelated to surgery

## RISK FACTORS

| Patient factors | Surgical factors |
| --- | --- |
| Increasing age | Thoracic surgery |
| History of prior stroke or TIA | Transplant surgery |
| Hypertension | Endocrine surgery |
| History of atrial fibrillation | Burn surgery |
| Valvular disease | Otolaryngology surgery |
| Cardiovascular disease | Hemicolectomy |
| Renal disease | |
| Diabetes mellitus | |
| Smoker or COPD | |
| Patent foramen ovale | |
| Migraine with or without aura | |

# PREVENTION

### CAROTID STENOSIS

- Evaluate patients for general risk factors for stroke, including carotid stenosis
- Consider carotid endarterectomy for patients with symptomatic high-grade (50-99%) stenosis
- Carotid stenting may be considered in selected high-risk patients

### PERIOPERATIVE ANTICOAGULATION MANAGEMENT

- Avoid bridging of warfarin therapy in patients with atrial fibrillation
- Do not continue or start aspirin

### PERIOPERATIVE BETA-BLOCKER THERAPY MANAGEMENT

- Maintain chronic beta-blocker therapy
- Avoid initiation of beta-blocker therapy immediately before surgery

### PERIOPERATIVE ATRIAL FIBRILLATION MANAGEMENT

- Continue antiarrhythmic or rate-controlling agents
- Correct postoperative electrolyte imbalances and fluid volume

### INTRAOPERATIVE BLOOD PRESSURE MANAGEMENT

- Avoid hypotension
- Avoid metoprolol
- Maintain blood pressure within 20% of baseline

### TIMING OF SURGERY

- Patients with a history of previous stroke are at high risk of perioperative stroke
- Delaying surgery decreases the risk (lowest risk 9 months after stroke)
- Delay elective surgery at least 6 months and ideally 9 months after stroke, if possible
- Balance the increased risk of stroke with the risks of delaying surgery
- Do not delay emergency surgery

### OTHER CONTRIBUTING FACTORS

- Avoid severe hypo- and hyperglycemia
- Continue statin therapy
- Avoid hypocarbia

# POSTOPERATIVE EVALUATION

- The modified National Institutes of Health Stroke Scale (NIHSS) can be used to assess patients with suspected perioperative stroke
  - 0 = no stroke
  - 1–4 = minor stroke
  - 5–15 = moderate stroke
  - 15–20 = moderate/severe stroke
  - 21–42 = severe stroke

| Item | Score |
|---|---|
| Level of consciousness questions | 0 = Answers both correctly<br>1 = Answers one correctly<br>2 = Answers neither correctly |
| Level of consciousness commands | 0 = performs both tasks correctly<br>1 = performs one task correctly<br>2 = perform neither task |
| Gaze | 0 = Normal<br>1 = Partial gaze palsy<br>2 = Total gaze palsy |
| Visual fields | 0 = No visual loss<br>1 = Partial hemianopsia<br>2 = Bilateral hemianopsia |
| Left arm | 0 = No drift<br>1 = Drift before 10 s<br>2 = Fails before 10 s<br>3 = No effort against gravity<br>4 = No movement |

| Item | Score |
|---|---|
| Right arm | Same scoring as left arm |
| Left leg | Same scoring as left arm |
| Right leg | Same scoring as left arm |
| Sensory | 0 = Normal<br>1 = Abnormal |
| Language | 0 = Normal<br>1 = Mild aphasia<br>2 = Severe aphasia<br>3 = Mute |
| Neglect | 0 = Normal<br>1 = Mild<br>3 = Severe |

## MANAGEMENT

- Early diagnosis is key (< 25 min after symptom onset)
  - Emergency non-contrast CT scan to discriminate between ischemic stroke from intracranial hemorrhage and nonvascular causes of neurologic symptoms (e.g., tumors)
  - Multimodal CT and MRI may provide additional information
- Emergency treatment (< 60 min after symptom onset):
  - Move the patient to acute stroke unit
  - Correction of postoperative causes of hypotension (volume depletion, blood loss, myocardial ischemia or arrhythmias)
  - Treat fever
  - Cardiac monitoring and treatment of arrhythmias if they occur
  - Intravenous thrombolysis may be beneficial
  - Intraarterial thrombolysis can be administered within 6 hours of symptom onset, either alone or in conjunction with intravenous thrombolysis
  - Aspirin can be used when deemed safe
  - Mechanical thrombectomy in patients with large vessel occlusion, between 6 and 24 hours after symptom onset

### SUGGESTED READING

- Benesch C, Glance LG, Derdeyn CP, Fleisher LA, Holloway RG, Messé SR, et al. Perioperative Neurological Evaluation and Management to Lower the Risk of Acute Stroke in Patients Undergoing Noncardiac, Nonneurological Surgery: A Scientific Statement From the American Heart Association/American Stroke Association. Circulation. 2021;143(19):e923-e46.
- Lindberg AP, Flexman AM. Perioperative stroke after non-cardiac, non-neurological surgery. BJA Educ. 2021;21(2):59-65.
- Ng JLW, Chan MTV, Gelb Adrian W, Warner David S. Perioperative Stroke in Noncardiac, Nonneurosurgical Surgery. Anesthesiology. 2011;115(4):879-90.

# POSTOPERATIVE DELIRIUM (POD)

## LEARNING OBJECTIVES

- Recognize the signs of POD
- Identify risk factors for POD
- Reduce the risk of POD in susceptible patients
- Manage POD occurrence

## DEFINITION AND MECHANISM

- Postoperative delirium (POD) is defined as an acute onset fluctuating change in mental status characterized by reduced awareness of the environment and disturbance of attention
- It is a temporary neurocognitive syndrome observed after surgery
- Incidence in older surgical patients varies from 7% to 53%
- POD prolongs postoperative ventilation, intensive care, length of stay, increases costs, and negatively impacts functional outcome and survival

## SIGNS

**3 subtypes:**
- Hyperactive: Restlessness, agitation, and hypervigilance, often hallucinations and delusions
- Hypoactive: Lethargy and sedation, slow response to questioning, little spontaneous movement
- Mixed: Both hyperactive and hypoactive features

## RISK FACTORS

| Predisposing | Precipitating |
|---|---|
| Advanced age | ICU admission |
| Male sex | High-risk surgical procedure |
| Low body mass index | Sleep deprivation |
| Sight/hearing loss | Polypharmacy |
| Social isolation | Medications |
| Multimorbidity | Severe illness (e.g., infection, fracture, stroke) |
| Prior cognitive impairment | Hyper- or hypothermia |
| Malnutrition | Sensory deprivation |
| Low serum albumin | Increasing duration of surgery |
| Frailty | Urgency of surgery |

## PREVENTION

- Identify risk factors
- Frailty assessment
- Bispectral index (BIS) monitoring (Target BIS 40-60)
- Avoid benzodiazepines
- Multi-component interventions (visual and hearing aids, sleep promotion, minimalization of catheters/cannulae...)
- Regional anesthesia instead of general
- Treat pain (multimodal strategy)
- Prehabilitation programs that improve physical and cognitive capacity

Preventative measures requiring further investigation:
- Total intravenous anesthesia (TIVA)
- Lighter sedation
- Dexmedetomidine
- Melatonin
- Steroids
- Cholinergic stimulation

## MANAGEMENT

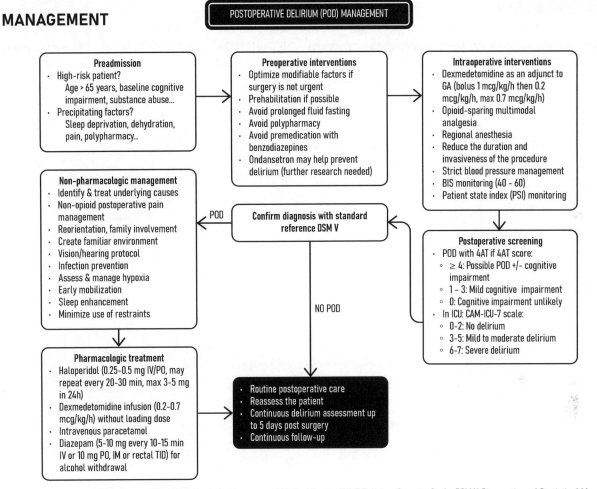

POSTOPERATIVE DELIRIUM (POD) MANAGEMENT

**Preadmission**
- High-risk patient?
  Age > 65 years, baseline cognitive impairment, substance abuse...
- Precipitating factors?
  Sleep deprivation, dehydration, pain, polypharmacy...

**Preoperative interventions**
- Optimize modifiable factors if surgery is not urgent
- Prehabilitation if possible
- Avoid prolonged fluid fasting
- Avoid polypharmacy
- Avoid premedication with benzodiazepines
- Ondansetron may help prevent delirium (further research needed)

**Intraoperative interventions**
- Dexmedetomidine as an adjunct to GA (bolus 1 mcg/kg/h then 0.2 mcg/kg/h, max 0.7 mcg/kg/h)
- Opioid-sparing multimodal analgesia
- Regional anesthesia
- Reduce the duration and invasiveness of the procedure
- Strict blood pressure management
- BIS monitoring (40 - 60)
- Patient state index (PSI) monitoring

**Non-pharmacologic management**
- Identify & treat underlying causes
- Non-opioid postoperative pain management
- Reorientation, family involvement
- Create familiar environment
- Vision/hearing protocol
- Infection prevention
- Assess & manage hypoxia
- Early mobilization
- Sleep enhancement
- Minimize use of restraints

POD

**Confirm diagnosis with standard reference DSM V**

**Postoperative screening**
- POD with 4AT if 4AT score:
  - ≥ 4: Possible POD +/- cognitive impairment
  - 1 – 3: Mild cognitive impairment
  - 0: Cognitive impairment unlikely
- In ICU: CAM-ICU-7 scale:
  - 0-2: No delirium
  - 3-5: Mild to moderate delirium
  - 6-7: Severe delirium

NO POD

**Pharmacologic treatment**
- Haloperidol (0.25-0.5 mg IV/PO, may repeat every 20-30 min, max 3-5 mg in 24h)
- Dexmedetomidine infusion (0.2-0.7 mcg/kg/h) without loading dose
- Intravenous paracetamol
- Diazepam (5-10 mg every 10-15 min IV or 10 mg PO, IM or rectal TID) for alcohol withdrawal

- Routine postoperative care
- Reassess the patient
- Continuous delirium assessment up to 5 days post surgery
- Continuous follow-up

BIS, bispectral index; 4AT, 4 A's test; CAM-ICU-7, Confusion Assessment Method for the ICU-7 Delirium Severity Scale; DSM V, Diagnostic and Statistical Manual of Mental Disorders, Fifth edition; TID, three times a day.

## SUGGESTED READING

- Chan MT, Cheng BC, Lee TM, Gin T; CODA Trial Group. BIS-guided anesthesia decreases postoperative delirium and cognitive decline. J Neurosurg Anesthesiol. 2013;25(1):33-42.
- Fong TG, Tulebaev SR, Inouye SK. Delirium in elderly adults: diagnosis, prevention and treatment. Nat Rev Neurol. 2009;5(4):210-220.
- Haque N, Naqvi RM, Dasgupta M. Efficacy of Ondansetron in the Prevention or Treatment of Post-operative Delirium-a Systematic Review. Can Geriatr J. 2019;22(1):1-6. Published 2019 Mar 30.
- Hoogma, Danny Feike; Milisen, Koen; Rex, Steffen; Al tmimi, Layth. Postoperative delirium: identifying the patient at risk and altering the course: A narrative review. European Journal of Anaesthesiology and Intensive Care 2(3):p e0022, June 2023.
- Khan BA, Perkins AJ, Gao S, et al. The Confusion Assessment Method for the ICU-7 Delirium Severity Scale: A Novel Delirium Severity Instrument for Use in the ICU. Crit Care Med. 2017;45(5):851-857.
- Mossie A, Regasa T, Neme D, Awoke Z, Zemedkun A, Hailu S. Evidence-Based Guideline on Management of Postoperative Delirium in Older People for Low Resource Setting: Systematic Review Article. Int J Gen Med. 2022;15:4053-4065.
- Robinson TN, Eiseman B. Postoperative delirium in the elderly: diagnosis and management. Clin Interv Aging. 2008;3(2):351-355.
- Subramaniam B, Shankar P, Shaefi S, et al. Effect of Intravenous Acetaminophen vs Placebo Combined With Propofol or Dexmedetomidine on Postoperative Delirium Among Older Patients Following Cardiac Surgery: The DEXACET Randomized Clinical Trial [published correction appears in JAMA. 2019 Jul 16;322(3):276]. JAMA. 2019;321(7):686-696.
- Swarbrick CJ, Partridge JSL. Evidence-based strategies to reduce the incidence of postoperative delirium: a narrative review. Anaesthesia. 2022;77 Suppl 1:92-101.

# 145

# POSTOPERATIVE NAUSEA AND VOMITING (PONV)

## LEARNING OBJECTIVES

- Prevent and treat postoperative nausea and vomiting (PONV)

## DEFINITION AND MECHANISM

- Postoperative nausea and vomiting (PONV) is the second most common postoperative complication after pain

## SCORING

- Scoring systems like the Apfel simplified risk score can help raise awareness of PONV and thus increase prophylaxis use. The incidence of PONV, with the presence of 0, 1, 2, 3, and 4 risk factors is approximately 10%, 20%, 40%, 60%, and 80%, respectively.

| Risk factor | Points |
|---|---|
| Female gender | 1 |
| Non-smoker | 1 |
| History of PONV and/or motion sickness | 1 |
| Postoperative opioids | 1 |
| Sum of points | 0-4 |

## MANAGEMENT

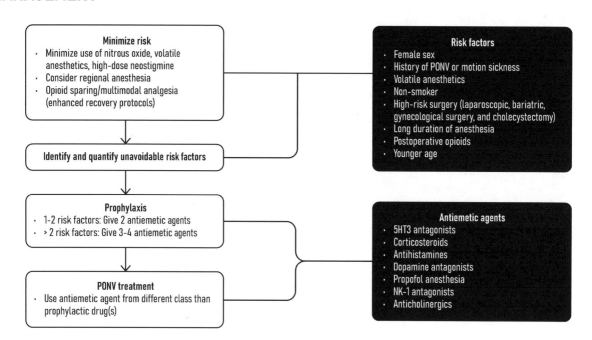

## PONV IN CHILDREN

- Children have different risk factors for PONV than adults:
  - Age ≥ 3 years
  - History of PONV/motion sickness
  - Family history of PONV
  - Post-pubertal female
  - High-risk surgeries (strabismus, adenotonsillectomy, otoplasty)
  - Surgery < 30 minutes
  - Volatile anesthetics

- Dexamethasone and 5HT3 antagonists are the antiemetics of choice in children:
  - 0 risk factors
    - No prophylaxis or dexamethasone or 5HT3 antagonist
  - 1-2 risk factors
    - Dexamethasone and 5HT3 antagonist
  - > 2 risk factors
    - Dexamethasone and 5HT3 antagonist + consider total intravenous anesthesia

## KEEP IN MIND

- Do not underestimate the severity of PONV, patients report that it's a worse experience than pain
- PONV can lead to decreased patient satisfaction, aspiration, dehydration, increased length of stay and higher medical costs

## SUGGESTED READING

- Gan TJ, Belani KG, Bergese S, et al. Fourth Consensus Guidelines for the Management of Postoperative Nausea and Vomiting [published correction appears in Anesth Analg. 2020 Nov;131(5):e241]. Anesth Analg. 2020;131(2):411-448.
- Shaikh SI, Nagarekha D, Hegade G, Marutheesh M. Postoperative nausea and vomiting: A simple yet complex problem. Anesth Essays Res. 2016 Sep-Dec;10(3):388-396.
- Weibel S, Rücker G, Eberhart LHJ, et al. Drugs for preventing postoperative nausea and vomiting in adults after general anaesthesia: a network meta -analysis. Cochrane Database of Systematic Reviews. 2020;(10)

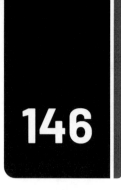

# POSTOPERATIVE NERVE INJURIES

## LEARNING OBJECTIVES

- Describe the mechanisms, risk factors, and symptoms of postoperative nerve injuries
- Diagnose postoperative nerve injuries
- Prevent and manage postoperative nerve injuries

## DEFINITION AND MECHANISM

- Postoperative peripheral nerve injuries are complications of both general and regional anesthesia
- Third-most common cause of anesthesia-related medical litigation
- Very rare
- Potentially results in significant morbidity for the patient
- Direct nerve damage from surgery, needle trauma, or secondary to regional anesthesia or peripheral catheter
- Stretch and compression: Poor padding and positioning of limbs, use of tourniquets and surgical retractors
- Ischemia: Caused primarily by tourniquets, prolonged immobility, hematoma surrounding a nerve, and local anesthetic agents
- Local anesthetic toxicity: High concentrations and prolonged exposure increase risk
- Double crush syndrome: Decreased tolerance of a nerve to compression after previous compression
- Idiopathic
- Combination of mechanisms

## RISK FACTORS

| | |
|---|---|
| Surgical | Neurosurgery<br>Cardiac surgery<br>Gastrointestinal surgery |
| Patient-specific | Hypertension<br>Diabetes mellitus<br>Smoking<br>Double crush syndrome<br>Preexisting peripheral neuropathy<br>Anatomical abnormalities |
| Anesthetic | General anesthesia<br>Epidural anesthesia |
| Perioperative | Hypovolemia<br>Dehydration<br>Hypotension<br>Hypoxia<br>Electrolyte disturbance<br>Hypothermia |

## SYMPTOMS

- Sensory
  - Anesthesia
  - Paresthesia
  - Hypoesthesia
  - Hyperesthesia
  - Pain in the areas supplied by the affected nerves
- Motor
  - Paresis
  - Paralysis
- Autonomic dysfunction
- Trophic changes

# CLASSIFICATION

| Seddon | Sunderland | Pathophysiology |
|---|---|---|
| Neuropraxia (compression) | Type 1 | Local myelin damage with the nerve still intact |
| Axonotmesis (crush) | Type 2 | Continuity of axons is lost<br>Endoneurium, perineurium, and epineurium remain intact<br>Loss of continuity of axons with Wallerian degeneration due to disruption of axoplasmic flow |
| | Type 3 | Type 2 with endoneurial injury |
| | Type 4 | Type 2 with endoneurial and perineurial injury but an intact epineurium |
| Neurotmesis (transection) | Type 5 | Complete physiological disruption of the entire nerve trunk<br>Early surgical intervention necessary<br>Prognosis guarded |

## Upper extremity nerve injuries

| Affected nerve(s) | Mechanism of injury | Clinical presentation |
|---|---|---|
| Ulnar nerve | Direct pressure on the ulnar groove<br>Prolonged forearm flexion | Tingling or numbness along the little finger<br>Weakness of abduction/adduction of the fingers |
| Brachial plexus | Compression, stretching, or direct injury resulting from a regional technique | C5-6 lesion: Arm hangs by side, medially rotated and pronated<br>C8-T1 lesion: Claw hand and numbness in the ulnar distribution |
| Radial nerve | Tourniquet/arterial pressure cuffs<br>Compression against a patient screen<br>Arm board at incorrect height | Wrist drop<br>Numbness along posterior surface of the lower arm and a variable area of the dorsum of the hand and lateral fingers |
| Median nerve | Direct nerve damage from regional techniques<br>Invasive procedures around the elbow<br>Compression in the carpal tunnel | Paresthesia along the palmar aspect of the lateral fingers<br>Weakness of abduction and opposition of the thumb<br>Weak wirst flexion<br>Forearm kept in supination<br>Hand appears flattened |
| Axillary (C5-6) and musculocutaneous nerve (C5-7) | Shoulder surgery or shoulder dislocation | Weakness of shoulder abduction and anesthesia along upper lateral border of the arm (axillary nerve)<br>Weakness of elbow flexion and numbness along the lateral border of the forearm (musculocutaneous nerve) |

## Lower extremity nerve injuries

| Affected nerve(s) | Mechanism of injury | Clinical presentation |
|---|---|---|
| Sciatic nerve (L4-S3) | Stretch, compression, ischemia, direct damage<br>Lithotomy, frog leg, and sitting positions<br>Regional techniques | Paralysis of the hamstring muscles and all the muscles below the knee<br>Weak knee flexion and foot drop<br>Impaired sensation below the knee except the medial aspect of the leg and foot |
| Femoral nerve (L2-4) | Compression at the pelvic brim by retractors<br>Ischemia associated with aortic cross-clamp<br>Lithotomy position<br>Invasive procedures to access the femoral vessels<br>Hip arthroplasty | Loss of sensation at the front of the thigh and medial aspect of the leg<br>Weak hip flexion<br>Loss of knee extension<br>Decreased or absent knee jerk reflex |
| Superficial peroneal nerve (L4-5, S1-2) | Lithotomy<br>Lateral position | Loss of dorsiflexion and eversion of the foot<br>Loss of sensation along the anterolateral border of the leg and dorsum of the digits except those supplied by the saphenous and sural nerves |

## DIAGNOSIS

- Thorough history and clinical examination to localize the lesion and identify preexisting peripheral neuropathy
- Electromyography
- Nerve conduction studies
- Imaging: MRI, high-resolution ultrasound
- Early consultation with a neurologist

## PREVENTION

**Preoperative history and physical assessment**
- Identify body habitus, preexisting neurologic symptoms, diabetes mellitus, peripheral vascular disease, alcohol dependency, arthritis, and sex
- Assess whether patients can comfortably tolerate the anticipated operative position

**Positioning strategy for upper extremities**
- Limit arm abduction in a supine patient to 90°
- Prone position may allow patients to comfortably tolerate abduction greater than 90°
- Avoid flexion of the elbow or limit flexion/extension to 90°
- Keep forearm in supine or neutral position

**Positioning strategy for lower extremities**
- Limit hip flexion/extension
- Avoid prolonged pressure on the peroneal nerve at the fibular head
- Position patients with preoperative mobility limitations while they are still fully awake

**Documentation**
- Carefully document specific perioperative positioning actions that may be useful for continuous improvement

**Protective padding**
- Padded armboards and padding at the elbow to decrease the risk of upper extremity neuropathy
- Chest rolls in the laterally positioned patient to decrease the risk of upper extremity neuropathy
- Specific padding to prevent pressure of a hard surface against the peroneal nerve at the fibular head to decrease the risk of peroneal neuropathy
- Avoid inappropriate use of padding (e.g., padding too tight)

**Equipment**
- Avoid improper use of automated blood pressure cuffs on the arm (e.g., placed below the antecubital fossa)
- Avoid the use of shoulder braces in a steep head-down position

**Postoperative physical assessment**
- Simple assessment of peripheral nerve function for early detection of peripheral neuropathies

Postoperative nerve injuries

# MANAGEMENT

- Correct underlying pathology and alleviate symptoms
- Consult neurology
- Surgical correction is rarely indicated
- Physiotherapy
- Orthotic measures (foot care, splints, and limb supports)

━━ **SUGGESTED READING** ━━

- Chui J, Murkin JM, Posner KL, Domino KB. Perioperative Peripheral Nerve Injury After General Anesthesia: A Qualitative Systematic Review. Anesth Analg. 2018;127(1):134-143.
- Hewson DW, Bedforth NM, Hardman JG. Peripheral nerve injury arising in anaesthesia practice. Anaesthesia. 2018;73(S1):51-60.
- Lalkhen AG, Bhatia K. Perioperative peripheral nerve injuries. Continuing Education in Anaesthesia Critical Care & Pain. 2012;12(1):38-42.
- Practice Advisory for the Prevention of Perioperative Peripheral Neuropathies 2018: An Updated Report by the American Society of Anesthesiologists Task Force on Prevention of Perioperative Peripheral Neuropathies*. Anesthesiology. 2018;128(1):11-26.

# POSTOPERATIVE NEUROCOGNITIVE DISORDER

## LEARNING OBJECTIVES

- Define and diagnose postoperative neurocognitive disorders (pNCD)
- Identify patients at risk of pNCD
- Prevent pNCD

## DEFINITION AND MECHANISM

- Cognition is defined as 'the mental action or process of acquiring knowledge and understanding through thought, experience, and the senses'
- Six domains:
  - Perceptual–motor function
  - Language
  - Learning and memory
  - Social cognition
  - Complex attention
  - Executive function
- Can be influenced by endogenous and exogenous conditions (stress, inflammation, hormonal balance, disease)
- Changes physiologically through aging
- Surgery is associated with a (temporary) decline in cognitive function due to the physical and psychological stresses

## DEFINITION

- pNCD is not yet defined by the Diagnostic and Statistical Manual of Mental Disorders, 5th Edition
- Described in the literature as a postoperative decline in cognitive function that can potentially last from months to years
- Different grades:
  - Mild neurocognitive disorder: Noticeable decline in cognitive function, requiring adjustment to maintain independence in daily activities that extends beyond the regular changes of aging
  - Major neurocognitive disorder: Significant burden of cognitive impairment that results in impaired activities of daily living
- Can be detected from 7 days after surgery, and is different from transient cognitive deficits immediately after surgery (e.g., postoperative delirium)

## RISK FACTORS

- Advanced age
- Disabilities
- Frailty
- Major surgery
- History of alcohol abuse
- Lower educational status
- History of stroke
- Longer duration of anesthesia
- Postoperative infection
- Respiratory complications
- Anticholinergic medication
- Sevoflurane use for anesthesia
- Reoperation

## DIAGNOSIS

- Diagnosis of pNCD is complex and requires neuropsychometric testing
- Cognitive domains that are evaluated:
  - Learning and memory
  - Language
  - Perceptual motor
  - Social cognition
  - Complex attention
  - Executive function
  - Delirium
- In practice, several validated short-form tests are used

| Test | Description | Advantages | Disadvantages |
|------|-------------|------------|---------------|
| MiniCog | Very short test consisting of a three-word registration, a clock drawing test and the three-word recall | Easy to administer, available in many languages, results independent from language skills and education, parallel versions available | Not sensitive for mild cognitive dysfunction |
| IQ-CODE (Informant Questionnaire on Cognitive Decline in the Elderly), short form | Questionnaire addressing change in everyday activities in 7 aspects (short-term and long-term memory, temporal and spatial orientation, learning, managing financial issues) in five gradations, to be filled-out by relatives or friends | Questionnaire that can be handed out to relatives, no patient participation required, easy to administer, easy evaluation | Only subjective estimation of cognitive function, limited scientific usability |
| MMSE (Mini Mental State Examination) | Widely-used cognition test designed in 1975 for Alzheimer's Disease detection, takes 10 min to administer | Easy to administer, already widely introduced into clinical routine, good data availability | Low sensitivity for mild and medium cognitive dysfunction, primarily sensitive for dementia detection |
| Clock-drawing test | Patient is asked to draw a clock showing a defined time. Detects impairment in visio-spacial and problem-solving abilities | Short and easy to administer, no license or template required | There are different approaches to evaluate the results. Conflicting database on sensitivity for mild cognitive impairment and generalization of the results on different domains of cognition |
| MoCA (Montreal Cognitive Assessment) | Detailed cognition test, sensitive to detect even mild cognitive impairments, takes 10-15 min to administer | Covers many cognitive domains, sensitive for mild cognitive impairment, easy interpretation of results Available in many languages and parallel versions | Requires operator training, time-consuming administration makes it unsuitable for clinical routine |

# PREVENTION

- Carefully prepare high-risk patients and inform the patient, relatives or confidantes about the procedure
- Do not exceed the minimum required time of preoperative fasting
- Avoid unnecessary postponement of surgery
- Avoid routine benzodiazepine administration
- Perioperative sensory orientation: Encourage patients to wear their glasses, hearing aids, and dentures until anesthesia induction
- Limit opioid use
- Perioperative warming
- Adequate analgesia
- Avoid deep sedation
- Continuously monitor depth of sedation/anesthesia (EEG)
- Maintain homeostasis and hemodynamics
- Facilitate early postoperative mobilization and re-orientation
- Propofol total IV anesthesia and dexmedetomidine were found to be protective, but further research is needed
- Moderate evidence indicates that dexmedetomidine reduces the risk of postoperative neurocognitive disorder

## SUGGESTED READING

- Brodier EA, Cibelli M. Postoperative cognitive dysfunction in clinical practice. BJA Educ. 2021;21(2):75-82.
- Olotu C. Postoperative neurocognitive disorders. Curr Opin Anaesthesiol. 2020;33(1):101-108.
- Shoair OA, Grasso Ii MP, Lahaye LA, Daniel R, Biddle CJ, Slattum PW. Incidence and risk factors for postoperative cognitive dysfunction in older adults undergoing major noncardiac surgery. A prospective study. J Anaesthesiol Clin Pharmacol. 2015;31(1):30-36.

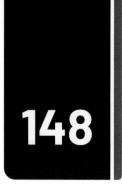

# POSTOPERATIVE PAIN MANAGEMENT

**148**

## LEARNING OBJECTIVES

- Describe the importance of postoperative pain management
- Assess postoperative pain
- Manage postoperative pain

## DEFINITION AND MECHANISM

- Adequate postoperative pain management is essential to enable a quick return to normal function
- Uncontrolled pain increases sympathetic activity and the stress response, leading to multisystem consequences (e.g., hyperglycemia, immunosuppression, increased risk of myocardial ischemia)
- Pain after abdominal or thoracic surgery can lead to splinting of the diaphragm and chest wall, resulting in decreased lung volumes, atelectasis, poor cough, sputum retention, infection, and hypoxia
- Pain can reduce mobility and increase the risk of thromboembolism
- Psychological effects: anxiety, feeling of helplessness
- Untreated or inadequately treated postoperative pain can lead to chronic pain
- Traditionally, opioids were the standard treatment for postoperative pain
- Today, multimodal approaches for pain management are the treatment of choice

## PAIN ASSESSMENT

- Perform pain assessment at regular, frequent intervals and after every intervention
- The severity of pain and the effectiveness of analgesia determine the frequency
- Record pain as the fifth vital sign
- Assessment includes:
  - Site, circumstances associated with onset
  - Character
  - Intensity (at rest and on movement)
  - Associated symptoms (e.g., nausea)
  - Effect on activity and sleep
  - Relevant medical history
  - Other factors influencing the patient's treatment
  - Current and previous medications and analgesic strategies
- Severity scales:
  - Unidimensional
    - Numeric (numeric rating scales, visual analog scale)
    - Categorical (verbal descriptor scale)
  - Multidimensional (less useful in acute postoperative pain)
    - McGill Pain Questionnaire
    - Leeds Assessment of Neuropathic Symptoms and Signs (LANSS) can be used to identify those at risk of developing chronic neuropathic pain
  - Pictorial and behavioral scales may be needed for children or cognitively impaired patients
    - Face, Legs, Activity, Cry, Consolability (FLACC) scale
    - Abbey pain scale

# PAIN MANAGEMENT STRATEGY

## POSTOPERATIVE PAIN MANAGEMENT

### PLANNING
- Multiple factors affect postoperative pain (e.g., type of surgery, pain threshold, patient age, chronic pain, opioid tolerance)
- Identify patients at high risk of postoperative pain and discuss analgesic strategy before surgery
- Educate patient on home pain relief
- Administer first postoperative analgesia before intraoperative analgesia and local anesthesia wear off

### PHARMACOLOGICAL ANALGESIA
- Paracetamol: Mild analgesic with few side-effects
- Non-steroidal anti-inflammatory drugs (NSAIDs): Administer preoperatively or early during surgery to account for long onset of action
- Opioids: Balance the analgesic effect against side-effects (nausea and vomiting, sedation, pruritus, respiratory depression, constipation, urinary retention)
- Adjuvants (e.g., gabapentinoids, N-methyl-D-aspartate receptor antagonists, alpha-2 adrenergic agonists): Reduce pain and opioid requirements as part of a balanced multimodal analgesic strategy
- IV clonidine and dexmedetomidine reduce pain intensity, opioid consumption, and postoperative nausea
- Low-dose IV ketamine reduces opioid requirements, nausea, and vomiting
- Dexamethasone > 0.1 mg/kg has intrinsic analgesic effects

## PAIN IN SPECIAL CIRCUMSTANCES

- Opioid-dependent patients (long-term opioids for chronic pain, opioids for cancer pain, recreational use)
  - Manage patient expectations
  - Provide adequate analgesia
  - Prevent or manage withdrawal symptoms
- Acute neuropathic pain after surgery
  - Incidence depends on type of surgery (e.g., 85% following limb amputation)
  - Pre-emptive analgesia (regional techniques, ketamine, administration before start of surgery) may be helpful
  - Maintain a high index of suspicion for patients at high risk
  - Treatment is extrapolated from chronic neuropathic pain treatment: Tricyclic antidepressants, ketamine, anticonvulsants, lidocaine, and tramadol may have a role

### REGIONAL ANESTHESIA
- Excellent pain relief, often eliminates opioid requirement
- Better patient satisfaction and possible reduction in length of stay
- Local anesthetic infiltration
- Peripheral nerve blocks (single injection or continuous)

### NEURAXIAL ANESTHESIA
- Epidural block
- Spinal anesthesia
- Commence oral analgesia before return of sensation

### Example of pain management strategy (modification of WHO pain ladder)

| Anticipated pain | Mild | Moderate | Severe |
|---|---|---|---|
| Pain score | 1-3 | 4-7 | 7-10 |
| Regular (at timed intervals) | Simple analgesics: Paracetamol and/or low-dose weak opioids Use local infiltration or regional blocks when possible | Add NSAIDs +/- weak opioids Use local infiltration or regional blocks when possible | Add strong opioid Replace weak opioids with strong opioids Consider epidural block/ patient-controlled analgesia |
| As required | NSAIDs or weak opioids | Short-acting opioids (e.g., morphine oral/IV/IM) | Short-acting opioids (e.g., morphine oral/IV/IM) Patient-controlled (epidural) analgesia |

## SUGGESTED READING

- Horn R, Kramer J. Postoperative Pain Control. [Updated 2022 Sep 19]. In: StatPearls [Internet]. Treasure Island (FL): StatPearls Publishing; 2022 Jan-. Available from: https://www.ncbi.nlm.nih.gov/books/NBK544298/
- Pollard BJ, Kitchen, G. Handbook of Clinical Anaesthesia. Fourth Edition. CRC Press. 2018. 978-1-4987-6289-2.
- Tharakan L, Faber P. Pain management in day-case surgery. BJA Education. 2015;15(4):180-3.

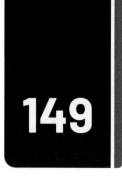

# PRONE POSITION

## LEARNING OBJECTIVES

- Describe the physiological effects and possible complications of prone positioning
- Manage patients presenting for surgery in the prone position

## DEFINITION AND MECHANISM

- Prone positioning is commonly used for access to the posterior head, neck, and spine during spinal surgery, access to the retroperitoneum and upper urinary tracts, and access to posterior structures when required during plastic surgery
- Prone surgery is associated with a variety of complications and requires specific considerations

## PHYSIOLOGY

| Physiology | |
|---|---|
| Respiratory | Increased functional residual capacity<br>Increased arterial oxygen pressure<br>Chest wall and lung compliance remain unchanged |
| Cardiovascular | Reduced stroke volume<br>Compensatory sympathetic tachycardia and increase in peripheral vascular resistance<br>Increased pulse pressure and stroke volume variation |
| Cerebral blood flow | Reduced cerebral blood flow<br>Increased intracranial pressure<br>Vessel distension |
| Renal function | Slight increase in urine output |

## COMPLICATIONS

- Pressure injuries

| Pressure injuries | |
|---|---|
| Direct pressure injuries | Skin necrosis<br>Contact dermatitis<br>Tracheal compression<br>Salivary gland swelling<br>Breast injury<br>Injury to the genitalia<br>Compression of the pinna<br>Compression of the femoral neurovascular bundle |
| Indirect pressure injuries | Macroglossia and oropharyngeal swelling<br>Mediastinal compression<br>Visceral ischemia (liver, pancreas)<br>Avascular necrosis of femoral head<br>Peripheral vessel occlusion<br>Limb compartment syndrome and rhabdomyolysis |

- Ophthalmic complications ranging from corneal abrasions to postoperative visual loss
  - Direct pressure on the eye: central retinal artery occlusion
  - No direct pressure on the eye: Ischemic optic neuropathy
  - Risk factors: Atherosclerosis, diabetes, hypertension, male gender, blood loss, long duration of the procedure
  - Prevention: Avoid direct ocular pressure
- Peripheral nerve injuries
  - All superficial peripheral nerves should be considered at risk
  - Usually does not present in the recovery room, 90% present within 7 days
  - Can be sensory or mixed motor/sensory
  - Risk factors: Male gender, prolonged hospital stay, diabetes, advanced age, extremes in BMI
  - Prevention: Place arms at side, < 90° at elbow or shoulder if arms are abducted, avoid direct pressure in the axilla, pad the elbows

# MANAGEMENT

### POSITIONING

- Six staff members are needed to position the patient: One at the head, one at the feet and two on either side of the patient
- Additional staff members may be needed for obese patients or patients with unstable spines requiring log-rolling
- Alternatively, specialized equipment (e.g., the Jackson table) can be used to turn the patient
- It may be helpful to disconnect monitoring, infusions and breathing system while turning the patient to prevent accidental dislodging

### AIRWAY MANAGEMENT

- Securely fastened reinforced cuffed tracheal tube
- Note the supine airway pressures to check for bronchospasm or endobronchial intubation with sustained or significant increases in pressure
- The bed should not leave the room until correct tube position and ventilation has been confirmed
- Perform a 'leak test' before extubation

### EMERGENCY MANAGEMENT

Accidental extubation
- Immediately check security and patency of the airway
- If dislodged, turn patient supine and reintubate without delay
- Check the tracheal tube after every repositioning of the patient or their head
- Consider laryngeal mask airway placement for airway rescue
- Alternative: Fiberoptic reintubation in prone position

Cardiac arrest
- Chest compressions with hands over both scapula or the thoracic spine or open cardiac compressions if during thoracotomy
- Defibrillation with pads anteroposterior, posterolateral, or on the right axilla and cardiac apex
- Consider placing pads before turning prone in high-risk patients
- Support the head/neck during shock

# SUGGESTED READING

- Feix B, Sturgess J. Anaesthesia in the prone position. Continuing Education in Anaesthesia Critical Care & Pain. 2014;14(6):291-7.
- Edgcombe H, Carter K, Yarrow S. Anaesthesia in the prone position. BJA: British Journal of Anaesthesia. 2008;100(2):165-83.
- Kwee MM, Ho YH, Rozen WM. The prone position during surgery and its complications: a systematic review and evidence-based guidelines. Int Surg. 2015;100(2):292-303.

# SUCCINYLCHOLINE MYALGIAS

## LEARNING OBJECTIVES

- Describe the mechanism of action of succinylcholine
- Describe the side effects of succinylcholine
- Prevent and manage succinylcholine-induced myalgias

## DEFINITION AND MECHANISM

- Succinylcholine is a depolarizing neuromuscular blocking agent
- It is considered the standard drug for rapid sequence intubation
- Mechanisms
  - Acts as an acetylcholine receptor agonist
  - Not metabolized by acetylcholinesterase, leading to persistent depolarization of the muscle fibers
  - Effect: Desensitization of motor endplate to acetylcholine resulting in paralysis

## ADVERSE EFFECTS

- Paralysis of the diaphragm
- Arrhythmias
- Autonomic symptoms
- Hypotension
- Flushing
- Tachycardia
- Hyperkalemia
- Muscle fasciculation
- Jaw rigidity
- Apnea
- Bradycardia
- Increased intraocular pressure
- Excessive salivation
- Hypersensitivity reactions
- Malignant hyperthermia
- Myoglobinuria/myoglobinemia
- Myalgia
  - Myalgia has a high incidence (50-90%) and may last for several days, inducing significant discomfort

## RISK FACTORS

- Minor procedures
- Early ambulation

## PROTECTIVE FACTORS

- Children
- Age > 50
- Female
- Pregnancy
- Better muscular fitness

## PREVENTION

- Avoid succinylcholine use
- Use a higher dose of succinylcholine (1.5 mg/kg causes less myalgias than 1 mg/kg)
- Low-dose non-depolarizing muscle relaxants (e.g., 0.04 mg/kg rocuronium 2 min before succinylcholine), use cautiously (risk of potentially serious side effects)
- Lidocaine (1.5 mg/kg just before succinylcholine)
- Magnesium
- Non-steroidal anti-inflammatory drugs (e.g., 75 mg diclofenac 20 min before surgery)

## MANAGEMENT

- Postoperative muscle stretching exercises
- High-dose vitamin C

## SUGGESTED READING

- Gulenay M, Mathai JK. Depolarizing Neuromuscular Blocking Drugs. [Updated 2022 Nov 17]. In: StatPearls [Internet]. Treasure Island (FL): StatPearls Publishing; 2022 Jan-. Available from: https://www.ncbi.nlm.nih.gov/books/NBK532996/
- Schreiber JU, Lysakowski C, Fuchs-Buder T, Tramèr MR. Prevention of succinylcholine-induced fasciculation and myalgia: a meta-analysis of randomized trials. Anesthesiology. 2005;103(4):877-884.

# NEUROANESTHESIA

# ACUTE SPINAL CORD INJURY

## LEARNING OBJECTIVES

- Describe the mechanisms of and recognize acute spinal cord injury
- Classify spinal cord injury
- Manage patients with acute spinal cord injury

## DEFINITION AND MECHANISM

- Spinal cord injury (SCI) consists of damage to the spinal cord caused by an insult resulting in the transient or permanent loss of spinal motor, sensory, and autonomic function
- Approximately 14% of vertebral column fractures result in damage to the spinal cord

## ASSESSMENT

- Diaphragmatic breathing
- Hypotension without an obvious cause
- Bradycardia
- Priapism
- Flaccid areflexia
- Loss of pain response below a level

## PATHOPHYSIOLOGY

- Primary injury
  - Results from direct cord compression, hemorrhage, and traction forces
  - Mechanisms:
    - Subluxation of the vertebral elements causes a pincer-like direct damage to the cord
    - Hyperextension can cause compression of the cord between the ligamentum flavum and anterior osteophytes
    - Retropulsion of bone or disc fragments can cause either damage to the cord via direct cord compression or via impairment to the vascular supply
    - Penetrating injury can also cause direct compression and vascular injury
- Secondary injury
  - Within minutes after injury, secondary damage starts developing
  - Hemorrhage in the central grey matter damages neuronal cell membranes
  - Spinal cord edema and subsequent spinal cord ischemia
  - Ischemia extends bidirectionally, along the site of injury within hours
  - Systemic effects, local vasomotor changes, the release of free radicals, intracellular electrolyte shifts, neurotransmitters, cord edema, disruption of cell metabolism, and cell death are all thought to be involved in secondary injury
  - Prevention of secondary injury may make a dramatic difference to the quality of life of patients
- Neurogenic shock
  - Interruption of autonomic pathways leading to hypotension, bradycardia, and hypothermia
- Spinal shock
  - Loss of reflexes below the level of SCI
  - Gradual return of reflex activity when the reflex arcs below redevelop, often resulting in spasticity and autonomic hyperreflexia

# CLASSIFICATION

## American Spinal Injury (ASIA) impairment scale:

| | |
|---|---|
| A: Complete | No motor or sensory function is preserved in the sacral segments S4-5 |
| B: Sensory incomplete | Sensory but not motor function is preserved below the neurologic level & includes the sacral segments |
| C: Motor incomplete | Motor function is preserved below the neurologic level & more than half of key muscle functions below the neurologic level of injury have a muscle grade < 3 |
| D: Motor incomplete | Motor function is preserved below the neurologic level & at least half (half or more) of key muscle functions below the neurologic level of injury have a muscle grade ≥ 3 |
| E: Normal | Sensation & motor function are graded as normal in all segments |

# MANAGEMENT

### ACUTE SPINAL CORD INJURY MANAGEMENT

**Main goal: Minimize secondary injury**

→ Immobilize spine with hard collar

→ Keep patient well oxygenated

→ Prevent hypoxemia, hypotension, hyperglycemia, hyperthermia

**Airway considerations**
- Increased risk of regurgitation and pulmonary aspiration
- Minimize cervical spine movement during laryngoscopy using manual in-line stabilization
- Difficult airway equipment including a fiber-optic bronchoscope should be immediately available

**Cardiovascular considerations**
- Early catheterization is essential not only as a marker of renal perfusion but also to avoid bladder overdistension
- Maintain mean arterial pressure at 85-95 mmHg for 5-7 days (IV fluids, vasopressors)
- Avoid systemic blood pressure < 90 mmHg
- Avoid intraoperative blood loss

**Multimodal intraoperative monitoring**
- Somatosensory evoked potentials
- Motor evoked potentials
- Spontaneous EMG activity
- NOTE: volatile anesthetics interfere with motor evoked potential monitoring

EMG, Electromyography; SCI, Spinal cord injury

# SUGGESTED READING

- Bonner S, Smith C. Initial management of acute spinal cord injury. Continuing Education in Anaesthesia Critical Care & Pain. 2013;13(6):224-31.
- Dooney N, Dagal A. Anesthetic considerations in acute spinal cord trauma. Int J Crit Illn Inj Sci. 2011;1(1):36-43.

# ANEURYSM COILING

## LEARNING OBJECTIVES

- Describe the mechanisms of aneurysms and hemorrhage
- Describe the risk factors for aneurysms
- Recognize and treat aneurysmal hemorrhage
- Manage patients undergoing endovascular coiling

## DEFINITION AND MECHANISM

- Stroke is the second leading cause of death and the third most common cause of disability worldwide
- Hemorrhagic strokes account for about 32% of all strokes globally and can be caused by subarachnoid hemorrhage or intracerebral hemorrhage
- Most spontaneous (non-traumatic) subarachnoid hemorrhages are caused by ruptured saccular aneurysms
- Intracranial aneurysms are estimated to occur with a prevalence of 3.2% in the general population
- Aneurysmal subarachnoid hemorrhage accounts for approximately 5% of strokes and is caused by the rupture of an intracranial aneurysm, an acquired focal abnormal dilation of an arterial wall

## ANEURYSM RISK FACTORS

- Smoking
- Hypertension
- Connective tissue disorders
- Autosomal dominant polycystic kidney disease
- Ehlers–Danlos syndrome type IV

- Neurofibromatosis type 1
- Marfan syndrome
- Coarctation of the aorta
- Genetic predisposition

## HEMORRHAGE: SIGNS & SYMPTOMS

- Sudden onset of "worst headache of their life"
- Loss of consciousness
- Nausea and/or vomiting

- Nuchal rigidity
- Photophobia
- Seizure

## HEMORRHAGE TREATMENT

- Immediate management: Directed at stabilizing life-threatening conditions, minimizing neurologic injury, optimizing physiology and planning definitive care
  - Ensure a patent airway and adequate oxygenation and ventilation
  - Control acute hypertension
  - External ventricular drain
  - Control of headache with analgesics, anxiolysis, and bed rest
  - Stop and reverse anticoagulant therapy
  - Administer nimodipine (60 mg orally or by nasogastric tube every 4h, starting within 48h of hemorrhage and continued for 21 days)
- Definitive care
  - Surgical clipping or endovascular coiling

# MANAGEMENT

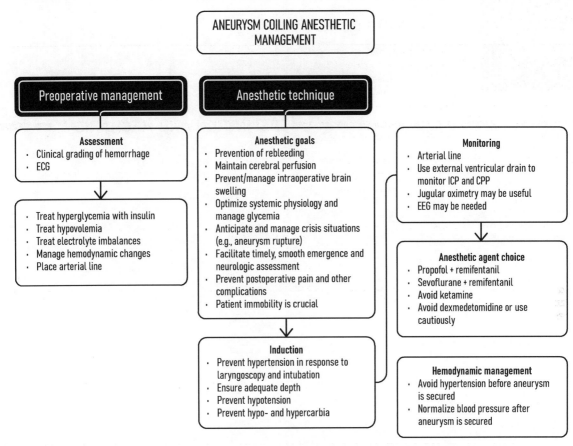

ICP, intracranial pressure; CPP, cerebral perfusion pressure

## KEEP IN MIND

- The optimal anesthetic technique depends on patient characteristics, severity of the aneurysm, and monitoring

## SUGGESTED READING

- Abd-Elsayed AA, Wehby AS, Farag E. Anesthetic management of patients with intracranial aneurysms. Ochsner J. 2014;14(3):418-425.
- Campos JK, Lien BV, Wang AS, Lin LM. Advances in endovascular aneurysm management: coiling and adjunctive devices. Stroke Vasc Neurol. 2020;5(1):14-21. Published 2020 Mar 15.
- Deepak Sharma; Perioperative Management of Aneurysmal Subarachnoid Hemorrhage: A Narrative Review. Anesthesiology 2020; 133:1283-1305

# AUTONOMIC DYSREFLEXIA

## LEARNING OBJECTIVES

- Define and describe autonomic dysreflexia
- Recognize signs and symptoms of autonomic dysreflexia
- Manage patients with autonomic dysreflexia

## DEFINITION AND MECHANISM

- Autonomic dysreflexia is a condition that emerges after a spinal cord injury, usually when the damage has occurred above the T6 level
- Dysregulation of the autonomic nervous system leads to an uncoordinated sympathetic response that may result in a potentially life-threatening hypertensive episode when there is a noxious stimulus below the level of the spinal cord injury
- Noxious stimuli consist usually of bladder or bowel distension
- The higher the injury, the greater the severity of the cardiovascular dysfunction
- Significantly increased risk of stroke by 300% to 400%

## SIGNS & SYMPTOMS

- Severe headache
- Hypertension
- Piloerection above the level of injury
- Bradycardia
- Facial flushing
- Pallor
- Cold skin

- Reduction in sweating below the level of the injury
- Visual disturbances
- Constricted pupils
- Nasal stuffiness
- Anxiety or feelings of doom
- Nausea and vomiting
- Dizziness

## EVALUATION

- Identify patients at risk (injury above T6)
- Document baseline blood pressure
- When severe headache occurs, measure blood pressure
- A systolic blood pressure > 150 mmHg or a diastolic blood pressure > 40 mmHg above baseline is indicative of autonomic dysreflexia

# ANESTHETIC MANAGEMENT

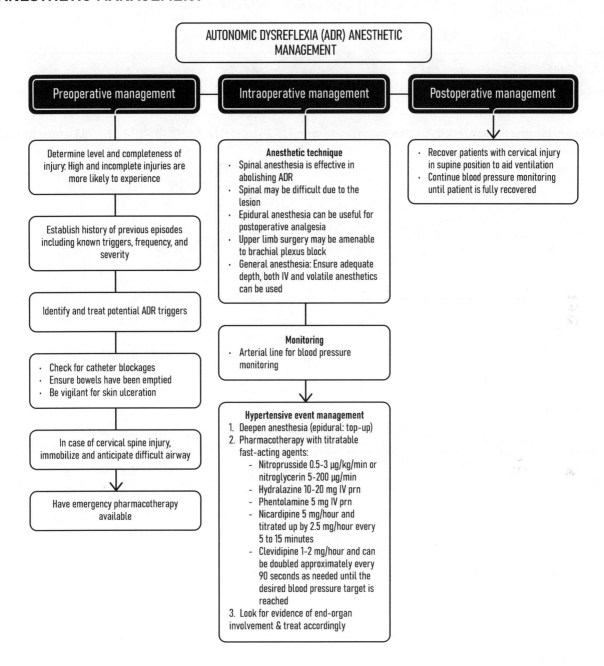

AUTONOMIC DYSREFLEXIA (ADR) ANESTHETIC MANAGEMENT

**Preoperative management**

- Determine level and completeness of injury. High and incomplete injuries are more likely to experience

- Establish history of previous episodes including known triggers, frequency, and severity

- Identify and treat potential ADR triggers

- Check for catheter blockages
- Ensure bowels have been emptied
- Be vigilant for skin ulceration

- In case of cervical spine injury, immobilize and anticipate difficult airway

- Have emergency pharmacotherapy available

**Intraoperative management**

**Anesthetic technique**
- Spinal anesthesia is effective in abolishing ADR
- Spinal may be difficult due to the lesion
- Epidural anesthesia can be useful for postoperative analgesia
- Upper limb surgery may be amenable to brachial plexus block
- General anesthesia: Ensure adequate depth, both IV and volatile anesthetics can be used

**Monitoring**
- Arterial line for blood pressure monitoring

**Hypertensive event management**
1. Deepen anesthesia (epidural: top-up)
2. Pharmacotherapy with titratable fast-acting agents:
   - Nitroprusside 0.5-3 µg/kg/min or nitroglycerin 5-200 µg/min
   - Hydralazine 10-20 mg IV prn
   - Phentolamine 5 mg IV prn
   - Nicardipine 5 mg/hour and titrated up by 2.5 mg/hour every 5 to 15 minutes
   - Clevidipine 1-2 mg/hour and can be doubled approximately every 90 seconds as needed until the desired blood pressure target is reached
3. Look for evidence of end-organ involvement & treat accordingly

**Postoperative management**

- Recover patients with cervical injury in supine position to aid ventilation
- Continue blood pressure monitoring until patient is fully recovered

## SUGGESTED READING

- Allen KJ, Leslie SW. Autonomic Dysreflexia. [Updated 2022 Nov 28]. In: StatPearls [Internet]. Treasure Island (FL): StatPearls Publishing; 2022 Jan-. Available from: https://www.ncbi.nlm.nih.gov/books/NBK482434/
- Petsas A, Drake J. Perioperative management for patients with a chronic spinal cord injury. BJA Education. 2015;15(3):123-30.

# CHIARI MALFORMATION

## LEARNING OBJECTIVES

- Types of a Chiari malformation
- Management of a Chiari malformation

## DEFINITION AND MECHANISM

- Chiari malformation is a structural defect in the cerebellum, characterized by a downward displacement of one or both cerebellar tonsils through the foramen magnum
- Occurs when part of the skull is misshapen or smaller than typical, pressing on the brain and forcing the brain downward
  - Congenital causes include hydrocephalus, craniosynostosis, hyperostosis, X-linked vitamin D-resistant rickets, and neurofibromatosis type I
  - Acquired disorders include space-occupying lesions due to brain tumors or hematomas and traumatic brain injury
- Most patients have no signs or symptoms and do not require treatment
- Other conditions associated with Chiari malformation include:
  - Hydrocephalus
  - Syringomyelia
  - Spina bifida
  - Spinal curvature
  - Tethered spinal cord syndrome
  - Ehlers-Danlos syndrome
  - Marfan syndrome

## TYPES OF CHIARI MALFORMATION

- The type depends on the anatomy of the brain tissue that is displaced and whether developmental problems are present:

| Type 1 | Type 2 |
|---|---|
| Occurs when the lower part of the cerebellum pushes into the foramen magnum<br>Signs or symptoms may not occur until late childhood or adulthood and is often first noticed by accident during an examination for another condition<br>Most common type and is not considered life-threatening | Congenital pediatric forms<br>A greater amount of cerebellum and brain stem tissue extends into the spinal compared with that in Chiari malformation type 1<br>The nerve tissue connecting both halves of the cerebellum may be missing or only partially formed<br>Nearly always accompanied by myelomeningocele, a form of spina bifida that occurs when the spinal canal and backbone do not close before birth<br>Often seen on ultrasound during pregnancy<br>Symptoms of Type II usually appear during childhood and are generally more severe than in Type 1<br>The term Arnold-Chiari malformation is specific to Type II malformations |
| **Type 3** | **Type 4** |
| Most serious form<br>A portion of the lower back part of the cerebellum or the brainstem extends through an abnormal opening in the back of the skull, possibly including the membranes surrounding the brain or spinal cord<br>Diagnosed with ultrasound during pregnancy or at birth<br>Can cause debilitating and life-threatening complications<br>Associated with severe neurological defects | An incomplete or underdeveloped cerebellum (cerebellar hypoplasia)<br>The cerebellum is in its normal position but parts are missing and portions of the skull and spinal cord may be visible |

# SIGNS AND SYMPTOMS

- Neurogenic dysphagia
- Cyanosis
- Weak crying
- Facial weakness
- Aspiration
- Headaches
- Tinnitus
- Lhermitte's sign
- Vertigo (dizziness)
- Nausea
- Schmahmann syndrome
- Nystagmus
- Facial pain
- Muscle weakness
- Impaired gag reflex
- Restless leg syndrome

- Sleep apnea
- Sleep disorders
- Impaired coordination
- Severe cases may develop all the symptoms and signs of a bulbar palsy
- Paralysis
- Papilledema on the fundoscopic exam due to increased intracranial pressure
- Pupillary dilation
- Dysautonomia:
  - Tachycardia
  - Syncope
  - Polydipsia
  - Chronic fatigue
- Opisthotonos
- Stridor

# DIAGNOSIS

- Patient history
- Neurological examination
- MRI/CT
- Ultrasound for Chiari II malformation

# MANAGEMENT

## Management of Chiari malformation

### Perioperative management

**Be aware of:**
- Difficult airway management
- Cervical spine fusion at the craniovertebral junction and thus a limited range of motion
- Autonomic dysfunction leading to unstable hemodynamics, lack of compensatory response to hyperthermia, hypotension, hypoxia, and hypocarbia
- Increased intracranial pressure (ICP) or hydrocephalus
- Increased ICP during head and neck movements and laryngoscopy
- Abnormal sensitivity to neuromuscular blocking agents

**Monitor:**
- Pulse oximetry
- Invasive arterial blood pressure
- Capnography
- Intracranial pressure
- Muscle relaxation
- Blood gases

**Maintain:**
- Normocapnia
- Normothermia

GA can lead to hypotension and if associated with increased ICP, leads to a decreased intracranial perfusion pressure

**Consider:**
- Nasal intubation topicalize with local anesthetic + use fiberoptic intubation
- The use of a videolaryngoscopy or awake fiberoptic intubation
- Regional anesthesia → to keep intracranial pressure and hemodynamics as stable as possible

**Avoid:**
- Flexion-extension of the neck to prevent further compression of the neural structure
- A sudden increase in ICP:
  Avoid high airway pressures
  Use intravenous anesthetics, except ketamine → more advantageous compared with volatile anesthetics to decrease ICP
- The use of succinylcholine
- Overdosing with non-depolarizing muscle relaxants

### Postoperative management

Carefully plan extubation

Consider postoperative respiratory support with slow weaning

Monitor the patient closely in the first 24 hours because of the risk of sudden apnea or cardiac arrest associated with autonomic dysfunction

## SUGGESTED READING

- Anesthetic management of a patient with Arnold-Chiari malformation type I with associated syringomyelia: A case report Anesth Pain Med. 2012;7(2):166-169.
- Coviello A, Golino L, Posillipo C, Marra A, Tognù A, Servillo G. Anesthetic management in a patient with Arnold-Chiari malformation type 1,5: A case report. Clin Case Rep. 2022;10(2):e05194.

# CRANIOTOMY

## LEARNING OBJECTIVES

- Describe the principle, indications and contraindications of craniotomy
- Manage patients undergoing craniotomy

## DEFINITION AND MECHANISM

- Craniotomy is a surgical procedure in which a part of the skull is temporarily removed to expose the brain and perform an intracranial procedure

## INDICATIONS

- Brain aneurysm
- Vascular malformations (arterio-venous malformation, cavernous angioma, arterio-venous fistula)
- Brain tumors (meningioma, high-grade and low-grade glioma, epidermoid, ependymoma, oligodendroglioma, gliobastoma multiforme, diffuse midline glioma, metastases)
- Orbital tumors
- Pituitary adenomas
- Cerebellopontine angle tumors
- Pain treatment (microvascular decompression)
- Brain abscess
- Subdural empyema
- Hematomas (intracerebral, epidural, subdural)
- Decompressive craniectomy
- Lobectomy
- Epilepsy surgery
- Craniosynostosis
- Depressed skull fractures
- Intracranial foreign bodies
- Cerebrospinal fluid leak repair

## CONTRAINDICATIONS

- Advanced age/frailty
- Poor functional status (< 4 METS)
- Severe cardiopulmonary disease
- Severe systemic collapse (sepsis, multiorgan failure)
- Pathologies that can be addressed by a single burr hole
- Altered preoperative coagulation parameters
- Uncorrected bleeding disorders

# MANACEMENT

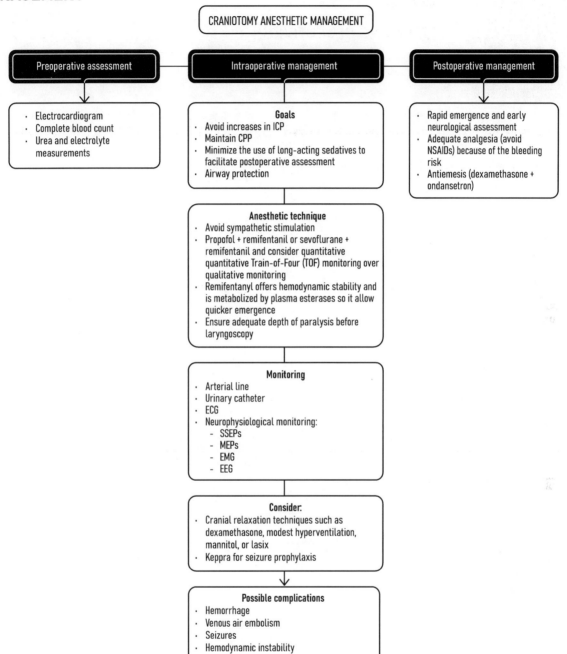

**CRANIOTOMY ANESTHETIC MANAGEMENT**

**Preoperative assessment**
- Electrocardiogram
- Complete blood count
- Urea and electrolyte measurements

**Intraoperative management**

**Goals**
- Avoid increases in ICP
- Maintain CPP
- Minimize the use of long-acting sedatives to facilitate postoperative assessment
- Airway protection

**Anesthetic technique**
- Avoid sympathetic stimulation
- Propofol + remifentanil or sevoflurane + remifentanil and consider quantitative quantitative Train-of-Four (TOF) monitoring over qualitative monitoring
- Remifentanyl offers hemodynamic stability and is metabolized by plasma esterases so it allow quicker emergence
- Ensure adequate depth of paralysis before laryngoscopy

**Monitoring**
- Arterial line
- Urinary catheter
- ECG
- Neurophysiological monitoring:
  - SSEPs
  - MEPs
  - EMG
  - EEG

**Consider:**
- Cranial relaxation techniques such as dexamethasone, modest hyperventilation, mannitol, or lasix
- Keppra for seizure prophylaxis

**Possible complications**
- Hemorrhage
- Venous air embolism
- Seizures
- Hemodynamic instability

**Postoperative management**
- Rapid emergence and early neurological assessment
- Adequate analgesia (avoid NSAIDs) because of the bleeding risk
- Antiemesis (dexamethasone + ondansetron)

SSEP, somatosensory evoked potential; MEP, motor evoked potential; EMG, electromyography, EEG, electroencephalography

# SUGGESTED READING

- Dinsmore J. Anaesthesia for elective neurosurgery. BJA: British Journal of Anaesthesia. 2007;99(1):68-74.
- Fernández-de Thomas RJ, De Jesus O. Craniotomy. [Updated 2022 Apr 9]. In: StatPearls [Internet]. Treasure Island (FL): StatPearls Publishing; 2022 Jan-. Available from: https://www.ncbi.nlm.nih.gov/books/NBK560922/
- Keown, T., Bhangu, S. and Solanki3, S. (2022) Anaesthesia for craniotomy and brain tumour resection, WFSA. Available at: https://resources.wfsahq.org/atotw/anaesthesia-for-craniotomy-and-brain-tumour-resection/ (Accessed: January 18, 2023).

# EPILEPSY

## LEARNING OBJECTIVES

- Definition of epilepsy
- Anesthetic management of epilepsy

## DEFINITION AND MECHANISM

- Epilepsy is a central nervous system (neurological) disorder in which brain activity becomes abnormal, causing seizures or periods of unusual behavior, sensations, and sometimes loss of awareness
- It is characterized by recurrent (2 or more) seizures which means that having a single seizure does not mean that a patient also has epilepsy
- Normal regulatory functions are altered in epileptogenic disorders
- The standard treatment for adults with epilepsy is antiepileptic drug (AED) therapy
- Approximately 20-30% of patients remain refractory to drug therapy or develop intolerable side effects and resective surgery may be considered
- Epilepsy occurs in approximately 1 in 200 of the general population

## SIGNS AND SYMPTOMS

- Seizures
- Temporary confusion
- A staring spell
- Stiff muscles

- Uncontrollable jerking movements of the arms and legs
- Loss of consciousness or awareness
- Psychological symptoms such as fear, anxiety, or deja vu

## CLASSIFICATION

- Generalized epilepsy
  - Tonic-clonic
  - Absence
  - Myoclonic
  - Clonic
  - Tonic
  - Atonic

- Focal seizures
  - Simple
  - Complex
  - Evolving to generalized
- Mixed seizures (focal and generalized)
- Unclassified

## CAUSES

- Most cases are idiopathic and a definite cause is only found in 25%-35%
- Specific causes include:
  - Genetic: juvenile myoclonic epilepsy
  - Trauma: depressed skull fractures or intracranial hemorrhage
  - Tumors: particularly slow-growing frontal tumors

  - Infection: meningitis or encephalitis
  - Cerebrovascular disease: 6%-15% of stroke patients
  - Alcohol: lowers the seizure threshold
  - Others: dementia, multiple sclerosis, metabolic disorders

## RISK FACTORS

- Young or older age
- Familial history
- Head injury
- Stroke and other vascular diseases

- Dementia
- Infection (e.g., meningitis)
- Seizures in childhood

# COMPLICATIONS

- Status epilepticus
- Sudden unexpected death in epilepsy

# DIAGNOSIS

- At least two unprovoked (or reflex) seizures occurring more than 24 hours apart
- One unprovoked (or reflex) seizure and a probability of further seizures similar to the general recurrence risk (at least 60%) after two unprovoked seizures, occurring over the next 10 years
- Witnessed seizures
- Tests:
  - EEG
  - CT, MRI
  - Blood glucose
  - ECG

# ANTI-EPILEPTIC AGENTS

- The aim is to achieve a seizure-free patient with minimal drug-related side-effects
- Consider the seizure type and history, patient age, and side effects to choose the correct anticonvulsant
- Monotherapy will control seizures in many patients but some require the addition of second or third-line agents

| Agent | Side-effects |
|---|---|
| Phenytoin | Skin rash, drowsiness, ataxia, slurred speech, gingival hypertrophy, excess hair growth, anemias, neuropathy |
| Sodium Valproate | Tremor, drowsiness, weight gain, alopecia, raised hepatic transaminase, thrombocytopenia |
| Carbamazepine | Rash, double vision, ataxia, hyponatremia, thrombocytopenia |
| Phenobarbital | Drowsiness, rash, osteomalacia, anaemia, folate deficiency |
| Ethosuximide | Nausea, drowsiness, anorexia, photophobia |
| Lamotrigine | Rash, drowsiness, double vision, headache, insomnia, tremor, flu-like symptoms |
| Levetiracetam | Dizziness, drowsiness, insomnia, ataxia, tremor, headache, behavioral problems |
| Primidone | Nausea, nystagmus, sedation, anemias, ataxia |
| Vigabatrin | Visual field defects, drowsiness, psychotic reactions |
| Gabapentin | Drowsiness, dizziness, headache |
| Clobazam | Drowsiness, tolerance |

# MANAGEMENT

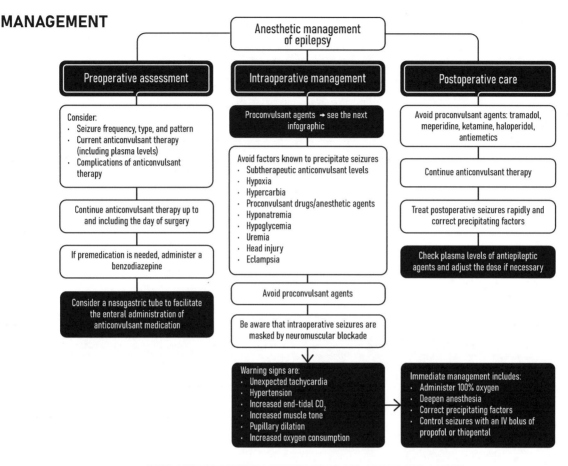

## Anesthetic management of epilepsy

### Preoperative assessment

Consider:
- Seizure frequency, type, and pattern
- Current anticonvulsant therapy (including plasma levels)
- Complications of anticonvulsant therapy

Continue anticonvulsant therapy up to and including the day of surgery

If premedication is needed, administer a benzodiazepine

Consider a nasogastric tube to facilitate the enteral administration of anticonvulsant medication

### Intraoperative management

Proconvulsant agents → see the next infographic

Avoid factors known to precipitate seizures
- Subtherapeutic anticonvulsant levels
- Hypoxia
- Hypercarbia
- Proconvulsant drugs/anesthetic agents
- Hyponatremia
- Hypoglycemia
- Uremia
- Head injury
- Eclampsia

Avoid proconvulsant agents

Be aware that intraoperative seizures are masked by neuromuscular blockade

Warning signs are:
- Unexpected tachycardia
- Hypertension
- Increased end-tidal $CO_2$
- Increased muscle tone
- Pupillary dilation
- Increased oxygen consumption

Immediate management includes:
- Administer 100% oxygen
- Deepen anesthesia
- Correct precipitating factors
- Control seizures with an IV bolus of propofol or thiopental

### Postoperative care

Avoid proconvulsant agents: tramadol, meperidine, ketamine, haloperidol, antiemetics

Continue anticonvulsant therapy

Treat postoperative seizures rapidly and correct precipitating factors

Check plasma levels of antiepileptic agents and adjust the dose if necessary

## INTERACTIONS BETWEEN ANTIEPILEPTIC AND ANESTHETIC AGENTS

### INTRAVENOUS INDUCTION AGENTS

- Propofol is an anticonvulsant at anesthetic doses and is safe to use
- Thiopental is an anticonvulsant at anesthetic doses and is safe to use
- Most barbiturates are anticonvulsant at normal clinical doses and are safe to use
- Ketamine is an anticonvulsant at anesthetic doses and is safe to use
- Benzodiazepines (e.g., midazolam) are all potent anticonvulsants and are safe to use
- Avoid etomidate as it prolongs seizures and is frequently associated with postoperative seizures

### INHALATIONAL AGENTS AND NITROUS OXIDE

- Most inhalation agents are safe to use
- Avoid enflurane as it causes postoperative seizures
- Nitrous oxide is safe to use

### OPIOIDS

- Most opioids are safe to use because of their long history of safe use
- Remifentanil is safe to use
- Avoid tramadol as this lowers the seizures threshold
- Avoid meperidine as this is a potent proconvulsant
- Avoid alfentanil as this is a potent enhancer of EEG activity

### NEUROMUSCULAR BLOCKERS

- Non-depolarizing neuromuscular blockers (NMBs) are safe to use
- However, use them with caution as they may mask seizure activity
- Avoid succinylcholine → hyperkalemia, especially in status epilepticus patients
- Apply neuromuscular monitoring as the dose and frequency of these drugs may need to be adjusted

### ANTIEMETICS

Dopamine antagonists are particulary associated with extrapyramidal effects and acute dystonic reactions
Which might be confused with seizure activity
- Avoid phenothiazines (e.g., prochlorperazine)
- Avoid benzamides (e.g., metoclopramide)
- Avoid bytorophenones (e.g., droperidol)

### LOCAL ANESTHETICS

- Can readily cross the blood-brain barrier
- Result in seizures if plasma levels are too high
- Avoid high plasma levels of lidocaine as it provokes seizures

## SUGGESTED READING

- Carter, E.L., Adapa, R.M., 2015. Adult epilepsy and anaesthesia. BJA Education 15, 111–117.
- Pollard BJ, Kitchen, G. Handbook of Clinical Anaesthesia. Fourth Edition. CRC Press. 2018. 978-1-4987-6289-2.

Epilepsy

# 157

# HYDROCEPHALUS

## LEARNING OBJECTIVES

- Define hydrocephalus
- Describe the age-related signs and symptoms of hydrocephalus
- Anesthetic management of a patient with hydrocephalus

## DEFINITION AND MECHANISM

- Hydrocephalus is the excess accumulation of cerebrospinal fluid (CSF) in the ventricular system of the brain, resulting in increased intracranial pressure (ICP)
- It is caused by obstruction to CSF flow in the ventricles or subarachnoid space, or by excess CSF production from a congenital malformation blocking normal drainage or from complications of head injuries or infections
- Hydrocephalus can happen at any age but occurs more frequently among infants and older adults (> 60 years)

## SIGNS AND SYMPTOMS

The signs and symptoms vary by the age of onset

### Infants

- Changes in the head
  □ Unusually large head
  □ Rapid increase in the size of the head
  □ Bulging or tense soft spot (fontanel) on the top of the head
- Physical signs and symptoms
  □ Nausea and vomiting
  □ Sleepiness or lethargy
  □ Irritability
  □ Poor eating
  □ Seizures
  □ Reduced upward gaze (Parinaud's syndrome)
  □ Problems with muscle tone and strength

### Toddlers and older children

- Physical signs and symptoms
  □ Headache
  □ Blurred or double vision
  □ Abnormal eye movements
  □ Abnormal enlargement of the head
  □ Sleepiness or lethargy
  □ Nausea or vomiting
  □ Unstable balance
  □ Poor coordination
  □ Poor appetite
  □ Loss of bladder control or frequent urination

- Behavioral and cognitive changes
  □ Irritability
  □ Change in personality
  □ Decline in school performance
  □ Delays or problems with previously acquired skills (e.g., walking, talking)

### Young and middle-aged adults

- Headache
- Lethargy
- Loss of coordination or balance
- Loss of bladder control or frequent urination
- Vision problems
- Decline in memory, concentration, and other thinking skills

### Older adults (> 60 years)

- Loss of bladder control or frequent urination
- Memory loss
- Progressive loss of other thinking or reasoning skills
- Gait disturbance
- Poor coordination or balance

## CAUSES

Noncommunicating hydrocephalus: Obstruction of CSF outflow
- Space-occupying lesion
- Subarachnoid or intraventricular hemorrhage
- Spina bifida
- Arnold-Chiari malformation
- Dandy-Walker malformation
- Head injury
- Aqueductal stenosis
- Tumors

Communicating hydrocephalus: Failure of absorption of CSF by the arachnoid villi

- Subarachnoid or intraventricular hemorrhage
- Meningitis
- Head injury
- Achondroplasia
- Craniofacial syndromes
- Other skull base deformities
- Choroid plexus papilloma or carcinoma

Hydrocephalus

# RISK FACTORS

## Newborns

- Abnormal development of the central nervous system that obstructs the CSF flow
- Bleeding within the ventricles (i.e., intraventricular hemorrhage), a possible complication of premature birth
- Infection in the uterus (e.g., rubella or syphilis) during pregnancy may cause inflammation in the fetal brain tissues

## Other contributing factors

- Lesions or tumors of the brain or spinal cord
- Central nervous system infections (e.g., bacterial meningitis or mumps)
- Bleeding in the brain from a stroke or head injury
- Other traumatic injury to the brain

# TREATMENT

- **Short-term (acute and emergency situations)**: External ventricular drain or ventriculostomy
  - Inserted into the frontal horn of the lateral ventricle
  - Drain reduces the ICP and allows to measure ICP
  - Only short-term management due to the risk of infection

- **Long-term**: Cerebral shunt
  - Allows drainage of CSF to distal sites
  - Placement of a ventricular catheter into the cerebral ventricles to bypass the flow obstruction/malfunctioning arachnoid villi and drain the excess CSF into other body cavities from where it can be resorbed
  - Most shunts drain fluid into the peritoneal cavity (ventriculoperitoneal shunt), alternative sites include the right atrium (ventriculoatrial shunt), pleural cavity (ventriculopleural shunt), and gallbladder
  - The shunt can also be placed in the lumbar space of the spine to redirect the CSF to the peritoneal cavity (lumboperitoneal shunt)

# MANAGEMENT

```
                          HYDROCEPHALUS
         ┌──────────────────────┼──────────────────────┐
  Preoperative         Intraoperative management      Postoperative
  management                                           management
```

**Preoperative management**

- Standard anesthetic history and examination
- Assess patients for signs of raised ICP (i.e., headache, vomiting, and altered level of consciousness)
- Vomiting can lead to dehydration and electrolyte imbalance
- Emergency patients are often already intubated and ventilated in ICU or arrive as an emergency transfer
- Blocked shunts can present as acute cases where patients may have a full stomach or decreased consciousness level

**Intraoperative management**

- Routine anesthetic monitoring
- Inhalational or intravenous induction if a full stomach is not a consideration
- Rapid sequence induction may be required in the emergency situation (full stomach or vomiting)
- Patients are typically placed in the supine position; lateral position is required for a lumboperitoneal shunt
- The head may be held in the three-point pin system to facilitate some shunt and endoscopic procedures
- Bolus doses of opioids to cover the period of subcutaneous tunneling during shunt surgery as it is highly stimulating
- Complications
  - Hypotension following the release of CSF and reduction in ICP
  - Bradycardia
  - Subcutaneous tunneling of the distal portion of the shunt may cause pneumothorax or hemothorax
  - Significant risk of air embolism during ventriculoatrial shunt creation

**Postoperative management**

- Wake patients with minimal coughing and straining
- Some emergency cases should be kept intubated and ventilated
- Analgesia with paracetamol and NSAIDs; morphine may be required for the first 24 hours
- New focal neurological signs prompt an urgent CT scan to rule out intracranial hematoma

ICP, intracranial pressure; ICU, intensive care unit; CSF, cerebrospinal fluid; NSAIDs, nonsteroidal anti-inflammatory drugs.

# SUGGESTED READING

- Krovvidi H, Flint G, Williams AV. Perioperative management of hydrocephalus. BJA Educ. 2018;18(5):140-146.
- Pollard BJ, Kitchen G. Handbook of Clinical Anaesthesia. 4th ed. Taylor & Francis group; 2018. Chapter 14 Neurosurgery, Chapman E.

# 158

# MÉNIÈRE'S DISEASE

## LEARNING OBJECTIVES

- Describe the clinical features of Ménière's disease
- Diagnose Ménière's disease
- Treat Ménière's disease

## DEFINITION AND MECHANISM

- Ménière's disease is an inner ear disorder characterized by intermittent, spontaneous episodes of vertigo, tinnitus, and hearing loss
- Possibly caused by the accumulation of endolymphatic fluid in the cochlea and vestibular organ (endolymphatic hydrops)
- Often progresses slowly, leading to end-organ damage
- The exact etiology remains unknown
- Significantly impacts the social functioning of the affected patient

## DIAGNOSIS

- A full and accurate diagnosis may take months to attain
- Diagnostic criteria:
  - Two or more spontaneous attacks of vertigo, each lasting 20 minutes to 12 hours
  - Audiometrically documented fluctuating low- to medium-frequency sensorineural hearing loss in the affected ear on at least 1 occasion before, during, or after one of the episodes of vertigo
  - Fluctuating aural symptoms (hearing loss, tinnitus, or fullness) in the affected ear
  - Other causes excluded by other tests
- Probable Ménière's disease can include:
  - At least 2 episodes of vertigo or dizziness lasting 20 minutes to 24 hours
  - Fluctuating aural symptoms (hearing loss, tinnitus, or fullness) in the affected ear
  - Other causes excluded by other tests
- Differentiation between vertigo of central, peripheral, and cardiovascular origin
- Full otologic history
- Question the patient about the characteristics of vertigo, hearing loss, and earlier episodes of these symptoms
- Note the duration of vertigo and hearing loss episodes, as well as any potential triggers
- Evaluate family history of hearing and balance problems
- Complete physical examination including a comprehensive neurological examination
- Document peripheral sensation in all extremities
- Examine gait
- Cerebellar diagnostic tests
- Conduct Romberg, Fukuda, and pronator drift tests
- Perform the Dix-Hallpike maneuver with Frenzel goggles
- Document orthostatic blood pressures
- MRI
- Audiometric evaluation

| Condition | Clinical presentation | Differentiation from Ménière's disease |
|---|---|---|
| Autoimmune (e.g., multiple sclerosis) | Often progressive, fluctuating bilateral hearing loss that is responsive to steroid | May present with vision, skin, and joint problems |
| Benign paroxysmalpositional vertigo | Positional vertigo lasting less than a minute | Not associated with hearing loss, tinnitus, or aural fullness; short duration of vertigo episodes |
| Infectious (e.g., Lyme disease) | Viral (e.g., adenovirus) or bacterial (e.g., staphylococcus/streptococcus); can lead to complete hearing loss and vestibular crisis event with prolonged vertigo and/or hearing loss | Losses are often permanent and do not fluctuate; can present with severe otalgia and fever |
| Otosyphilis | Sudden unilateral or bilateral sensorineural fluctuating hearing loss, tinnitus, and/or vertigo | Vertigo attacks not typically accompanied by aural symptoms immediately before or after attacks |
| Stroke/ischemia | Vertigo may last for minutes with nausea, vomiting, and severe imbalance; may also include visual blurring and drop attacks | Insults are often permanent and do not fluctuate<br>May be comorbid with dysphagia, dysphonia, or other neurologic symptoms and signs<br>Usually no associated hearing loss or tinnitus |
| Vestibular migraine | Present with attacks lasting from minutes to over 24 hours, though they typically last for hours | Timing of attacks may be shorter or longer<br>Hearing loss less likely<br>Patients often have a migraine history<br>More photophobia than visual aura |
| Vestibular schwannoma | May present with vertigo, but the majority present with chronic imbalance, asymmetric hearing loss, and tinnitus | Chronic imbalance is more likely than profound episodic vertigo<br>Hearing loss does not typically fluctuate |
| Labyrinthitis | Sudden severe vertigo with profound hearing loss and prolonged vertigo (e.g., 24 hours) | Vertigo, nausea with hearing loss<br>Not episodic, not fluctuating |
| Vestibular neuritis | Viral infection of vestibular system; leads to acute prolonged vertigo with prolonged nausea, vomiting without hearing loss, tinnitus, or aural fullness<br>Severe rotational vertigo lasts 12 to 36 hours with decreasing disequilibrium for the next 4 to 5 days | Vertigo, nausea without hearing loss |

## RISK FACTORS

- Migraine
- Autoimmune diseases (rheumatoid arthritis, systemic lupus erythematosus, ankylosing spondylitis)
- Genetic component

## TREATMENT

- Thiazide diuretics
- Vestibular suppressants
- Betahistine
- Intratympanic steroid injection
- Intratympanic gentamycin injection
- Vestibular nerve section or labyrinthectomy
- Sodium restriction diet
- Caffeine restriction/elimination

## ANESTHETIC CONSIDERATIONS

- Surgical treatments can be performed under either local or general anesthesia
- Based on clinical experience, patients may not be able to lie down; in this case, general anesthesia is preferred

## SUGGESTED READING

- Basura GJ, Adams ME, Monfared A, Schwartz SR, Antonelli PJ, Burkard R, et al. Clinical Practice Guideline: Ménière's Disease. Otolaryngology-Head and Neck Surgery. 2020;162(2_suppl):S1-S55.
- Kersbergen CJ, Ward BK. A Historical Perspective on Surgical Manipulation of the Membranous Labyrinth for Treatment of Meniere's Disease. Frontiers in Neurology. 2021;12.
- Koenen L, Andaloro C. Meniere Disease. [Updated 2022 Sep 30]. In: StatPearls [Internet]. Treasure Island (FL): StatPearls Publishing; 2022 Jan-. Available from: https://www.ncbi.nlm.nih.gov/books/NBK536955/

# PITUITARY SURGERY

## LEARNING OBJECTIVES

- Describe the common indications for pituitary surgery
- Manage patients undergoing pituitary surgery

## DEFINITION AND MECHANISM

- Pituitary adenomas are common in clinical practice
- Pituitary adenomas can be classified as either functioning or nonfunctioning, depending on whether they secrete hormones
- Patients with functioning adenomas frequently present with symptoms of hormone excess
- Patients with nonfunctioning adenomas often present later and have symptoms resulting from the mass effect of the tumor, such as headaches, visual loss due to compression of the optic chiasm, and hypopituitarism due to compression of the anterior pituitary
- Common clinical conditions resulting from pituitary adenomas: Cushing's disease, acromegaly, prolactin overproduction, panhypopituitarism
- Surgical resection has become the primary therapy when medical treatment fails, with transsphenoidal pituitary surgery being the most common technique
- Transsphenoidal pituitary surgery presents unique challenges for anesthesia due to both the endocrine and neurosurgical management

### PITUITARY SURGERY: PREOPERATIVE ASSESSMENT

**Respiratory system**

- Excess growth hormone in acromelagics can lead to thickening of pharyngeal and laryngeal soft tissues, macroglossia, reduction in the size of the rima glottidis, and hypertrophy of the ariepiglottic folds, soft palate and epiglottis
- A hoarse voice or stridor may indicate recurrent laryngeal nerve palsy or laryngeal stenosis
- Acromegalics may have an enlarged thyroid which may cause tracheal compression
- Spirometry and indirect laryngoscopy may be of additional value
- Obstructive sleep apnea is common in acromegaly and Cushing's disease, identify and treat accordingly

**Cardiovascular**

- Routinely perform ECG in all patients
- Inverted T waves and high voltage QRS complexes are common in Cushing's disease
- Left ventricular hypertrophy, heart failure, arrythmias and ischemic heart disease are common in Cushing's disease and acromegaly patients
- Patients with chronic obstructive sleep apnea may be at increased risk of cor pulmonale
- Hypertension is common, should be controlled pharmacologically

**Neurological**

- Perform a thorough cranial nerve examination, with particular emphasis on visual acuity and visual fields
- Tumors compressing the optic chiasma can cause a bi-temporal hemianopia
- Identify symptoms of raised intracranial pressure
- Perform a pituitary MRI in all patients

**Endocrine**

- Diabetes mellitus and impaired glucose tolerance are common, a sliding scale insulin regime may be useful
- Measure T3, T4 and TSH and normalize thyroid function
- Measure basal prolactin and serum cortisol, many patients require perioperative glucocorticoid
- Assess hormone imbalance treatment

**Diagnostic investigations**

- Perform full blood count, urea and electrolytes and blood glucose
- Deranged sodium levels may indicate diabetes insipidus or inappropriate ADH secretion
- Chest X-ray, lateral view of X-ray neck, ECG, echocardiography, pulmonary function tests, hormonal assays and coagulation profile should be performed depending on the clinical condition
- Arterial blood gas analysis is essential in patients with sleep apnea syndrome and impaired pulmonary function

**Premedication**

- Continue antihypertensive, heart failure, bronchodilator and antacid medications
- Stop angiotensin converting enzyme inhibitors and diuretics
- Treat patients prone to gastro-esophageal reflux with an H2-receptor agonist and proton pump inhibitor (e.g., ranitidine. omeprazole)
- Initiate insulin sliding scale therapy for diabetic patients when appropriate
- Start glucocorticoid replacement when appropriate: 100 mg hydrocortisone at induction
- Avoid benzodiazepines and other sedatives to facilitate rapid emergence

T3, triiodothyronine; T4, thyroxine; TSH, thyroid-stimulating hormone; ADH, antidiuretic hormone

Pituitary surgery

# PITUITARY SURGERY: INTRAOPERATIVE MANAGEMENT

### Positioning

- Usually supine position with the head up and neck extended
- Head is held in position with a clamp and the pituitary region visualized via image intensifier
- Check all connections to the circuit prior to the start of surgery
- Protect pressure points and routinely pad the eyes

### Anesthetic technique

- Goals: Facilitate surgical exposure, preserve cerebral perfusion, avoid hypertensive surges and facilitate rapid emergence
- Any anesthetic technique suitable for intracranial surgery is acceptable, depending on the condition of each individual patient
- Take raised intracranial pressure into special consideration if present
- Fiber-optic intubation may be necessary if difficult intubation is suspected
- Propofol, sevoflurane or desflurane to facilitate rapid emergence
- Neuromuscular blocking (atracurium, vecuronium) is essential and needs to be continuously monitored to prevent coughing
- Remifentanil is valuable in periods of intense surgical stimulation

### Monitoring

- Routine monitoring: Pulse oximetry, ECG, temperature and capnography
- Invasive arterial blood pressure monitoring and large bore IV access
- Patients with acromegaly may have compromised ulnar blood flow, assess blood flow in radial and ulnar arteries prior to cannulation

### Surgical approach and surgical field

- Most common approach: Transsphenoidal
- Minimize bleeding from the nasal mucosa: Infiltration with xylometazoline or 1% lidocaine with epinephrine 1:200,000 for vasoconstriction
- Treat exaggerated hypertensive responses with phentolamine, beta-blockers, or short-acting opioids
- Insert a lumbar drain for tumors with significant suprasellar extension: Standard 16g epidural catheter at L3/L4

# PITUITARY SURGERY: POSTOPERATIVE MANAGEMENT

### Airway

- Increased risk of airway obstruction
- Ensure throat packs are removed
- Ideally, extubate in awake state to avoid aspiration of blood
- Oropharyngeal airway patency is essential
- Use continuous positive airway pressure only as a last resort and in a critical area
- Overnight pulse oximetry monitoring and supplementary oxygen for the postoperative nights

### Neurological assessment

- Smooth and rapid emergence to facilitate early neurological assessment
- Assessment of the integrity of the cranial nerves, particularly CN II-VI

### Analgesia

- Patients usually complain of a frontal headache postoperatively
- Codeine or stronger opioids when required
- Prophylactic antiemetics

### Possible complications & treatment

- Bleeding: venous bleeding may require packing, stop arterial bleeding by pharmacological reduction of blood pressure with IV induction agent or alpha- and beta-blockers. Postpone further surgery and transfer patient to ICU when arterial bleeding occurs
- CSF leak: leave the lumbar drain in place for 24-48 hours
- Diabetes insipidus: Provide access to free fluids and monitor electrolytes and urine
- Innapropriate ADH production syndrome: Restrict fluids, cautious use of hypertonic saline may be required

ADH, antidiuretic hormone

## SUGGESTED READING

- Dunn LK, Nemergut EC. Anesthesia for transsphenoidal pituitary surgery. Curr Opin Anaesthesiol. 2013;26(5):549-554.
- Griffiths S, Perks A. The Hypothalamic Pituitary Axis Part 2: Anaesthesia For Pituitary Surgery. WFSA. Published July 26, 2010. Accessed January 19, 2023. https://resources.wfsahq.org/atotw/the-hypothalamic-pituitary-axis-part-2-anaesthesia-for-pituitary-surgery/

# POSTERIOR FOSSA SURGERY

## LEARNING OBJECTIVES

- Describe the posterior fossa
- Describe the indications for posterior fossa surgery
- Manage patients undergoing posterior fossa surgery

## DEFINITION AND MECHANISM

- The posterior fossa is the deepest cranial fossa
- Surrounded by:
  - Anteriorly: The dorsum sellae and basilar portion of the occipital bone (clivus)
  - Laterally: The petrosal and mastoid components of the temporal bone
  - Superiorly: The dural layer (tentorium cerebelli)
  - Inferiorly and posteriorly: The occipital bone
- Contains many important structures: the brainstem, cerebellum and lower cranial nerves
- The cerebrospinal fluid pathway is very narrow through the cerebral aqueduct, and any obstruction can cause hydrocephalus which can result in a significant increase in intracranial pressure

## PATHOLOGIES

- Tumors are the most common pathologies of the posterior fossa
- Pathologies which require surgical intervention:

| Tumors | Axial tumors | Medulloblastoma (most common) |
|---|---|---|
| | | Cerebellar astrocytoma |
| | | Brainstem glioma |
| | | Ependymoma |
| | | Choroid plexus papilloma |
| | | Dermoid tumours |
| | | Hemangioblastoma |
| | | Metastatic tumours |
| | Cerebellopontine angle tumours | Schwannoma |
| | | Meningioma |
| | | Acoustic neuroma |
| | | Glomus jugulare tumour |
| Vascular malformations | | Posterior cerebellar artery aneurysm |
| | | Vertebral/vertebrobasillar aneurysm |
| | | Basillar tip aneurysm |
| | | AV malformations |
| | | Cerebellar hematoma |
| | | Cerebellar infarction |
| Cysts | | Epidermoid cyst |
| | | Arachnoid cyst |
| Cranial nerve lesions | | Trigeminal neuralgia (cranial nerve V) |
| | | Hemifacial spasm (cranial nerve VII) |
| | | Glossopharyngeal neuralgia (cranial nerve IX) |
| Craniocervical abnormalities | Atlanto-occipital instability | Congenital |
| | | Acquired |
| | Atlanto-axial instability | Congenital |
| | | Acquired |
| | Arnold-Chiarri malformation | |

# MANAGEMENT

## POSTERIOR FOSSA SURGERY MANAGEMENT

### Preoperative assessment

- Thorough evaluation of the neurological and cardiorespiratory status
- Routine assessment and optimization of coexisting conditions
- Evaluation for cerebellar and cranial nerve dysfunction
- Testing for presence of elevated ICP
- Evaluation of hydration status and electrolyte disturbance
- Airway evaluation
- Evaluation for intraoperative positioning

### Intraoperative management

**Monitoring**
- Routine: Pulse oximetry, ECG, capnography and temperature
- Invasive arterial blood pressure monitoring
- Central venous catheter
- Venous air embolism monitoring: Precordial Doppler
- Neurological monitoring: EEG, SSEPs, BAEPs, EMG

**Anesthetic goals**
- Avoid significant increase in ICP
- Maintain CPP
- Avoid hemodynamic instability
- Enable neurological monitoring
- Ensure early detection and management of complications

**Anesthetic technique**
- Remifentanil in patients with elevated ICP
- Either inhalation or IV technique
- Avoid nitrous oxide
- Immediately notify surgeon of unexpected hemodynamic change
- Careful observation of volume status

### Postoperative management

- Presence of lower cranial nerve dysfunction and potential for aspiration pneumonia: Postoperative mechanical ventilation
- Extensive intraoperative dissection: Possible airway compromise after extubation
- Possible airway edema and tongue swelling after prolonged prone positioning
- Consider ICP monitoring if ventilation is required
- Carefully manage postoperative hypertension
- Prophylactic antiemetics
- Adequate analgesia (opioids)

ICP, intracranial pressure; ECG, electrocardiography; EEG, electroencephalography; SSEP, somatosensory evoked potential; BAEP, brainstem auditory evoked potential; EMG, electromyography; CPP, cerebral perfusion pressure

# KEEP IN MIND

- Maintain consistent and modest levels of inhalation or IV anesthetic agents to minimize interference during somatosensory evoked potential (SSEP) monitoring
- Avoid neuromuscular blocking agents during motor evoked potential (MEP) monitoring.
- Use total IV anesthesia during motor evoked potential monitoring
- Intraoperative positioning
  - The sitting position improves surgical access to the posterior fossa, but is associated with several potential complications:

| Complication | Management |
|---|---|
| Cardiovascular instability | Notify the surgeon of their proximity to vital structures |
| Venous air embolism | Administer high-concentration oxygen, discontinue nitrous oxide, maintain cardiovascular stability, central venous catheter to aspirate air from right atrium, immediate initiation of chest compression in the event of a massive air embolism with cardiac arrest |
| Pneumocephalus | High-flow oxygen, burr hole and aspiration of air in severe cases |
| Macroglossia | Ensure airway clearance |
| Quadriplegia | Avoid this complication by paying close attention to positioning and avoiding prolonged hypotension |

## SUGGESTED READING

- Jagannathan S, Krovvidi H. Anaesthetic considerations for posterior fossa surgery. Continuing Education in Anaesthesia Critical Care & Pain. 2014;14(5):202-6.
- Sandhu K, Gupta N. Chapter 14 - Anesthesia for Posterior Fossa Surgery. In: Prabhakar H, editor. Essentials of Neuroanesthesia: Academic Press; 2017. p. 255-76.

Posterior fossa surgery

# SPINA BIFIDA

## LEARNING OBJECTIVES

- Types of spina bifida
- Perioperative management of spina bifida

## DEFINITION AND MECHANISM

- Refers to a congenital neural tube defect
- Results from the failure of the fetal neural tube to close within the first three weeks of gestation
- This leads to the incomplete fusion of the posterior lamina and pines of the vertebral column, and most commonly in the lumbosacral segments
- The incidence is approximately 1:1000 live births, however, it is decreasing due to folate supplementation
- Often no symptoms and often discovered as an incidental finding on radiographic examination
- Dimpling of the skin or a hairy patch at the base of the spine may be present in up to 70% of the patients with cord abnormalities

## TYPES OF SPINA BIFIDA

| Spina bifida occulta (closed spina bifida) | Meningocele | Myelomeningocele |
| --- | --- | --- |
| The most common and mildest type<br>A midline defect of the spinal column without protrusion of the spinal cord or meninges and intact overlying skin<br>No associated hydrocephalus or hindbrain herniation<br>One or more vertebrae do not form properly, but the gap is very small<br>Most affected individuals are asymptomatic and lack neurological signs<br>In some cases, it may be associated with patches of hair, a lipoma, discoloration of the skin, or a dermal sinus in the midline of the low back | The least common form of spina bifida<br>A single developmental defect allows the meninges to herniate between the vertebrae<br>But the spinal cord assumes a normal position in the spinal canal<br>Cases of tethered cord have been reported | Various amounts of neural tissue and meninges herniate through the defect to form a cerebrospinal fluid (CSF)-filled sac structure covered by a thin layer of skin tissue<br>May rupture and leak cerebrospinal fluid<br>The extent of the neurological deficit depends greatly on the location of the meningomyelocele, it most commonly occurs in the lumbosacral region<br>Clinical features:<br>- Flaccid paralysis of the lower limbs, absence of deep tendon reflexes, lack of response to touch and pain, kyphosis, scoliosis, and urinary and fecal incontinence<br>- Postural abnormalities of the lower limbs including clubfeet and subluxation of the hip<br>- Lesions above T4 generally result in paraplegia, whereas lesions below S1 allow ambulation<br>Associated with hydrocephalus and type II Arnold-Chiari malformation<br>Hydrocephalus is typically managed with a ventriculoperitoneal shunt |

## RISK FACTORS

- Deficiency of folic acid before and in the early stages of pregnancy
- Family history of spina bifida
- Medication intake during pregnancy: valproic acid, calcium-channel blockers, carbamazepine, cytochalasins

Spina bifida

## CONDITIONS ASSOCIATED WITH SPINA BIFIDA

- Attention and learning difficulties
- Bladder function problems
- Bowel function problems
- Depression
- Epilepsy and seizures
- Hip displacement
- Hydrocephalus
- Latex allergy

- Vision problems
- Lymphedema
- Obesity
- Pressure injury
- Scoliosis
- Sleep apnea
- Tethered spinal cord
- Weakness or paralysis

## DIAGNOSIS

- X-ray
- CT and MRI

## PRENATAL DIAGNOSIS

- Ultrasound
- Detection of alpha-fetoprotein in amniotic fluid

## MANAGEMENT

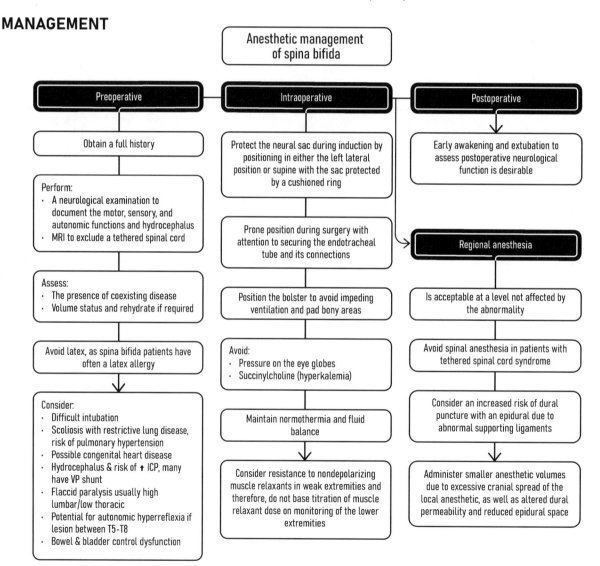

ICP, intracranial pressure; VP, ventricular peritoneal

Spina bifida

# PREGNANCY

- Neuraxial is generally safe
- Consider:
  - Difficulty locating the epidural space
  - An asymmetric block likely related to scarring
  - Dural punctures
  - The need for multiple operator attempts to place the anesthesia
  - A higher risk of post dural puncture headache

- The conus medullaris will likely be in an abnormal low position
- Scoliosis can further complicate the spine anatomy
- Use imaging to locate the best level for neuraxial anesthesia
- Attempt a block at the level where the cord is not too posteriorly located and the epidural space is likely to be normal
- Meningocele & myelomeningocele:
  - If spinal level involvement T11 or higher, likely will have painless labor

# OPEN SURGERY

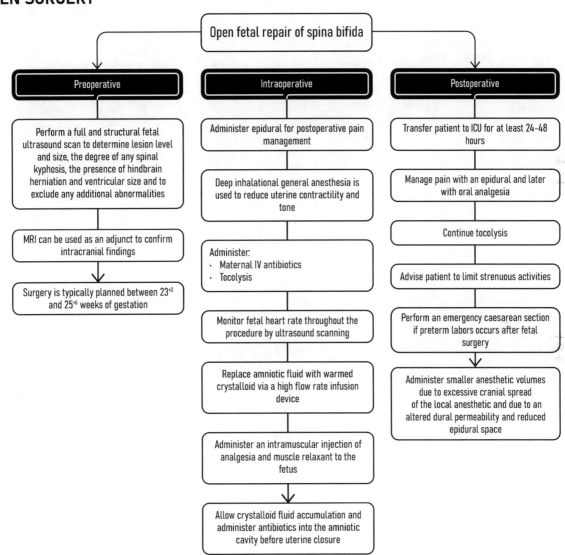

**Open fetal repair of spina bifida**

**Preoperative**

- Perform a full and structural fetal ultrasound scan to determine lesion level and size, the degree of any spinal kyphosis, the presence of hindbrain herniation and ventricular size and to exclude any additional abnormalities
- MRI can be used as an adjunct to confirm intracranial findings
- Surgery is typically planned between 23$^{+0}$ and 25$^{+6}$ weeks of gestation

**Intraoperative**

- Administer epidural for postoperative pain management
- Deep inhalational general anesthesia is used to reduce uterine contractility and tone
- Administer:
  - Maternal IV antibiotics
  - Tocolysis
- Monitor fetal heart rate throughout the procedure by ultrasound scanning
- Replace amniotic fluid with warmed crystalloid via a high flow rate infusion device
- Administer an intramuscular injection of analgesia and muscle relaxant to the fetus
- Allow crystalloid fluid accumulation and administer antibiotics into the amniotic cavity before uterine closure

**Postoperative**

- Transfer patient to ICU for at least 24-48 hours
- Manage pain with an epidural and later with oral analgesia
- Continue tocolysis
- Advise patient to limit strenuous activities
- Perform an emergency caesarean section if preterm labors occurs after fetal surgery
- Administer smaller anesthetic volumes due to excessive cranial spread of the local anesthetic and due to an altered dural permeability and reduced epidural space

## SUGGESTED READING

- Griffiths, S., Durbridge, J.A., 2011. Anaesthetic implications of neurological disease in pregnancy. Continuing Education in Anaesthesia Critical Care & Pain 11, 157-161.
- O'Neal MA. A Pregnant Woman with Spina Bifida: Need for a Multidisciplinary Labor Plan. Front Med (Lausanne). 2017;4:172.
- Sacco, A., Ushakov, F., Thompson, D., Peebles, D., Pandya, P., De Coppi, P., Wimalasundera, R., Attilakos, G., David, A.L., Deprest, J., 2019. Fetal surgery for open spina bifida. The Obstetrician & Gynaecologist 21, 271-282.
- Spina Bifida. In: Bissonnette B, Luginbuehl I, Marciniak B, Dalens BJ. eds. Syndromes: Rapid Recognition and Perioperative Implications. Mgraw Hill; 2006.

# SPINE SURGERY

## LEARNING OBJECTIVES

- Anesthetic management of spine surgery

## DEFINITION AND MECHANISM

- The scope of spine surgery is extensive
- Patients usually present with one of five pathologies at any site from cervical to lumbosacral:
  - Trauma (unstable vertebral fractures)
  - Infection (epidural abscess)
  - Malignancy (either primary or metastatic)
  - Congenital (scoliosis)
  - Degenerative
- Major spinal surgery is often associated with major bleeding, infection, and postoperative respiratory complications
- 1% incidence of spinal cord damage

## OPEN SURGERY

- The majority of spinal procedures are performed in the prone position
  - Exceptions: anterior cervical surgery, thoracic discectomies
  - Complications of the prone position:
    - Accidental extubation
    - Ophthalmic complications (corneal abrasions, postoperative visual loss)
    - Peripheral nerve injury (ulnar nerve at the elbow, brachial plexus)
    - Pressure injuries (skin necrosis, breast/genital injury)
    - Abdominal compression (venous congestion in epidural veins, organ ischemia, impaired ventilation, lower limb thrombosis, and reduced cardiac output)
  - Support the patient with pillow, gel pads, and foam bolsters to ensure that:
    - The abdomen is free
    - The head is at or above the level of the heart in a neutral position using a headrest or a Mayfield head fixator
    - The eyes are taped closed, without padding, and free from external pressure, regularly checked where possible
    - The arms are in a natural position no more than 90° abduction with slight internal rotation paying particular attention to the ulnar nerve at the elbow
  - Specific devices are available to facilitate proning: Montreal mattress, Jackson operating table, Wilson Frame, and the Andrews operating table

# MANAGEMENT

## Intraoperative management of spine surgery

### Monitoring

- ECG
- Noninvasive blood pressure monitoring
- Pulse oximetry
- Capnography
- Temperature
- Urine output
- Serial blood gas and arterial blood pressure if substantial blood loss is anticipated
- Central venous catheter in case of fluid balance management or delivery of inotropes/vasopressors

### Blood loss

Note that massive blood loss can occur during spinal surgery, particularly in scoliosis surgery and extensive stabilization

↓

Provide adequate large-bore venous access, rapid transfusers, cell salvage, readily available blood and blood products, and antifibrinolytics (tranexamic acid)

↓

Secure all vascular cannulae to prevent dislodgement in the prone position

### Airway management

Consider:
- Difficult laryngoscopy in patients with disease of the upper three cervical vertebrae
- Poor mouth opening in patients with limited extension at the craniocervical junction

↓

Use an alternative technique such as awake fiber-optic intubation

↓

Fix the tracheal tube (TT) in place securely. Intraoperative displacement of the TT is very difficult to manage

### Temperature

Maintain normothermia with forced warm air blankets and heated fluids

### Anesthesia

Do not use anesthetic vapors as intraoperative spinal cord monitoring is required

↓

TIVA with propofol is preferred

↓

Remifentanil is safe to use

### Analgesia

Opiates remain the mainstay, however, a multimodal approach is most effective
- IV adjuvants paracetamol and tramadol
- Ketamine 1 mg/kg bolus followed by 1–2 mg/kg/24 hours
- Avoid NSAIDs because of hematoma formation and spinal cord compression

↓

Start with adequate pain management (gabapentin or pregabalin) perioperatively

↓

Administer additional analgesia such as ketamine or clonidine intraoperatively

# Management of spine surgery

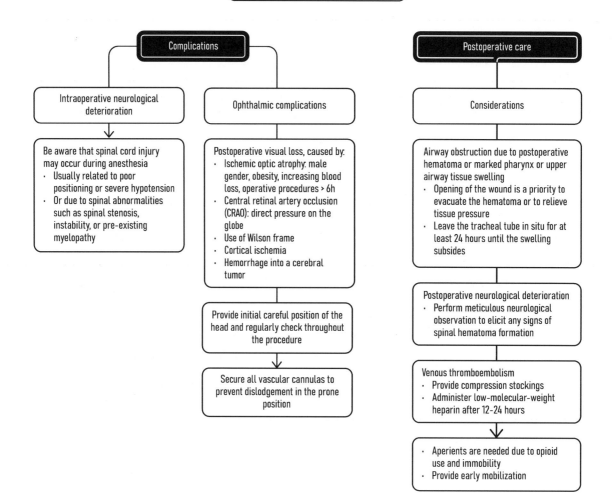

**Complications**

**Intraoperative neurological deterioration**

Be aware that spinal cord injury may occur during anesthesia
- Usually related to poor positioning or severe hypotension
- Or due to spinal abnormalities such as spinal stenosis, instability, or pre-existing myelopathy

**Ophthalmic complications**

Postoperative visual loss, caused by:
- Ischemic optic atrophy: male gender, obesity, increasing blood loss, operative procedures > 6h
- Central retinal artery occlusion (CRAO): direct pressure on the globe
- Use of Wilson frame
- Cortical ischemia
- Hemorrhage into a cerebral tumor

Provide initial careful position of the head and regularly check throughout the procedure

Secure all vascular cannulas to prevent dislodgement in the prone position

**Postoperative care**

**Considerations**

Airway obstruction due to postoperative hematoma or marked pharynx or upper airway tissue swelling
- Opening of the wound is a priority to evacuate the hematoma or to relieve tissue pressure
- Leave the tracheal tube in situ for at least 24 hours until the swelling subsides

Postoperative neurological deterioration
- Perform meticulous neurological observation to elicit any signs of spinal hematoma formation

Venous thromboembolism
- Provide compression stockings
- Administer low-molecular-weight heparin after 12-24 hours

- Aperients are needed due to opioid use and immobility
- Provide early mobilization

# MANAGEMENT OF AIRWAY COMPROMISE FOLLOWING CERVICAL SPINAL SURGERY

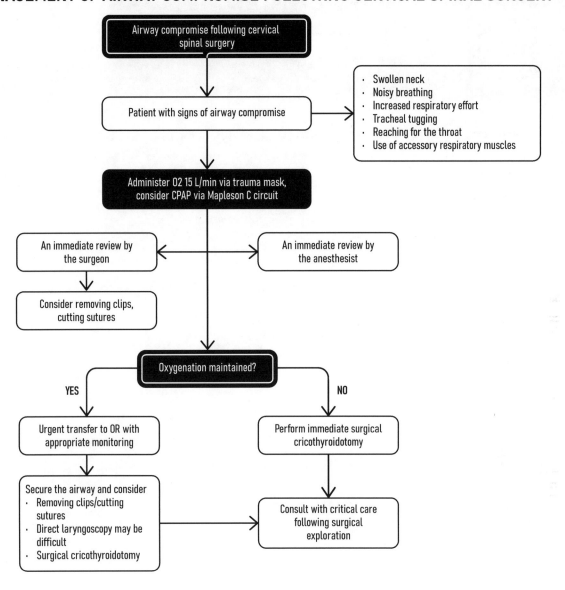

**Airway compromise following cervical spinal surgery**

↓

Patient with signs of airway compromise →

- Swollen neck
- Noisy breathing
- Increased respiratory effort
- Tracheal tugging
- Reaching for the throat
- Use of accessory respiratory muscles

↓

**Administer O2 15 L/min via trauma mask, consider CPAP via Mapleson C circuit**

An immediate review by the surgeon ← → An immediate review by the anesthesist

↓

Consider removing clips, cutting sutures

↓

**Oxygenation maintained?**

YES ↓

Urgent transfer to OR with appropriate monitoring

NO ↓

Perform immediate surgical cricothyroidotomy

↓

Secure the airway and consider
- Removing clips/cutting sutures
- Direct laryngoscopy may be difficult
- Surgical cricothyroidotomy

→

Consult with critical care following surgical exploration

## SUGGESTED READING

- Nowicki R. 2014. Anaesthesia for major spinal surgery. Continuing Education in Anaesthesia Critical Care & Pain. 14;4:147-152.
- Pollard BJ, Kitchen, G. Handbook of Clinical Anaesthesia. Fourth Edition. CRC Press. 2018. 978-1-4987-6289-2.

# SUBARACHNOID HEMORRHAGE

**163**

## LEARNING OBJECTIVES

- Describe the pathophysiology and symptoms of a subarachnoid hemorrhage
- Diagnose and clinically grade a subarachnoid hemorrhage
- Manage patients presenting with a subarachnoid hemorrhage

## DEFINITION AND MECHANISM

- Subarachnoid hemorrhage accounts for 5% of all strokes
- Mortality rate ~50%
- One-third of survivors need lifelong care
- Prompt diagnosis and early treatment are critical

## PATHOPHYSIOLOGY

- Etiology
  - Intracranial aneurysm (85% of cases)
  - Arteriovenous malformations
  - Trauma
  - Moyamoya disease
- Risk factors
  - Hypertension
  - Atherosclerosis
  - Cocaine use
  - Alcohol abuse
  - Smoking
  - Connective tissue disorders
  - Coarctation of the aorta
  - Congenital conditions (autosomal-dominant polycystic kidney disease, Ehlers Danlos Type 4, familial intracerebral aneurysms)
- Cause
  - Hemodynamically induced shear stress (sudden increase in cerebrovascular arterial pressure)
- Aneurysmal rupture leads to blood quickly traversing through the intracranial cisterns and subarachnoid space (within seconds)
- Global cerebral ischemia resulting from increased intracranial pressure, decreased cerebral perfusion, and reduced cerebral blood flow
- Intraventricular bleeding can cause acute ventricular dilatation and hydrocephalus
- Brain tissue oxygen pressure and pH are reduced
- Compensatory hypertension occurs within minutes to hours
- Blood-brain barrier disruption, cerebral edema, and a thromboinflammatory cascade

## SIGNS & SYMPTOMS

- Sudden onset of "worst headache of life"
- Loss of consciousness
- Nausea and/or vomiting
- Nuchal rigidity
- Photophobia
- Seizures
- Comatose and hypertensive at presentation

## COMPLICATIONS

- Re-bleeding
- Seizures
- Hydrocephalus
- Vasospasm

## DIAGNOSIS

- Non-contrast cranial CT
- Lumbar puncture in patients with a high index of suspicion and a normal CT scan (red blood cell count, bilirubin level, and xanthochromia)
- CT angiogram and/or digital subtraction angiography to identify the cause

# CLINICAL GRADING

| Grade | World Federation of Neurologic Surgeons | Hess and Hunt | Fisher (CT scan apperience) |
|-------|-----------------------------------------|---------------|-----------------------------|
| 1 | Glasgow Coma Scale score 15, no motor deficit | Asymptomatic or minimal headache and slight nuchal rigidity | No blood detected |
| 2 | Glasgow Coma Scale score 13-14, no motor deficit | Moderate to severe headache nuchal rigidity, no neurological deficit other than cranial nerve palsy | Diffuse thin layer of subarachnoid blood (vertical layers < 1 mm thick) |
| 3 | Glasgow Coma Scale score 13-14 with motor deficit | Drowsy, confusion, or mild neurological deficit | Localized clot or thick layer of subarachnoid blood (vertical layers ≥ 1 mm thick) |
| 4 | Glasgow Coma Scale score 7-12, with or without motor deficit | Stupor, moderate-to-severe hemiparesis, possibly early decerebrate rigidity and vegetative disturbances | Diffuse or no subarachnoid blood but intracerebral or intraventricular clots |
| 5 | Glasgow Coma Scale score 3-6, with or withour motor deficit | Deep coma, decerebrate rigidity, moribund appearance | |

# MANAGEMENT

## SUBARACHNOID HEMORRHAGE ACUTE MANAGEMENT

OXYGENATION AND VENTILATION
- Secure airway
- Provide oxygenation and ventilation (tracheal intubation)
- Patients who regain consciousness may only require supplemental oxygen

RESTORATION OF CEREBRAL PERFUSION
- Early placement of an external ventricular drain
- Avoid excessive or rapid loss of cerebrospinal fluid during drain placement

PREVENTION OF RE-BLEEDING
- Control acute hypertension
- Control headache with analgesics, anxiolysis and bed rest
- Maintain systolic blood pressure at < 160 mmHg (nicardipine, esmolol, clevidipine)
- Stop and reverse anticoagulants if the patients uses them
- Use antifribrinolytics only in patients at high risk of re-bleeding in whom definitive treatment is delayed

SEIZURE PROPHYLAXIS
- Initiate seizure prophylaxis only in patients with a poor neurologic grade, unsecured aneurysm, and associated intracerebral hemorrhage

NIMODIPINE
- Administer 60 mg nimodipine orally or by nasogastric tube every 4h, starting within 48h of subarachnoid hemorrhage
- Continue for 21 days
- The dose may need to be reduced or discontinued in patients with higher grades of subarachnoid hemorrhage experiencing hypotension (treat hypotension with vasopressors first)

PLANNING DEFINITIVE TREATMENT
- Obliteration of the ruptured aneurysm has to be performed as early as possible
- Transfer patient to an experienced center with multidisciplinary teams if necessary

- Treatment options
  - Endovascular coiling: Preferred in geriatric patients, particularly those with high-grade aneurysmal subarachnoid hemorrhage from the rupture of basilar apex aneurysm
  - Surgical clipping: Preferred in patients with large intraparenchymal hematomas, aneurysm of the middle cerebral artery, and in those not likely to be compliant with long-term follow-up

## SUBARACHNOID HEMORRHAGE DEFINITIVE TREATMENT: ANESTHETIC MANAGEMENT I

### PREOPERATIVE ASSESSMENT
- Clinical grading of hemorrhage
- Evaluate and manage pulmonary, cardiovascular, neurologic and endocrine complications

### ANESTHETIC GOALS
- Facilitate timely definitive treatment
- Prevention of re-bleeding
- Maintain cerebral perfusion
- Prevent/manage intraoperative brain swelling to facilitate surgical exposure
- Facilitate neurophysiological monitoring
- Facilitate temporary clipping
- Optimize systemic physiology and manage glycemia
- Anticipate and manage crisis situations (e.g., aneurysm rupture)
- Facilitate timely, smooth emergence and neurologic assessment
- Prevent postoperative pain and other complications

### INDUCTION
- Rapid sequence induction in patients who are nauseous or vomiting
- Ensure adequate depth
- Succinylcholine can be used safely after ensuring adequate depth
- Avoid hyper- and hypotension: Have antihypertensive and vasopressor agents available
- Avoid hypo- and hypercarbia

### MONITORING
- Arterial line
- ECG
- Intracranial pressure and cerebral perfusion pressure when external ventricular drain is placed
- Jugular venous oximetry (not routinely used)
- Electroencephalogram
- Somatosensory-evoked and motor-evoked potentials

### ANESTHETIC AGENTS
- Based on patient's neurologic status, procedure, coexisting disease, and need for neurophysiological monitoring
- TIVA strategy: propofol + short-acting opioids: Remifentanyl
- Use isoflurane, desflurane and sevoflurane in concentrations > 1.0 MAC
- High-dose desflurane (1.5 MAC) increases brain oxygenation and improves acidosis, but can worsen brain swelling
- Vasodilatory effect of inhalational agents can be minimized by hyperventilation
- Both IV and inhalational anesthetics can effectively provide optimal surgical conditions
- Avoid nitrous oxide
- Dexmedetomidine is a useful adjunct
- Ketamine may be used as an adjunct, but avoid bolus doses

### HEMODYNAMIC MANAGEMENT
- Avoid hypertension before aneurysm is secured
- Induce brief periods of hypertension during temorary clipping
- Normalize blood pressure after aneurysm is secured

# SUBARACHNOID HEMORRHAGE DEFINITIVE TREATMENT: ANESTHETIC MANAGEMENT II

### INTRACRANIAL PRESSURE MANAGEMENT AND BRAIN RELAXATION

- Maintain adequate depth of anesthesia
- Optimize hemodynamic parameters
- Optimal positioning (head elevation, avoid excessive flexion or rotation of the neck)
- Maintain normocarbia/moderate hypocarbia
- IV mannitol, hypertonic saline, furosemide
- Cerebrospinal fluid drainage
- Burst suppression with IV bolus of propofol/thiopental
- Timing of hyperventilation is important (after opening of the dura)

### TEMPORARY CLIPPING AND NEUROPROTECTION

- A temporary clip may be placed on the parent vessel to reduce blood flow through the aneurysm
- Avoid prolonged clipping (> 10 min)
- Neurophysiological monitoring to detect ischemia and guide reperfusion
- Reduce cerebral metabolic demand during clipping (burst suppression, hypothermia) (cautiously, only in selected cases)
- Induce hypertension to recruit collateral flow

### ADENOSINE-INDUCED TEMPORARY FLOW ARREST

- Can be used when temporary clipping is not feasible
- Administer in close communication with the surgeon and minimize duration
- Avoid in patients with coronary artery disease, cardiac conduction abnormalities, or reactive airways disease

### RAPID VENTRICULAR PACING

- Technique to control complex aneurysms during clipping
- Induction of ventricular tachycardia using a bipolar pacing electrode introduced through the internal jugular vein into the right ventricle
- Place external defibrillating pads
- Minimize duration to avoid cerebral ischemia
- Not suitable for patients with coronary artery disease and cardiac arrhythmias

### VASOSPASM & DELAYED CEREBRAL ISCHEMIA

- Cerebral vasospasm can lead to delayed cerebral ischemia
- Treatment for vasospasm: Perform resuscitation to avoid hypovolemia and administer vasopressors or inotropes to induce hypertension
- Oral nimodipine to reduce delayed cerebral ischemia

### POSTOPERATIVE MANAGEMENT

- Grade 1 or 2 patients with uneventful surgery can be extubated in the operating room
- Grade 4 or 5 patients are usually kept electively intubated and ventilated
- Extubate grade 3 patients in coordination with the surgical team
- Coughing can be prevented with IV lidocaine 1.5 mg/kg
- Treat excessive increases in blood pressure with esmolol 0.1-0.5 mg/kg or labetalol 5-10 mg boluses
- Keep patient in ICU with close monitoring of neurological status, hemodynamic status and fluid status
- In patients with multiple aneurysms, systemic blood pressure must be maintained within 20% of baseline

## SUGGESTED READING

- Claassen J, Park S. Spontaneous subarachnoid haemorrhage. Lancet. 2022;400(10355):846-862
- Deepak Sharma; Perioperative Management of Aneurysmal Subarachnoid Hemorrhage: A Narrative Review. Anesthesiology 2020; 133:1283-1305
- Luoma A, Reddy U. Acute management of aneurysmal subarachnoid haemorrhage. Continuing Education in Anaesthesia Critical Care & Pain. 2013;13(2):52-8.
- Kundra S, Mahendru V, Gupta V, Choudhary AK. Principles of neuroanesthesia in aneurysmal subarachnoid hemorrhage. J Anaesthesiol Clin Pharmacol. 2014;30(3):328-337.
- Robba C, Busl KM, Claassen J, et al. Contemporary management of aneurysmal subarachnoid haemorrhage. An update for the intensivist. Intensive Care Med. 2024;50(5):646-664.

# TRAUMATIC BRAIN INJURY

## LEARNING OBJECTIVES

- Describe and classify traumatic brain injury
- Describe the acute management goals for traumatic brain injury patients
- Manage traumatic brain injury patients

## DEFINITION AND MECHANISM

- Traumatic brain injury is the leading cause of death and disability in young adults in the developed world
- Heterogeneous condition in terms of etiology, severity, and outcome
- Can be divided into primary and secondary brain injury
  □ Primary injury occurs as a consequence of the initial physical insult (skull fracture, contusions, intracranial hematoma, cerebral edema, diffuse brain injury)
  □ Secondary injury results from inflammatory and neurotoxic processes: Increased intracranial pressure, hypoperfusion, cerebral ischemia

| Component | | Score |
|---|---|---|
| Eye opening | Spontaneous | 4 |
| | To speech | 3 |
| | To pain | 2 |
| | None | 1 |
| Best verbal response | Orientated | 5 |
| | Confused | 4 |
| | Inappropriate | 3 |
| | Incomprehensible | 2 |
| | None | 1 |
| Best motor response | Obeying | 6 |
| | Localizing | 5 |
| | Withdrawing | 4 |
| | Flexing | 3 |
| | Extending | 2 |
| | None | 1 |

## CLASSIFICATION

Glasgow Coma Scale (GCS) re-evaluate every 30 min:
- 15-13: Mild
- 13-9: Moderate
- < 8: Severe

## IMMEDIATE MANAGEMENT

| System | Management goals |
|---|---|
| Airway | Early tracheal intubation if GCS ≤ 8 or unable to maintain respiratory goals |
| Respiratory | Avoid hypoxia, maintain $SaO_2$ > 97%, $PaO_2$ > 11 kPa<br>Maintain a $PaCO_2$ value of 4.5 – 5.0 kPa<br>Hyperventilation, a $PaCO_2$ value of 4.0 – 4.5 kPa reserved for impending herniation |
| Cardiovascular | Avoid hypotension, maintain MAP > 80 mmHg<br>Replace intravascular volume, avoid hypotonic and glucose-containing solutions<br>Use blood as necessary, reverse existing coagulopathy<br>Vasopressor agents as necessary to maintain cerebral perfusion pressure (CPP) |
| Brain | Monitor intracranial pressure (ICP), avoid ICP > 20 mmHg<br>Maintain CPP > 60 mmHg<br>Adequate sedation and analgesia<br>Hyperosmolar therapy, keep $Na^+$ < 155 mmol/L, Posm < 320 mosm/L<br>CSF drainage<br>Treat seizures<br>Barbiturate coma, decompressive craniectomy, hypothermia, all reserved for elevated ICP refractory to standard medical care |
| Metabolic | Monitor blood glucose, aim for blood glucose 6 – 10 mmol/L<br>Avoid hyperthermia<br>DVT thromboprophylaxis |

# MANAGEMENT

## TRAUMATIC BRAIN INJURY ANESTHETIC MANAGEMENT

### ANESTHETIC GOALS

- Maintain CPP
- Treat increased ICP
- Provide optimal surgical conditions (adequate muscle relaxation, avoiding hypertension, propofol TIVA to reduce ICP during surgery)
- Avoid secondary insults such as hypoxemia, hyper- and hypocarbia, hypo- and hyperglycemia
- Provide adequate analgesia and amnesia

### ANESTHETIC TECHNIQUE

- Avoid nitrous oxide
- Either IV or volatile anesthetic agents
- Avoid hypotension, hypoxia
- Raised ICP: Mannitol 0.25-1.0 g/kg
- Maintain CPP at 50-70 mmHg
- Avoid high-dose methylprednisolone in patients with moderate to severe traumatic brain injury

### MONITORING

- Arterial line for blood pressure, blood gas and blood glucose monitoring
- Central venous pressure monitoring may be useful
- ICP monitoring in patients with severe traumatic brain injury
- Cerebral oxygenation monitoring may be useful

### IV FLUIDS AND BLOOD PRESSURE MANAGEMENT

- Warm, non-glucose containing isotonic crystalloid solution IV
- Vasopressors can be used to treat hypotension or to augment CPP (norepinephrine, dopamine, phenylephrine)

### GLYCEMIC CONTROL

- Intensive insulin therapy remains controversial
- Target glucose range of 80-180 mg/dL

### THERAPEUTIC HYPOTHERMIA AND STEROIDS

- Hypothermia reduces cerebral metabolism during stress, reduces excitatory neurotransmitters release, and attenuates blood-brain barrier permeability
- Use hypothermia optionally and cautiously (risk of pneumonia)
- Steroids do not improve outcomes or lower ICP

### BLOOD TRANSFUSION

- A liberal transfusion strategy is not recommended, keep the transfusion threshold identical to other critically ill patients

CPP, cerebral perfusion pressure; ICP, intracranial pressure

## SUGGESTED READING

- Claassen J, Park S. Spontaneous subarachnoid haemorrhage. Lancet. 2022;400(10355):846-862
- Curry P, Viernes D, Sharma D. Perioperative management of traumatic brain injury. Int J Crit Illn Inj Sci. 2011;1(1):27-35.
- Dinsmore J. Traumatic brain injury: an evidence-based review of management. Continuing Education in Anaesthesia Critical Care & Pain. 2013;13(6):189-95.
- Moppett IK. Traumatic brain injury: assessment, resuscitation and early management. Br J Anaesth. 2007;99(1):18-31.
- Robba C, Busl KM, Claassen J, et al. Contemporary management of aneurysmal subarachnoid haemorrhage. An update for the intensivist. Intensive Care Med. 2024;50(5):646-664.

# NEUROMUSCULAR DISEASES

# AMYOTROPHIC LATERAL SCLEROSIS (ALS)

## LEARNING OBJECTIVES

- Describe the pathophysiology of Amyotrophic lateral sclerosis (ALS)
- Signs and symptoms of ALS
- Anesthetic management of ALS

## DEFINITION AND MECHANISM

- Amyotrophic lateral sclerosis (ALS), also known as Lou Gehrig's Disease, is a rare and progressive nervous system disease that affects nerve cells in the brain and spinal cord
- Resulting in the progressive loss of motor neurons that control voluntary muscles
- ALS often begins with muscle twitching and weakness in a limb, or slurred speech
- Eventually, ALS affects the control of the muscles needed to move, speak, eat, and breathe
- The most common cause of death for patients with ALS is respiratory failure
- On average, patients die within 3-5 years after symptoms begin
- There is no cure for this fatal disease
- Most ALS cases are considered sporadic, about 5-10% of all ALS cases are familial

## SIGNS AND SYMPTOMS

- Difficulty walking or doing normal daily activities
- Tripping and falling
- Weakness in the legs, feet, or ankles
- Hand weakness or clumsiness
- Slurred speech or trouble swallowing
- Muscle cramps and twitching (fasciculations) in the arms, shoulders, and tongue
- Inappropriate crying, laughing, or yawning
- Cognitive and behavioral changes
- Pulmonary/breathing problems:
  □ Shortness of breath
  □ Weak cough
  □ Difficulty clearing the throat and lungs
  □ Extra saliva
  □ Inability to lie flat in bed
  □ Repeated chest infections and pneumonia
  □ Respiratory failure

Symptoms with the progression of the disease:
- Not be able to stand or walk, get in or out of bed on their own
- Dysphagia
- Dysarthria
- Dyspnea
- Weight loss
- Malnourishment
- Muscle cramps and neuropathy
- Anxiety and depression
- Dementia

## RISK FACTORS

- Age: increases with age and is most commonly between 40 and 70
- Gender: males are more likely to develop ALS before the age of 65
- Race and ethnicity: Caucasians and non-Hispanics are most likely to develop the disease
- Heredity: in 5-10% of the cases
- Smoking
- Environmental toxin exposure: lead, pesticides such as Aldrin, Dieldrin, and DDT
- Military service

## COMPLICATIONS

- Breathing problems requiring BiPAP or tracheostomy
- Difficulty with speaking
- Malnutrition and dehydration
- Dementia

# DIAGNOSIS

- EMG
- A nerve conduction study
- MRI

- Blood and urine tests
- Muscle biopsy (altough this is routinely peformed)

# TREATMENT

The goal of treatment is to improve symptoms:
- Supportive health care:
  - Physical therapy
  - Nutritional counseling
  - Speech therapy
  - Assistive devices: splints, braces, grab bars,...
- Non-invasive ventilation

- Medications to manage symptoms including muscle cramps, stiffness, excess saliva, phlegm, unwanted episodes of crying and/or laughing, or other emotional displays
- FDA-approved medications:
  - Riluzole (Rilutek)
  - Edaravone (Radicava)

# MANAGEMENT

## *Preoperative and perioperative management*

**Anesthetic management of Amyotrophic lateral sclerosis**

**Preoperative management**

Obtain:
- A medical history
- A preoperative examination
- Respiratory function test
- Blood test

Prepare for a difficult airway due to spasticity and cramps, tracheal constriction, or scar after tracheotomy

Use video laringoscopy or the use of a fiberoptic scope as laryngoscopy and intubation may be challenging

Consider:
- An aspiration risk due to bulbar dysfunction
- Frequent pulmonary dysfunction with restricted pattern

Avoid depolarizing neuromuscular blocking agents (succinylcholine)

Administer non-depolarizing neuromuscular blocking agents (rocuronium) in reduced doses

Use opioids with caution as they can decrease the post-operative respiratory function

Administer an infusion of lidocaine, ketamine, glutamate or magnesium sulphate, perioperatively to reduce the opioid requirement

Patient position:
- The prone position is possible but should be considered carefully in awake ALS patients without airway protection
- The supine position may be stressful for the ALS patient
- The upper/semi-sitting position may help to relieve respiration

**Perioperative management**

Be aware that:
- General anesthesia causes aspiration or ventilatory depression due to abnormal response of muscle relaxants and rhabdomyolysis
- The use of regional central neuraxial block may exacerbate the preexisting neurological diseases
- There is the risk of postoperative ventilation and subsequent weaning difficulties, infection, and atelectasis due to respiratory complications
- ALS patients are vulnerable to hyperkalemia following the administration of succinylcholine
- That vessel cannulation might be difficult due to cramps or spasticity

General anesthesia with propofol and fentanyl is considered to be safe

Total Intravenous Anesthesia (TIVA) is safe; however, volatile anesthetics should be used with caution.

Treat hypovolemia which is apparent primarily after induction due to malnutrition/dehydration

Apply lung protective ventilation

Amyotrophic lateral sclerosis (ALS)

## Postoperative management

- Transfer patient to ICU
- Administer paracetamol or NSAIDs postoperatively for pain management
  - Avoid opioids because of respiratory depression
- Respiratory distress may require prolonged mechanical ventilation as well as re-intubation
  - Be aware that weaning is often prolonged and difficult
- Consider that bulbar symptoms like dysphagia or dysarthria as well as cognitive impairment may lead to malnutrition and require intravenous or tube feeding

## SUGGESTED READING

- Gaik C, Wiesmann T. 2021Anaesthesia recommendations for Amyotrophic lateral sclerosis. Orphananesthesia.https://www.orphananesthesia.eu/en/rare-diseases/published-guidelines/amyotrophic-lateral-sclerosis/1684-amyotrophic-lateral-sclerosis-2/file.html
- Marsh, S., Pittard, A., 2011. Neuromuscular disorders and anaesthesia. Part 2: specific neuromuscular disorders. Continuing Education in Anaesthesia Critical Care & Pain 11, 119-123.
- Sarna R, Gupta A, Arora G. Amyotrophic lateral sclerosis and anaesthetic challenges: Perioperative lignocaine infusion-an aid. Indian J Anaesth. 2020;64(5):448-449.
- Thampi SM, David D, Chandy TT, Nandhakumar A. Anesthetic management of a patient with amyotrophic lateral sclerosis for transurethral resection of bladder tumor. Indian J Anaesth. 2013;57(2):197-199.

# GUILLAIN-BARRÉ SYNDROME

## LEARNING OBJECTIVES

- Describe the etiology and symptoms of Guillain-barré syndrome
- Diagnose and treat Guillain-barré syndrome
- Manage patients with Guillain-barré syndrome presenting for surgery

## DEFINITION AND MECHANISM

- Guillain-Barré syndrome (GBS) is an acute demyelinating polyneuropathy typically occurring as an autoimmune response following a gastrointestinal or respiratory infection
- Most common cause of acute, flaccid, neuromuscular paralysis in the United States
- Potentially severely debilitating disorder
- Mortality rate ~10%
- Initial presentation is often misdiagnosed as hysteria

## ETIOLOGY

- Affects all ages, but a tendency towards young adults and the elderly
- Slightly more prevalent in men
- Children are less severely affected
- Usually occurs within a month of a respiratory or gastrointestinal infection
- Common pathogens causing GBS:
  - Campylobacter jejuni (associated with axonal degeneration in addition to primary demyelination)
  - Epstein Barr virus
  - Mycoplasma pneumonia
  - Cytomegalovirus

## SIGNS & SYMPTOMS

- Clinical signs
  - Acute inflammatory demyelinating polyradiculopathy
  - Acute motor axonal neuropathy
  - Acute motor sensory axonal neuropathy
  - Miller Fisher syndrome (ataxia, areflexia, and ophthalmoplegia, possibly with limb weakness, ptosis, and facial and bulbar palsy)
- Symptoms
  - Motor weakness that can be mild, but also so severe that it causes complete paralysis
  - Areflexia
  - Facial palsy and bulbar weakness
  - Ophthalmoplegia
  - Sensory symptoms
  - Severe pain, often affecting the girdle area
  - Weakness of the respiratory musculature leading to respiratory failure
  - Autonomic dysfunction causing under- or overactivity of the sympathetic and parasympathetic systems leading to arrhythmias, fluctuations in blood pressure and pulse, urinary retention, ileus, and excessive sweating

## DIAGNOSIS

- Physical findings: Progressive muscle weakness and areflexia over the course of few days to a few weeks
- When GBS is suspected, monitor for arrhythmias and respiratory muscle weakness
- Further investigations:
  - Blood testing: Full blood count, urea and electrolytes, liver and renal function tests, clotting screen, calcium levels, antibody tests, blood cultures, and inflammatory markers
  - ECG
  - Head CT
  - Lumbar puncture and CSF analysis
  - Electrophysiological studies
  - Gadolinium-enhanced MRI of the spinal cord

Guillain-barré syndrome

# TREATMENT

- Supportive therapy
  - Physiotherapy and occupational therapy
  - Counseling
  - Nutritional support
  - Analgesia
  - Thromboembolic prophylaxis
  - Respiratory support
    - Indications for intubation and ventilation:
      - Vital capacity < 20 mL/kg
      - Maximal inspiratory pressure (MIP) < 30 cmH$_2$O
      - Maximal expiratory pressure (MEP) < 40 cmH$_2$O
      - Decrease of > 30% in vital capacity, MIP or MEP
- Specific therapy
  - Treatment of choice: IV immunoglobulins (0.4 g/kg bodyweight daily, 5 days) but be aware of potential side effects such as hyperviscosity syndrome (myocardial infarction, stroke), hypotension, transfusion reactions
  - Plasmapheresis, up to 5 exchanges of 250 mL/kg of plasma with 4.5% human albumin solution (more difficult to administer, more side-effects and contraindications)
  - CSF filtration (rarely performed)

# ANESTHETIC CONSIDERATIONS

- Preoperative
  - Many patients are ventilated in the ICU
  - Assess bulbar and ventilatory function to predict the need for postoperative ventilation
  - Ileus increases the risks of aspiration
- Induction
  - Rapid sequence induction with rocuronium as succinylcholine is contraindicated (potentially fatal hyperkalemia)
  - Autonomic dysfunction can complicate induction and intubation by resulting in a labile pulse and blood pressure
- Intraoperative
  - Controlled ventilation if respiratory function is impaired
  - Avoid non-depolarizing neuromuscular blockers
  - Consider extubating when fully recovered or once bulbar reflexes have returned
- Postoperative
  - Ventilation is often required
  - Careful monitoring of respiratory function
  - Adequate analgesia

═══ SUGGESTED READING ═══

- Nguyen TP, Taylor RS. Guillain Barre Syndrome. [Updated 2022 Jul 4]. In: StatPearls [Internet]. Treasure Island (FL): StatPearls Publishing; 2022 Jan-. Available from: https://www.ncbi.nlm.nih.gov/books/NBK532254/
- Pollard BJ, Kitchen, G. Handbook of Clinical Anaesthesia. Fourth Edition. CRC Press. 2018. 978-1-4987-6289-2.
- Richards KJC, Cohen AT. Guillain-Barré syndrome. BJA CEPD Reviews. 2003;3(2):46-9.

# LAMBERT-EATON MYASTHENIC SYNDROME (LEMS)

## LEARNING OBJECTIVES

- Definition of Lambert-Eaton myasthenic syndrome (LEMS)
- Treatment and anesthetic management of LEMS

## DEFINITION AND MECHANISM

- Lambert-Eaton myasthenic syndrome (LEMS) is a very rare condition in which the immune system attacks the neuromuscular junctions of voltage-gated calcium channels, thereby interfering with the ability of nerve cells to send signals to muscle cells
- A miscommunication between the nerve cell and the muscles that leads to the gradual onset of muscle weakness and autonomic nervous system dysfunction
- Two types of LEMS:
  - Paraneoplastic LEMS is often associated (50-60%) with small-cell lung cancer
    - Treat underlying cancer as this may improve symptoms from this condition
    - Characterized by an older age of onset (average 60 years)
    - Caused by an accidental attack by the immune system as it attempts to fight the cancer
  - LEMS may also be associated with:
    - Endocrine diseases such as hypothyroidism or diabetes mellitus type 1
    - It may have a genetic component linked to autoimmunity
    - Younger age of onset (on average 35 years)
- Myasthenia gravis has very similar symptoms to Lambert-Eaton syndrome
- In contrast to myasthenia gravis, the weakness in Eaton–Lambert syndrome usually improves with exercise

## SIGNS & SYMPTOMS

- Primary clinical manifestation: muscle weakness and muscle fatigue
- Trouble walking
- Muscle pain or stiffness
- Tingling sensation in your hands or feet
- Droopy eyelids (ptosis)
- Double vision (diplopia)
- Dry mouth and dry eyes
- Constipation
- Decreased sweating

- Weight loss
- Difficulty peeing
- Erectile dysfunction
- Dysarthria and dysphagia are late-stage symptoms
- Dyspnea and respiratory failure
- Lambert-Eaton myasthenic syndrome typically affects upper leg muscle strength first, followed by shoulder muscles, muscles of the hands and feet, muscles affecting speech and swallowing, and eye muscles
- Symptoms develop gradually over weeks or months

## DIAGNOSIS

- Blood tests to detect antibodies
- Electromyography
- Screening for malignancy: CT, MRI, PET

## TREATMENT

- Treatment for underlying malignancy: surgery, radiation, or chemotherapy
- Improve muscle strength: amifampridine, guanidine
- Acetylcholinesterase inhibitors: pyridostigmine (30-120 mg every 3-6 hours) or 3,4-diaminopyridine
- Intravenous immune globulin
- Immunosuppression: prednisolone, azathioprine, methotrexate, cyclosporine
- Plasmapheresis
- Rituximab

Lambert-Eaton myasthenic syndrome (LEMS)

# MANAGEMENT

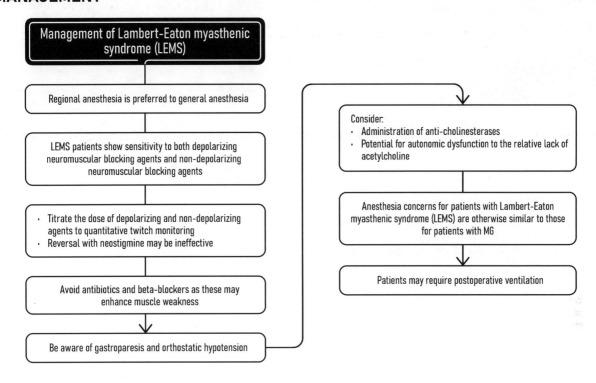

**Management of Lambert-Eaton myasthenic syndrome (LEMS)**

Regional anesthesia is preferred to general anesthesia

LEMS patients show sensitivity to both depolarizing neuromuscular blocking agents and non-depolarizing neuromuscular blocking agents

- Titrate the dose of depolarizing and non-depolarizing agents to quantitative twitch monitoring
- Reversal with neostigmine may be ineffective

Avoid antibiotics and beta-blockers as these may enhance muscle weakness

Be aware of gastroparesis and orthostatic hypotension

Consider:
- Administration of anti-cholinesterases
- Potential for autonomic dysfunction to the relative lack of acetylcholine

Anesthesia concerns for patients with Lambert-Eaton myasthenic syndrome (LEMS) are otherwise similar to those for patients with MG

Patients may require postoperative ventilation

## SUGGESTED READING

- Kesner VG, Oh SJ, Dimachkie MM, Barohn RJ. Lambert-Eaton Myasthenic Syndrome. Neurol Clin. 2018;36(2):379-394.
- Marsh, S., Pittard, A., 2011. Neuromuscular disorders and anaesthesia. Part 2: specific neuromuscular disorders. Continuing Education in Anaesthesia Critical Care & Pain 11, 119-123.
- Weingarten TN, Araka CN, Mogensen ME, Sorenson JP, Marienau ME, Watson JC, Sprung J. 2014. Lambert-Eaton myasthenic syndrome during anesthesia: a report of 37 patients. Journal of Clinical anesthesia. 26;8:648-653.

# MULTIPLE SCLEROSIS

## LEARNING OBJECTIVES

- Knowing the challenges in the perioperative management of patients with multiple sclerosis

---

- Multiple sclerosis is a chronic disabling demyelinating inflammatory disease of the central nervous system
- It involves demyelination in scattered areas of the central nervous system
- This leads to the slowing of conduction along the affected neural pathway
- More often in women, it usually presents its first symptoms between the ages of 20 and 40
- Cause is unknown, the most widely accepted theory is of an inflammatory immune-mediated disorder
- There are different types:
  - Primary-progressive MS
  - Secondary-progressive MS
  - Relapsing-remitting MS

## DEFINITION AND MECHANISM

- Diagnosis is based on McDonald's criteria
- Management is multidirectional
  - Therapy of exacerbations:
    - Corticosteroids
  - Prevention of exacerbations:
    - Immunomodulatory therapy: interferon beta, glatiramer, Alemtuzumab
  - Therapy of chronic symptoms:
    - E.g., spasticity: baclofen
    - E.g., pain: anticonvulsants
    - E.g., urinary incontinence: oxybutynin

## PHYSIOLOGICAL CHANGES

- Symptoms vary depending on the nerve fibers affected:

| Physiological changes | |
|---|---|
| Respiratory | FRC ↓, diaphragmatic paralysis, central control of ventilation is altered, risk of chronic aspiration (due to cranial nerve involvement with impaired control of pharyngeal and laryngeal muscles) Increased incidence of obstructive sleep apnea |
| Autonomic nervous system | Hemodynamic instability Syncope, impotence, bladder and bowel dysfunction, vasomotor instability, orthostasis |
| Neurological | Sensory deficits: numbness, tingling, itching of the extremities or trunk. Impairment of facial sensation, trigeminal neuralgia, hemifacial spasms, facial myokymia Cerebellar involvement: tremor, scanning speech, coordination defects, nystagmus, unsteady gait Motor deficits: paraparesis, paraplegia, spasticity, increased deep tendon reflexes Cognitive impairment Increased incidence of epilepsy Fatigue Depression, bipolar disease Pain Lhermitte's sign |
| Visual | Optic neuritis: (unilateral) scotoma, painful eye movements, double or blurred vision |
| Urological | Bladder dysfunction |

# MANAGEMENT

- Perioperative stress or anesthesia are often implicated as causes of exacerbation of the disease
- Infection, emotional lability, and hyperpyrexia may explain the increased frequency of multiple sclerosis exacerbation postoperatively

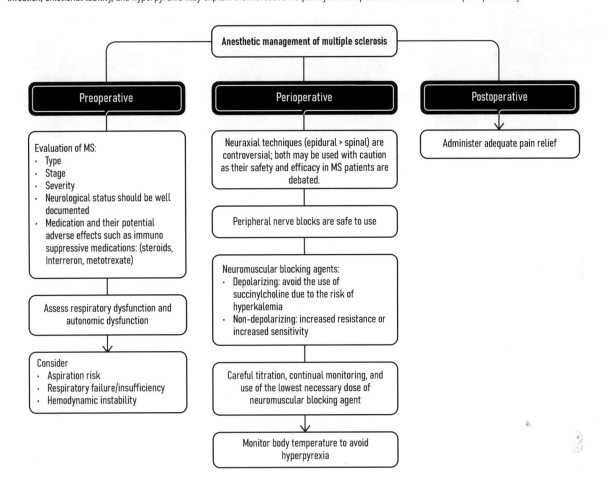

## SUGGESTED READING

- A. R. Doratta and A. Schubert. Multiple sclerosis and anesthetic implications. 2002 Curr Opin Anesthesiol 15:365-370.
- Makris A, Piperopoulos A, Karmaniolou I. Multiple sclerosis: basic knowledge and new insights in perioperative management. J Anesth. 2014;28(2):267-278.

# MYASTHENIA GRAVIS

## LEARNING OBJECTIVES

- Know the challenges in the perioperative management of these patients
- Recognise a myasthenic or cholinergic crisis

## DEFINITION AND MECHANISM

- Myasthenia Gravis (MG) is an autoimmune disease of the neuromuscular junction at the postsynaptic membrane
- Autoantibodies to acetylcholine receptor (AchR) disrupt its function by receptor blockade and conformational change leading to increased degradation which results in decreased motor end-plate potential amplitude and failure in the initiation of muscle contraction
- It is the most common disorder of the neuromuscular junction

## SIGNS AND SYMPTOMS

- Muscle weakness and fatigue of:

| Extraocular muscle group | Ptosis<br>Diplopia |
|---|---|
| Bulbar muscle group | Dysarthria<br>Dysphagia<br>Dysphonia |
| Axial-limb muscle group | Symmetrical, more often in proximal muscles |
| Respiratory muscles | Dyspnea |

- Symptoms vary over the day and from day to day, often with normal or near-normal muscle strength in the morning
- Clinical presentation varies from mild and localized to severe, generalized weakness of multiple muscle groups

Myasthenic crisis is a life-threatening condition in which severe respiratory muscle insufficiency leads to respiratory failure
- Precipitants
  - Infection
  - Surgery
  - Residual neuromuscular block
  - Pain
  - Hypo- and hyperthermia
  - Reduction or withdrawal of treatment
  - Pregnancy
  - Stress
  - Sleep deprivation

# PRECIPITANTS

| | |
|---|---|
| Antibiotics | Aminoglycoside<br>Fluoroquinolones<br>Tetracycline<br>Macrolides<br>Sulfonamides<br>Penicillin<br>Vancomycin<br>Clindamycin<br>Ketolides |
| Non-depolarizing neuromuscular-blocking agents | Pancuronium<br>Vecuronium<br>Atracurium |
| Cardiovascular agents | Beta-blockers<br>Calcium channel blockers<br>Procainamide<br>Quinidine<br>Beryllium |
| Anesthetic agents | Local: procaine, lidocaine, bupivacaine<br>Inhalation: halothane, isoflurane<br>Neuromuscular blockers |
| Anticonvulsants | Carbamazepine<br>Gabapentine<br>Phenobarbital<br>Phenytoin<br>Ethosuximide |
| Other agents | Botulinum toxin<br>Chloroquine<br>Hydroxychloroquine<br>Magnesium (Causes a significant decrease of acetylcholine release)<br>Penicillamine<br>Quinine<br>Iodinated contrast agents, although modern contrast agents should be safe<br>Cisplatinum<br>Riluzole<br>Interferon-alfa<br>Interleukin-2<br>High-dose corticosteroids |

Treatment
- Respiratory support
- Urgent neurological input
- High-dose steroids/intravenous immunoglobulins

# MANAGEMENT

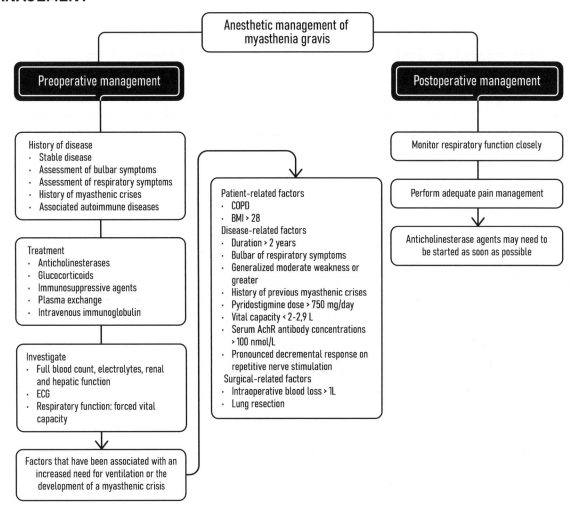

**Anesthetic management of myasthenia gravis**

**Preoperative management**

History of disease
- Stable disease
- Assessment of bulbar symptoms
- Assessment of respiratory symptoms
- History of myasthenic crises
- Associated autoimmune diseases

Treatment
- Anticholinesterases
- Glucocorticoids
- Immunosuppressive agents
- Plasma exchange
- Intravenous immunoglobulin

Investigate
- Full blood count, electrolytes, renal and hepatic function
- ECG
- Respiratory function: forced vital capacity

Factors that have been associated with an increased need for ventilation or the development of a myasthenic crisis

Patient-related factors
- COPD
- BMI > 28

Disease-related factors
- Duration > 2 years
- Bulbar of respiratory symptoms
- Generalized moderate weakness or greater
- History of previous myasthenic crises
- Pyridostigmine dose > 750 mg/day
- Vital capacity < 2-2,9 L
- Serum AchR antibody concentrations > 100 nmol/L
- Pronounced decremental response on repetitive nerve stimulation

Surgical-related factors
- Intraoperative blood loss > 1L
- Lung resection

**Postoperative management**

Monitor respiratory function closely

Perform adequate pain management

Anticholinesterase agents may need to be started as soon as possible

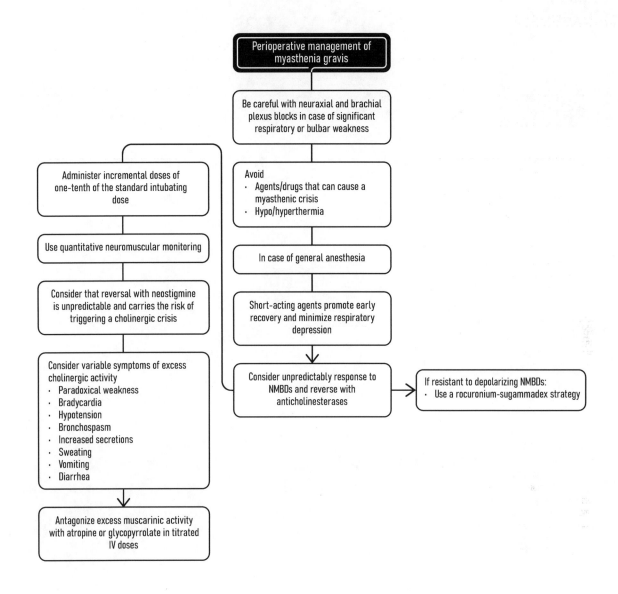

**Perioperative management of myasthenia gravis**

- Be careful with neuraxial and brachial plexus blocks in case of significant respiratory or bulbar weakness

- Avoid
  - Agents/drugs that can cause a myasthenic crisis
  - Hypo/hyperthermia

- In case of general anesthesia

- Short-acting agents promote early recovery and minimize respiratory depression

- Consider unpredictably response to NMBDs and reverse with anticholinesterases

- If resistant to depolarizing NMBDs:
  - Use a rocuronium-sugammadex strategy

- Administer incremental doses of one-tenth of the standard intubating dose

- Use quantitative neuromuscular monitoring

- Consider that reversal with neostigmine is unpredictable and carries the risk of triggering a cholinergic crisis

- Consider variable symptoms of excess cholinergic activity
  - Paradoxical weakness
  - Bradycardia
  - Hypotension
  - Bronchospasm
  - Increased secretions
  - Sweating
  - Vomiting
  - Diarrhea

- Antagonize excess muscarinic activity with atropine or glycopyrrolate in titrated IV doses

---

**SUGGESTED READING**

- Dhallu MS, Baiomi A, Biyyam M, Chilimuri S. Perioperative Management of Neurological Conditions. Health Serv Insights. 2017;10:1178632917711942.
- Dillon FX. Anesthesia issues in the perioperative management of myasthenia gravis. Semin Neurol. 2004;24(1):83-94.
- P. Daum, J. Smelt and I.R. Ibrahim. Perioperative management of myasthenia gravis. 2021, BJA Education, 21(11): 414-429.

# MYOTONIC DYSTROPHY

## LEARNING OBJECTIVES

- Describe the causes and symptoms of myotonic dystrophy
- Diagnose and treat myotonic dystrophy
- Manage myotonic dystrophy patients presenting for surgery

## DEFINITION AND MECHANISM

- Myotonic dystrophy (DM) is an autosomal dominant disorder characterized by muscle dystrophy starting in early adulthood
- Myotonic dystrophy type I (DM1, Steinert disease) and type II (DM2, proximal myotonic myopathy, milder form of type I)
- Multisystem disorder affecting somatic and smooth muscle, as well as ophthalmological, cardiovascular, endocrine, and central nervous systems

## ETIOLOGY

- Genetic disorder caused by an expansion of DNA tandem repeats, resulting in an RNA gain of function mutation
- DM1 is caused by an expansion of a CTG repeat in the 3'-untranslated region of the DM1 protein kinase gene
- DM2 is caused by the expansion of a CCTG repeat in the intron of the CCHC-type zinc finger nucleic aced-binding protein gene
- DM is the most common muscular dystrophy in the European population
- DM1 is more common than DM2

## SIGNS & SYMPTOMS

- Can range from potentially lethal in infancy to mild in late adulthood
- DM1 is classified into three types:
  - Congenital myotonic dystrophy
    - Fetal-onset involvement of muscle and central nervous system
    - Reduced fetal movement and polyhydramnios
    - Equinovarus and ventriculomegaly on fetal ultrasound
    - Neonatal mortality rate ~18%
    - Childhood/adulthood: Characteristic tented appearance of the upper lip that results from facial diplegia, marked dysarthria, expressive aphasia, hypotonia rather than myotonia
    - Frequent respiratory involvement
  - Mild myotonic dystrophy
    - Mild muscle weakness, myotonia and cataracts
    - Onset between 20-70 years of age (typically after 40)
    - Usually normal lifespan
  - Classic myotonic dystrophy
    - Onset during the second, third or fourth decade of life
    - Myotonia is the primary initial symptom
    - Characterized by "warm-up phenomenon": Symptoms appear more pronounced after rest and improve with muscle activity
    - Distal muscle weakness is the main symptom, leading to impairment of fine motor tasks with the hands and impaired gait
    - "Myopathic face": due to weakness and wasting of facial, levator palpebrae and masticatory muscles
    - Cardiac conduction abnormalities are common
    - Reduced lifespan
- DM2:
  - Manifests in adulthood (median age 48 years) with a variable presentation
  - Early-onset cataract, varying grip myotonia, proximal muscle weakness or stiffness, hearing loss, myofascial pain
  - Weakness and/or myalgias are the most common initial symptoms
  - Mostly axial and proximal muscle weakness affecting the neck flexors, long finger flexors, hip flexors, and hip extensors
  - Abdominal, musculoskeletal and exercise-related pain
  - Sometimes misdiagnosed as fibromyalgia

# DIAGNOSIS

- Genetic testing
- Elevations in alkaline phosphatase, gamma-glutamyl transferase, serum aspartate aminotransferase, and serum alanine aminotransferase in 30-50% of patients
- Electrodiagnostic testing:
  - Motor nerve conduction studies: Decreased amplitude with normal latency and normal conduction velocity
  - Sensory nerve conduction studies: Typically normal
  - Electromyography:
    - Sustained runs of positive sharp waves
    - Trains of negative spikes
    - Fluctuating amplitude and frequencies
- Muscle biopsy: Type I fiber atrophy, Type 2 fiber hypertrophy, irregular fiber size, rows of internal nuclei, fibrosis, myofibrils oriented perpendicular to muscle fiber

# DIFFERENTIAL DIAGNOSIS

- Schwartz-Jampel Syndrome
- Duchenne muscular dystrophy
- Hyperkalemic Periodic Paralysis (HPP)
- Paramyotonia Congenita (PC)
- Myotonia Congenita
- Myotubular myopathy
- Acid maltase deficiency
- Debrancher deficiency
- Inflammatory myopathies
- Hypothyroid myopathy
- Chloroquine myopathy
- Statin myopathy
- Cyclosporine myopathy

# TREATMENT

- No curative treatment, therapy is supportive and consists of monitoring and treating the issues associated with DM

| Treatment | |
|---|---|
| Cardiovascular | Annual ECG monitoring for cardiac conduction disturbances<br>Baseline cardiac imaging every 1 to 5 years |
| Pulmonary | Obtaining baseline and serial pulmonary function testing to monitor for neuromuscular respiratory failure |
| Daytime somnolence and obstructive sleep apnea | Evaluate for sleep apnea and treat if necessary<br>Consider neurostimulants (e.g., methylphenidate) for excessive sleepiness |
| Ocular involvement | Annual eye exam<br>Surgical removal of cataracts |
| Obstetrics and gynecology | High-risk obstetrics evaluation for patients who are pregnant or considering pregnancy |
| Endocrine issues | Baseline and annual fasting blood glucose and hemoglobin A1C<br>Screening for hypothyroidism<br>Treat erectile dysfunction if necessary |
| Myotonia | Medications such as mexiletine, tricyclic antidepressants, benzodiazepines, or calcium antagonists reduce sustained myotonia<br>Sodium channel blockers are contraindicated in patients with second and third-degree heart block |
| Muscle weakness | Physical and occupational therapy to strengthen muscles |

## Complications

| | |
|---|---|
| Central nervous system | Intellectual disabilities<br>Cerebrovascular accidents<br>Anxiety and depression<br>Hypersomnia and sleep apnea<br>Ventriculomegaly |
| Ophtalmologic | Cataracts<br>Hyperopia<br>Astigmatism |
| Cardiac | Atrial arrhythmias<br>Conduction system slowing<br>Ventricular arrhythmias<br>Cardiomyopathy<br>Early-onset heart failure |
| Pulmonary | Pneumonia<br>Increased risk of anesthesia-related pulmonary complications |
| Gastrointestinal | Dysphagia<br>Gallstones and cholecystitis<br>Transaminitis and liver enzyme elevations<br>Increased risk of post-anesthesia aspiration |
| Endocrine | Insulin insensitivity<br>Testicular atrophy and male infertility<br>Increased risk of abortion, miscarriage, pre-term birth, dysmenorrhea |
| Dermatologic | Androgenic alopecia<br>Increased risk of basal cell carcinoma and pilomatrixomas |
| Musculoskeletal | Progressive loss of motor function<br>Myalgias |

Myotonic dystrophy

# MANAGEMENT

## Preoperative management

### History
- Review of respiratory disease
- Swallowing difficulties
- Cardiovascular history
- Medications for myotonia

### Investigations
- Assess respiratory function
- Arterial blood gases
- Chest X-ray
- Fluoroscopy to detect diaphragmatic myotonia
- Echocardiography if there is significant cardiovascular system involvement
- Liver Function Tests

### Premedication
- Avoid respiratory depressants
- Aspiration prophylaxis
- IV potassium supplementation may exacerbate myotonia

## Intraoperative management

### Monitoring
- Arterial line for blood pressure and blood gas monitoring
- Invasive cardiovascular monitoring if there is significant cardiovascular involvement
- Peripheral nerve stimulator (may give false sense of security regarding muscle power)
- Temperature
- Glycemic control

### Induction & maintenance
- Use a minimal dose of induction agents
- Inhalational induction is preferred
- Intubation can usually be performed without muscle relaxation due to muscle atrophy
- Avoid depolarizing neuromuscular blocking agents (e.g., succinylcholine)
- Avoid long acting non depolarizing neuromuscular blocking agents or use short-acting ones
- Spontaneous reversal of the neuromuscular block is the safest, avoid neostigmine
- Although suggamadex is coming up as a reversal agent in patient with neuromuscular disorders
- Minimize opioids
- Maintain normothermia
- Treat myotonia with IV procainamide (may cause heart block) or phenytoin

### Regional techniques
- Do not eliminate myotonia
- Paralysis of the abdominal muscles may precipitate respiratory failure
- Epidural block may be helpful for analgesia
- Local infiltration of the muscle relieves myotonia

## Postoperative management
- Closely monitor the patient in the ICU
- Postoperative ventilation
- Controlled oxygen therapy in patients with chronic hypoxic drive
- Early physiotherapy
- Tracheostomy may be required if bronchial secretions are a cause for concern
- Continue ECG monitoring

# SUGGESTED READING

- Gurunathan U, Kunju SM, Stanton LML. Use of sugammadex in patients with neuromuscular disorders: a systematic review of case reports. BMC Anesthesiol. 2019;19(1):213.
- Marsh S, Pittard A. Neuromuscular disorders and anaesthesia. Part 2: specific neuromuscular disorders. Continuing Education in Anaesthesia Critical Care & Pain. 2011;11(4):119-23.
- Pollard BJ, Kitchen, G. Handbook of Clinical Anaesthesia. Fourth Edition. CRC Press. 2018. 978-1-4987-6289-2.
- Vydra DG, Rayi A. Myotonic Dystrophy. [Updated 2022 Jun 27]. In: StatPearls [Internet]. Treasure Island (FL): StatPearls Publishing; 2022 Jan-. Available from: https://www.ncbi.nlm.nih.gov/books/NBK557446/

# PARKINSON'S DISEASE

## LEARNING OBJECTIVES

- Describe the clinical presentation of Parkinson's disease
- Diagnose and treat Parkinson's disease
- Manage Parkinson's disease patients presenting for surgery

## DEFINITION AND MECHANISM

- Parkinson's disease (PD) is an idiopathic neurodegenerative disorder, characterized by bradykinesia, muscle rigidity and asymmetric resting tremor
- Most common movement disorder (~1% prevalence in the population > 65 years of age)
- Loss of dopaminergic neurons in the pars compacta region of the substantia nigra

## ETIOLOGY

- The etiology of PD is unknown but may be induced by genetic, environmental or infectious factors
- Increasing age is the most consistent risk factor

| Clinical features | | Timing |
|---|---|---|
| Primary motor features | Resting tremor (usually asymmetrical) | Usually at diagnosis |
| | Bradykinesia | |
| | Rigidity | |
| Early non-motor features | Fatigue | May precede diagnosis |
| | Depression/anxiety | |
| | Sleep disturbance | |
| | Constipation | |
| Later features | Gait change: Stooped posture, shuffling gait with small steps, loss of arm-swing | 5–10 years after onset of symptoms |

## SIGNS & SYMPTOMS

| Clinical features | | Timing |
|---|---|---|
| | Dysphagia | |
| | Expressionless face | |
| | Small handwriting | |
| | Soft speech | |
| | Postural instability | |
| | Cognitive disturbance, slowed cognitive speed, inattention, poor problem solving | Increasing likelihood as time from diagnosis increases |
| | Dementia | › 80% at 20 years after diagnosis |
| Autonomic | Postural hypotension | 5-10 years after onset of symptoms |
| | Sialorrhea | |
| | Urinary dysfunction | |
| | Sexual dysfunction | |

## DIAGNOSIS

- There are no specific diagnostic tests for PD
- Clinical diagnosis based on the hallmark symptoms (tremor at rest, muscle rigidity, bradykinesia)

# TREATMENT

- Treatment is symptomatic and usually pharmacological

| Medications | | Indication | Side-effects | Anesthetic implications |
|---|---|---|---|---|
| Dopamine agonists | Pramipexole, ropinirole | Monotherapy in early and established PD, adjunct to levodopa-DDI regime | Nausea, orthostatic hypotension, impulsive control disorders, somnolence | Risk of dopamine agonist withdrawal syndrome on acute withdrawal |
| | Rotigotine | 'Bridging' therapy in patients who are unable to take or absorb antiparkinsonian medication, adjuncts to levodopa-DDI regime | Nausea, orthostatic hypotension, impulsive control disorders, somnolence | Parenteral transdermal preparation |
| | Apomorphine | 'Bridging' therapy in patients who are unable to take or absorb antiparkinsonian medication, adjuncts to levodopa-DDI regime | Nausea, dyskinesias, cognitive impairment, postural instability | Subcutaneous infusion or injectable 'pen' for patients with troubling motor fluctuations, very emetogenic, risk of severe hypotension |
| Dopamine precursors with peripherally acting dopa decarboxylase inhibitor (DDI) | Levodopa-carbidopa, levodopa-benserazide | Motor symptoms in established PD | Nausea, orthostatic hypotension, dyskinesia, hallucinations | Risk of parkinsonism-hyperpyrexia syndrome on acute withdrawal; short halflife (1.5 h) - need to continue enteral administration in prolonged procedures |
| Monoamine oxidase B inhibitors | Selegiline, rasagiline | Used as monotherapy in early PD, or as adjunct to levodopa-DDI regime | Headache, arthralgia, exacerbation of levodopa side-effects when used as adjunct | Risk of serotonin syndrome (fever, hypertension, tachycardia, agitation) with meperidine |
| Catechol-O-methyl transferase inhibitors (COMTIs) | Entacapone, Tolcapone | Adjunct to levodopa-DDI regime | Dark-colored urine, exacerbation of levodopa side-effects | Reduce dose of other drugs metabolized by COMT pathways, e.g., epinephrine |

- Abrupt withdrawal of medications can result in withdrawal complications:
  - Parkinsonism-hyperpyrexia syndrome
    - Due to withdrawal of levodopa
    - Symptoms: Muscle rigidity, fever, cardiovascular instability, altered mental status (agitation, delirium, coma)
    - Significant mortality, up to 20% in untreated cases
  - Dopamine agonist withdrawal syndrome (DAWS)
    - Symptoms: Anxiety, nausea, depression, pain, orthostatic hypotension
    - Withdrawal of dopamine agonists should be planned electively and simultaneously replaced with levodopa therapy

Parkinson's disease

# MANAGEMENT

- Preoperative

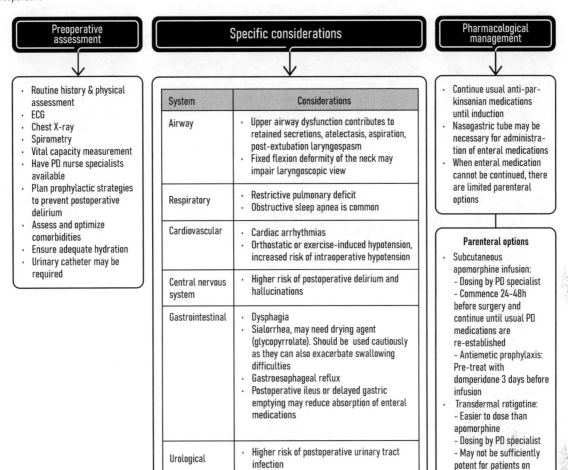

| Preoperative assessment |
|---|
| • Routine history & physical assessment |
| • ECG |
| • Chest X-ray |
| • Spirometry |
| • Vital capacity measurement |
| • Have PD nurse specialists available |
| • Plan prophylactic strategies to prevent postoperative delirium |
| • Assess and optimize comorbidities |
| • Ensure adequate hydration |
| • Urinary catheter may be required |

**Specific considerations**

| System | Considerations |
|---|---|
| Airway | • Upper airway dysfunction contributes to retained secretions, atelectasis, aspiration, post-extubation laryngospasm<br>• Fixed flexion deformity of the neck may impair laryngoscopic view |
| Respiratory | • Restrictive pulmonary deficit<br>• Obstructive sleep apnea is common |
| Cardiovascular | • Cardiac arrhythmias<br>• Orthostatic or exercise-induced hypotension, increased risk of intraoperative hypotension |
| Central nervous system | • Higher risk of postoperative delirium and hallucinations |
| Gastrointestinal | • Dysphagia<br>• Sialorrhea, may need drying agent (glycopyrrolate). Should be used cautiously as they can also exacerbate swallowing difficulties<br>• Gastroesophageal reflux<br>• Postoperative ileus or delayed gastric emptying may reduce absorption of enteral medications |
| Urological | • Higher risk of postoperative urinary tract infection |

**Pharmacological management**

- Continue usual anti-parkinsonian medications until induction
- Nasogastric tube may be necessary for administration of enteral medications
- When enteral medication cannot be continued, there are limited parenteral options

**Parenteral options**

- Subcutaneous apomorphine infusion:
  - Dosing by PD specialist
  - Commence 24-48h before surgery and continue until usual PD medications are re-established
  - Antiemetic prophylaxis: Pre-treat with domperidone 3 days before infusion
- Transdermal rotigotine:
  - Easier to dose than apomorphine
  - Dosing by PD specialist
  - May not be sufficiently potent for patients on higher-dose anti-parkinsonian medications

Parkinson's disease

- Intraoperative

# PARKINSON'S DISEASE (PD): INTRAOPERATIVE MANAGEMENT

**Anesthetic modality**

| Modality | Advantages | Disadvantages |
|---|---|---|
| Central neuraxial block | • Intraoperative monitoring of parkinsonian symptoms<br>• Enteral medication can be given intraoperatively<br>• Earlier return to postoperative oral intake<br>• Reduced use of systemic opioids<br>• No neuromuscular block required | • Muscle rigidity may make positioning difficult<br>• May be technically challenging with severe resting tremor<br>• Risk of hypotension<br>• Tremor is only eliminated in the areas with motor block, tremor elsewhere may hinder surgery |
| General anesthesia | • Tremor is eliminated | • Postoperative nausea and vomiting may hinder enteral dosing of medication<br>• Higher risk of postoperative pneumonia |

**Monitoring**

- Tremor may induce monitoring artifacts:
  - ECG may mimic atrial flutter or ventricular fibrillation
  - Non-invasive arterial pressure monitoring may be difficult
- Excessive sweating due to autonomic dysfunction may result in poor ECG electrode contact

**Intravascular volume**

- Arterial catheters (arterial pressure and pulse pressure variation)
- Transesophageal Doppler (stroke volume, flow time corrected)
- Devices utilizing pulse contour analysis to derive hemodynamic parameters (stroke volume, flow time corrected)
- Echocardiography (e.g., inferior vena cava diameter and collapsibility, left ventricular end diastolic area)
- Pulmonary artery catheters (cardiac output, central and pulmonary capillary wedge pressures)
- Central venous pressure does not correlate with volume status

**Neuromuscular blocking**

- Neuromuscular blocking agents can be safely used
- Residual block can mask parkinsonian symptoms postoperatively
- Use neostigmine cautiously (increases saliva viscosity)
- Rocuronium is preferred

**Airway management**

- Sialorrhea can be reduced with glycopyrrolate
- Consider intubation if dysphagia is suspected
- Rapid sequence induction may be necessary in patients with gastroparesis or gastroesophageal reflux
- Fixed flexion neck deformity may complicate laryngoscopy

**Antiemetics**

- Several antiemetics are contraindicated due to dopamine agonist effects
- Ondansetron and cyclizine have fewer side-effects
- Domperidone can be safely used as it does not cross the blood-brain-barrier

**Opioids**

- Meperidine is contraindicated in patients who take selegiline
- Other opioids can be used safely, although higher doses may cause rigidity

- Postoperative
  - Consider ICU admission
  - Assess the feasibility of enteral anti-parkinsonian medication
  - Adequate analgesia, tremor, and rigidity may hinder patient-controlled analgesia
  - Postoperative delirium: Non-pharmacological management is preferred, avoid haloperidol, benzodiazepines are safer
  - Physiotherapy facilitates early mobilization

# SUGGESTED READING

- Chambers DJ, Sebastian J, Ahearn DJ. Parkinson's disease. BJA Education. 2017;17(4):145-9.
- Pollard BJ, Kitchen, G. Handbook of Clinical Anaesthesia. Fourth Edition. CRC Press. 2018. 978-1-4987-6289-2.

# POLYMYOSITIS AND DERMATOMYOSITIS

## LEARNING OBJECTIVES

- Definition of polymyositis and dermatomyositis
- Management of polymyositis and dermatomyositis

## DEFINITION AND MECHANISM

- Myositis is the name for a group of rare conditions such as polymyositis and dermatomyositis, leading to weak, painful, or aching muscles
- Polymyositis and dermatomyositis are autoimmune myopathies characterized by inflammation and weakness of proximal skeletal muscles
- Characteristically there is a rise in serum enzymes derived from muscle, e.g., creatine phosphokinase (CPK) and myoglobin may be released leading to myoglobinuria
- Dermatomyositis, unlike polymyositis, is associated with a variety of characteristic skin manifestations
- The cause is unknown, likely an immune reaction triggered by a virus or tumor
- Both occur almost two times more often in women than in men
- It can occur at any age

## SIGNS AND SYMPTOMS

- Both polymyositis and dermatomyositis have symptoms in common with sclerosis or sometimes systemic lupus erythematosus:
  - Muscle weakness
  - Contraction of the arms and legs
  - Shortness of breath
  - Difficulty in swallowing
  - Muscle tenderness or pain
  - Raynaud's phenomenon
  - Fever
  - Fatigue
  - Weight loss
- If dermatomyositis occurs along with polymyositis, symptoms may also include:
  - Skin rash
  - Swelling around the eye
  - Swelling at the base and sides of the fingernails
  - Splitting of the skin of the fingers

## DIAGNOSIS

- Laboratory findings:
  - Elevations in serum creatine kinase, lactate dehydrogenase, aldolase, and aminotransferases
  - Myositis-specific autoantibodies
- Muscle biopsy
- Electromyogram
- MRI

## TREATMENT

- Corticosteroids
- Immunosuppressive drugs: methotrexate, cyclophosphamide, chlorambucil, azathioprine, cyclosporine
- Immunoglobulin therapy
- Exercise is important to reduce swelling and to build or restore muscle strength

Polymyositis and dermatomyositis

# MANAGEMENT

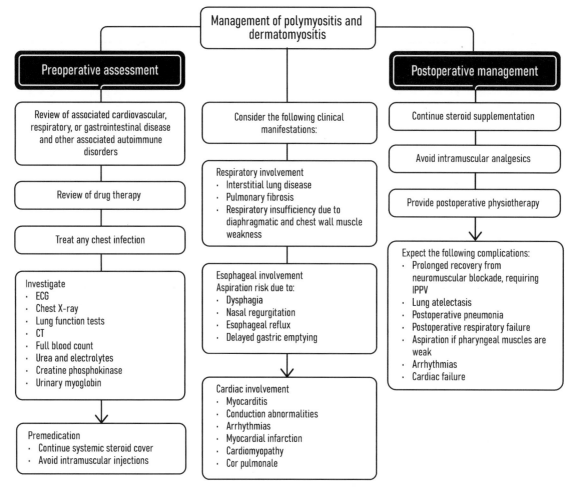

**Management of polymyositis and dermatomyositis**

## Preoperative assessment

Review of associated cardiovascular, respiratory, or gastrointestinal disease and other associated autoimmune disorders

Review of drug therapy

Treat any chest infection

Investigate
- ECG
- Chest X-ray
- Lung function tests
- CT
- Full blood count
- Urea and electrolytes
- Creatine phosphokinase
- Urinary myoglobin

Premedication
- Continue systemic steroid cover
- Avoid intramuscular injections

Consider the following clinical manifestations:

Respiratory involvement
- Interstitial lung disease
- Pulmonary fibrosis
- Respiratory insufficiency due to diaphragmatic and chest wall muscle weakness

Esophageal involvement
Aspiration risk due to:
- Dysphagia
- Nasal regurgitation
- Esophageal reflux
- Delayed gastric emptying

Cardiac involvement
- Myocarditis
- Conduction abnormalities
- Arrhythmias
- Myocardial infarction
- Cardiomyopathy
- Cor pulmonale

## Postoperative management

Continue steroid supplementation

Avoid intramuscular analgesics

Provide postoperative physiotherapy

Expect the following complications:
- Prolonged recovery from neuromuscular blockade, requiring IPPV
- Lung atelectasis
- Postoperative pneumonia
- Postoperative respiratory failure
- Aspiration if pharyngeal muscles are weak
- Arrhythmias
- Cardiac failure

IPPV, intermittent positive-pressure ventilation

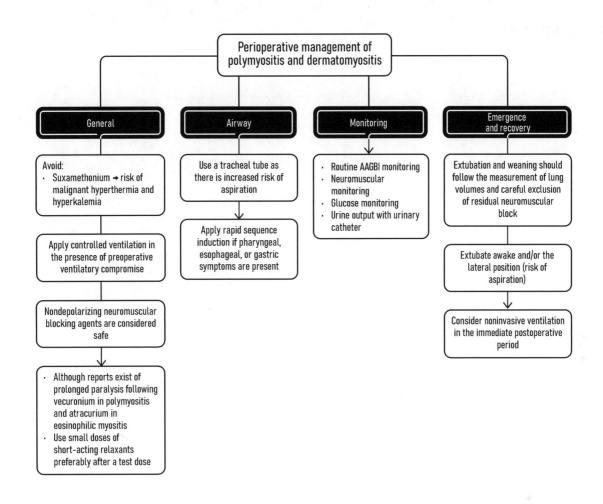

Perioperative management of polymyositis and dermatomyositis

**General**

Avoid:
- Suxamethonium → risk of malignant hyperthermia and hyperkalemia

Apply controlled ventilation in the presence of preoperative ventilatory compromise

Nondepolarizing neuromuscular blocking agents are considered safe

- Although reports exist of prolonged paralysis following vecuronium in polymyositis and atracurium in eosinophilic myositis
- Use small doses of short-acting relaxants preferably after a test dose

**Airway**

Use a tracheal tube as there is increased risk of aspiration

Apply rapid sequence induction if pharyngeal, esophageal, or gastric symptoms are present

**Monitoring**

- Routine AAGBI monitoring
- Neuromuscular monitoring
- Glucose monitoring
- Urine output with urinary catheter

**Emergence and recovery**

Extubation and weaning should follow the measurement of lung volumes and careful exclusion of residual neuromuscular block

Extubate awake and/or the lateral position (risk of aspiration)

Consider noninvasive ventilation in the immediate postoperative period

## SUGGESTED READING

- Christopher-Stine L, Vleugels An Amato AA. 2022 Clinical manifestations of dermatomyositis and polymyositis in adults. Up To Date.
- Dalakas MC, Hohlfeld R. Polymyositis and dermatomyositis. Lancet. 2003;362(9388):971-982.
- Pollard BJ, Kitchen, G. Handbook of Clinical Anaesthesia. Fourth Edition. CRC Press. 2018. 978-1-4987-6289-2.
- Raychaudhuri SP, Mitra A. Polymyositis and dermatomyositis: Disease spectrum and classification. Indian J Dermatol. 2012;57(5):366-370.

# OBSTETRICS

# AMNIOTIC FLUID EMBOLISM

## LEARNING OBJECTIVES

- Signs of amniotic fluid embolism (AFE)
- Management of AFE

## DEFINITION AND MECHANISM

- Amniotic fluid embolism (AFE) is one of the most catastrophic and life-threatening complications of pregnancy
- Occurs when amniotic fluid, fetal cells, hair, or other debris enters the maternal pulmonary circulation and causes cardiovascular collapse
- It is not a consequence of the "simple" mechanical respiratory obstruction, but a humoral effect causing anaphylactoid reactions or complement activation
- It can occur in:
  - Healthy women during labor
  - During cesarean section
  - After abnormal vaginal delivery
  - During the second trimester of pregnancy
  - 48 hours post delivery
  - During abortion
  - After abdominal trauma
  - During amnio-infusion
- Any breach of the barrier between maternal blood and amniotic fluid forces the entry of amniotic fluid into the systemic circulation and results in a physical obstruction of the pulmonary circulation
- The maternal prognosis after amniotic fluid embolism is very poor

## SIGNS AND SYMPTOMS

- Premonitory symptoms
  - Acute dyspnea
  - Sudden agitations
  - Sudden chills, shivering, sweating
  - Cough
  - Anxiety
  - Labored breathing
  - Tachypnea
- Altered mental status, seizures, and coma
- A rapid decline in pulse oximetry values or sudden absence or decrease in end-tidal carbon dioxide
- Hypotension
- Cyanosis: ventilation-perfusion mismatching as a result of pulmonary vascular constriction
- Fetal bradycardia
- Encephalopathy
- Uterine atony
- Acute pulmonary hypertension
- Coagulopathy/ severe hemorrhage

## DIAGNOSIS

- Four criteria must be present to make the diagnosis of AFE:
  - Acute hypotension or cardiac arrest
  - Acute hypoxia
  - Coagulopathy or severe hemorrhage in the absence of other explanations
  - All of these occur during labor, cesarean delivery, dilatation, and evacuation, or within 30 min postpartum with no other explanation of findings

## COURSE OF AFE

- Typical (classic) with three phases
  - Phase 1: Respiratory and circulatory disorders
  - Phase 2: Coagulation disturbances of maternal hemostasis
  - Phase 3: Acute renal failure and acute respiratory distress syndrome (ARDS)
  - Cardiopulmonary collapse
- Atypical
  - Life-threatening hemorrhage due to disseminated intravascular coagulation (DIC)

# DIFFERENTIAL DIAGNOSIS

- Anaphylaxis
- Aortic dissection
- Cholesterol embolism
- Myocardial infarction
- Pulmonary embolism
- Septic shock

- Air embolism
- Transfusion reaction
- Eclamptic convulsions and coma
- Convulsion from the toxic reaction to local anesthetic drugs
- Aspiration of gastric contents
- Hemorrhagic shock in an obstetric patient

# RISK FACTORS OR CAUSES

- Unpredictable – unpreventable

Risk factors:
- Older maternal age
- Multiparity
- Intense contractions during labor
- Abdominal trauma
- Cesarean section
- Induction of labor
- Placenta previa

- Eclampsia
- Multiple pregnancies
- Tears in the uterus or cervix
- Early separation of the placenta from the uterus wall
- Fetal factors:
  - Fetal distress
  - Fetal death
  - Male baby

---

**Management of amniotic fluid embolism (AFE)**

Key factors:
- Early recognition
- Prompt resuscitation
- Delivery of the fetus

Maintain vital signs:
- Perform oxygenation and control of the airway with ETT and $FiO_2$ 100%
- Perform arterial and CVP monitoring

Rapidly correct maternal hemodynamic instability
- Fluid resuscitation: isotonic crystalloid – colloid solutions – transfusion
- Vasopressors and inotropic support: epinephrine (first choice), phenylephrine, vasopressin
- Hydrocortisone: AFE is more similar to an anaphylactic reaction

Left uterine displacement is crucial in resuscitation efforts if the fetus remains in utero

Perform immediate cesarean section

Correct coagulopathy:
- Antifibrinolytic drugs
- Blood and blood products including FFP, platelets and cryoprecipitate
- Persistent uterine hemorrhage-hysterectomy is required

Other considerations:
- ECMO
- Cardiopulmonary bypass
- Right ventricular assist device
- Uterine artery embolization
- Intra-aortic balloon pump

ETT, endotracheal tube; CVP, central venous pressure; FFP, fresh frozen plasma

---

- Kaur K, Bhardwaj M, Kumar P, Singhal S, Singh T, Hooda S. Amniotic fluid embolism. J Anaesthesiol Clin Pharmacol. 2016;32(2):153-159.
- Pollard BJ, Kitchen, G. Handbook of Clinical Anaesthesia. Fourth Edition. CRC Press. 2018. 978-1-4987-6289-2.

Amniotic fluid embolism

# ANTEPARTUM BLEEDING

## LEARNING OBJECTIVES

- Definition of antepartum bleeding (APB)
- Causes and consequences of APB
- General management of APB

## DEFINITION AND MECHANISM

- Antepartum bleeding (APB) is defined as bleeding from the genital tract after 24 weeks of gestation and before the birth of the baby
- A relatively frequent problem, occurring in 5% to 6% of pregnant women
- It remains a major cause of perinatal mortality and maternal morbidity
- Four degrees of APB:
  - Spotting: stains, streaking, or spotting of blood
  - Minor hemorrhage: < 50 mL
  - Major hemorrhage: 50-1000mL without signs of circulatory shock
  - Massive hemorrhage: > 1000mL with or without signs of circulatory shock

## CAUSES

- Cervicitis
- Placenta abnormalities
  - Abruptio placentae
  - Placenta previa
  - Placenta accreta /increta/percreta
- Uterine rupture
- Vasa previa
- Amniotic fluid embolism

## COMPLICATIONS

| Maternal complications | Fetal complications |
|---|---|
| Perioperative anemia | Fetal hypoxia |
| Infection | Small for gestational age and fetal growth restriction |
| Maternal shock | Prematurity (iatrogenic and spontaneous) |
| Renal tubular necrosis | Fetal death |
| Consumptive coagulopathy | |
| Postpartum hemorrhage | |
| Prolonged hospital stay | |
| Psychological sequelae | |
| Complications of blood transfusion | |

# MANAGEMENT

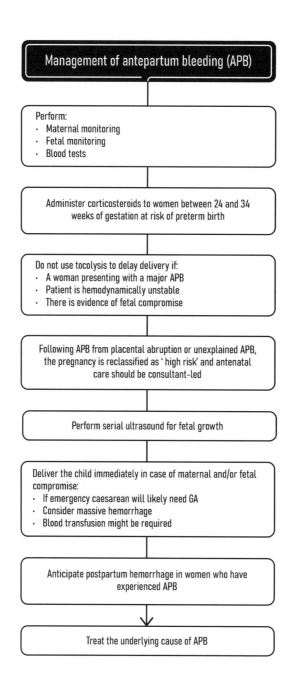

**Management of antepartum bleeding (APB)**

Perform:
- Maternal monitoring
- Fetal monitoring
- Blood tests

Administer corticosteroids to women between 24 and 34 weeks of gestation at risk of preterm birth

Do not use tocolysis to delay delivery if:
- A woman presenting with a major APB
- Patient is hemodynamically unstable
- There is evidence of fetal compromise

Following APB from placental abruption or unexplained APB, the pregnancy is reclassified as 'high risk' and antenatal care should be consultant-led

Perform serial ultrasound for fetal growth

Deliver the child immediately in case of maternal and/or fetal compromise:
- If emergency caesarean will likely need GA
- Consider massive hemorrhage
- Blood transfusion might be required

Anticipate postpartum hemorrhage in women who have experienced APB

Treat the underlying cause of APB

## SUGGESTED READING

- Antepartum haemorrhage Green-top Guideline No. 63 November 2011 royal College of obstreticans and gynaecologists. https://www.rcog.org.uk/media/pwdi1tef/gtg_63.pdf
- Mercier FJ, Van de Velde M. Major obstetric hemorrhage. Anesthesiol Clin. 2008;26(1):53-vi.
- Walfish, M., Neuman, A., Wlody, D., 2009. Maternal haemorrhage. British Journal of Anaesthesia 103, i47-i56.

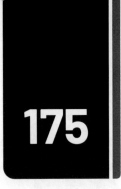

# BREASTFEEDING PATIENT

## LEARNING OBJECTIVES

- The presence of anesthetic agents in breastmilk
- The anesthetic management of breastfeeding patients

## DEFINITION AND MECHANISM

- Breastfeeding, or nursing, is the process by which human breast milk is fed to a child and is one of the most effective ways to ensure the health and survival of the infant
- Breastfeeding has many health benefits for the mother and infant
- Women who are breastfeeding may require anesthesia or sedation
- Concerns regarding the passage of medications into breast milk may lead to inconsistent advice resulting in:
  - Interruption of feeding for 24 hours or longer
  - Pumping and discarding of milk
  - Early cessation of breastfeeding
- All anesthetic and analgesic drugs transfer to breastmilk. However, only small amounts are present in very low concentrations and considered clinically insignificant
- It is safe to breastfeed as usual after anesthesia and surgery
- There is no need to express and discard breast milk ("pump and dump") after anesthesia

## ANESTHETIC AGENTS AND BREASTMILK

- Neonatal agent exposure is expressed by the relative infant dose (RID)
- The RID takes into account maternal and infant weight as well as the concentration of drug in breastmilk and indicates the percentage of drug in the baby relative to the mother
- RID levels < 10% are considered safe
- Nearly all anesthetic agents have RID values significantly less than 10%, except for morphine (9%)
- Certain opioids (i.e., codeine and tramadol) and drug classes (i.e., amphetamines, chemotherapy agents, ergotamines, and statins) are not recommended in breastfeeding mothers
- Due to pharmacogenetic variability in metabolizing codeine or tramadol, there is a risk of a neonatal opioid overdose if an "ultra-metabolizer" mother breastfeeds a "slow metabolizer" neonate

# MANAGEMENT

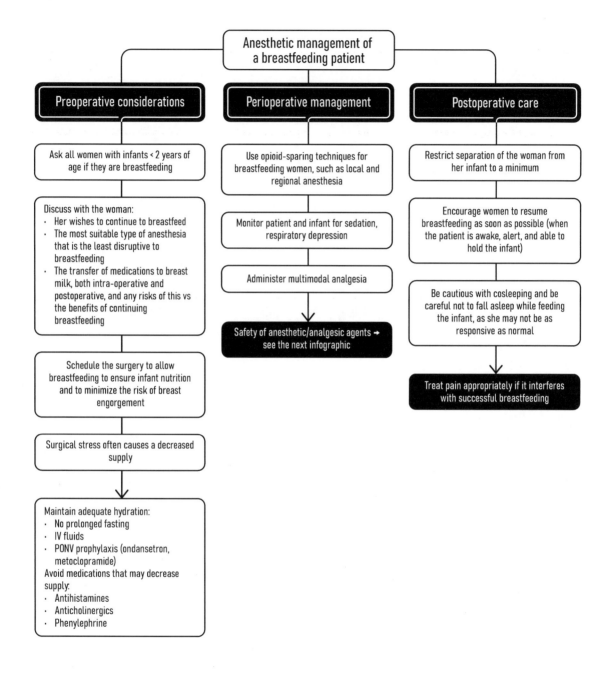

Anesthetic management of a breastfeeding patient

**Preoperative considerations**

Ask all women with infants < 2 years of age if they are breastfeeding

Discuss with the woman:
· Her wishes to continue to breastfeed
· The most suitable type of anesthesia that is the least disruptive to breastfeeding
· The transfer of medications to breast milk, both intra-operative and postoperative, and any risks of this vs the benefits of continuing breastfeeding

Schedule the surgery to allow breastfeeding to ensure infant nutrition and to minimize the risk of breast engorgement

Surgical stress often causes a decreased supply

Maintain adequate hydration:
· No prolonged fasting
· IV fluids
· PONV prophylaxis (ondansetron, metoclopramide)
Avoid medications that may decrease supply:
· Antihistamines
· Anticholinergics
· Phenylephrine

**Perioperative management**

Use opioid-sparing techniques for breastfeeding women, such as local and regional anesthesia

Monitor patient and infant for sedation, respiratory depression

Administer multimodal analgesia

Safety of anesthetic/analgesic agents ➜ see the next infographic

**Postoperative care**

Restrict separation of the woman from her infant to a minimum

Encourage women to resume breastfeeding as soon as possible (when the patient is awake, alert, and able to hold the infant)

Be cautious with cosleeping and be careful not to fall asleep while feeding the infant, as she may not be as responsive as normal

Treat pain appropriately if it interferes with successful breastfeeding

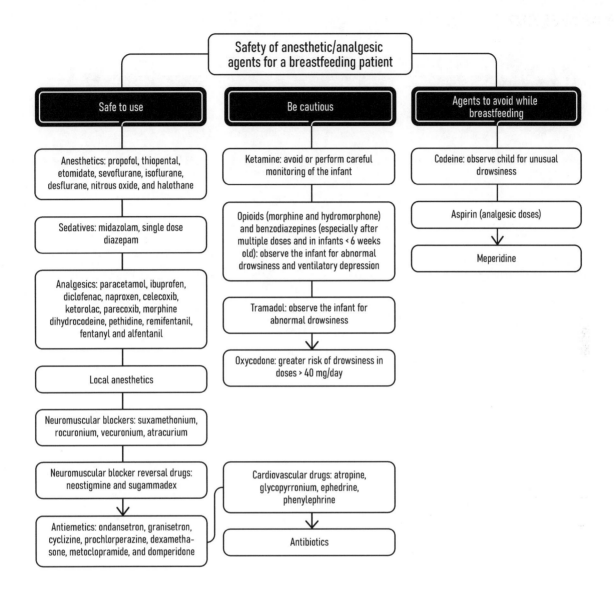

**Safety of anesthetic/analgesic agents for a breastfeeding patient**

**Safe to use**

- Anesthetics: propofol, thiopental, etomidate, sevoflurane, isoflurane, desflurane, nitrous oxide, and halothane
- Sedatives: midazolam, single dose diazepam
- Analgesics: paracetamol, ibuprofen, diclofenac, naproxen, celecoxib, ketorolac, parecoxib, morphine dihydrocodeine, pethidine, remifentanil, fentanyl and alfentanil
- Local anesthetics
- Neuromuscular blockers: suxamethonium, rocuronium, vecuronium, atracurium
- Neuromuscular blocker reversal drugs: neostigmine and sugammadex
- Antiemetics: ondansetron, granisetron, cyclizine, prochlorperazine, dexamethasone, metoclopramide, and domperidone

**Be cautious**

- Ketamine: avoid or perform careful monitoring of the infant
- Opioids (morphine and hydromorphone) and benzodiazepines (especially after multiple doses and in infants < 6 weeks old): observe the infant for abnormal drowsiness and ventilatory depression
- Tramadol: observe the infant for abnormal drowsiness
- Oxycodone: greater risk of drowsiness in doses > 40 mg/day
- Cardiovascular drugs: atropine, glycopyrronium, ephedrine, phenylephrine
- Antibiotics

**Agents to avoid while breastfeeding**

- Codeine: observe child for unusual drowsiness
- Aspirin (analgesic doses)
- Meperidine

## SUGGESTED READING

- General principles for anesthesia and perioperative management for a patient who is breastfeeding. Uptodate.com
- Mitchell, J., Jones, W., Winkley, E., Kinsella, S.M., 2020. Guideline on anaesthesia and sedation in breastfeeding women 2020. Anaesthesia 75, 1482–1493.
- Statement on resuming breastfeeding after anesthesia. 2019. American Society of Anesthesiologists
- Wanderer JP, Rathmell JP. 2017. Anesthesia & breastfeeding: more often than not, they are compatible. 127;4.

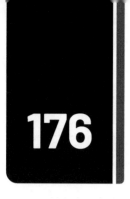

# 176

# BREECH PRESENTATION

## LEARNING OBJECTIVES

- Types of breech presentation
- Management of breech presentation

## DEFINITION AND MECHANISM

- Breech presentation refers to the fetus in the longitudinal lie with the buttocks or lower extremity entering the pelvis first
- Three types:
  - Frank breech: fetus has flexion of both hips, and the legs are straight with the feet near the fetal face, in a pike position
  - Complete breech: fetus sits with flexion of both hips and both legs in a tuck position
  - Incomplete breech: can have any combination of one or both hips extended, also known as footling (one leg extended) breech, or double footling breech (both legs extended)
- Occurs in 3-4% of all term pregnancies
  - A higher percentage of breech presentations occurs with less advanced gestational age
  - At 32 weeks, 7% of fetuses are breech
  - At 28 weeks or less, 25% are breech
- Clinical conditions associated with a breech presentation include those that may increase or decrease fetal motility, or affect the vertical polarity of the uterine cavity
- It is unsafe for a breech baby to be born vaginally due to the risk of injury (dislocated or broken bones) or umbilical cord problems (flattening or twisting)
- Turning the baby into the head-first position and/or a planned C-section are the safest option

## ETIOLOGY

- Prematurity
- Multiple gestation
- Aneuploidies
- Congenital anomalies: fetal sacrococcygeal teratoma, fetal thyroid goiter
- Mullerian anomalies
- Uterine leiomyoma

- Placental polarity as in placenta previa
- Polyhydramnios
- Oligohydramnios
- Previous history of breech presentation (recurrence rate is 10% for the second pregnancy and 27% in the third pregnancy)

## EVALUATION

- Physical exam: palpation of a hard, round, mobile structure at the fundus and the inability to palpate a presenting part in the lower abdomen superior to the pubic bone or the engaged breech in the same area, should raise suspicion of a breech presentation
- Cervical exam: the lack of a palpable presenting part, palpation of a lower extremity, usually a foot, or for the engaged breech, palpation of the soft tissue of the fetal buttocks may be noted
- Note that the soft tissue of the fetal buttocks may be interpreted as caput of the fetal vertex if the patient has been laboring
- Ultrasound confirms the diagnosis

# MANAGEMENT

**Urgent delivery is indicated if:**
- Abnormal cardiotocography
- Vaginal bleeding
- Unexplained pain

**Consider**
- An increased risk of maternal mortality, morbidity, & complications (infection, perineal trauma, hemorrhage)
- An increased risk of fetal complications:
  - Preterm delivery
  - Birth trauma
  - Major congenital anomalies
  - Umbilical cord prolapse
  - Hyperextension of the head
  - Spinal cord injuries with deflexion
  - Arrest of after-coming head
  - Intrapartum asphyxia
  - Intrapartum fetal death
- Pregnancy considerations (difficult intubation, aspiration, ↓ time to desaturation, aortocaval compression, 2 patients at once, mother and baby)

**Singleton birth**
**Four strategies have evolved:**
- External cephalic version (ECV) before labor, with a trial of labor if the version is successful and caesarean birth if unsuccessful
- ECV before labor, with a trial of labor if the version is successful. However, if the version is unsuccessful, a trial of labor and vaginal breech birth is offered to patients who have characteristics that are believed to place them at low risk of labor and delivery-related complications
- Caesarean birth is offered to higher-risk patients and any patient who declines to attempt a vaginal breech birth
- Planned caesarean birth for breech presentation, without an attempt at ECV
- A trial of labor and vaginal breech birth for patients who have characteristics that are believed to place them at low risk of labor and delivery-related complications, without an attempt at CV

**Epidural analgesia is preferred for vagina breech delivery**
- A vaginal breech is associated with a very high risk of umbilical cord compression and fetal head entrapment
- A sacral block may prevent premature maternal pushing and thus decrease the likelihood of fetal head entrapment
- Be ready to convert to general anesthesia
- General anesthesia can be required to relieve cervical entrapment

**Anesthesia for a caesarean delivery**
- Neuraxial or GA
- Possible need for uterine relaxation, have nitroglycerin available
- It may require a larger incision or a vertical incision

**Fetal head entrapment**
- Nitroglycerin IV 100-400mcg OR nitroglycerin SL 400-800mcg
- Likely need GA: RSI (propofol/succinylcholine) & start 2-3 MAC of volatile to relax the uterus
- Support hemodynamics, control hemorrhage

**Higher risk is expected if:**
- Hyperextended neck on ultrasound
- High estimated fetal weight (more than 3.8 kg)
- Low estimated weight (less than a tenth centile)
- Footling presentation
- Evidence of antenatal fetal compromise

**Twin gestation**
- The presentation of the fetuses may influence the mode of delivery
- Epidural analgesia is preferred for vaginal delivery
- Minimize the motor block if a spontaneous delivery is planned
- If an internal podalic version and extraction of twin B is planned, epidural anesthesia alone may be sufficient
- On occasion, general anesthesia is required for the delivery of the second twin
- Administration of a potent halogenated agent will relax the uterus and facilitate the delivery of the second twin

**Multiples**
- Delivery is generally performed via caesarean section via either regional or general anesthesia

# SUGGESTED READING

- Gray CJ, Shanahan MM. 2022. Breech presentation. StatPearls.
- Hofmeyer GD. 2022. Overview of breech presentation. Up to date.
- 2017. Management of Breech Presentation. BJOG: An International Journal of Obstetrics & Gynaecology 124, e151–e177.
- Stitely ML, Gherman RB. Labor with abnormal presentation and position. Obstet Gynecol Clin North Am. 2005;32(2):165-179.
- Pollack KL, Chestnut DH. 1990. Anesthesia for complicated vaginal deliveries. Anesthesiology clinics of North America. 8;1:115-129.
- Pratt SD. Anesthesia for breech presentation and multiple gestation. Clin Obstet Gynecol. 2003;46(3):711-729.

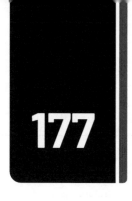

# 177

# CESAREAN DELIVERY

## LEARNING OBJECTIVES

- Indications for a cesarean delivery
- Benefits of regional versus general anesthesia
- Management of an elective cesarean section and operative vaginal delivery
- Management of an emergency cesarean section and operative vaginal delivery
- Patient position for epidural or spinal anesthesia for cesarean delivery

## DEFINITION AND MECHANISM

- A surgical procedure by which one or more babies are delivered through an incision in the mother's abdomen, often performed because vaginal delivery would put the baby or mother at risk
- Elective cesarean is the most common obstetric operation
- Planning for a cesarean section might be necessary if there are certain pregnancy complications
- Often performed as an urgent or emergency procedure

## INDICATIONS

- Breech
- Multiples
- Previous cesarean section
- Maternal high blood presure
- Cephalopelvic disproportion

- Malplacentation (minor or major placenta praevia) and morbidly adherent placenta (placenta accreta or perccreta)
- Prevention of transmission of HIV from mother to baby
- Maternal choice

## ANESTHESIA FOR CESAREAN SECTION

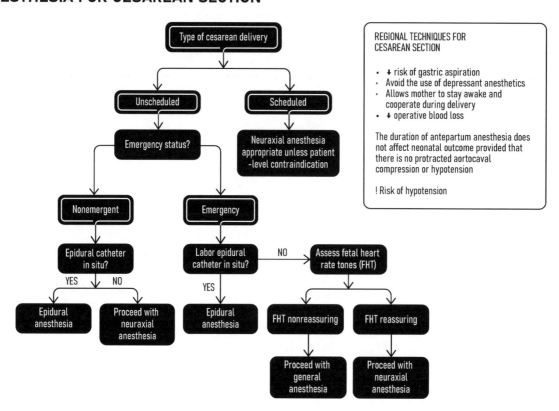

REGIONAL TECHNIQUES FOR CESAREAN SECTION

- ↓ risk of gastric aspiration
- Avoid the use of depressant anesthetics
- Allows mother to stay awake and cooperate during delivery
- ↓ operative blood loss

The duration of antepartum anesthesia does not affect neonatal outcome provided that there is no protracted aortocaval compression or hypotension

! Risk of hypotension

# BENEFITS OF REGIONAL VERSUS GENERAL ANESTHESIA

| Regional anesthesia | General anesthesia |
|---|---|
| Reduced blood loss<br>Improved pain relief postoperatively<br>Avoids the risk of failed intubation<br>The mother is awake when her baby is delivered<br>Facilitates the presence of birth partners at delivery<br>Supports skin-to-skin contact in the OR | Provides anesthesia when regional techniques are contraindicated, such as when the woman has:<br>- Abnormalities of clotting or recent thromboprophylaxis<br>- Significant cranial or spinal abnormalities (e.g, spina bifida, chiari malformation)<br>Alleviates profound anxiety of being awake during surgery<br>Facilitates the management of complex cases from the outset of the procedure<br>Eliminates any intraoperative sensation of tugging/stretching |

# MANAGEMENT OF AN ELECTIVE CESAREAN SECTION AND OPERATIVE VAGINAL DELIVERY

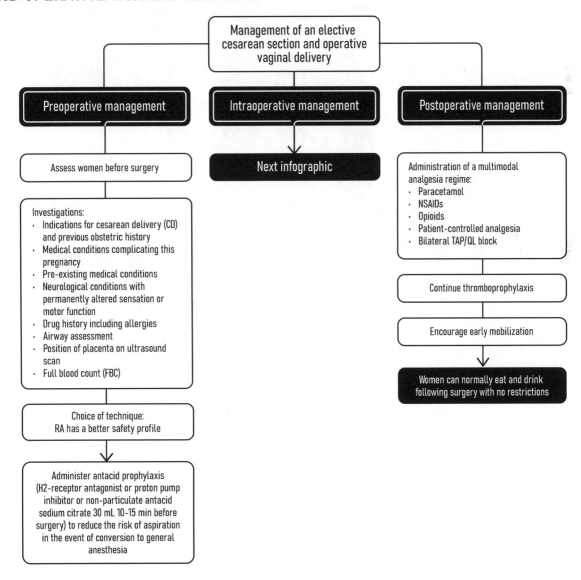

Cesarean delivery

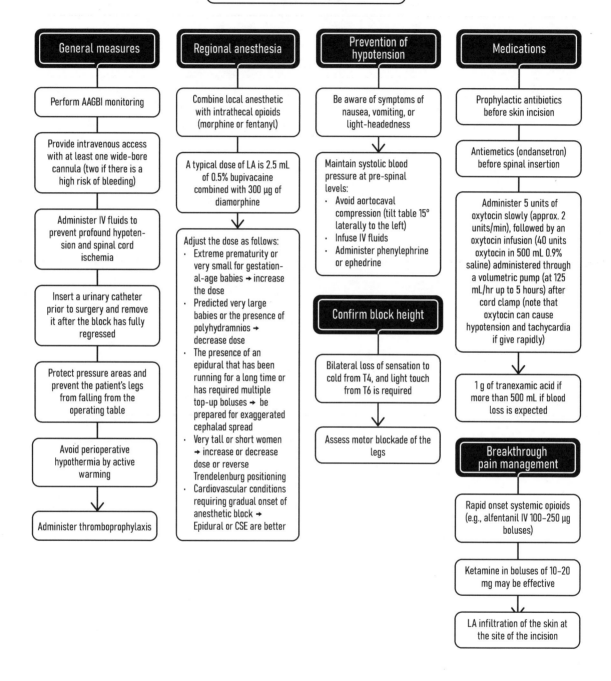

## Intraoperative care of an elective cesarean section and operative vaginal delivery

### General measures

Perform AAGBI monitoring

Provide intravenous access with at least one wide-bore cannula (two if there is a high risk of bleeding)

Administer IV fluids to prevent profound hypotension and spinal cord ischemia

Insert a urinary catheter prior to surgery and remove it after the block has fully regressed

Protect pressure areas and prevent the patient's legs from falling from the operating table

Avoid perioperative hypothermia by active warming

Administer thromboprophylaxis

### Regional anesthesia

Combine local anesthetic with intrathecal opioids (morphine or fentanyl)

A typical dose of LA is 2.5 mL of 0.5% bupivacaine combined with 300 μg of diamorphine

Adjust the dose as follows:
· Extreme prematurity or very small for gestational-age babies ➔ increase the dose
· Predicted very large babies or the presence of polyhydramnios ➔ decrease dose
· The presence of an epidural that has been running for a long time or has required multiple top-up boluses ➔ be prepared for exaggerated cephalad spread
· Very tall or short women ➔ increase or decrease dose or reverse Trendelenburg positioning
· Cardiovascular conditions requiring gradual onset of anesthetic block ➔ Epidural or CSE are better

### Prevention of hypotension

Be aware of symptoms of nausea, vomiting, or light-headedness

Maintain systolic blood pressure at pre-spinal levels:
· Avoid aortocaval compression (tilt table 15° laterally to the left)
· Infuse IV fluids
· Administer phenylephrine or ephedrine

### Confirm block height

Bilateral loss of sensation to cold from T4, and light touch from T6 is required

Assess motor blockade of the legs

### Medications

Prophylactic antibiotics before skin incision

Antiemetics (ondansetron) before spinal insertion

Administer 5 units of oxytocin slowly (approx. 2 units/min), followed by an oxytocin infusion (40 units oxytocin in 500 mL 0.9% saline) administered through a volumetric pump (at 125 mL/hr up to 5 hours) after cord clamp (note that oxytocin can cause hypotension and tachycardia if give rapidly)

1 g of tranexamic acid if more than 500 mL if blood loss is expected

### Breakthrough pain management

Rapid onset systemic opioids (e.g., alfentanil IV 100–250 μg boluses)

Ketamine in boluses of 10–20 mg may be effective

LA infiltration of the skin at the site of the incision

# MANAGEMENT OF AN EMERGENCY CESAREAN SECTION AND OPERATIVE VAGINAL DELIVERY

- Four groups according to the urgency of cesarean delivery

| Category | Risk to mother and/or baby | Indication | Target time for decision to delivery interval (DDI) |
|---|---|---|---|
| 1. Emergency | An immediate threat to life | An immediate threat to the life of the woman or fetus (e.g., severe fetal bradycardia, cord prolapse, uterine rupture, fetal blood sample pH ≤ 7.2) | ≤ 30 minutes |
| 2. Urgent | Maternal or fetal compromise | No immediate threat to life of woman or baby (e.g., antepartum haemorrhage APH, failure to progress) | ≤ 75 minutes |
| 3. Scheduled | Time for procedure to be scheduled | Requires early delivery (e.g., intrauterine growth retardation, failed induction of labor) | In the interests of mother and baby |
| 4. Elective (Management see above) | No maternal or fetal compromise | At a time to suit the woman and maternity services (breech, previous CD) | Usually after 39 weeks of gestation if possible |

# CESAREAN SECTION

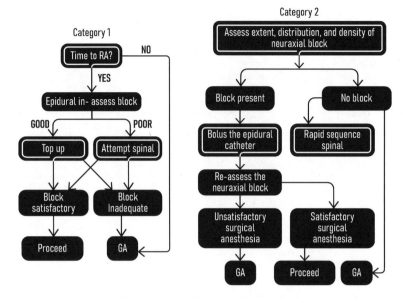

**Category 1**

Time to RA? — NO

YES

Epidural in- assess block

GOOD / POOR

Top up / Attempt spinal

Block satisfactory / Block Inadequate

Proceed / GA

**Category 2**

Assess extent, distribution, and density of neuraxial block

Block present / No block

Bolus the epidural catheter / Rapid sequence spinal

Re-assess the neuraxial block

Unsatisfactory surgical anesthesia / Satisfactory surgical anesthesia

GA / Proceed / GA

**INDICATIONS**
- Failure to progress
- Nonreassuring fetal status
- Cephalopelvic disproportion
- Malpresentation
- Prematurity prior uterine surgery involving the corpus
- Placenta praevia
- Certain maternal conditions

**IN TERMS OF URGENCY CESAREAN SECTION IS CLASSIFIED AS**
- **Category 1: Emergency** - Immediate threat to life of woman or fetus
- **Category 2: Urgent** - No immediate threat to life of woman or fetus but there is maternal or fetal compromise
- **Category 3: Scheduled** - No maternal or fetal compromise but early delivery is required
- **Category 4: Elective** - Delivery scheduled to suit mother or staff

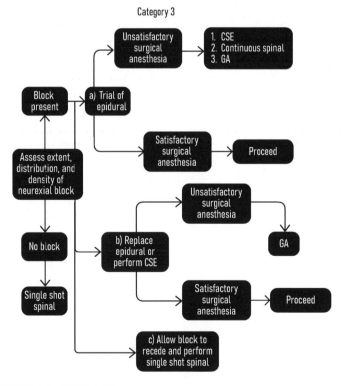

**Category 3**

Unsatisfactory surgical anesthesia → 1. CSE / 2. Continuous spinal / 3. GA

Block present — a) Trial of epidural

Satisfactory surgical anesthesia → Proceed

Assess extent, distribution, and density of neurexial block

No block — b) Replace epidural or perform CSE

Unsatisfactory surgical anesthesia → GA

Satisfactory surgical anesthesia → Proceed

Single shot spinal

c) Allow block to recede and perform single shot spinal

## EPIDURAL TOP-UP

- Can be used to provide anesthesia if there is a well-functioning epidural
- Can be administered in the delivery room if the anesthesiologist remains present at all times and vasopressors are immediately available
- Perform a block from sacral regions to T4 with 2 mL of LA
- Administration of the dose in 5–10 mL aliquots will help prevent hypotension or high block
- Adding opioids (fentanyl 100 μg or diamorphine 2.5-5 mg) will improve analgesia quality

Cesarean delivery

# INDICATIONS FOR GENERAL ANESTHESIA IN CESAREAN DELIVERY

- If RA is contraindicated
- If mothers decline RA
- Life-threatening conditions for the mother and/or baby
  - Prolonged fetal bradycardia
  - Umbilical cord prolapse
  - Major placental abruption (with maternal/fetal compromise)
  - Uterine rupture
  - Uncontrolled massive hemorrhage

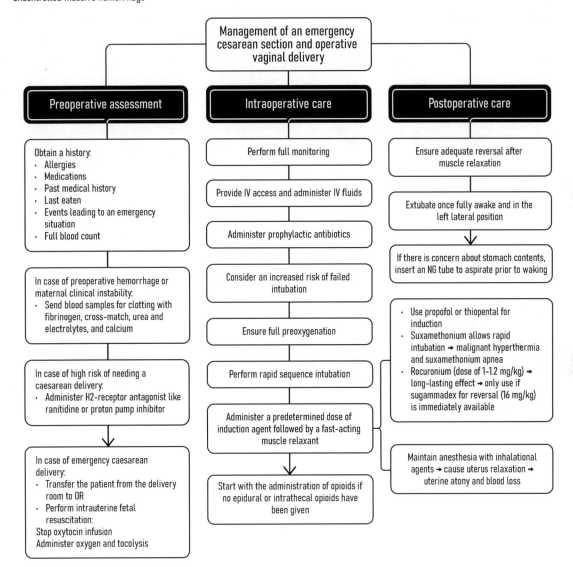

## PATIENT POSITION FOR EPIDURAL OR SPINAL ANESTHESIA FOR CESAREAN SECTION

### ABOUT
Pregnant women have an exaggerated lumbar lordosis, making it difficult to flex the lumbar spine. However, most pregnant women are young and have sufficient flexibility to facilitate insertion of a needle into the epidural or subarachnoid space.

### LATERAL DECUBITUS POSITION - ADVANTAGES
- Premedication can be used more liberally
- ↓ patient movement
- ↑ patient comfort
- Improved patient cooperation
- ↓ catheter displacement
- ↓ incidence of epidural vein cannulation
- ↓ incidence of vasovagal reactions
- More stable hemodynamics
- Bedside assistance easier or may not be required

### SITTING POSITION - ADVANTAGES
- Easier to identify the midline, particularly in obese and scoliotic patients
- Most practitioners have more experience with the sitting position
  - ↓ procedure time
  - ↓ distance from skin to the epidural space
- ! Caution
  - Greater cephalad spread of hypobaric solutions
  - May result in a low block with hyperbaric solutions

### TIPS
- Align the patient's back with the edge of the table or bed
- Align the coronal plane perpendicular to the floor with the tips of the spinous processes pointing toward the wall
- Flex thighs toward the abdomen and draw the knee to the chest
- The neck should be neutral or flexed so that the chin rests on the chest
- Ask the patient to assume the "fetal position" → may help to maximally flex the spine
- Align hips one above the other - Rest non-dependent arm on non-dependent hip
- Elevate the head with a pillow to avoid rotation of the spine

## SUGGESTED READING

- Adshead, D., Wrench, I., Woolnough, M., 2020. Enhanced recovery for elective Cesarean section. BJA Education 20, 354–357.
- Delgado C, Ring L, Mushambi MC. 2020. General anesthesia in obstetrics. BJA Education. 20;6:201-207.
- Mglennan A, Mustafa A. 2009. General anaesthesia for Cesarean section. Continuing Education in Anaesthesa Critical Care & Pain. 9;5:148-151.
- Neall G, Bampoe S, Sultan P. 2022. Analgesia for Cesarean section. BJA Education. 22;5:197-203.
- Pollard BJ, Kitchen, G. Handbook of Clinical Anaesthesia. Fourth Edition. CRC Press. 2018. 978-1-4987-6289-2.

# CERVICAL CERCLAGE

## LEARNING OBJECTIVES

- Describe the indications and risks for cervical cerclage
- Manage patients presenting for cervical cerclage

## DEFINITION AND MECHANISM

- Cervical cerclage is performed as an attempt to prolong pregnancy in women who are at high risk of preterm delivery due to cervical insufficiency
- Suturing of the cervix to prevent rupture of fetal membranes

## RISK FACTORS FOR CERVICAL INSUFFICIENCY

- Prior cervical procedures or trauma:
  - Loop electrode excisional procedure
  - Cone biopsy
  - Prior cervical lacerations
  - Repetitive cervical dilation and/or pregnancy terminations
- Maternal connective tissue diseases or abnormalities
- Congenital Mullerian anomalies
- Maternal exposure in utero to diethylstilbestrol

## INDICATIONS

- History-indicated: One or more second-trimester pregnancy losses related to painless cervical dilation and in the absence of labor or abruptio placentae, or prior cerclage placed due to cervical insufficiency in the second trimester
- Ultrasound-indicated: History of spontaneous loss or preterm birth at less than 34 weeks if the cervical length in a current singleton pregnancy is less than 25 mm before 24 weeks of gestation
- Rescue cerclage: Singleton pregnancy at less than 24 weeks with advanced cervical dilation in the absence of contractions, intraamniotic infection, or placental abruption
- Not recommended in pregnancies of multiple gestations

## TECHNIQUE

- Transvaginal
  - McDonald method: Simple purse-string suture at the cervicovaginal junction
  - Shirodkar method: Suturing anterior-posterior and posterior-anterior after an incision of the mucosa of the anterior cervix, with the aid of an Allis clamp
- Transabdominal
- Remove sutures between weeks 36-38 in women anticipating vaginal delivery:
  - McDonald cerclage requires no anesthesia
  - Shirodkar requires anesthesia (spinal, epidural)
  - Highly epithelialized sutures may require cesarean section

Cervical cerclage

# RISKS

- Rupture of fetal membranes
- Infection or sepsis
- Lacerations at the surgical site
- Anesthesia-related complications

# MANAGEMENT

### CONSIDERATIONS

- Aspiration risk in pregnancy
- Position in left uterine displacement when gestational age > 18-20 weeks
- Risk of membrane rupture and degree of cervical dilation may dictate anesthetic modality
- Possible need for uterine relaxation/reduction of fetal movements
- Avoid coughing, straining, position changes that provoke bulging and rupture of membranes
- Avoid contraindicated medications (e.g., NSAIDs) after 32 weeks
- Fetal monitoring may be necessary
- Pudendal nerve block is often inadequate

### SPINAL ANESTHESIA

- Sitting position: Risk of membrane bulging, rupture and fetal death
- Consider administering spinal anesthesia in the lateral position
- Avoid hypotension
- Cover T10-L1 as well as S2-S4

### GENERAL ANESTHESIA

- Indicated in bulging membranes to facilitate uterine relaxation with volatile anesthetics
- Avoid increases in intra-abdominal pressure (coughing, bucking, vomiting)
- Aspiration prophylaxis
- Left uterine displacement
- Maintain normocapnia
- Volatile anesthetics + opioid
- Fetal monitoring
- Avoid NSAIDs

### EPIDURAL ANESTHESIA

- Avoid hypotension
- Cover T10-L1 as well as S2-S4

====== **SUGGESTED READING** ======

- Bieber KB, Olson SM. Cervical Cerclage. [Updated 2022 Aug 1]. In: StatPearls [Internet]. Treasure Island (FL): StatPearls Publishing; 2022 Jan-. Available from: https://www.ncbi.nlm.nih.gov/books/NBK560523/
- Shennan, A, Story, L, Jacobsson, B, Grobman, WA; the FIGO Working Group for Preterm Birth. FIGO good practice recommendations on cervical cerclage for prevention of preterm birth. Int J Gynecol Obstet. 2021; 155: 19- 22.

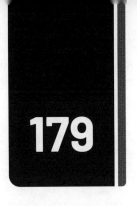

# CHALLENGES IN OBSTETRIC ANESTHESIOLOGY

## LEARNING OBJECTIVES

- Anesthetic management of medical problems in obstetric patients
- Safe obstetrical general anesthesia
- Methods of pain relief during labor

## DEFINITION AND MECHANISM

- Pregnant women may need anesthesia at any stage of gestation due to incidental surgery (e.g., appendicitis), trauma, delivery, or complications in the immediate postnatal period (e.g., bleeding, breast abscess)
- As pregnancy progresses, multisystemic physiological changes develop rapidly
- The obstetric anesthesiologist must understand these to provide optimum care to pregnant women
- Consider:
  - Significant cardiovascular or cerebrovascular disease
  - Significant respiratory disease, which may worsen throughout pregnancy
  - Morbid obesity (BMI > 40) or super morbid obesity (BMI > 50)
  - Significant hematological disease which may previously have resulted in failure to reach viable gestation
  - Corrected or palliated congenital heart disease
- Be aware that pregnant patients are more sensitive to the effects of general anesthesia than non-pregnant patients

## ANESTHETIC MANAGEMENT OF MEDICAL PROBLEMS IN OBSTETRIC PATIENTS

- **Acquired cardiac disease**
  - Ischaemic heart disease (obesity and advanced age is increasingly seen in the obstetric population)
  - Aortic dissection
  - Cardiomyopathy
  - Symptomatic valvular heart disease
  - Sudden adult death syndrome (SADS)
  - Antenatal management:
    - Assess symptoms and functional status (NYHA class)
    - Review recent ECG and echocardiography
    - Multidisciplinary planning for labor and delivery
  - Labor and delivery:
    - Perform continuous maternal monitoring with ECG and invasive blood pressure monitoring for high-risk patients
    - Provide epidural analgesia
    - Be aware of the hypertensive response to laryngoscopy in case of general anesthesia
    - Consider the administration of a bolus dose of labetalol, esmolol, nitroglycerin, sodium nitroprusside, or remifentanil to blunt the hemodynamic response to laryngoscopy
  - Postnatal management:
    - Be cautious with uterotonic agents due to side effects
    - Perform hemodynamic monitoring during the first 24 hours because of the risk of decompensation with autotransfusion postpartum
- **Congenital cardiac disease**
  - Maintain preload
    - Avoid prolonged fasting
    - Administer IV fluids
  - Maintain afterload
    - Avoid spinal anesthetic
    - Administer phenylephrine for hypotension (or noradrenaline in on-responders)
    - Administer oxytocin slowly (2 units/minute)
  - Avoid tachycardia
    - Administer effective analgesia
    - Perform early cardioversion for any tachyarrhythmia
  - Acyanotic congenital disease (ventricular septal defect, atrial septic defect, and patient ductus arteriosus)
    - Maintain systemic vascular resistance (SVR)
    - Avoid decrease in SVR
    - Maintain adequate intravascular volume
    - Avoid air bubbles
  - Cyanotic congenital heart disease (tetralogy od Fallot, tricupid atresia)
    - Maintain pulmonary vascular resistance (PVR)
    - Control SVR
    - Prevent hypoxia and acidosis
    - Maintain temperature
  - Maintain normothermia
- **Neurological disease**
  - Stroke
  - Subarachnoid hemorrhage
  - Epilepsy
  - Status epilepticus
    - Multiple sclerosis
      - Consider a theoretical risk of neurotoxicity to demyelinated nerves with regional anesthesia
    - Myasthenia gravis
      - Perform instrumental delivery as muscles fatigue quickly
      - Regional anesthesia is preferred over general anesthesia
      - Avoid magnesium as it can precipitate a myasthenic crisis
- **Respiratory disease**
  - Asthma
    - Screen for pulmonary hypertension
- **Hematological disease**
  - Increased risk of VTE, e.g., Factor V Leiden, antiphospholipid syndrome
  - Increased risk of bleeding, e.g., von Willebrand's disease, thrombocytopenias
  - Reduced oxygen-carrying capacity, e.g., sickle cell disease, thalassemia, spherocytosis

- Regional anesthesia is safe to use but pay attention to the timing of anticoagulant if used
- Therefore, perform a recent assessment of platelet count in thrombocytopenia
- **Back problems**
  - Spinal surgery
    - Regional anesthesia is safe to use in most types
    - Ultrasound can be used for assistance
    - Avoid scar sites
  - Scoliosis surgery
    - Avoid regional anesthesia in women with implanted rods
  - Spina bifida
    - Exclude tethered spinal cord
    - Regional anesthesia can be applied at an unaffected level if tethered spinal cord is excluded
    - Be cautious of accidental dural punctures
    - Reduce the epidural volume as dural permeability is reduced

## MATERNAL-TO-FETAL TRANSFER

| Medication class | Examples | Crossing of uteroplacental barrier |
|---|---|---|
| Intravenous agents | Thiopental<br>Propofol<br>Ketamine | Yes |
| Inhalational agents | Isoflurane<br>Sevoflurane<br>Desflurane | Yes |
| Benzodiazepines | Midazolam<br>Lorazepam | Yes |
| Opioids | Morphine<br>Fentanyl<br>Remifentanil | Yes |
| Neuromuscular blocking agents | Vecuronium<br>Rocuronium<br>Suxamethonium | No |
| Neuromuscular blocking reversal agents | Neostigmine<br>Sugammadex | Yes<br>Yes |
| Anticholinergic agents | Atropine<br>Glycopyrrolate | Yes<br>No |

## OBSTETRIC GENERAL ANESTHESIA

- Pre-OR preparation
  - Airway assessment
  - Fasting status
  - Antacid prophylaxis
  - Intrauterine fetal resuscitation if appropriate
- Rapid sequence induction
  - Check airway equipment and IV access
  - Optimize position: head up + left uterine displacement
  - Pre-oxygenate and consider nasal oxygenation
  - Perform cricoid pressure
  - Deliver appropriate induction and neuromuscular blocker doses
  - Consider facemask ventilation
- 1st intubation attempt:
  - If poor view of the larynx, optimize the attempt by:
    - Reducing/removing cricoid pressure
    - External laryngeal manipulation
    - Repositioning head/neck
    - Using bougie/stylet
  - Verify successful tracheal intubation or if the intubation attempt fails, ventilate with a facemask

- 2nd intubation attempt:
  - Consider:
    - Alternative laryngoscope
    - Remove cricoid pressure
  - Verify successful tracheal intubation or if the intubation attempt fails, ventilate with a facemask

- Declare failed intubation:
  - Priority is to maintain oxygenation
    - Supraglottic airway device
    - Facemask – oropharyngeal airway
- Further management: see non-obstetric surgery

# PAIN RELIEF DURING LABOR

- During the first and early second stages of labor, visceral pain (mediated by the T10 to L1 spinal segments) is experienced
  - This is usually felt in the abdomen, sacrum, and back
- In the latter part of the first stage and into the second stage, somatic pain (mediated via T12-L1 and S2-4) is experienced
  - This is located in the vagina, rectum, and perineum

# METHODS FOR PAIN RELIEF DURING LABOR

- See cesarean delivery for anesthesia

---

ENTONOX
- A 50:50 mixture of nitrous oxide and oxygen administered via a demand mouthpiece
- Rapid onset and offset
- Women are encouraged to breathe it during a contraction and to cease use in between them
- May cause drowsiness, nausea, and vomiting
- No effect on maternal or neonatal outcome

---

OPIOID ANALGESIA: PETHIDINE AND DIAMORPHINE
- Administered intramuscularly
- Cause sedation, nausea, and vomiting, therefore, administer an antiemetic
- Consider the risk of transfer to the fetus with consequent respiratory depression

---

PATIENT-CONTROLLED ANALGESIA
- Self-administration of small bolus doses (20-40 μg) of remifentanil with a lockout of 2–5 minutes
- Less effective than an epidural
- It is particularly advantageous when regional analgesia is contraindicated
- No adverse effects on labor or neonatal outcomes
- Consider a significant risk of respiratory depression and never leave the patient alone
- Keep naloxone and a self-inflating bag with oxygen immediately available

---

EPIDURAL ANALGESIA
- Is the most effective method of pain relief in labor
- Consider the following additional impact on labor:
  Increased length of the second stage (but not the first stage)
  Increased risk of instrumental delivery
  Increased levels of monitoring for both mother and baby which affects mobility in labor
- Perform a full assessment and check that there are no contraindications to the insertion
- Provide additionally:
  IV access
  CTG monitoring
  Vital sign monitoring
- Perform epidural analgesia in lateral or sitting position
- Watch carefully for an accidental dural puncture (ADP)
- If this occurs, insert the epidural catheter intrathecally or repeat the epidural procedure
- Combined spinal-epidural anesthesia can be used alternatively to epidural anesthesia alone
- Use a low dose spinal medication during spinal anesthesia

---

## SUGGESTED READING

- Delgado, C., Ring, L., Mushambi, M.C., 2020. General anaesthesia in obstetrics. BJA Education 20, 201–207.
- Pollard BJ, Kitchen, G. Handbook of Clinical Anaesthesia. Fourth Edition. CRC Press. 2018. 978-1-4987-6289-2.

# DYSPNEA DURING PREGNANCY

## LEARNING OBJECTIVES

- Describe the differences between physiological pregnancy-related dyspnea and pathological dyspnea
- Diagnose and treat underlying conditions of dyspnea during pregnancy

## DEFINITION AND MECHANISM

- Dyspnea is a common issue during pregnancy, caused by the physiological changes to the respiratory and cardiovascular systems
- 60 – 70% of pregnant women experience some form of dyspnea during the gestation period
- Most often first noticed while conversing, being unable to complete a sentence without pausing to breathe
- Distinguishing between physiological pregnancy-related dyspnea and pathological dyspnea can be challenging

## PHYSIOLOGICAL DYSPNEA

- Physiologically increased "need for breathing", possibly caused by progesterone-induced stimulation of the respiratory center in the brain, body habitus, anemia, and increased pulmonary blood flow
- Facilitates the increase in tidal volume needed due to the increased oxygen consumption

## PATHOLOGICAL DYSPNEA

- Key differences with physiological dyspnea:

|  | Physiological dyspnea | Pathological dyspnea |
|---|---|---|
| Mechanisms | Possibly progesterone-induced hyperventilation, body habitus, anemia, increased pulmonary blood flow | Due to etiology |
| Onset | Gradual | Acute |
| Timing | Starts earlier in first/second trimester | Usually starts in second trimester |
| Progression | Plateaus or improves near term | Progressively worsens near term |
| Positional symptoms | Worst in sitting position | May not tolerate supine position |
| Exercise tolerance | Not associated with exercise | May be unable to perform daily activities |
| Physical findings | No wheeze and chest clear to auscultation | Abnormal pulmonary and/or cardiac findings |

- Differential diagnosis:

| Cardiac | |
| --- | --- |
| ◦ Cardiomyopathy | ◦ Congenital heart disease |
| ◦ Valvular heart disease (Aortic regurgitation, aortic stenosis, mitral regurgitation, mitral stenosis) | ◦ Arrythmias/heart block |
| ◦ Pulmonary hypertension & right ventricular failure | ◦ Pericardial (pericarditis/tamponade) |
| ◦ Cardiac ischemia | |

| Respiratory | |
| --- | --- |
| ◦ Infections | ◦ Pneumothorax |
| ◦ Restrictive: interstitial lung disease, cystic fibrosis, neuromuscular disease, scoliosis | ◦ Anaphylaxis (bronchospasm) |
| ◦ Obstructive: asthma, COPD | |

| Pregnancy-specific | |
| --- | --- |
| ◦ Severe preeclampsia/eclampsia | ◦ Tocolytic induced pulmonary edema |
| ◦ Amniotic fluid embolism | ◦ Peripartum cardiomyopathy |
| ◦ Pulmonary embolism | ◦ High neuraxial blockade |

| Others |
| --- |
| ◦ Anemia |
| ◦ Hypothyroidism |
| ◦ Hepatic dysfunction |

## DIAGNOSIS & TREATMENT

| Cause of dyspnea | Clinical signs | Diagnostic investigations | Treatment |
| --- | --- | --- | --- |
| Physiological | Need to take a deep breath intermittently, or when unable to get a deep enough breath | None | Reassurance |
| Asthma/airway disease | Dyspnea with chest tightness or wheezing | Spirometry pre- and postbronchodilator | Inhaled beta-agonists ± inhaled steroids |
| Cardiac disease | Myocardial/valvular dysfunction: progressive orthopnea or orthopnea with paroxysmal nocturnal dyspnea Often present at end of second trimester or in early postpartum period when fluid shifts occur | Echocardiogram | Diuretics, beta-blockers as indicated, ACE inhibitors contraindicated in pregnancy |
| Arrhythmia | Sudden onset and cessation, associated sensation of palpitations or chest discomfort | Electrocardiogram, Holter or event monitor | Beta-blockers, calcium channel blockers |
| Venous thromboembolism | Sudden onset, any trimester May have associated deep venous thrombosis features | Computerized tomography pulmonary angiogram, V/Q scan, lower-extremity Dopplers | Anticoagulation with injectable heparins in pregnancy, warfarin in the postpartum period |

## SUGGESTED READING

- Hegewald MJ, Crapo RO. Respiratory physiology in pregnancy. Clin Chest Med.
- Mehta N, Chen K, Hardy E, Powrie R. Respiratory disease in pregnancy. Best Pract Res Clin Obstet Gynaecol. 2015;29(5):598-611.

# EXTERNAL CEPHALIC VERSION

## LEARNING OBJECTIVES

- Definition of external cephalic version (ECV)
- Procedure to perform ECV

## DEFINITION AND MECHANISM

- Is a procedure to change the presentation of the fetus from breech, transverse, or oblique to vertex by applying pressure externally to the fetus through the gravid abdomen in order to enable vaginal delivery
  - In contrast to the internal cephalic version, in which a hand is inserted through the cervix to turn the baby
- About 3% of the babies are in a breech position after 36 weeks of pregnancy
- Typically performed around 37 weeks but can even be performed in early labor
- The procedure is done externally by applying firm pressure to the patient's abdomen
- This pressure lasts several minutes and can cause the uterus to cramp

- The success rate is about 58%, tends to be the best at 37 weeks, and depends on:
  - Practitioner experience
  - Maternal weight
  - Uterine relaxation
  - A palpable fetal head
  - A non-engaged breech
  - Non-anterior placenta
  - An amniotic fluid index above 7-10 cm
- Only a small chance (5%) that the baby will turn spontaneously to breech again

| Factors that may increase the success | Factors associated with a decreased success |
|---|---|
| Multiparity<br>Transverse or oblique presentation<br>Complete breech<br>Adequate amniotic fluid | Nulliparity<br>Advanced dilation<br>Estimated fetal weight < 2500 g<br>Anterior, lateral, or cornual placenta<br>Decreased amniotic fluid or rupture of membranes<br>Maternal obesity<br>Frank breech<br>Fetal spine in the posterior position |

## CONTRAINDICATIONS

- Reduced amniotic fluid
- Vaginal bleeding
- Multiples
- Abnormal fetal monitoring
- Ruptured membranes
- Placenta praevia
- Vasa previa
- Irregularly shaped uterus

- Maternal hypertension
- Preeclampsia
- Diabetes mellitus
- Cesarean section
- Oligohydramnios
- Hyperextended fetal head
- Significant fetal or uterine anomaly
- Fetal growth restriction

## COMPLICATIONS

- Premature rupture of the membranes
- Placental abruption
- Preterm labor
- Fetal distress

- Vaginal bleeding
- Umbilical cord entanglement
- Severe maternal discomfort

# MANGEMENT

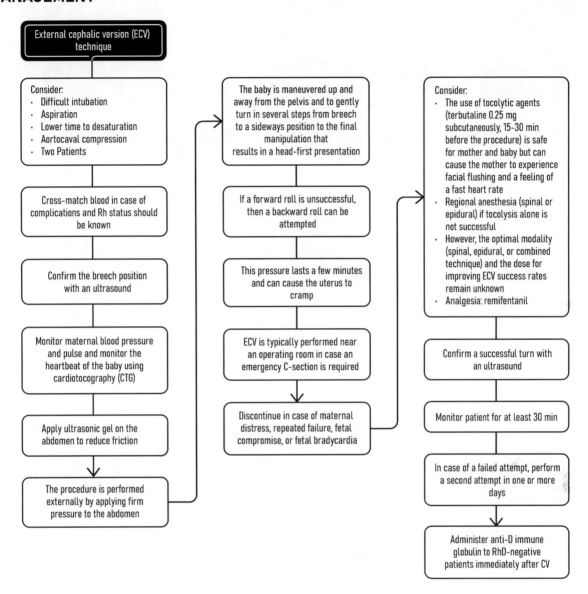

**External cephalic version (ECV) technique**

Consider:
- Difficult intubation
- Aspiration
- Lower time to desaturation
- Aortocaval compression
- Two Patients

↓

Cross-match blood in case of complications and Rh status should be known

↓

Confirm the breech position with an ultrasound

↓

Monitor maternal blood pressure and pulse and monitor the heartbeat of the baby using cardiotocography (CTG)

↓

Apply ultrasonic gel on the abdomen to reduce friction

↓

The procedure is performed externally by applying firm pressure to the abdomen

→

The baby is maneuvered up and away from the pelvis and to gently turn in several steps from breech to a sideways position to the final manipulation that results in a head-first presentation

↓

If a forward roll is unsuccessful, then a backward roll can be attempted

↓

This pressure lasts a few minutes and can cause the uterus to cramp

↓

ECV is typically performed near an operating room in case an emergency C-section is required

↓

Discontinue in case of maternal distress, repeated failure, fetal compromise, or fetal bradycardia

→

Consider:
- The use of tocolytic agents (terbutaline 0.25 mg subcutaneously, 15-30 min before the procedure) is safe for mother and baby but can cause the mother to experience facial flushing and a feeling of a fast heart rate
- Regional anesthesia (spinal or epidural) if tocolysis alone is not successful
- However, the optimal modality (spinal, epidural, or combined technique) and the dose for improving ECV success rates remain unknown
- Analgesia: remifentanil

↓

Confirm a successful turn with an ultrasound

↓

Monitor patient for at least 30 min

↓

In case of a failed attempt, perform a second attempt in one or more days

↓

Administer anti-D immune globulin to RhD-negative patients immediately after CV

## SUGGESTED READING

- Rosman AN, Guijt A, Vlemmix F, Rijnders M, Mol BW, Kok M. Contraindications for external cephalic version in breech position at term: a systematic review. Acta Obstet Gynecol Scand. 2013;92(2):137-142.
- Weiniger, C.F., Rabkin, V., 2020. Neuraxial block and success of external cephalic version. BJA Education 20, 296–297.
- Weiniger CF. Analgesia/anesthesia for external cephalic version. Curr Opin Anaesthesiol. 2013;26(3):278-287.

# FETAL DISTRESS

## LEARNING OBJECTIVES

- Definition and causes of fetal distress
- Fetal monitoring
- Treatment and anesthetic management of fetal distress

## DEFINITION AND MECHANISM

- Fetal distress is a broad term to define a compromised fetus due to hypoxia
- Subclasses of fetal distress are:
  - Fetal asphyxia: a non-reassuring fetal status due to a diminished but persistant gas exchange
  - Fetal anoxia: complete cessation of gas exchange, which can be fatal in less than ten minutes

## CAUSES OF ASPHYXIA

- Inadequate perfusion on the maternal side
  - Maternal hypotension
  - Aortocaval compression
- Interruption of gas exchange across the placenta
  - Placental abruption
- Interruption of umbilical blood flow
  - Cord compression
- Transient intermittent hypoxia caused by uterine contractions of normal labor

## FETAL MONITORING

- Fetal monitoring aids in detecting fetal distress through alterations in the fetal heart rate or scalp blood gases
- Modalities of fetal monitoring are:
  - External heart rate monitoring
    - Ultrasound scanning
    - Doppler ultrasound
    - Cardiotocography
  - Internal heart rate monitoring
    - Fetal scalp electrodes
  - Fetal acid-base status
- Fetal heart rate, baseline variability, and decelerations are used to assess characteristic pattern changes in the fetal heart rate
  - The normal fetal heart rate is between 110 and 160 beats per minute
    - Persistent fetal tachycardia and bradycardia can be associated with fetal hypoxia, however, fetal bradycardia is most commonly seen
    - Possible causes of tachycardia are fever, chorioamnionitis, anticholinergic agents, beta-sympathomimetics, or fetal anemia
    - Possible causes of bradycardia are congenital heart block or beta-adrenergic blocking agents

  - Early decelerations occur simultaneously with uterine contractions and usually are less than 20 bpm below the baseline
    - Early decelerations are not ominous
  - Late decelerations begin 10 to 30 seconds after the beginning of a uterine contraction and end 10-30 seconds after the end of the uterine contraction
    - Late decelerations represent a response to hypoxia
- Fetal acid-base status can be obtained from the scalp
  - It is used to exclude or confirm fetal acidosis
  - A pH of 7.2 is considered abnormal and urgent delivery should be arranged
  - Relative contra-indications for fetal scalp blood pH sampling are intact membranes, infections (HIV, herpes, herpes simplex), and fetal coagulopathy

## SIGNS OF FETAL DISTRESS

- A nonreassuring fetal heart rate pattern
  - Repetitive late decelerations
  - Loss of fetal beat-to-beat variability
  - Sustained fetal heart rate < 80/min
- Fetal scalp pH < 7.0
- Meconium-stained amniotic fluid
- Intrauterine growth restriction

# MANAGEMENT

- 4 categories were defined to classify an emergency cesarean section:

| Category | Risk to mother and/or baby | Indication | Target time for decision to delivery interval (DDI) |
|---|---|---|---|
| 1. Emergency | An immediate threat to life | An immediate threat to the life of the mother or fetus (e.g., severe foetal bradycardia, cord prolapse, uterine rupture, foetal blood sample pH ≤ 7.2) | ≤ 30 minutes |
| 2. Urgent | Maternal or fetal compromise | No immediate threat to life of woman or baby (e.g., antepartum haemorrhage (APH), failure to progress) | ≤ 75 minutes |
| 3. Scheduled | Time for procedure to be scheduled | Requires early delivery (e.g., intrauterine growth retardation, failed induction of labor) | In the interests of mother and baby |
| 4. Elective (Management see above) | No maternal or fetal compromise | At a time to suit the woman and maternity services (breech, previous caesarean delivery (CD)) | Usually after 39 weeks of gestation if possible |

- General anesthesia is the preferred anesthetic technique for life-threatening conditions (category 1) unless epidural anesthesia can be established by using a pre-existing epidural catheter
- Regional anesthesia is preferred if there is an urgent but non-life-threatening condition (category 2-4)
- See also cesarean delivery

## SUGGESTED READING

- Cesarean birth NICE guidelines (2021). Available at: https://www.nice.org.uk/guidance/ng192.
- Morgan and Mikhail's clinical anesthesiology (2022). Mgraw Hill Medical. Chapter 41.
- Omotayo, Rotimi & Akinsowon, OR & Bello, EO & Olumide, Akadiri & Akintan, AL & Omotayo, SE. (2019). Fetal distress, options of anesthesia, and immediate postdelivery outcome at state specialist hospital Akure. Tropical Journal of Obstetrics and Gynaecology. 36. 424.

# GESTATIONAL DIABETES

**183**

## LEARNING OBJECTIVES

- Define gestational diabetes
- Describe the complications associated with gestational diabetes
- Management of gestational diabetes

## DEFINITION AND MECHANISM

- Gestational diabetes is diabetes diagnosed for the first time during pregnancy, resulting in hyperglycemia affecting the pregnancy and baby's health
- It can happen at any stage of pregnancy but most commonly develops in the second or third trimester
- Usually improves after giving birth
- Occurs when the body cannot produce enough insulin to meet the extra needs in pregnancy

## SIGNS AND SYMPTOMS

Gestational diabetes does not usually cause any noticeable signs or symptoms
- Hyperglycemia
- Antenatal glycosuria
- Increased thirst
- More frequent urination
- Dry mouth
- Tiredness
- Blurred eyesight
- Genital itching or thrush

## COMPLICATIONS

Maternal
- Gestational hypertension and preeclampsia
- Cesarean section
- Gestational diabetes in future pregnancies
- Type 2 diabetes

Fetal
- Excessive birth weight (i.e., > 4.1 kg)
- Preterm birth
- Respiratory distress syndrome
- Hypoglycemia or jaundice
- Obesity and type 2 diabetes later in life
- Polyhydramnios
- Stillbirth

## RISK FACTORS

- Age > 40 years
- Increased BMI (BMI > 30 kg/m2)
- Prediabetes
- Gestational diabetes during a previous pregnancy
- Polycystic ovary syndrome
- Family history of diabetes
- Previously delivered a baby weighing $\geq$ 4.1 kg
- Black, Hispanic, American Indian, and Asian American ethnicity

## TREATMENT

- Control blood glucose levels
  - Changes in diet and exercise to lower blood glucose
  - Medicine (i.e., tablets or insulin injections) if dietary management is inadequate
- Blood glucose testing kit to monitor the effects of treatment
- Close monitoring during pregnancy and birth to check for any potential complications
- Ideal to give birth before 41 weeks → induction of labor or cesarean section may be recommended if labor does not start naturally by this time
- Early delivery may also be recommended if there are health concerns for the mother or baby, or if the blood glucose levels are not well controlled

Gestational diabetes

# MANAGEMENT

- Goal: Avoid maternal hypoglycemia or hyperglycemia (which can increase the risk of neonatal hypoglycemia), safe management of glycemic control, effective analgesia for labor
- Availability of appropriate equipment to monitor and treat hypoglycemia or hyperglycemia (e.g., glucometer, infusion pumps, 20% glucose) in the delivery units and obstetric theaters

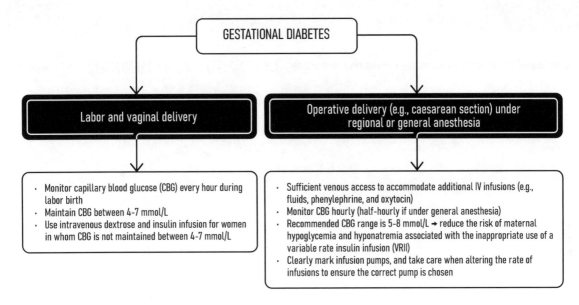

Variable rate intravenous insulin infusion (VRII) to maintain glycemic control
- Used when the target CBG range is not achieved by modification of the patient's usual medications
- Glucose-containing substrate fluid alongside the IV insulin infusion to prevent gluconeogenesis, lipolysis, and ketoacidosis
  - 5% glucose in 0.9% saline with premixed 0.15% (20 mmol/L) KCl or 0.30% (40 mmol/L) KCl to reduce the risk of developing hypokalemia
- Continue basal insulin after starting a VRII

See also preeclampsia considerations
See also cesarean section considerations

# PREVENTION

- Eat healthy food (high in fiber, low in fat and calories)
- Stay active
- Start pregnancy at a healthy weight
- Do not gain more weight than recommended during pregnancy

═══ SUGGESTED READING ═══

- Yap Y, Modi A, Lucas N. The peripartum management of diabetes. BJA Educ. 2020;20(1):5-9.

# HYSTERECTOMY

## LEARNING OBJECTIVES

- Define and classify the different types of hysterectomy
- Describe the complications that are associated with hysterectomy
- Management of a patient undergoing a hysterectomy

## DEFINITION AND MECHANISM

- A hysterectomy is the partial (cervix preserved) or total (cervix removed) surgical removal of the uterus
- It may also involve the removal of the cervix, ovaries (oophorectomy), fallopian tubes (salpingectomy), and other surrounding structures
- The woman can no longer get pregnant or menstruate after surgery

### Classification

- **Total or complete hysterectomy:** Removal of the uterus and cervix, preserving the ovaries
- **Supracervical or partial hysterectomy:** Removal of just the upper part of the uterus while preserving the cervix
- **Total hysterectomy with bilateral salpingo-oophorectomy:** Removal of the uterus, cervix, fallopian tubes, and ovaries
- **Radical hysterectomy with bilateral salpingo-oophorectomy:** Removal of the uterus, cervix, fallopian tubes, ovaries, upper vagina, and some surrounding tissue (i.e., parametrium) and lymph nodes (cancer)

## INDICATIONS

- Abnormal or heavy vaginal bleeding that is not managed by other treatments
- Severe pain with menstruation that is not managed by other treatments
- Leiomyomas or uterine fibroids (noncancerous tumors)
- Cervical or uterine malignancy or pre-malignant lesions
- Uterine prolapse
- Uterine hyperplasia, recurrent uterine polyps, endometriosis, or adenomyosis
- Postpartum to remove placenta praevia or placenta percreta
- As a last resort in case of excessive postpartum hemorrhage
- Chronic pelvic pain related to the uterus but not managed by other treatments

## COMPLICATIONS

- Blood clots (venous thromboembolism [VTE])
- Infection
- Heavy bleeding
- Urinary incontinence and vaginal prolapse
- Adhesion formation and bowel obstruction
- Torn internal stitches
- Urinary tract injury
- Vaginal problems
- Ovary failure
- Early menopause symptoms (e.g., hot flashes, vaginal dryness, loss of libido, insomnia)
- Issues related to anesthesia

# MANAGEMENT

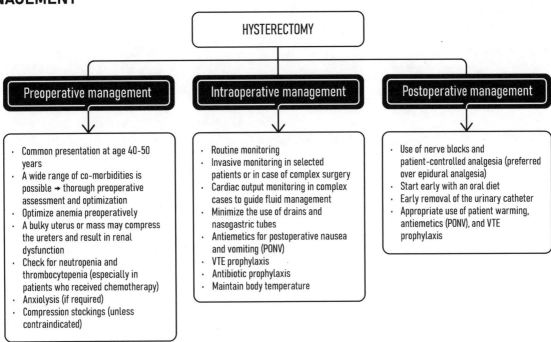

**HYSTERECTOMY**

**Preoperative management**

- Common presentation at age 40-50 years
- A wide range of co-morbidities is possible → thorough preoperative assessment and optimization
- Optimize anemia preoperatively
- A bulky uterus or mass may compress the ureters and result in renal dysfunction
- Check for neutropenia and thrombocytopenia (especially in patients who received chemotherapy)
- Anxiolysis (if required)
- Compression stockings (unless contraindicated)

**Intraoperative management**

- Routine monitoring
- Invasive monitoring in selected patients or in case of complex surgery
- Cardiac output monitoring in complex cases to guide fluid management
- Minimize the use of drains and nasogastric tubes
- Antiemetics for postoperative nausea and vomiting (PONV)
- VTE prophylaxis
- Antibiotic prophylaxis
- Maintain body temperature

**Postoperative management**

- Use of nerve blocks and patient-controlled analgesia (preferred over epidural analgesia)
- Start early with an oral diet
- Early removal of the urinary catheter
- Appropriate use of patient warming, antiemetics (PONV), and VTE prophylaxis

# TECHNIQUES

| Technique | Advantages | Disadvantages |
|---|---|---|
| Abdominal hysterectomy | Not limited by the size of the uterus<br>Combination with reduction and incontinence surgery possible<br>No increase in postsurgical complications compared to vaginal technique | Longest recovery period<br>Higher risk of bleeding compared to laparoscopic surgery<br>Vaginal or laparoscopic techniques are preferred in obese patients |
| Vaginal hysterectomy | Shortest surgery time<br>Short recovery period and discharge from hospital<br>Less analgesic requirements compared to laparoscopic technique | Limited by the size of the uterus and previous surgery<br>Limited ability to evaluate the fallopian tubes and ovaries |
| Laparoscopic-assisted vaginal hysterectomy | Possible with a larger uterus, depending on the surgeon's skills<br>Combination with reduction operations are possible | Malignancies can only be removed by this approach if they are intact<br>Not suggested for patients with cardiopulmonary disease |
| Total laparoscopic hysterectomy | Short inpatient treatment duration compared to abdominal technique<br>Possiblity to diagnose and treat other pelvic diseases<br>Early recovery compared to abdominal technique<br>Less bleeding and post operative infections compared to abdominal technique | Increased length of surgery<br>Requires a high degree of laparoscopic surgical skills<br>Higher risk of bladder or ureter injury |

## Abdominal hysterectomy

- Trendelenburg position
- Transverse Pfannenstiel incision, occasionally midline incision
- General anesthesia or neuraxial block
  - General anesthesia
    - Muscle relaxation and controlled ventilation
    - Adjustment of ventilation parameters due to diaphragmatic splinting caused by Trendelenburg position
    - Multimodal analgesia with paracetamol, NSAIDs, opioids, and local blocks (e.g., TAP block for transverse incision, rectus sheath block for midline incisions)
  - Neuraxial block
    - Add an intrathecal opioid
    - Block height to at least T4
    - Do not position the patient for surgery too soon → Trendelenburg position will increase the cephalad spread of the spinal block
    - Manage hypotension with vasopressors
- Transfusion in patients with preoperative anemia
- Postoperative: Gabapentin, paracetamol, NSAIDs, opioids, patient-controlled analgesia, antiemetics, and VTE prophylaxis

## Vaginal hysterectomy

- Lithotomy position → take precautions to avoid nerve injuries
- General anesthesia or neuraxial block
  - General anesthesia
    - Spontaneous breathing or mechanical ventilation → anticipate potential respiratory changes when the patient is moved into the Trendelenburg position
    - Multimodal analgesia with paracetamol, NSAIDs, opioids, and local anesthetic infiltration
  - Neuraxial block
    - Consider adding an intrathecal opioid for postoperative analgesia
    - Block height to at least T8
    - Do not position the patient for surgery too soon → lithotomy and Trendelenburg position will increase the cephalad spread of the spinal block
    - Manage hypotension with vasopressors
    - Supplemental sedation (if required)
- Less postoperative pain compared to abdominal technique
- Postoperative: Paracetamol, NSAIDs, oral opioids, antiemetics, and VTE prophylaxis

## Laparoscopic hysterectomy

- Lithotomy position with steep Trendelenburg
- Consider the risk of pneumoperitoneum
- Large bore venous access to anticipate intraoperative cardiovascular complications or intraperitoneal injury
- Uterine manipulator is inserted through the cervix → may provoke vagal stimulation and bradycardia
- The uterus is removed vaginally (laparoscopic-assisted vaginal hysterectomy) or through an abdominal incision (total laparoscopic hysterectomy)
- General anesthesia
  - Muscle relaxation, tracheal intubation, and controlled ventilation
  - Pneumoperitoneum and steep Trendelenburg position will alter lung mechanics, and $CO_2$ can accumulate from insufflation → adjust parameters to ensure adequate ventilation
  - Multimodal analgesia with paracetamol, NSAIDs, opioids, and local infiltration
- Transfusion in patients with preoperative anemia
- Less postoperative pain compared to abdominal technique
- Postoperative: Paracetamol, NSAIDs, oral opioids, antiemetics, and VTE prophylaxis

### SUGGESTED READING

- Pollard BJ, Kitchen G. Handbook of Clinical Anaesthesia. 4th ed. Taylor & Francis group; 2018. Chapter 11 Gynaecological surgery, Hobbs A and Craig SK.

# MULTIPLE GESTATION

## LEARNING OBJECTIVES

- Define the signs and symptoms of multiple gestation
- Describe the complications associated with multiple gestation
- Management of multiple gestation

## DEFINITION AND MECHANISM

- Multiple gestation is a pregnancy with more than one fetus at a time, occurring in approximately 3% of all pregnancies
- Examples include pregnancy with twins, triplets or quadruplets
- High-risk pregnancy requiring extra care
- Most women have multiple births via cesarean section
- Babies are often born prematurely and with a low birth weight → may need NICU care
- The goal is to complete 37 weeks (is considered as full term) in twin pregnancies → increases the chance of survival of both babies with adequate weight

## SIGNS AND SYMPTOMS

- Exaggerated signs of pregnancy (e.g., extreme nausea and fatigue, severe vomiting)
- Faster than usual weight gain in the first semester of pregnancy
- Sore or very tender breasts
- Higher than normal levels of pregnancy hormones (i.e., human chorionic gonadotrophin)
- Higher than normal levels of protein alpha-fetoprotein in the mother's blood
- Larger than usual belly compared to most women at a similar stage of pregnancy
- More than one fetal heartbeat

## CAUSES

- One fertilized egg (ovum) splits before it implants in the uterine lining → monozygotic or identical twins
- Two (or more) separate eggs are fertilized by different sperm at the same time → dizygotic or fraternal twins
- Fraternal twins are more common than identical twins
- In a pregnancy with triplets or more, the babies could all be identical, all fraternal, or a mixture of both

## COMPLICATIONS

Maternal

- Anemia
- Increased aortocaval compression
- Rapid desaturation
- Preterm prelabor rupture of membranes
- Preterm labor
- Prolonged labor
- Gestational hypertension
- Preeclampsia/eclampsia
- Gestational diabetes
- Placental abruption
- Disseminated intravascular coagulation
- Operative delivery
- Uterine atony
- Antepartum and postpartum hemorrhage

Fetal

- Preterm delivery
- Low birth weight
- Congenital anomalies (e.g., cerebral palsy)
- Polyhydramnios
- Cord entanglement
- Umbilical cord prolapse
- Fetal growth restriction, intrauterine growth restriction (IUGR), or small for gestational age
- Malpresentation (e.g., breech presentation)
- Increased mortality (i.e., miscarriage, stillbirth)
- Monochorionic twins (one placenta) risks that are unique to them
  - Twin-twin transfusion syndrome
  - Twin anemia polycythemia sequence
  - Selective intrauterine growth restriction (IUGR)

## RISK FACTORS

- Family history of twins, triplets, or more increases the chance of multiple gestation pregnancy
- Infertility treatments
- Age ≥ 35 years (women are more likely to release more than one egg per cycle)

## MANAGEMENT

- All obstetric patients are considered to have a full stomach and are at risk for gastric reflux and possible pulmonary aspiration, regardless of the time of last oral intake

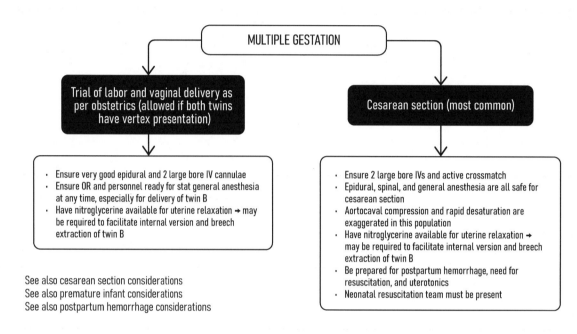

MULTIPLE GESTATION

**Trial of labor and vaginal delivery as per obstetrics (allowed if both twins have vertex presentation)**

- Ensure very good epidural and 2 large bore IV cannulae
- Ensure OR and personnel ready for stat general anesthesia at any time, especially for delivery of twin B
- Have nitroglycerine available for uterine relaxation → may be required to facilitate internal version and breech extraction of twin B

See also cesarean section considerations
See also premature infant considerations
See also postpartum hemorrhage considerations

**Cesarean section (most common)**

- Ensure 2 large bore IVs and active crossmatch
- Epidural, spinal, and general anesthesia are all safe for cesarean section
- Aortocaval compression and rapid desaturation are exaggerated in this population
- Have nitroglycerine available for uterine relaxation → may be required to facilitate internal version and breech extraction of twin B
- Be prepared for postpartum hemorrhage, need for resuscitation, and uterotonics
- Neonatal resuscitation team must be present

## SUGGESTED READING

- Frölich M.A. (2022). Obstetric anesthesia. Butterworth IV J.F., & Mackey D.C., & Wasnick J.D.(Eds.), Morgan & Mikhail's Clinical Anesthesiology, 7e. Mgraw Hill. https://accessanesthesiology.mhmedical.com/content.aspx?bookid=3194&sectionid=266522956
- Rédai I (2013). Chapter 196. twin pregnancy, breech presentation, trial of labor after cesarean birth: anesthetic considerations for patients attempting vaginal birth. Atchabahian A, & Gupta R(Eds.), The Anesthesia Guide. Mgraw Hill. https://accessanesthesiology.mhmedical.com/content.aspx?bookid=572&sectionid=42543788

# NON-OBSTETRIC SURGERY

## LEARNING OBJECTIVES

- Describe the physiological changes associated with pregnancy and their anesthetic implications
- Describe the anesthetic implications of commonly used medications
- Manage obstetric patients presenting for non-obstetric surgery

## DEFINITION AND MECHANISM

- Non-obstetric emergency surgery may be required at any trimester during pregnancy, which carries the unique challenge of caring simultaneously for two patients
- An understanding of the physiological changes of pregnancy is essential for safe anesthesia
- Most common indications: Acute appendicitis, cholecystitis, trauma, and surgery for maternal malignancies
- Main risks: Fetal loss, premature labor, and delivery

## PHYSIOLOGICAL CHANGES & IMPLICATIONS

| System | Physiological change | Anesthetic amplications |
|---|---|---|
| Cardiovascular | Increased cardiac output by up to 50%<br>Increased uterine perfusion up to 10% of cardiac output<br>Decreased systemic vascular resistance, pulmonary vascular resistance, and arterial pressure<br>Aortocaval compression from 13 weeks | Uterine perfusion not autoregulated<br>Hypotension common under regional and general anesthesia<br>Supine hypotensive syndrome requires left lateral tilt |
| Respiratory | Increased minute ventilation<br>Respiratory alkalosis<br>Decreased expiratory reserve volume, residual volume, and functional residual capacity<br>Ventilation/perfusion mismatch<br>Increased oxygen consumption<br>Upward displacement of diaphragm<br>Increased thoracic diameter<br>Mucosal edema | Potential hypoxemia in the supine and Trendelenburg positions<br>Breathing more diaphragmatic than thoracic<br>Difficult laryngoscopy and intubation; bleeding during attempts |
| Central nervous system | Epidural vein engorgement<br>Decreased epidural space volume<br>Increased sensitivity to opioids and sedatives | More extensive local anesthetic spread |
| Hematological | 30% red cell volume increase<br>Increased white blood cell count<br>50% plasma volume increase<br>Increased coagulation factors<br>Decreased albumin and colloid osmotic pressure | Dilutional anemia<br>Thromboembolic complications<br>Edema, decreased protein binding of drugs |
| Gastrointestinal | Increased intragastric pressure<br>Decreased barrier pressure | Increased aspiration risk<br>Antacid prophylaxis, RSI after 18 weeks gestation |
| Renal | Increased renal plasma flow and glomerular filtration rate<br>Decreased reabsorptive capacity | Normal urea and creatinine may mask impaired renal function<br>Glycosuria and proteinuria |

# MEDICATION SIDE-EFFECTS & ANESTHETIC IMPLICATIONS

| Medication | Side-effects and anesthetic implications |
|---|---|
| Volatile agents | Decreased MAC, reduced uterine tone, hypotension |
| Nitrous oxide | Prolonged exposure may inhibit DNA synthesis; avoid in the first trimester |
| Succinylcholine | Reduced plasma cholinesterase may cause prolonged action |
| Non-depolarizing neuromuscular blocking agents | Quaternary ammonium compounds do not cross the placenta |
| Local anaesthetics | Reduced protein-binding, increased risk of toxicity; use lower intrathecal doses in late pregnancy |
| Opioids | Increased maternal sensitivity, fetal withdrawal, intrauterine growth restriction with chronic use |
| Non-steroidal anti-inflammatory drugs | Premature ductus arteriosus closure, avoid after 28 weeks; ketorolac contraindicated |
| Warfarin | Teratogenic, crosses the placenta |
| Heparin | Does not cross the placenta |
| Atropine | Fetal tachycardia, crosses the placenta |
| Glycopyrrolate | Quaternary ammonium compound, does not cross the placenta |
| Phenytoin, carbamazepine, sodium valproate | Congenital malformations (neural tube defects) |
| Magnesium sulphate | Muscle weakness, interaction with neuromuscular blocking agents |
| ACE inhibitors | Intrauterine growth restriction, oligohydramnios, renal impairment |
| Beta-blockers | Intrauterine growth restriction, neonatal hypoglycemia, bradycardia |
| Thiazides | Neonatal thrombocytopenia |
| Beta-2-agonists: ritodrine, terbutaline, salbutamol | Tachyarrhythmias, pulmonary edema, hypokalemia, hyperglycemia |
| Oxytocin receptor antagonists: atosiban | Nausea, vomiting, fewer side-effects than beta-2-agonists |
| Calcium-channel blockers: nifedipine | Hypotension, fewer side-effects than beta-2-agonists |

# MANAGEMENT

**ABOUT**
- **Incidence of non-obstetric surgery during pregnancy:** 1-2%
- **Anesthesia management objective:** Prevention of intrauterine fetal hypoxia and acidosis
- Elective procedures should always be delayed until after pregnancy
- **Optimal time for intervention:** Second trimester - lowest risk of preterm labor
- Laparoscopy is considered safe during any trimester and the indications are the same as for nonpregnant patients

**CRITERIA**
- Surgery should be done at an institution with neonatal and pediatric services
- Obstetric provider with caesarean delivery privileges should be readily available
- Qualified individual should be readily available to interpret the fetal heart rate
- Fetal monitoring should be available at all times

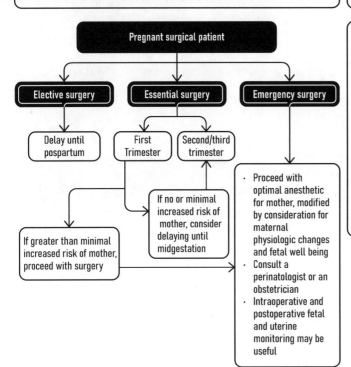

**MANAGEMENT OF ANESTHESIA**
- Plan for fetal monitoring, potential maternal arrest, urgent cesarean delivery
- Regional techniques are preferred
- Aspiration prophylaxis
- Left uterine displacement
- Maintain eucarbia
- Adequate uterine perfusion with fluids and vasopressors
- $O_2$ inhaled concentrations at least 50%
- **Postoperative:** Deep venous thrombosis prophylais, fetal heart rate and uterine activity monitoring (at least 24 hrs)
- **Postoperative analgesia:** Paracetamol - ! AVOID ibuprofen (3rd trimester) and metamizol (ALL trimesters)

**[Flowchart content:]**

Pregnant surgical patient

- Elective surgery
  - Delay until pospartum
    - If greater than minimal increased risk of mother, proceed with surgery
- Essential surgery
  - First Trimester
    - If no or minimal increased risk of mother, consider delaying until midgestation
  - Second/third trimester
- Emergency surgery
  - Proceed with optimal anesthetic for mother, modified by consideration for maternal physiologic changes and fetal well being
  - Consult a perinatologist or an obstetrician
  - Intraoperative and postoperative fetal and uterine monitoring may be useful

## SUGGESTED READING

- Haggerty E, Daly J. Anaesthesia and non-obstetric surgery in pregnancy. BJA Education. 2021;21(2):42-3.
- Nejdlova M, Johnson T. Anaesthesia for non-obstetric procedures during pregnancy. Continuing Education in Anaesthesia Critical Care & Pain. 2012;12(4):203-6.

# PERIPARTUM CARDIAC ARREST

## LEARNING OBJECTIVES

- Identify and treat underlying causes of peripartum cardiac arrest
- Manage patients presenting with peripartum cardiac arrest

## DEFINITION AND MECHANISM

- Peripartum cardiac arrest is a rare event with an incidence of one in 12,000 – 36,000 women per year
- A prompt, coordinated response by a multidisciplinary team is essential
- Need to consider two patients: The mother and the fetus
- The maternal cardiac arrest response team and should have regular updated training through didactics and simulation sessions and the response protocols should be reviewed periodically
- Strong leadership and teamwork are essential

## CAUSES & TREATMENTS

| Cause of cardiac arrest | | Treatment |
|---|---|---|
| Complications of anesthesia | High neuraxial block | Treat hypotension aggressively (e.g., low-dose adrenaline)<br>Support airway and breathing |
| | Loss of airway, aspiration, respiratory depression | Support airway and breathing<br>Difficult airway algorithm |
| | Hypotension | Treat with vasopressors<br>Lower head of bed to improve cerebral perfusion<br>Volume replacement<br>Obtain more intravenous access |
| | Local anesthetic systemic toxicity (LAST) | Give intralipid<br>Consider cardiopulmonary bypass or ECMO |

| Cause of cardiac arrest | | Treatment |
|---|---|---|
| Bleeding | Coagulopathy | Fibrinogen replacement<br>Fresh frozen plasma<br>Cryoprecipitate<br>Platelets<br>Consider tranexamic acid 1 g IV |
| | Uterine atony | Give uterotonics<br>Bakri balloon<br>Compression suture<br>Uterine artery embolisation<br>Hysterectomy |
| | Placenta accreta | Consider uterine artery embolisation<br>Consider hysterectomy |
| | Placental abruption | Delivery if indicated<br>Monitor for coagulopathy |
| | Placenta previa | Delivery if indicated<br>Prepare for lower uterine segment atony |
| | Uterine rupture | Uterine repair or hysterectomy |
| | Trauma | Call general surgeon<br>Activate massive transfusion |
| | Transfusion reaction | Stop transfusion<br>Notify blood bank<br>Adrenaline<br>Steroids<br>Send tryptase |

Peripartum cardiac arrest

| Cause of cardiac arrest | | Treatment |
|---|---|---|
| Cardiovascular | Cardiomyopathy | Inotrope infusion<br>Call for ECMO |
| | Myocardial infarction | Inotrope infusion<br>Call for ECMO<br>Call for cardiac surgeon<br>Call cardiac catheterization laboratory<br>Send cardiac enzymes |
| | Aortic dissection | Call cardiac surgeon<br>Activate massive transfusion |
| | Arrhythmias | Ventricular fibrillation: Defibrillate<br>Unstable ventricular tachycardia:<br>Amiodarone, lidocaine<br>Torsade de pointes: Defibrillate,<br>magnesium<br>Stable ventricular tachycardia:<br>Amiodarone, lidocaine<br>Supraventricular tachycardia: Adenosine<br>Atrial fibrillation: Amiodarone,<br>cardioversion |
| Medications | Anaphylaxis | Adrenaline<br>Steroids<br>Diphenhydramine<br>Ranitidine |
| | Illicit | Opioid overdose: Naloxone<br>Benzodiazepine overdose: Flumazenil<br>Cocaine coronary vasospasm: Oxygen, aspirin, nitrates,<br>thrombolytic therapy, or acute percutaneous coronary<br>intervention |
| | Drug error | Identify, discontinue agent and treat |
| | Magnesium toxicity | Stop magnesium<br>Give calcium chloride 10 mL in 10%<br>solution or calcium gluconate 30 mL in<br>10% solution |
| | Insulin overdose | Give glucose/dextrose<br>Glucagon |
| | Oxytocin overdose | Treat hypotension |

Peripartum cardiac arrest

| Cause of cardiac arrest | | Treatment |
|---|---|---|
| Embolic | Pulmonary embolus | Call Interventional radiology<br>Call cardiac surgeon<br>Prepare catheterisation laboratory<br>Echocardiography<br>Start heparin IV<br>Consider thrombolytics in cardiac arrest<br>Nitric oxide |
| | Coronary thrombus | Call cardiac surgeon<br>Catheterisation laboratory<br>Nitroglycerine |
| | Amniotic fluid embolism/Anaphylactoid syndrome of pregnancy | Adrenaline<br>Initiate cardiopulmonary resuscitation<br>Call for extracorporeal membrane oxygenator<br>Call for transesophageal echocardiography<br>Prepare for coagulopathy and need for massive transfusion protocol<br>Consider unproven 'A-OK' therapy: atropine, ondansetron, ketorolac<br>Consider steroids<br>Consider nitric oxide |
| | Venous air embolism | Flood field if uterine venous sinuses open<br>Internalise uterus |
| Fever | Infection, sepsis | Give broad spectrum antibiotics<br>Fluids, volume replacement<br>Vasopressors<br>Place arterial line<br>Perform echocardiogram<br>Inotrope if low cardiac output |
| General non-obstetric causes of cardiac arrest | Hypotension | Treat with vasopressors<br>Lower head of bed to improve cerebral perfusion<br>Fluids, volume replacement<br>Obtain more intravenous access<br>Call for transthoracic echocardiography |
| | Hypoxia | Airway control<br>100% oxygen |
| | Hypothermia | Warm patient<br>Warm fluids<br>Blankets<br>Increase room temperature |

| Cause of cardiac arrest | | Treatment |
|---|---|---|
| | Hyperkalemia | Calcium<br>Insulin and glucose<br>Furosemide<br>Albuterol<br>Sodium bicarbonate to correct acidosis<br>Intubate and hyperventilate<br>Polystyrene sulphonate (potassium binder)<br>Consider hemodialysis |
| | Hypoglycemia | Give glucose/dextrose<br>Glucagon |
| | Hypercarbia/acidosis | Intubate trachea and optimize ventilation<br>Determine cause of acidosis<br>Sodium bicarbonate |
| | Thrombus | See pulmonary embolus above |
| | Trauma | Call general or trauma surgeon |
| | Toxin | Give antidote if agent known |
| | Tension pneumothorax | Needle decompression<br>Insert chest tube |
| | Tamponade | Call for ECMO<br>Call cardiac surgeon |
| Hypertension | Pre-eclampsia/eclampsia/HELLP | Antihypertensive agents: labetalol (avoid in asthmatics), hydralazine, nicardipine<br>Magnesium |
| | Intracranial hemorrhage with increased intracranialpressure | Call neurosurgeon<br>Blood pressure goal: systolic < 140 mmHg<br>Elevate head of bed 30°<br>Reverse coagulopathy if present<br>Hypertonic saline/mannitol |

ECMO, extracorporeal membrane oxygenation; HELLP, hemolysis, elevated liver enzymes, low platelet count.

Peripartum cardiac arrest

# MANAGEMENT

### Call maternal cardiac arrest team
- Obstetrician with scalpel
- Obstetric & cardiac anesthesiologists
- Neonatologist
- Adult cardiac arrest team
- ECMO team if available
- Consider transesophageal/transthoracic echocardiogram

### Chest compressions and manual left uterine displacement
- Chest compressions: 100/min, 5 cm
- Hand placement: Lower sternum
- Use backboard
- Swap/change providers every 2 min
- Manual left uterine displacement

### Defibrillate
- Defibrillate if indicated
- Energy requirements are unaltered in pregnancy
- Resume compressions after defibrillation

### Airway & breathing
- Ventilate with 100% oxygen, 500-700 mL at 10 bpm
- Bag-mask ventilation until endotracheal intubation
- Place laryngeal mask airway in event of failed intubation
- Monitor end-tidal $CO_2$ (> 1,3 kPa or 10 mmHg suggests quality chest compressions)

### Access, medications, fluids, laboratory tests
- Intravenous or intraosseous (humerus) access above diaphragm
- Give resuscitation medications in standard doses
- Rapid intravascular volume repletion
- Fluid warmer, massive transfusion blood products as needed
- Send laboratory tests as indicated

### Resuscitative hysterotomy and differential diagnosis
- Perform resuscitative hysterotomy (perimortem caesarean delivery) by 5 min if no return of spontaneous circulation at 4 min, if ≥ 20 weeks of gestation to improve maternal outcome, or in case of maternal fatal injuries
- Perform hysterotomy at the site of arrest
- Consider differential diagnosis, stop offending agents, treat etiology

### Post-resuscitation care
- Start when spontaneous circulation has returned
- Patients may require further surgery to repair or close the resuscitative hysterotomy
- Follow appropriate hemostasis, antibiotics, and intensive care protocols
- Avoid hypothermia

ECMO, extracorporeal membrane oxygenation.

## SUGGESTED READING

- Jeejeebhoy FM, Zelop CM, Lipman S, Carvalho B, Joglar J, Mhyre JM, et al. Cardiac Arrest in Pregnancy. Circulation. 2015;132(18):1747-73.
- Madden AM, Meng ML. Cardiopulmonary resuscitation in the pregnant patient. BJA Educ. 2020;20(8):252-258.

# PERIPARTUM CARDIOMYOPATHY

## LEARNING OBJECTIVES

- Describe the risk factors and symptoms of peripartum cardiomyopathy
- Diagnose peripartum cardiomyopathy
- Manage patients with peripartum cardiomyopathy

## DEFINITION AND MECHANISM

- Peripartum cardiomyopathy (PPCM) is a rare cause of cardiomyopathy occurring during late pregnancy or in the early postpartum period
- Characterized by significant left ventricular dysfunction and heart failure in the peripartum period in the absence of other identifiable causes of heart failure
- Potentially life-threatening condition
- Left ventricle ejection fraction is nearly always less than 45%
- Etiology is unclear but likely multifactorial (hormonal, inflammatory, genetic,...)

## RISK FACTORS

- African descent
- Increasing age
- Pregnancy-related hypertension
- Multiparity
- Multiple gestations
- Obesity
- Chronic hypertension
- Chronic tocolytics use
- Cocaine use

## SIGNS & SYMPTOMS

- Paroxysmal nocturnal dyspnea
- Pedal edema
- Orthopnea
- Dyspnea on exertion
- Dry cough
- Palpitations
- Increase in abdominal girth
- Lightheadedness
- Chest pain
- Jugular venous distentions
- Displaced apical impulse
- Third heart sound
- Mitral regurgitation murmurs

## DIAGNOSIS

- Diagnosis is based on exclusion
- Differential diagnoses:
  - Pulmonary embolism
  - Severe sepsis
  - Amniotic fluid embolism
  - Preeclampsia/pregnancy-induced hypertensive disease
  - Arrhythmias
  - Severe anemia
  - Myocardial infarction
  - Dilated cardiomyopathy of other etiologies
  - Pre-existing valvular disease
- Diagnostic tests:
  - Routine blood tests
    - Evaluate for anemia, electrolyte abnormalities, endocrine conditions, renal or liver dysfunction
    - Brain natriuretic peptide (BNP) is commonly elevated in patients with heart failure and PPCM
  - Chest radiography if pulmonary edema is suspected as PPCM can typically be diagnosed without one
    - Cardiomegaly and/or pulmonary edema are suggestive of heart failure but nonspecific to PPCM
  - ECG
    - Sinus tachycardia, supraventricular tachycardia, ventricular tachycardia, ST segment and T wave abnormalities, dilation of chambers, and QRS prolongation may be observed but are nonspecific
    - A normal ECG does not exclude PPCM
  - Echocardiography
    - Left ventricular ejection fraction < 45%: Requirement for PPCM diagnosis
    - Evaluation of other etiologies such as valvular diseases or structural abnormalities
    - Ventricle/atrium dilation and left ventricular thrombus or atrial thrombosis may be present
  - Cardiac MRI
    - Evaluation of other causes of heart failure
  - Cardiac catheterization
    - Only for selected patients
    - Left heart catheterization is indicated in patients with suspected ischemic cardiomyopathy

# MANAGEMENT

Management is similar to that of other causes of heart failure
- Pharmacological
  - Angiotensin-converting enzyme (ACE) inhibitors: First-line treatment postpartum, contraindicated during pregnancy
  - Hydrazaline and nitrate therapy can be used safely during pregnancy
  - Beta-blockers
  - Digoxin (carefully monitor plasma levels)
  - Loop diuretics (e.g., furosemide)
  - Avoid calcium channel blockers and aldosterone antagonists
  - Thromboprophylactic low molecular weight heparin
- Non-pharmacological:
  - Non-invasive ventilation or intubation
  - Inotropic support: e.g., norepinephrine, milrinone, and levosimendan
  - Intra-aortic balloon pump, left ventricular assist device or extracorporeal membrane oxygenation may be required in severe cases
  - Heart transplantation in severe cases who do not respond to therapy
  - Implantable defibrillator or cardiac resynchronization in patients with chronic functional impairment
- Key objectives of care for PPCM:
  - Heart failure (HF) goal-directed medical therapy
  - Alleviate symptoms and reduce pulmonary congestion
  - Optimize preload and afterload, including appropriate reduction of afterload
  - Provide hemodynamic support with inotropes and vasopressors if necessary
  - When peripartum cardiomyopathy (PPCM) is identified during labor, optimize medical management before delivery whenever feasible
  - Facilitate multidisciplinary team planning for labor, delivery, and postpartum care

# PROGNOSIS

| | |
|---|---|
| Good prognosis | Small left ventricular diastolic dimension (less than 5.5cm)<br>Left ventricular ejection fraction greater than 30% to 35% and fractioning of shortening greater than 20% at the time of diagnosis<br>Absence of troponin elevation<br>Absence of left ventricular thrombus<br>Non-African ethnicity |
| Poor prognosis | QRS greater than 120 ms<br>Delayed diagnosis<br>High New York Heart Association (NYHA) class<br>Multiparity<br>African descent<br>Age > 30-35<br>LVEF < 25% |

# COMPLICATIONS

- Thromboembolism
- Arrhythmias
- Progressive heart failure
- Misdiagnosis as preeclampsia
- Fetal distress from hypoxia
- Progressive pump failure
- Sudden death

# ANESTHETIC MANAGEMENT

## PERIPARTUM CARDIOMYOPATHY (PPCM) ANESTHETIC MANAGEMENT

### CONSIDERATIONS

- Planning of labor and delivery must be a multidisciplinary approach with Anesthesiologist and OBGYN
- Decide on mode of delivery based on patient's past obstetric history, current hemodynamic status, and response to medical management
- Consider including a vaginal delivery as an option if the PPCM is compensated
- Monitoring: ECG, oxygen saturations, blood pressure, low threshold for invasive arterial blood pressure monitoring
- Postpartum care: ICU, ongoing (invasive) hemodynamic monitoring, careful fluid management, adequate analgesia

### VAGINAL DELIVERY

- Consider techniques to limit the increase in plasma catecholamines, systemic vascular resistance, and myocardial workload associated with labor
- Prevent aorto-caval compression by avoiding supine positioning without uterine displacement
- Consider early labour epidural anesthesia to limit cardiovascular stress
- Manage the second stage of labor with instrumental assistance to reduce myocardial workload and the detrimental cardiovascular effects of prolonged Valsalva maneuvers

### CAESAREAN SECTION

**Goals**
- Maintain myocardial perfusion by avoiding arrhythmias and episodes of hypotension or tachycardia
- Optimize cardiac output by maintaining preload and contractility and preventing increased afterload
- Invasive arterial blood pressure monitoring is necessary

**Neuraxial anesthesia**
- Titrated by incremental top-up of epidural or combined epidural and low-dose spinal anesthesia
- Avoid significant falls in systemic vascular resistance
- Pay attention to the timing of anticoagulation administration

**General anesthesia**
- Smooth induction
- Fast-acting opioid (alfentanil, remifentanil) to attenuate the pressor response to laryngoscopy and intubation
- Inotropes (dobutamine, calcium sensitizers, phosphodiesterase inhibitors) may be needed to offset the myocardial depression of anesthetic agents
- Vasopressors may be necessary
- Maintain preload
- Use uterotonic medication cautiously
- Consider using videolaryngoscopy for intubation as a first choice to reduce airway related complications

## SUGGESTED READING

- Honigberg MC, Givertz MM. Peripartum cardiomyopathy. BMJ. 2019;364:k5287. Published 2019 Jan 30. doi:10.1136/bmj.k5287
- Putra ICS, Irianto CB, Raffaello WM, Suciadi LP, Prameswari HS. Pre-pregnancy obesity and the risk of peripartum cardiomyopathy: A systematic review and meta-analysis. Indian Heart J. 2022;74(3):235-238.
- Rodriguez Ziccardi M, Siddique MS. Peripartum Cardiomyopathy. [Updated 2022 Jul 19]. In: StatPearls [Internet]. Treasure Island (FL): StatPearls Publishing; 2022 Jan-. Available from: https://www.ncbi.nlm.nih.gov/books/NBK482185/
- Thompson L, Hartsilver E. Peripartum cardiomyopathy. WFSA. https://resources.wfsahq.org/atotw/peripartum-cardiomyopathy/#:~:text=Titrated%20neuraxial%20anaesthesia%2C%20by%20incremental,agents%20that%20reduce%20myocardial%20contractility. Published February 24, 2015. Accessed February 13, 2023.

# PHYSIOLOGICAL CHANGES DURING PREGNANCY

## LEARNING OBJECTIVES

- Describe the major physiological changes during pregnancy
- Describe the anesthetic implications of the physiological changes during pregnancy

## DEFINITION AND MECHANISM

- Every major organ system is affected by substantial physiological changes during pregnancy
- Many of these changes significantly affect the pharmacokinetic and pharmacodynamic properties of different therapeutic agents, including anesthetics
- Understanding these changes and their effects is essential to optimize therapy and anesthesia in obstetric patients
- Consider adding a 'P' designation to ASA physical status classifications for parturients, such as ASA 1 P for a healthy parturient and ASA 2 P for a parturient with mild systemic disease, etc.

---

### PHYSIOLOGICAL CHANGES DURING PREGNANCY

**ABOUT**
- Significant anatomical and physiological changes take place to nurture and accommodate the developing fetus
- Begin after conception and affect every organ system in the body
- Result of:
  - Altered hormonal activity
  - Biochemical changes associated with ↑ metabolic demands of a growing fetus, placenta, and uterus
  - Mechanical displacement by an enlarging uterus

| | |
|---|---|
| **Blood chemistry** | ↑ Number of blood cells<br>↑ Clotting factors<br>↑ Fibrinolytic activity<br>Iron deficiency and anemia |
| **Cardiac system** | · ↑ CO, ↑ SV, ↑ HR, ↓ SVR<br>· Left ventricular hypertrophy<br>· Regurgitant murmurs |
| **Respiratory system** | · ↑ MV (↑ TV and ↑ RR)<br>· ↓ $PaCO_2$<br>· ↑ $PaO_2$<br>· ↓ FRC<br>· ↓ Functional reserve capacity<br>· ↑ Risk of apnea and dyspnea<br>· Hyperventilation |
| **Gastrointestinal system** | · Nausea and vomiting<br>· Mechanical displacement due to growing uterus<br>· Gastroesophageal reflux |

| | |
|---|---|
| **General changes** | Mood and behavioral changes<br>↑ nutritional demands |
| **Neurological system** | · ↑ CSF pressure<br>· Engorgement of epidural veins<br>· ↓ MAC<br>· ↓ LA volumes required |
| **Renal system** | · ↑ Renal blood flow<br>· ↑ GFR<br>· ↓ Plasma, urea and creatinine<br>· ↑ Risk of UTI<br>· ↑ Urinary protein & glucose |
| **Musculoskeletal system** | · Reversible bone loss<br>· Exaggerated lordosis in the lower back<br>· Joint laxity<br>· ↑ Mobility in sacroiliac joint and pubic symphysis |

CSF, cerebrospinal fluid; MAC, minimum alveolar concentration; LA, local anesthetic; MV, minute ventilation; TV, tidal volume; RR, respiratory rate; $PaCO_2$, partial pressure of carbon dioxide; $PaO_2$, partial pressure of oxygen; FRC, functional residual capacity; CO, cardiac output; SV, stroke volume; HR, heart rate; SVR, systemic vascular resistance; GFR, glomerular filtration rate; UTI, urinary tract infection

## ANESTHETIC IMPLICATIONS

| Anesthetic implications | |
|---|---|
| Cardiovascular | Uterine perfusion not autoregulated<br>Hypotension common under regional and general anesthesia<br>Supine hypotensive syndrome requires left lateral tilt |
| Respiratory | Potential hypoxemia in the supine and Trendelenburg positions<br>Breathing more diaphragmatic than thoracic<br>Difficult laryngoscopy and intubation; bleeding during attempts |
| Central nervous system | More extensive local anesthetic spread |
| Hematological | Dilutional anemia<br>Thromboembolic complications<br>Edema, decreased protein binding of drugs |
| Gastrointestinal | Increased aspiration risk<br>Antacid prophylaxis, RSI after 18 weeks gestation |
| Renal | Normal urea and creatinine may mask impaired renal function<br>Glycosuria and proteinuria |

## SUGGESTED READING

- Costantine M. Physiologic and pharmacokinetic changes in pregnancy. Frontiers in Pharmacology. 2014;5.
- Nejdlova M, Johnson T. Anaesthesia for non-obstetric procedures during pregnancy. Continuing Education in Anaesthesia Critical Care & Pain. 2012;12(4):203-6.

Physiological changes during pregnancy

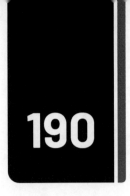

# PLACENTA ACCRETA

## LEARNING OBJECTIVES

- Definition of placenta accreta spectrum
- Anesthetic management of placenta accreta

## DEFINITION AND MECHANISM

- Refers to a severe pregnancy complication that occurs when the placenta grows too deeply into the uterine wall
- With placenta accreta, part or all of the placenta remains attached after delivery, thereby possibly leading to severe blood loss after delivery
- Is considered a high-risk pregnancy complication
- Three types:
  - Placenta accreta:
    - Placental villi adhere to the myometrium
    - Placenta does not pass through the wall of the uterus and does not impact the uterine muscles
    - Majority of cases
  - Placenta increta:
    - Invasion of the myometrium
    - Placenta does not pass through the uterine wall
    - 15-18% of cases
  - Placenta percreta:
    - Invasion through the myometrium to the serosa and surrounding organs
    - Might impact other organs such as the bladder or intestines
    - Most severe
    - 5-7% of cases

## SIGNS AND SYMPTOMS

- Often no signs or symptoms
- Although vaginal bleeding during the third trimester might occur

## RISK FACTORS

- Previous uterine surgery or cesarean section
- Placenta position: if the placenta partially or totally covers the cervix (placenta previa) or sits in the lower portion of the uterus
- Maternal age > 35 years
- Multiparity
- IVF

## COMPLICATIONS

- Major vaginal bleeding
- Thromboembolism
- Coagulopathy
- Anemia
- Premature birth
- Amniotic fluid embolism
- Damage to the uterus and surrounding organs
- Loss of fertility due to a hysterectomy
- Acute transfusion reaction
- Acute respiratory distress syndrome (ARDS)
- Acute kidney injury
- Infection
- Multisystem organ failure

## DIAGNOSIS

- Ultrasound
- MRI

# MANAGEMENT

Planning for delivery
- Obstetricians will plan delivery between 35+0 and 36+6 weeks gestation in women stringy suspected to have placenta accreta
- Administer a single course of antenatal glucocorticoids between 34 and 36 weeks of gestation
- Symptoms of bleeding or preterm labor may hasten the need for delivery

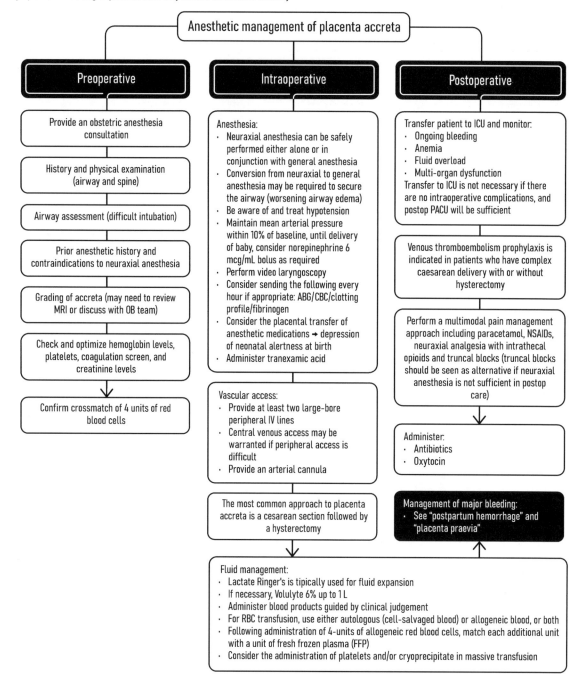

**Anesthetic management of placenta accreta**

**Preoperative**

- Provide an obstetric anesthesia consultation
- History and physical examination (airway and spine)
- Airway assessment (difficult intubation)
- Prior anesthetic history and contraindications to neuraxial anesthesia
- Grading of accreta (may need to review MRI or discuss with OB team)
- Check and optimize hemoglobin levels, platelets, coagulation screen, and creatinine levels
- Confirm crossmatch of 4 units of red blood cells

**Intraoperative**

Anesthesia:
- Neuraxial anesthesia can be safely performed either alone or in conjunction with general anesthesia
- Conversion from neuraxial to general anesthesia may be required to secure the airway (worsening airway edema)
- Be aware of and treat hypotension
- Maintain mean arterial pressure within 10% of baseline, until delivery of baby, consider norepinephrine 6 mcg/mL bolus as required
- Perform video laryngoscopy
- Consider sending the following every hour if appropriate: ABG/CBC/clotting profile/fibrinogen
- Consider the placental transfer of anesthetic medications → depression of neonatal alertness at birth
- Administer tranexamic acid

Vascular access:
- Provide at least two large-bore peripheral IV lines
- Central venous access may be warranted if peripheral access is difficult
- Provide an arterial cannula

The most common approach to placenta accreta is a cesarean section followed by a hysterectomy

Fluid management:
- Lactate Ringer's is tipically used for fluid expansion
- If necessary, Volulyte 6% up to 1 L
- Administer blood products guided by clinical judgement
- For RBC transfusion, use either autologous (cell-salvaged blood) or allogeneic blood, or both
- Following administration of 4-units of allogeneic red blood cells, match each additional unit with a unit of fresh frozen plasma (FFP)
- Consider the administration of platelets and/or cryoprecipitate in massive transfusion

**Postoperative**

Transfer patient to ICU and monitor:
- Ongoing bleeding
- Anemia
- Fluid overload
- Multi-organ dysfunction
Transfer to ICU is not necessary if there are no intraoperative complications, and postop PACU will be sufficient

Venous thromboembolism prophylaxis is indicated in patients who have complex caesarean delivery with or without hysterectomy

Perform a multimodal pain management approach including paracetamol, NSAIDs, neuraxial analgesia with intrathecal opioids and truncal blocks (truncal blocks should be seen as alternative if neuraxial anesthesia is not sufficient in postop care)

Administer:
- Antibiotics
- Oxytocin

Management of major bleeding:
- See "postpartum hemorrhage" and "placenta praevia"

## SUGGESTED READING

- Reale, S.C., Farber, M.K., 2022. Management of patients with suspected placenta accreta spectrum. BJA Education 22, 43-51.
- Silver RM, Barbour KD. Placenta accreta spectrum: accreta, increta, and percreta. Obstet Gynecol Clin North Am. 2015;42(2):381-402.

# PLACENTA PRAEVIA

## LEARNING OBJECTIVES

- Description of placenta praevia
- Management of placenta praevia

## DEFINITION AND MECHANISM

- When the placenta attaches inside the uterus near or over the cervical opening
- Classified as a complication of pregnancy
- Commonly occurs around 32 weeks of gestation, however, placenta praevia should be suspected if there is bleeding after 24 weeks of gestation
- Affects approximately 0.5% of pregnancies
- A cesarean section is often required because of the high bleeding risk
- The cause is unknown, however, is thought to be related to abnormal vascularisation of the endometrium caused by scarring or atrophy from previous trauma, surgery, or infection

## CLASSIFICATION

- Minor
  - Placenta is in the lower uterine segment, but the lower edge does not cover the internal os
- Major
  - Placenta is in the lower uterine segment, and the lower edge covers the internal os

- Other than that placenta previa can also be classified as:
  - Complete:
    - The placenta completely covers the cervix, blocking the vagina
  - Partial:
    - The placenta partially covers the cervix
  - Marginal:
    - Placenta is positioned at the edge of the cervix
    - Touching but not covering the cervix
    - More likely to resolve on its own

## COMPLICATIONS

| Maternal | Fetal |
|---|---|
| Placenta accreta | Intrauterine growth restriction |
| Hypotension | Hypoxia |
| Antepartum bleeding | Premature infant |
| Placental abruption | Low birth weight |
| Postpartum hemorrhage | |
| Abnormal placentation | |

## RISK FACTORS

- Previous placenta previa, cesarean delivery, myomectomy, or endometrium damage caused by dilation and curettage
- Younger than 20 or older than 35
- Multiparity
- Smoking or cocaine use during pregnancy
- Pregnant with twins, triplets, or more
- Previous surgery on the uterus
- History of uterine fibroids

## DIAGNOSIS

- Ultrasound

# MANAGEMENT

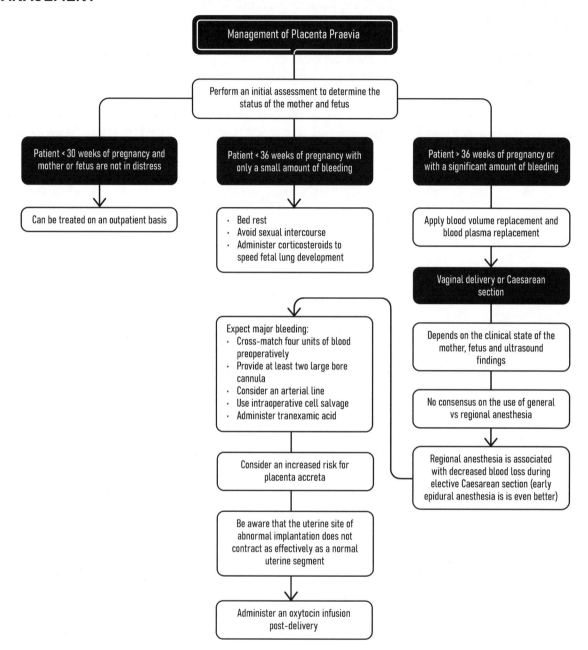

**Management of Placenta Praevia**

Perform an initial assessment to determine the status of the mother and fetus

**Patient < 30 weeks of pregnancy and mother or fetus are not in distress**
→ Can be treated on an outpatient basis

**Patient < 36 weeks of pregnancy with only a small amount of bleeding**
→
- Bed rest
- Avoid sexual intercourse
- Administer corticosteroids to speed fetal lung development

Expect major bleeding:
- Cross-match four units of blood preoperatively
- Provide at least two large bore cannula
- Consider an arterial line
- Use intraoperative cell salvage
- Administer tranexamic acid

Consider an increased risk for placenta accreta

Be aware that the uterine site of abnormal implantation does not contract as effectively as a normal uterine segment

Administer an oxytocin infusion post-delivery

**Patient > 36 weeks of pregnancy or with a significant amount of bleeding**
→ Apply blood volume replacement and blood plasma replacement

**Vaginal delivery or Caesarean section**

Depends on the clinical state of the mother, fetus and ultrasound findings

No consensus on the use of general vs regional anesthesia

Regional anesthesia is associated with decreased blood loss during elective Caesarean section (early epidural anesthesia is is even better)

## SUGGESTED READING

- Plaat F, shonfeldd A. 2015. Major obstetric hemorrhage. BJA education. 15;4:190-193.
- Pollard BJ, Kitchen, G. Handbook of Clinical Anaesthesia. Fourth Edition. CRC Press. 2018. 978-1-4987-6289-2.
- Walfish, M., Neuman, A., Wlody, D., 2009. Maternal haemorrhage. British Journal of Anaesthesia 103, i47–i56.

# PLACENTAL ABRUPTION

## LEARNING OBJECTIVES

- Signs of placental abruption
- Degrees of placental abruption
- Management of placental abruption

## DEFINITION AND MECHANISM

- Hemorrhage arising from the premature separation of a normally situated placenta
- Separation of the placental bed from the decidua basalis before delivery of the fetus
- Occurs in 1% of pregnancies
- Leading cause of vaginal bleeding in the latter half of pregnancy
- Emergency with high maternal and fetal morbidity/mortality
- Major complications:
  - Hemorrhagic shock
  - Acute kidney injury
  - Coagulopathy
  - Fetal demise
  - Maternal death
  - Delivering premature infant
  - Transfusion-associated complications
  - Hysterectomy
  - Recurrence has been reported in 4 to 12% of cases

## SIGNS AND SYMPTOMS

- Key diagnostic factors:
  - Vaginal bleeding (although about 20% of cases have no bleeding)
  - Uterine tenderness
  - Rapid contractions
  - Abdominal pain
  - Fetal heart rate abnormalities
- The clinical implications of a placental abruption vary based on the extent of the separation and the location of the separation
- Placental abruption can be complete or partial and marginal or central
- The classification of placental abruption is based on the following clinical findings:

| Class 0: asymptomatic | Class 1: Mild | Class 2: Moderate | Class 3: Severe |
|---|---|---|---|
| Discovery of a blood clot on the maternal side of a delivered placenta<br>Diagnosis is made retrospectively | No sign of vaginal bleeding or a small amount of vaginal bleeding<br>Slight uterine tenderness<br>Maternal blood pressure and heart rate within normal limits<br>No signs of fetal distress | No sign of vaginal bleeding to a moderate amount of vaginal bleeding<br>Significant uterine tenderness with tetanic contractions<br>Change in vital signs: maternal tachycardia, orthostatic changes in blood pressure<br>Evidence of fetal distress<br>Clotting profile alteration: hypofibrinogenemia | No sign of vaginal bleeding to heavy vaginal bleeding<br>Tetanic uterus/board-like consistency on palpation<br>Maternal shock<br>Clotting profile alteration: hypofibrinogenemia and coagulopathy<br>Fetal death |

- Classification of 0 or 1 is usually associated with a partial, marginal separation
- Whereas, classification of 2 or 3 is associated with complete or central separation

Placental abruption

*Stages of hypovolemic shock*

| | I Compensated | II Mild | III Moderate | IV Severe |
|---|---|---|---|---|
| Blood loss | < 15%; 750–1000 ml | 15–30%; 1000–1500 ml | 30–40%; 1500–2000 ml | > 40%; ≥ 2000 ml |
| Heart rate (beats/min) | > 100 | > 100 | > 120 | > 140 |
| Arterial pressure | Normal; vasoconstriction redistributes blood flow, slight increase in diastolic pressure | Orthostatic changes in arterial pressure, vasoconstriction intensifies in non-critical organs (skin, muscle, gut) | Markedly decreased (systolic arterial pressure < 90 mm Hg); vasoconstriction decreases perfusion to abdominal organs | Profoundly decreased (systolic arterial pressure < 80 mm Hg); decreased perfusion to vital organs (brain, heart) |
| Respiration | Normal | Mild increase | Moderate tachypnea | Marked tachypnea—respiratory failure |
| Mental status | Normal, slightly anxious | Mildly anxious, agitated | Confused, agitated | Obtunded |
| Urine output (ml/h) | > 30 | 20–30 | < 20 | None (anuria) |
| Capillary refill | Normal (< 2 s) | > 2 s; clammy skin | Usually > 3 s; cool, pale skin | > 3 s; cold, mottled skin |

# RISK FACTORS

- Health history and past obstetrical events:
  - Smoking
  - Cocaine use
  - Maternal age over 35 years
  - Hypertension
  - Placental abruption in a prior pregnancy
- Current pregnancy:
  - Multiple gestation pregnancies
  - Polyhydramnios
  - Preeclampsia
  - Sudden uterine decompression
  - Short umbilical cord
- Unexpected trauma

# CAUSES

- The exact etiology is unknown
- Specific cause is often unknown
- Trauma or injury to the abdomen
- Rarely a short umbilical cord or rapid loss of amniotic fluid

# DIAGNOSIS

- Clinical signs/symptoms
- Ultrasound (however low sensitivity)

Placental abruption

# MANAGEMENT

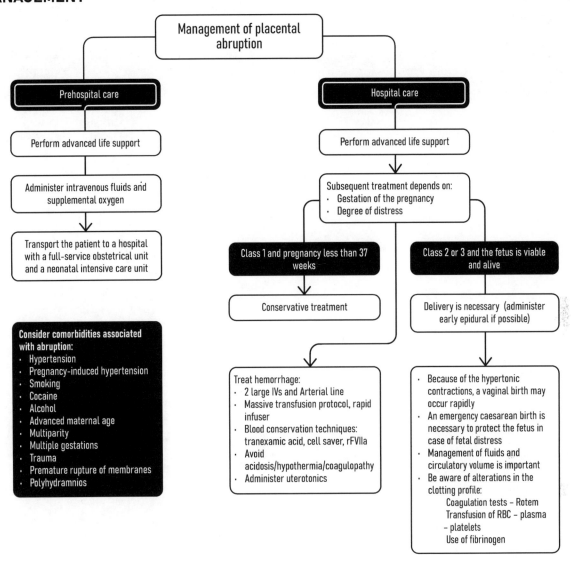

Management of placental abruption

**Prehospital care**

Perform advanced life support

Administer intravenous fluids and supplemental oxygen

Transport the patient to a hospital with a full-service obstetrical unit and a neonatal intensive care unit

**Consider comorbidities associated with abruption:**
- Hypertension
- Pregnancy-induced hypertension
- Smoking
- Cocaine
- Alcohol
- Advanced maternal age
- Multiparity
- Multiple gestations
- Trauma
- Premature rupture of membranes
- Polyhydramnios

**Hospital care**

Perform advanced life support

Subsequent treatment depends on:
- Gestation of the pregnancy
- Degree of distress

**Class 1 and pregnancy less than 37 weeks**

Conservative treatment

**Class 2 or 3 and the fetus is viable and alive**

Delivery is necessary (administer early epidural if possible)

Treat hemorrhage:
- 2 large IVs and Arterial line
- Massive transfusion protocol, rapid infuser
- Blood conservation techniques: tranexamic acid, cell saver, rFVIIa
- Avoid acidosis/hypothermia/coagulopathy
- Administer uterotonics

- Because of the hypertonic contractions, a vaginal birth may occur rapidly
- An emergency caesarean birth is necessary to protect the fetus in case of fetal distress
- Management of fluids and circulatory volume is important
- Be aware of alterations in the clotting profile:
    Coagulation tests – Rotem
    Transfusion of RBC – plasma – platelets
    Use of fibrinogen

## SUGGESTED READING

- Schmidt P, Skelly CL, Raines DA. Placental Abruption. In: StatPearls. Treasure Island (FL): StatPearls Publishing; April 1, 2022.
- Walfish, M., Neuman, A., Wlody, D., 2009. Maternal haemorrhage. British Journal of Anaesthesia 103, i47–i56.

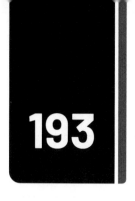

# POST-DURAL PUNCTURE HEADACHE (PDPH)

**193**

## LEARNING OBJECTIVES

- Recognize the risk factors for PDPH
- Recognize signs and symptoms of PDPH
- Take measures to reduce the risk of PDPH
- Make diagnostic assessments for PDPH
- Manage PDPH occurrence

## DEFINITION AND MECHANISM

- Post-dural puncture headache (PDPH) is a headache occurring within 5 days of a dural puncture, caused by cerebrospinal fluid leakage through the puncture
- It is usually accompanied by neck stiffness and/or subjective hearing symptoms
- PDPH usually remits spontaneously within 2 weeks
- It is recommended to place intrathecal catheters selectively (e.g., after a difficult epidural procedure), to reduce the need for multiple epidural attempts and the risk of subsequent dural puncture

## RISK FACTORS

- Patient-related:
  - Age: Uncommon in patients less than 10 years of age; peak incidence is in the teens and early 20s
  - Gender: Nonpregnant females have twice the risk compared to age-matched men
- Equipment related:
  - Needle gauge (larger > smaller)
  - Needle tip design (cutting > noncutting)

## RISK MANAGEMENT AFTER ACCIDENTAL DURAL PUNCTURE

- Reinsert the stylet
- Subarachnoid saline (although lack of evidence)
- Consider administration of intravneous cosyntropin (although only tested in small trials)
- Limiting/avoiding pushing during labor
- Epidural opiates
- Prophylactic epidural blood patch

## SIGNS & SYMPTOMS

- Most cases of PDPH will be typical in
  - Onset—often delayed, but within 48 hours
  - Presentation—symmetric, bilateral headache
  - Associated symptoms—more likely with severe headache
- Symptoms:
  - Headache accompanied by at least one of these symptoms:
  - Neck stiffness
  - Tinnitus
  - Hypoacusia
  - Photophobia
  - Nausea

## DIAGNOSIS

- PDPH diagnosis remains a diagnosis of exclusion, it is critical to rule out other etiologies
  - Benign etiologies
    - Nonspecific headache
    - Exacerbation of chronic headache (e.g., tension-type headache)
    - Hypertensive headache
    - Pneumocephalus
    - Sinusitis
    - Drug-related side effect
    - Spontaneous intracranial hypotension
    - Other
  - Serious etiologies
    - Meningitis
    - Subdural hematoma (SDH)
    - Subarachnoid hemorrhage
    - Preeclampsia/eclampsia
    - Intracranial venous thrombosis (ICVT)
    - Other

Post-dural puncture headache

# MANAGEMENT

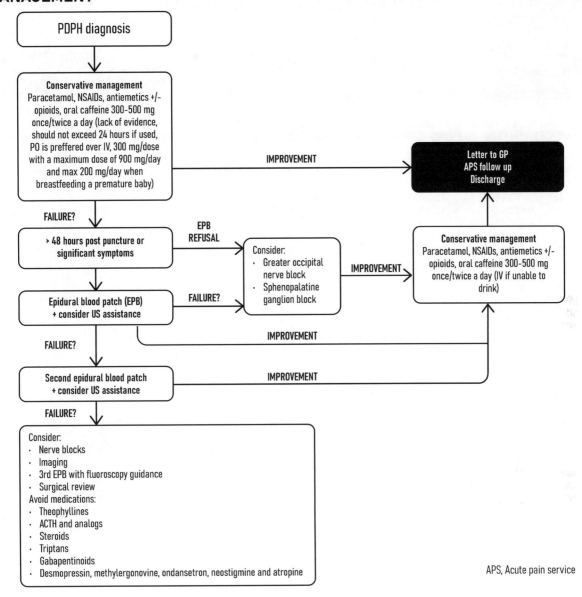

**PDPH diagnosis**

**Conservative management**
Paracetamol, NSAIDs, antiemetics +/- opioids, oral caffeine 300-500 mg once/twice a day (lack of evidence, should not exceed 24 hours if used, PO is preffered over IV, 300 mg/dose with a maximum dose of 900 mg/day and max 200 mg/day when breastfeeding a premature baby)

IMPROVEMENT →

**Letter to GP
APS follow up
Discharge**

**FAILURE?**

**> 48 hours post puncture or significant symptoms**

EPB REFUSAL →

**Consider:**
· Greater occipital nerve block
· Sphenopalatine ganglion block

IMPROVEMENT →

**Conservative management**
Paracetamol, NSAIDs, antiemetics +/- opioids, oral caffeine 300-500 mg once/twice a day (IV if unable to drink)

**Epidural blood patch (EPB)
+ consider US assistance**

FAILURE? →

IMPROVEMENT

**FAILURE?**

**Second epidural blood patch
+ consider US assistance**

IMPROVEMENT →

**FAILURE?**

**Consider:**
· Nerve blocks
· Imaging
· 3rd EPB with fluoroscopy guidance
· Surgical review
**Avoid medications:**
· Theophyllines
· ACTH and analogs
· Steroids
· Triptans
· Gabapentinoids
· Desmopressin, methylergonovine, ondansetron, neostigmine and atropine

APS, Acute pain service

## KEEP IN MIND

- There is no evidence to support the common practice of recommending bed rest (can delay the proper treatment) and aggressive hydration in the prevention of PDPH
- PDPH may carry a risk of medicolegal liability
- Accidental dural puncture (ADP) may result in chronic headache and back pain
- Anesthetic procedures with risk of PDPH require proper informed consent

## SUGGESTED READING

- Jagannathan DK, Arriaga AF, Elterman KG, et al. Effect of neuraxial technique after inadvertent dural puncture on obstetric outcomes and anesthetic complications. Int J Obstet Anesth 2016; 25:23.
- Russell R, Laxton C, Lucas DN, Niewiarowski J, Scrutton M, Stocks G. Treatment of obstetric post-dural puncture headache. Part 2: epidural blood patch. Int J Obstet Anesth. 2019;38:104-118
- Statement on post-dural puncture headache management. American Society of Anesthesiologists (ASA). https://www.asahq.org. Published October 13, 2021. Accessed December 14, 2022.

Post-dural puncture headache (PDPH)

# POSTPARTUM HEMORRHAGE

**194**

## LEARNING OBJECTIVES

- Understand the common causes of postpartum hemorrhage (PPH)
- Management of PPH

## DEFINITION AND MECHANISM

- Postpartum hemorrhage (PPH) is defined as excessive bleeding within 24 hours after childbirth, although it can less frequently occur up to 6 weeks postpartum
  - Vaginal delivery: estimated blood loss (EBL) > 500 mL
  - Post-C-section: EBL > 1000 mL
  - PPH is the leading cause of maternal mortality in low-income countries and the primary cause of nearly one-quarter of all maternal deaths globally

## SIGNS AND SYMPTOMS

- EBL > 500
- Tachycardia
- Hypotension
- Delayed capillary refill
- Decreased urine output (oliguria or anuria)
- Pallor
- Lightheadedness
- Palpitations

- Confusion
- Syncope
- Fatigue
- Air hunger
- Diaphoresis
- Cold & clammy skin
- Restlessness and anxiety
- Nausea and vomiting

## RISK FACTORS

However, 20% of postpartum hemorrhage occurs in women with no identifiable risk factors

| Risk factors | |
| --- | --- |
| Medical or surgical history | Previous postpartum hemorrhage<br>Leiomyomata (Fibroids)<br>Previous caesarean delivery or other uterine instrumentation<br>Advanced maternal age (> 35 years)<br>Obesity<br>Grand multiparity |
| Other | Prolonged use of uterotonic agents (e.g., oxytocin)<br>Use of anticoagulant medications<br>Rapid delivery |
| Fetal issues | Multifetal gestation<br>Polyhydramnios<br>Large-for-gestational-age fetus<br>Fetal macrosomia |
| Maternal issues | Hypertensive disorders of pregnancy<br>Perioperative anemia<br>Inherited coagulopathy such as Von Willebrand's Disease (VWD)<br>Acquired coagulopathy such as HELLP syndrome |
| Labor & delivery issues | Trial of labor after caesarean delivery<br>Prolonged labor<br>Induction and augmentation of labor<br>Arrest of progress during the second stage of labor<br>Prolonged third stage of labor<br>Instrumentation during delivery (forceps or vacuum-assisted) |
| Placental/uterine issues | Placental abruption<br>Placenta praevia<br>Retained placenta<br>Chorioamnionitis<br>Acute uterine inversion<br>Subinvolution of the uterus |

# CAUSES

| The four T's mnemonic of postpartum hemorrhage: | | |
|---|---|---|
| Tonus | Atonic uterus | 70-80% |
| Tissue | Retained placenta, invasive placenta | 10-20% |
| Trauma | Laceration, hematoma, uterine inversion, rupture | 10-20% |
| Thrombin | Coagulopathy | 1% |

# MANAGEMENT

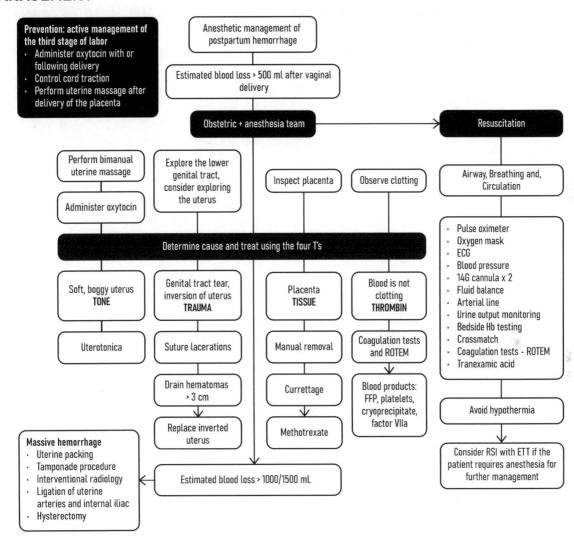

ROTEM, rotational thromboelastometry; FFP, fresh frozen plasma; RSI, rapid sequence induction; ETT, endotracheal tube

# SUGGESTED READING

- Anderson JM, Etches D. Prevention and management of postpartum hemorrhage. Am Fam Physician. 2007;75(6):875-882.
- Evensen A, Anderson JM, Fontaine P. Postpartum hemorrhage: prevention and treatment. Am Fam Physician. 2017; 95(7): 442-449.
- 2017. Prevention and Management of Postpartum Haemorrhage. BJOG: An International Journal of Obstetrics & Gynaecology 124, e106-e149.
- E. Mavrides, S. Allard, E. Chandraharan, P. Collins, L. Green, BJ. Hunt, S. Riris. AJ. Thomason on behalf of the Royal college of obstetricians and gynaecologists. Prevention and management of postpartum haemorrhage. BJOG 2016; 124:e 106-e149
- Watkins EJ, Stem K. Postpartum hemorrhage. JAAPA. 2020;33(4):29-33.
- WHO recommendations for the prevention and treatment of postpartum haemorrhage.

# PREECLAMPSIA

## LEARNING OBJECTIVES

- Definition, signs, and symptoms of preeclampsia
- Management of preeclampsia

## DEFINITION AND MECHANISM

- Preeclampsia is defined as new onset hypertension (systolic blood pressure ≥ 140 mmHg, diastolic blood pressure ≥ 90 mmHg, or both) accompanied by one or more of the following features at or after 20 weeks of gestation:
  - Proteinuria:
    - Spot urinary protein-to-creatinine ratio > 30 mg/mmoL or a 24-hour urine collection with > 300 mg of protein
  - Other maternal organ dysfunction, including:
    - Acute kidney injury
    - Liver involvement
    - Neurological complications: seizures, severe headaches, persistent visual scotomata, clonus, blindness, altered mental status, or stroke
  - Hematological complications:
    - Thrombocytopenia
    - Disseminated intravascular coagulation (DIC)
    - Hemolysis
- Preeclampsia can also be superimposed on women who have hypertension or proteinuria before 20 weeks of gestation, making the diagnosis more challenging/problematic in these patients
- Preeclampsia represents a potentially progressive clinical condition; the sub-categories 'mild' and 'severe' are no longer used
- HELLP syndrome (hemolysis, elevated liver enzymes, and low platelets) representing a severe form of preeclampsia, can be potentially life-threatening to both mother and the baby
- Women may present critically, with complications such as placental abruption or DIC
- Left untreated, preeclampsia can lead to serious, even fatal, complications for both the mother and the baby
  - Early delivery of the baby is often recommended
- Preeclampsia affects 2–8% of pregnancies worldwide

## SIGNS AND SYMPTOMS

- Proteinuria or other signs of kidney problems
- Thrombocytopenia
- Increased liver enzymes
- Severe headaches
- Visual changes, including temporary loss of vision, blurred vision, or light sensitivity
- Shortness of breath
- Abdominal pain
- Nausea or vomiting

## SEVERE PREECLAMPSIA

- Severe features associated with preeclampsia that warrant consideration of planned early birth before 37 weeks of gestation:
  - Inability to control maternal blood pressure despite using 3 or more classes of antihypertensives in appropriate doses
  - Progressive deterioration in liver function, renal function, hemolysis, or platelet count
  - Maternal pulse oximetry less than 90% on room air
  - Ongoing neurological features, such as severe intractable headache, repeated visual scotomata, or eclampsia
  - Placental abruption
  - Reversed end-diastolic flow in the umbilical artery on Doppler velocimetry, a non-reassuring cardiotocograph, or stillbirth

# CAUSES

- Abnormal placentation
- Immunological factors
- Prior or existing maternal pathology (see risk factors)
- Dietary factors, such as low dietary calcium intake
- Environmental factors, such as air pollution

# RISK FACTORS

| High risk factors | Moderate risk factors |
|---|---|
| Hypertensive disease in previous pregnancy | First pregnancy |
| Chronic kidney disease | Age ≥ 40 years |
| Autoimmune disease (e.g., antiphospholipid syndrome) | Pregnancy interval ≥ 10 yr |
| Type 1 or type 2 diabetes mellitus | Family history of preeclampsia |
| Chronic hypertension | Multiple pregnancy |

# PREVENTION

- Daily intake of 75-150 mg aspirin from 12 weeks until 36-37 weeks of gestation for woman with one high-risk, or more than two moderate-risk factors
- Calcium supplementation (> 1 g/day) for women with low dietary calcium intake

# DIAGNOSIS

- Blood pressure ≥ 140 mmHg systolic or ≥ 90 mmHg diastolic on two separate readings taken at least four to six hours apart after 20 weeks of gestation in an individual with previously normal blood pressure
- An increase in systolic blood pressure of ≥ 30 mmHg or an increase in diastolic blood pressure of ≥ 15 mmHg in a woman with essential hypertension that began before 20 weeks of gestation
- Proteinuria ≥ 0.3 grams (300 mg) or more of protein in a 24-hour urine sample or a spot urinary protein-to-creatinine ratio ≥ 0.3
- Blood and urine analysis
- Fetal ultrasound

# MANAGEMENT

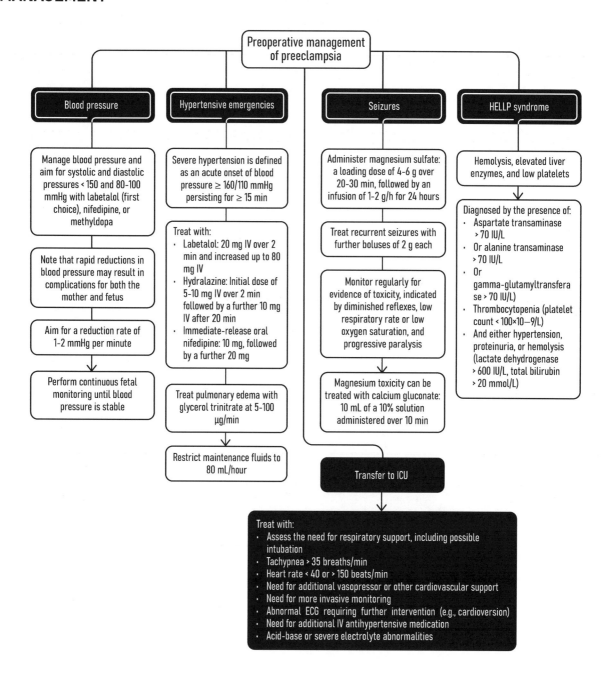

**Preoperative management of preeclampsia**

**Blood pressure**

Manage blood pressure and aim for systolic and diastolic pressures < 150 and 80-100 mmHg with labetalol (first choice), nifedipine, or methyldopa

Note that rapid reductions in blood pressure may result in complications for both the mother and fetus

Aim for a reduction rate of 1-2 mmHg per minute

Perform continuous fetal monitoring until blood pressure is stable

**Hypertensive emergencies**

Severe hypertension is defined as an acute onset of blood pressure ≥ 160/110 mmHg persisting for ≥ 15 min

Treat with:
- Labetalol: 20 mg IV over 2 min and increased up to 80 mg IV
- Hydralazine: Initial dose of 5-10 mg IV over 2 min followed by a further 10 mg IV after 20 min
- Immediate-release oral nifedipine: 10 mg, followed by a further 20 mg

Treat pulmonary edema with glycerol trinitrate at 5-100 µg/min

Restrict maintenance fluids to 80 mL/hour

**Seizures**

Administer magnesium sulfate: a loading dose of 4-6 g over 20-30 min, followed by an infusion of 1-2 g/h for 24 hours

Treat recurrent seizures with further boluses of 2 g each

Monitor regularly for evidence of toxicity, indicated by diminished reflexes, low respiratory rate or low oxygen saturation, and progressive paralysis

Magnesium toxicity can be treated with calcium gluconate: 10 mL of a 10% solution administered over 10 min

**HELLP syndrome**

Hemolysis, elevated liver enzymes, and low platelets

Diagnosed by the presence of:
- Aspartate transaminase > 70 IU/L
- Or alanine transaminase > 70 IU/L
- Or gamma-glutamyltransferase > 70 IU/L)
- Thrombocytopenia (platelet count < 100×10−9/L)
- And either hypertension, proteinuria, or hemolysis (lactate dehydrogenase > 600 IU/L, total bilirubin > 20 mmol/L)

**Transfer to ICU**

Treat with:
- Assess the need for respiratory support, including possible intubation
- Tachypnea > 35 breaths/min
- Heart rate < 40 or > 150 beats/min
- Need for additional vasopressor or other cardiovascular support
- Need for more invasive monitoring
- Abnormal ECG requiring further intervention (e.g., cardioversion)
- Need for additional IV antihypertensive medication
- Acid-base or severe electrolyte abnormalities

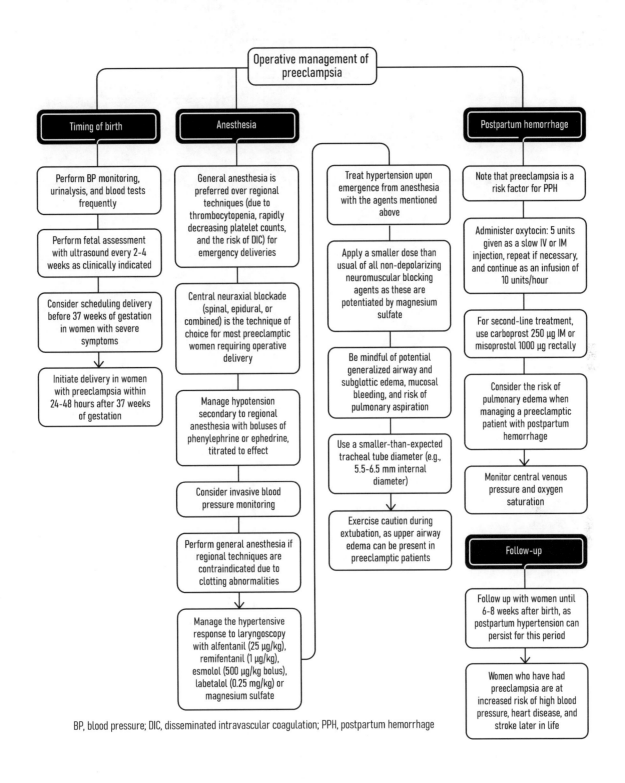

**Operative management of preeclampsia**

**Timing of birth**

Perform BP monitoring, urinalysis, and blood tests frequently

Perform fetal assessment with ultrasound every 2-4 weeks as clinically indicated

Consider scheduling delivery before 37 weeks of gestation in women with severe symptoms

Initiate delivery in women with preeclampsia within 24-48 hours after 37 weeks of gestation

**Anesthesia**

General anesthesia is preferred over regional techniques (due to thrombocytopenia, rapidly decreasing platelet counts, and the risk of DIC) for emergency deliveries

Central neuraxial blockade (spinal, epidural, or combined) is the technique of choice for most preeclamptic women requiring operative delivery

Manage hypotension secondary to regional anesthesia with boluses of phenylephrine or ephedrine, titrated to effect

Consider invasive blood pressure monitoring

Perform general anesthesia if regional techniques are contraindicated due to clotting abnormalities

Manage the hypertensive response to laryngoscopy with alfentanil (25 µg/kg), remifentanil (1 µg/kg), esmolol (500 µg/kg bolus), labetalol (0.25 mg/kg) or magnesium sulfate

Treat hypertension upon emergence from anesthesia with the agents mentioned above

Apply a smaller dose than usual of all non-depolarizing neuromuscular blocking agents as these are potentiated by magnesium sulfate

Be mindful of potential generalized airway and subglottic edema, mucosal bleeding, and risk of pulmonary aspiration

Use a smaller-than-expected tracheal tube diameter (e.g., 5.5-6.5 mm internal diameter)

Exercise caution during extubation, as upper airway edema can be present in preeclamptic patients

**Postpartum hemorrhage**

Note that preeclampsia is a risk factor for PPH

Administer oxytocin: 5 units given as a slow IV or IM injection, repeat if necessary, and continue as an infusion of 10 units/hour

For second-line treatment, use carboprost 250 µg IM or misoprostol 1000 µg rectally

Consider the risk of pulmonary edema when managing a preeclamptic patient with postpartum hemorrhage

Monitor central venous pressure and oxygen saturation

**Follow-up**

Follow up with women until 6-8 weeks after birth, as postpartum hypertension can persist for this period

Women who have had preeclampsia are at increased risk of high blood pressure, heart disease, and stroke later in life

BP, blood pressure; DIC, disseminated intravascular coagulation; PPH, postpartum hemorrhage

═══ **SUGGESTED READING** ═══

- Goddard, J., Wee, M.Y.K., Vinayakarao, L., 2020. Update on hypertensive disorders in pregnancy. BJA Education 20, 411–416.
- Leslie, D., Collis, R., 2016. Hypertension in pregnancy. BJA Education 16, 33–37.

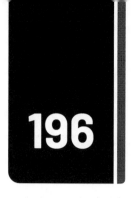

# 196

# PRELABOR RUPTURE OF MEMBRANES (PROM)

## LEARNING OBJECTIVES

- Define prelabor rupture of membranes
- Complications of prelabor rupture of membranes
- Management of prelabor rupture of membranes

## DEFINITION AND MECHANISM

- Previously known as premature rupture of membranes, PROM refers to the breakage of the amniotic sac before the onset of labor
- It can occur at term ($\geq$ 37 weeks of gestation) or preterm (< 37 weeks of gestation), the latter is preterm PROM (PPROM)
- Occurs in approximately 8% of term pregnancies and 30% of preterm pregnancies
- About 50% of patients with PROM will deliver within one week

### Classification

- **PROM:** Rupture happens early, at least one hour before labor begins
- **Prolonged PROM:** More than 18 hours have passed between rupture and the onset of labor
- **Preterm PROM (PPROM):** Rupture occurs before 37 weeks of gestation
- **Midtrimester PPROM or previable PPROM (< 1%):** Rupture occurs before 24 weeks of gestation, the fetus cannot survive outside the uterus before this age

## SIGNS AND SYMPTOMS

- Painless gush or steady leakage of fluid from the vagina
- Loss of fluid may be associated with the fetus becoming easier to feel through the abdomen, decreased uterine size, or the presence of meconium in the fluid

## COMPLICATIONS

Maternal
- Placental abruption
- Infection (e.g., chorioamnionitis)
- Postpartum endometritis
- Future PROM in later pregnancies

Fetal
- Premature birth and related complications (e.g., bronchopulmonary dysplasia, necrotizing enterocolitis, intraventricular hemorrhage, and cerebral palsy)
- Umbilical cord compression or umbilical cord prolapse
- Infection (e.g., sepsis)
- Abnormal fetal presentation (e.g., breech presentation)

## RISK FACTORS

- Infection: Amniotic fluid infection (chorioamnionitis), urinary tract infections, sexually transmitted diseases, lower genital tract infections (e.g., bacterial vaginosis)
- Prior PROM or preterm delivery in previous pregnancies
- Polyhydramnios
- Multiple gestation
- Vaginal bleeding
- Maternal smoking
- Maternal drug use
- Maternal underweight or nutritional deficits
- Invasive procedures (e.g., amniocentesis)
- Cervical insufficiency (i.e., short or prematurely dilated cervix during pregnancy)

## TREATMENT

Treatment depends on the gestational age of the pregnancy, health status of the fetus, and whether complications are present
- **Delivery:** Indicated for fetal compromise, infection, or evidence of fetal lung maturity or gestational age $\geq$ 34 weeks
- **Expectant management:** Involves strategies to delay labor, including to delay labor including bed rest, medications (i.e., antibiotics, corticosteroids, and magnesium sulfate), and frequent monitoring for infection or fetal distress

# MANGEMENT

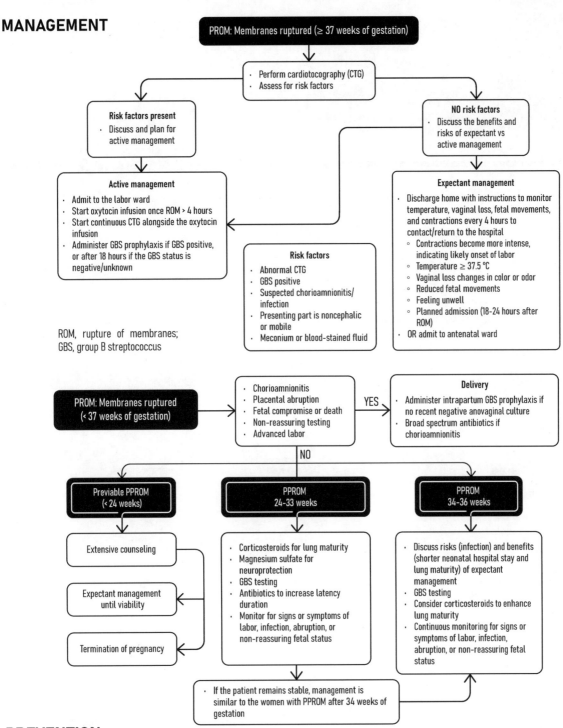

**PROM: Membranes ruptured (≥ 37 weeks of gestation)**

- Perform cardiotocography (CTG)
- Assess for risk factors

**Risk factors present**
- Discuss and plan for active management

**NO risk factors**
- Discuss the benefits and risks of expectant vs active management

**Active management**
- Admit to the labor ward
- Start oxytocin infusion once ROM > 4 hours
- Start continuous CTG alongside the oxytocin infusion
- Administer GBS prophylaxis if GBS positive, or after 18 hours if the GBS status is negative/unknown

**Risk factors**
- Abnormal CTG
- GBS positive
- Suspected chorioamnionitis/infection
- Presenting part is noncephalic or mobile
- Meconium or blood-stained fluid

**Expectant management**
- Discharge home with instructions to monitor temperature, vaginal loss, fetal movements, and contractions every 4 hours to contact/return to the hospital
  - Contractions become more intense, indicating likely onset of labor
  - Temperature ≥ 37.5 °C
  - Vaginal loss changes in color or odor
  - Reduced fetal movements
  - Feeling unwell
  - Planned admission (18-24 hours after ROM)
- OR admit to antenatal ward

ROM, rupture of membranes; GBS, group B streptococcus

**PROM: Membranes ruptured (< 37 weeks of gestation)**

- Chorioamnionitis
- Placental abruption
- Fetal compromise or death
- Non-reassuring testing
- Advanced labor

**YES**

**Delivery**
- Administer intrapartum GBS prophylaxis if no recent negative anovaginal culture
- Broad spectrum antibiotics if chorioamnionitis

**NO**

**Previable PPROM (< 24 weeks)**

Extensive counseling

Expectant management until viability

Termination of pregnancy

**PPROM 24-33 weeks**
- Corticosteroids for lung maturity
- Magnesium sulfate for neuroprotection
- GBS testing
- Antibiotics to increase latency duration
- Monitor for signs or symptoms of labor, infection, abruption, or non-reassuring fetal status

**PPROM 34-36 weeks**
- Discuss risks (infection) and benefits (shorter neonatal hospital stay and lung maturity) of expectant management
- GBS testing
- Consider corticosteroids to enhance lung maturity
- Continuous monitoring for signs or symptoms of labor, infection, abruption, or non-reassuring fetal status

- If the patient remains stable, management is similar to the women with PPROM after 34 weeks of gestation

# PREVENTION

- Women with a history of preterm delivery (with or without PROM) are recommended to receive progesterone supplementation to help prevent recurrence

# SUGGESTED READING

- Dayal S, Hong PL. Premature Rupture Of Membranes. [Updated 2022 Jul 18]. In: StatPearls [Internet]. Treasure Island (FL): StatPearls Publishing; 2022 Jan. Available from: https://www.ncbi.nlm.nih.gov/books/NBK532888/

# UMBILICAL CORD PROLAPSE

## LEARNING OBJECTIVES

- Define umbilical cord prolapse
- Describe the risk factors for developing umbilical cord prolapse
- Umbilical cord prolapse management

## DEFINITION AND MECHANISM

- Umbilical cord prolapse is an obstetric emergency in which the umbilical cord descends through the cervix alongside (occult) or past (overt) the fetal presenting part
- It can occur before or during the delivery of the baby, usually close to the end of pregnancy (after 37 weeks)
- Compression of, or vasospasm of, the umbilical cord impairs the blood flow between the placenta and fetus, leading to fetal hypoxia and bradycardia
- Fetal hypoxia may result in fetal death or permanent disability if not rapidly diagnosed and managed
- Early recognition and intervention are important to reduce the adverse outcomes in the fetus

### Classification

- **Overt prolapse:** Cord exits the cervix before the fetal presenting part
- **Occult prolapse:** Cord exits the cervix with the fetal presenting part

## COMPLICATIONS

- Surviving infants may develop complications secondary to asphyxia (i.e., neonatal encephalopathy and cerebral palsy)
- Stillbirth

## RISK FACTORS

- Maternal age ≥ 35 years
- Premature rupture of membranes
- Preterm delivery
- Low birth weight
- Multiple gestation pregnancies
- Placenta praevia
- Polyhydramnios
- Fetal malpresentation (i.e., breech presentation)
- External cephalic version procedure
- Intrauterine growth restriction
- Fetal and cord abnormalities

## DIAGNOSIS

- Fetal bradycardia (< 120 bpm) in the setting of ruptured membranes should prompt immediate evaluation for potential cord prolapse
- Umbilical cord prolapse is diagnosed by seeing or palpating the prolapsed cord on pelvic examination

| Overt prolapse | Occult prolapse |
| --- | --- |
| Diagnosis is clinical and made by palpation of a pulsating structure in the vaginal vault or visibly protruding from the vaginal introitus Typically accompanied by fetal bradycardia or severe variable decelerations | Only fetal bradycardia may appear The cord is not visible or palpable ahead of the fetal presenting part |

# MANAGEMENT

**Goal:** Avoid cord compression and vasospasm
- Call for help
- Establish an intravenous line (if not already placed)
- Ensure continuous fetal monitoring
- Administer oxygen via a face mask (if needed)
- Administer aspiration prophylaxis
- Umbilical cord prolapse is an acute obstetric emergency requiring immediate delivery of the baby, usually via cesarean section
  - Allow instrumental/vaginal delivery if considered quicker
  - Inform the anesthesiologist, pediatrician, and OR staff
  - Patient consent
- Funic decompression: Elevating the fetal presenting part to aid cord decompression
  - Two fingers/hand in the vagina – manual elevation of the presenting part
  - Steep Trendelenburg or knee-chest position, lying on the left side is preferred
  - Bladder filling with a Foley catheter (≥ 500 mL of normal saline)
- Funic reduction (rarely used): Replacement of the umbilical cord into the uterus
- Tocolysis in case of fetal distress or if prolonged interval to delivery is expected
- Keep the cord warm and moist if it is protruding from the vagina and delivery is not imminent
- Avoid aortocaval compression
- Minimize handling of the cord outside of the vagina to prevent vasospasm

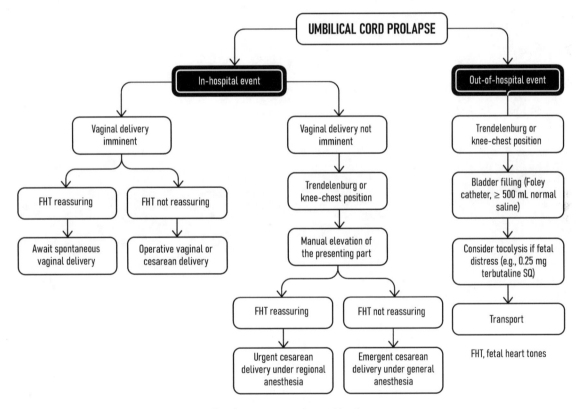

See also cesarean section considerations

## SUGGESTED READING

- Boushra M, Stone A, Rathbun KM. Umbilical Cord Prolapse. [Updated 2022 Jun 5]. In: StatPearls [Internet]. Treasure Island (FL): StatPearls Publishing; 2022 Jan. Available from: https://www.ncbi.nlm.nih.gov/books/NBK542241/
- Sayed Ahmed WA, Hamdy MA. Optimal management of umbilical cord prolapse. Int J Womens Health. 2018;10:459-465.

# UTERINE INVERSION

## LEARNING OBJECTIVES

- Description and four degrees of uterine inversion
- Signs and symptoms of uterine inversion
- Management of uterine inversion

## DEFINITION AND MECHANISM

- Uterine inversion is a rare complication when the uterine fundus collapses into the endometrial cavity, turning the uterus partially or completely inside out
- A life-threatening obstetric emergency as it can lead to severe blood loss, shock, and even maternal death
- In extremely rare cases (5% of uterine inversions), fibroids or tumors cause uterine inversion
- Four degrees of uterine inversion:
  - 1st degree (incomplete): the fundus is within the endometrial cavity
  - 2nd degree (complete): the fundus protrudes through the cervical os
  - 3rd degree (prolapsed): the fundus protrudes to or beyond the introitus
  - 4th degree (total): both the uterus and vagina are inverted and protrudes outside the vagina

- Time of occurrence:
  - Acute: within 24 hours of delivery
  - Subacute: more than 24 hours but less than four weeks postpartum
  - Chronic: ≥ 1 month postpartum
- The incidence ranges from 1 in 3500 to 20,000 deliveries

## SIGNS AND SYMPTOMS

- Postpartum bleeding
- Abdominal pain
- A smooth, round mass protruding from the cervix or vagina
- Urinary retention
- Hypotension
- Hemodynamic shock
- Bradycardia

## RISK FACTORS

- Short umbilical cord
- Rapid or prolonged labor and delivery
- Use of uterine relaxants
- Nulliparity
- Fetal macrosomia
- Retained placenta
- Severe preeclampsia
- Uterine atony
- Placenta accreta spectrum
- Uterine anomalies or tumors (leiomyoma)

## COMPLICATIONS

- Major hemorrhage
- Multi-organ damage
- Shock
- Sheehan syndrome
- Hysterectomy

## CAUSES

- Mismanagement of the third stage of labor such as:
  - Fundal pressure
  - Excess cord traction during the third stage of labor
- Other natural causes can be:
  - Uterine weakness
  - Precipitate delivery
  - Short umbilical cord
- It is more common in multiple gestations than in singleton pregnancies

## DIAGNOSIS

- Clinical findings
- Ultrasound examination shows an abnormal uterine fundal contour with a homogenous globular mass within the uterus

## MANAGEMENT

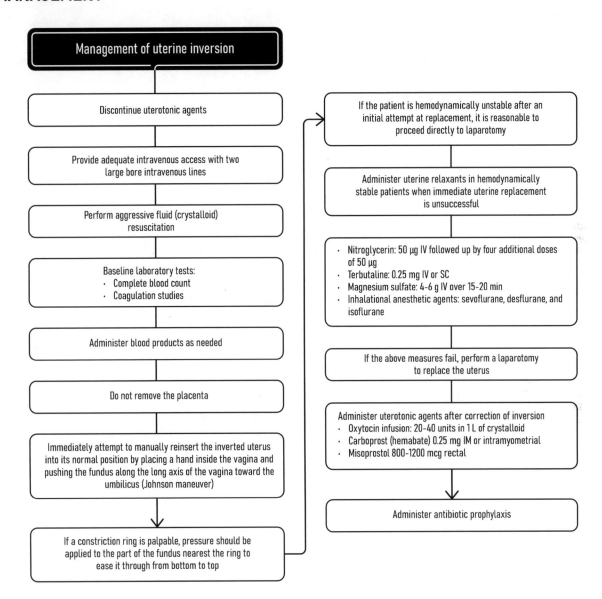

**Management of uterine inversion**

Discontinue uterotonic agents

Provide adequate intravenous access with two large bore intravenous lines

Perform aggressive fluid (crystalloid) resuscitation

Baseline laboratory tests:
- Complete blood count
- Coagulation studies

Administer blood products as needed

Do not remove the placenta

Immediately attempt to manually reinsert the inverted uterus into its normal position by placing a hand inside the vagina and pushing the fundus along the long axis of the vagina toward the umbilicus (Johnson maneuver)

If a constriction ring is palpable, pressure should be applied to the part of the fundus nearest the ring to ease it through from bottom to top

If the patient is hemodynamically unstable after an initial attempt at replacement, it is reasonable to proceed directly to laparotomy

Administer uterine relaxants in hemodynamically stable patients when immediate uterine replacement is unsuccessful

- Nitroglycerin: 50 µg IV followed up by four additional doses of 50 µg
- Terbutaline: 0.25 mg IV or SC
- Magnesium sulfate: 4-6 g IV over 15-20 min
- Inhalational anesthetic agents: sevoflurane, desflurane, and isoflurane

If the above measures fail, perform a laparotomy to replace the uterus

Administer uterotonic agents after correction of inversion
- Oxytocin infusion: 20-40 units in 1 L of crystalloid
- Carboprost (hemabate) 0.25 mg IM or intramyometrial
- Misoprostol 800-1200 mcg rectal

Administer antibiotic prophylaxis

## SUGGESTED READING

- Macones G. 2022. Peurperal uterine inversion. Up to date.
- Shepherd LJ, Shenassa H, Singh SS. Laparoscopic management of uterine inversion. J Minim Invasive Gynecol. 2010;17(2):255-257.
- Wendel MP, Shnaekel KL, Magann EF. Uterine Inversion: A Review of a Life-Threatening Obstetrical Emergency. Obstet Gynecol Surv. 2018;73(7):411-417.

# UTERINE RUPTURE

## LEARNING OBJECTIVES

- Description of uterine rupture
- Management of uterine rupture

---

## DEFINITION AND MECHANISM

- Uterine rupture refers to a complete division of all three layers of the uterus: the endometrium (inner epithelial layer), myometrium (smooth muscle layer), and perimetrium (serosal outer surface)
- Typical rupture occurs during labor, but it may occasionally happen earlier in pregnancy
- The fetus is left without the protection of the uterus, potentially leading to oxygen deprivation and a slowing of the fetal heart rate
- Suspect uterine rupture based on a rapid drop in the baby's heart rate during labor
- The cardinal sign of uterine rupture is loss of fetal station on a manual vaginal exam
- The maternal mortality rate is < 1%, while the fetal mortality rate is between 2-6 %
- Incomplete rupture:
  - Peritoneum is still intact
- Complete rupture:
  - All three layers are ruptured
  - The contents of the uterus spill into the peritoneal cavity or the broad ligament
- Bladder injury is not uncommon with uterine rupture
- A cesarean section is recommended in women who have had a prior rupture

## SIGNS AND SYMPTOMS

- Vaginal bleeding
- Abdominal pain and tenderness
- Chest pain, pain between the scapulae, or pain on inspiration
- Hypovolemic shock
- Signs associated with fetal oxygenation:
  - Late deceleration
  - Reduced variability
  - Tachycardia
  - Bradycardia
- Absent fetal heart sounds
- Cessation of uterine contractions
- Palpation of the fetus outside the uterus (usually occurs only with a large, complete rupture)

## RISK FACTORS

- History of uterine surgery
- Previous uterine rupture
- Uterine trauma
- Congenital uterine anomalies such as septate uterus or bicornuate uterus
- Vaginal birth after cesarean section
- Trauma
- Cocaine use
- Stretch uterus (multiples or too much amniotic fluid)
- A breech position requiring external cephalic version
- Prolonged labor

## COMPLICATIONS

| Maternal | Fetal |
|---|---|
| Major maternal blood loss | Intraventricular hemorrhage |
| A higher risk of coagulopathy | Seizures |
| Longer fetal exposure to hypoxia | Brain ischemia |
| Hysterectomy | Death |

# DIAGNOSIS

- Laboratory tests:
  - Hemoglobin or hematocrit
  - Coagulation tests (prothrombin time, activated partial thromboplastin time, fibrinogen, thromboelastogram)
- Ultrasound
  - To rule out placenta praevia, placental abruption, or spontaneous abortion
  - To support the diagnosis: abnormality in the uterine wall, a hematoma next to hysterotomy scar, free fluid in the peritoneum, anhydramnios or fetal parts outside the uterus

# MANAGEMENT

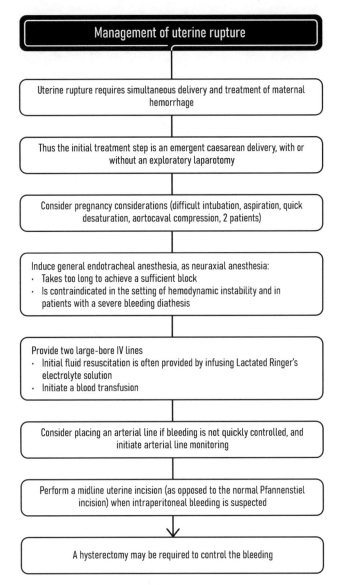

**Management of uterine rupture**

Uterine rupture requires simultaneous delivery and treatment of maternal hemorrhage

Thus the initial treatment step is an emergent caesarean delivery, with or without an exploratory laparotomy

Consider pregnancy considerations (difficult intubation, aspiration, quick desaturation, aortocaval compression, 2 patients)

Induce general endotracheal anesthesia, as neuraxial anesthesia:
- Takes too long to achieve a sufficient block
- Is contraindicated in the setting of hemodynamic instability and in patients with a severe bleeding diathesis

Provide two large-bore IV lines
- Initial fluid resuscitation is often provided by infusing Lactated Ringer's electrolyte solution
- Initiate a blood transfusion

Consider placing an arterial line if bleeding is not quickly controlled, and initiate arterial line monitoring

Perform a midline uterine incision (as opposed to the normal Pfannenstiel incision) when intraperitoneal bleeding is suspected

A hysterectomy may be required to control the bleeding

## SUGGESTED READING

- Gibbins KJ, Weber T, Holmgren CM, Porter TF, Varner MW, Manuck TA. Maternal and fetal morbidity associated with uterine rupture of the unscarred uterus. Am J Obstet Gynecol. 2015;213(3):382.e1-382.e3826.
- Guiliano M, Closset E, Therby D, LeGoueff F, Deruelle P, Subtil D. Signs, symptoms and complications of complete and partial uterine ruptures during pregnancy and delivery. Eur J Obstet Gynecol Reprod Biol. 2014;179:130-134.
- Plaat F, Shonfeld A. 2015. Major obstetric haemorrhage. BJA Education. 15;4:190-193.
- Walfish M, Neuman A, Wlody D. 2009. Maternal haemorrhage. BJA:: British Journal of Anaesthesia. 103;1:47-56.

# PEDIATRICS

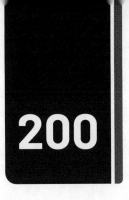

# BRONCHOPULMONARY DYSPLASIA

**200**

## LEARNING OBJECTIVES

- Describe bronchopulmonary dysplasia
- Understand the pathophysiology of bronchopulmonary dysplasia
- Recognize the risk factors for developing bronchopulmonary dysplasia
- Anesthetic management of a pediatric patient with bronchopulmonary dysplasia

## DEFINITION AND MECHANISM

- Bronchopulmonary dysplasia (BPD) is a chronic lung disease in preterm infants who require long-term oxygen because the alveoli that are present, are not mature enough to function properly
- Babies are not born with BPD, the condition results from damage to the lungs, usually caused by mechanical ventilation and long term use of oxygen at a higher concentration
- BPD is more common in infants with a low birth weight and those who receive prolonged mechanical ventilation to treat respiratory distress syndrome
- BPD develops most commonly in the first 4 weeks after birth

| Criteria for BPD diagnosis | |
| --- | --- |
| Infants requiring supplemental oxygen with $FiO_2$ > 0.21 and more than 28 days of life, are diagnosed via an assessment at 36 weeks postmenstrual age, as having: | |
| Mild BPD | Infant breathing room air |
| Moderate BPD | Infant requiring < 30% $FiO_2$ |
| Severe BPD | Infant requiring > 30% $FiO_2$ or positive pressure ventilation |

## SIGNS AND SYMPTOMS

- Hypoxemia
- Hypercapnia
- Crackles, wheezing, and decreased breath sounds
- Increased bronchial secretions
- Hyperinflation
- Feeding problems due to prolonged intubation (oral-tactile hypersensitivity/oral aversion)
- Need for continued oxygen therapy after the gestational age of 36 weeks
- Repeated lower respiratory infections that may require hospitalization
- Delayed growth and development

## CAUSES

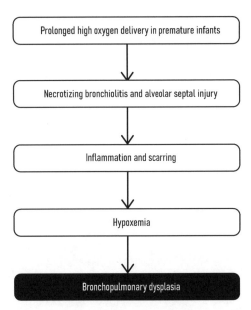

# RISK FACTORS

- Antenatal factors
  - Intrauterine growth restriction
  - Genetic predisposition
  - Maternal smoking
  - Chorioamnionitis
  - Pregnancy-induced hypertensive disorders
- Prematurity
- Postnatal factors
  - Mechanical ventilation
  - Sepsis
  - Oxygen toxicity
  - Patent ductus arteriosus

# COMPLICATIONS

- Airway disease and respiratory morbidity due to prolonged tracheal intubation and mechanical ventilation
  - Development of tracheomalacia and bronchomalacia
  - BPD spells: Acute cyanotic events caused by increases in central airway compliance
  - Subglottic stenosis
  - Airway granulomas
  - Pseudopolyps
  - Persistent airway obstruction and hyperreactivity
- Pulmonary hypertension
- Cor pulmonale

# PATHOPHYSIOLOGY

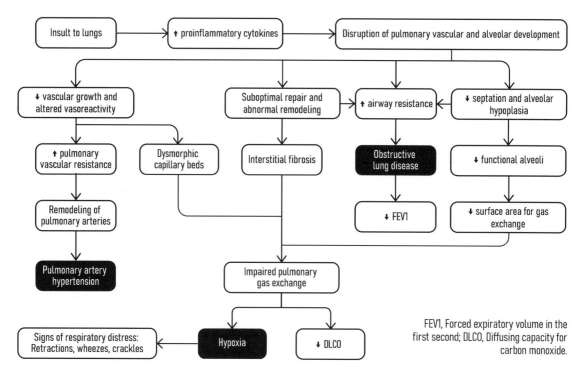

FEV1, Forced expiratory volume in the first second; DLCO, Diffusing capacity for carbon monoxide.

# TREATMENT

- There is no cure for BPD, treatment focuses on minimizing further lung damage and providing support for the infant's lungs
- Oxygen therapy
  - Nasal continuous positive airway pressure (NCPAP)
  - Bilevel positive airway pressure (BiPAP)
- Medications
  - **Diuretics:** Decrease fluid in and around the alveoli
  - **Bronchodilators:** Relax the muscles around the air passages, widening the airway openings and making breathing easier
  - **Corticosteroids:** Reduce and/or prevent inflammation within the lungs, reduce swelling in the trachea, and decrease the mucus production
  - **Viral immunization:** Prevent infection (i.e., respiratory syncytial virus)

Bronchopulmonary dysplasia

# MANAGEMENT

## BRONCHOPULMONARY DYSPLASIA

### Preoperative management

**PREANESTHETIC EVALUATION**
- Review medical history and perform a detailed physical examination to minimize the risk of perioperative respiratory and cardiac complications
  - **Preoperative history:** Prior anesthetic history, current medications, allergies, cough or sputum production, prior hospitalizations (including the need for tracheal intubation or IV infusions), and exercise tolerance
  - **Physical examination:** Assessment of vital signs, type of breath sounds, presence of wheezing or cough, use of accessory muscles, cyanosis, altered mental state, and hydration status
- Evaluate possibility of pulmonary hypertension and right ventricular dysfunction via ECG or echocardiography
- Oxygen should be made available for OR transport (BPD patients require long-term oxygen supplementation)
- Administer nebulized β2-adrenergic agonists 1-2 hours before anesthesia induction in patients with reactive airway disease and bronchospasm
- Several days of preoperative inhaled or oral steroid administration might be needed in patients with more severe airway disease
- Do not anesthetize BPD patients for elective surgery during an acute respiratory infection due to the high risk of bronchospasm → postpone surgery 4-6 weeks in case of active upper or lower respiratory tract infection
- Correct fluid and electrolyte imbalances due to chronic diuretic administration

**PREANESTHETIC PREPARATION**
- Oral midazolam (0.5-1 mg/kg) to reduce anxiety-induced acute bronchospasm → caution in children with pulmonary hypertension and upper airway disease
- Stress-dose steroid administration in children with a history of systemic corticosteroid use in the last 6 months

### Postoperative management

- Postoperative care needed depends on the severity of the disease, pulmonary hypertension, type of procedure, and opioid requirements
- Admit patients requiring mechanical ventilation or CPAP and further diuretic administration to the pediatric ICU

CPAP, continuous positive airway pressure

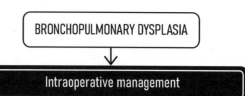

## Induction of anesthesia

| Intravenous induction | · Etomidate in patients with limited hemodynamic reserve<br>· Thiopental may induce bronchospasm and systemic hypotension<br>· Ketamine maintains arterial pressure and systemic vascular resistance while enhancing smooth muscle relaxation and bronchodilation → but associated with ↑ in pulmonary vascular resistance (PVR) and pulmonary artery pressure<br>· Propofol results in lower rates of wheezing after tracheal intubation than thiopental, agent of choice in hemodynamically stable patients with reactive airway disease |
|---|---|
| Inhalational induction | · Volatile anesthetics mitigate hypoxic pulmonary vasoconstriction → ↓ ventilation-perfusion mismatch<br>· Sevoflurane ↓ the incidence of laryngospasm and cardiac dysrhythmias, and has bronchodilating effects → agent of choice for mask induction<br>· Titrate volatile anesthetics in patients with pulmonary hypertension due to concerns for dose-dependent depression of cardiac contractility and reductions in systemic vascular resistance (SVR) |

## Anesthetic management

- **Goal:** Provide adequate anesthesia and analgesia while avoiding bronchospasm, ↑ in PVR, or ↓ in cardiac contractility
- Ventilatory settings for asthma (longer expiratory time, slow-normal respiratory rate)
- Maintain oxygen saturation > 90% to avoid pulmonary hypertension and cor pulmonale
- Hypercapnia is acceptable as long as the arterial pH > 7.25
- Consider laryngeal mask airway to avoid tracheal intubation (biggest risk factor for bronchospasm)
- Ensure a deep level of inhalation anesthesia before tracheal intubation to ↓ the risk of ↑ airway resistance and bronchospasm occurring with airway manipulation
- IV glycopyrrolate or atropine after induction can ↓ secretions and provide additional bronchodilation before tracheal intubation
- Use properly sized cuffed tracheal tubes for lower fresh gas flows, avoidance of multiple intubations for air leak, and more accurate $ETCO_2$ waveform tracings compared to uncuffed tracheal tubes
- Humify gases to prevent inspissation of dried secretions
- Suction the trachea only while the patient is deeply anesthetized
- Deep extubation to avoid the risk of bronchospasm from coughing on the tracheal tube → does not protect the airway from aspiration
- Treat and optimize any acute respiratory decompensation
- Avoid hypoxia, hypercapnia, acidosis, sympathetic surges, ↑ in airway pressures, and hypothermia to avoid ↑ in PVR and pulmonary hypertensive crisis
- Regional anesthesia avoids airway manipulation but may not be feasible for pediatric patients or for certain sites of surgery

## Neuromuscular blocking drugs

- Avoid histamine-releasing neuromuscular blocking drugs
- Use acetylcholinesterase inhibitors with caution due to the risk of muscarinic receptor activation and resultant bronchospasm

## PREVENTION

- Antenatal steroid administration
- Surfactant therapy
- Improved ventilator strategies to minimize lung injury

## KEEP IN MIND

- BPD is one of the most common pulmonary disorders encountered by pediatric anesthesiologists
- BPD, a common sequela of preterm birth, is associated with persistent airway disease and pulmonary hypertension
- Anesthetic effects might have life-threatening consequences in BPD patients (limited respiratory reserve)
  - Intraoperative bronchospasms or airway collapse → hypoxemia, acute pulmonary hypertension, right-sided heart failure, arrhythmias, and death
  - Effects on myocardial contractility can impair right ventricular function → reduction in cardiac output and cardiovascular compromise → cor pulmonale
- Respiratory infections (i.e., pneumonia) can further complicate the perioperative course

## SUGGESTED READING

- Lauer R, Vadi M, Mason L. Anaesthetic management of the child with co-existing pulmonary disease. BJA. 2012;109(1):i47-i59.
- Leslie V, Jivan K. Bronchopulmonary Dysplasia. In: Freeman BS, Berger JS. eds. Anesthesiology Core Review: Part Two Advanced Exam. McGraw-Hill Education; 2016.
- Schmidt AR, Ramamoorthy C. Bronchopulmonary dysplasia. Paediatr Anaesth. 2022;32(2):174-180.

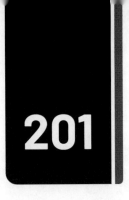

# CEREBRAL PALSY

## LEARNING OBJECTIVES

- Describe cerebral palsy
- Recognize the symptoms and signs of cerebral palsy
- Outline the anticipated challenges for airway management in patients with cerebral palsy
- Identify common intraoperative complications associated with cerebral palsy

## DEFINITION AND MECHANISM

- Cerebral palsy (CP) is a group of permanent neurodevelopmental disorders that affects an individual's muscle tone, motor functions, movement, and posture
- CP is attributed to non-progressive disturbances that occur in the developing fetal or infant brain
- CP is the most common motor disability in childhood

## SIGNS AND SYMPTOMS

- Signs and symptoms vary among patients
- CP can affect the whole body or might be limited primarily to one or two limbs, or one side of the body
- Symptoms get more noticeable over the first few years of life, but underlying problems do not worsen over time

### Movement and coordination

- Stiff muscles and exaggerated reflexes (spasticity)
- Variations in muscle tone (too stiff or floppy)
- Stiff muscles with normal reflexes (rigidity)
- Lack of balance and muscle coordination (ataxia)
- Tremors or jerky involuntary movements
- Favoring one side of the body (e.g., only reaching with one hand or dragging a leg while crawling)
- Difficulty walking (e.g., walking on toes, crouched gait, scissors-like gait with knees crossing, wide gait, or asymmetrical gait)
- Difficulty with fine motor skills

### Speech and eating

- Delays in speech development
- Difficulty speaking
- Difficulty with sucking, chewing, or eating
- Excessive drooling or problems with swallowing

### Development

- Delays in reaching motor skills milestones (babies with CP do not roll over, sit, crawl, or walk as early as other children of their age)
- Learning disability
- Intellectual disability
- Delayed growth (smaller size than expected)

### Other problems

- Epilepsy
- Difficulty hearing
- Problems with vision and abnormal eye movements
- Abnormal touch or pain sensations
- Bladder and bowel problems (e.g., constipation and urinary incontinence)
- Mental health conditions (e.g., emotional disorders and behavioral problems)

## RISK FACTORS

- Fetal pathogenic factors
  - Vascular maldevelopments
  - Congenital genetic/metabolic disorders
  - Microcephaly
  - Fetal trauma
  - Neonatal asphyxia in the peripartum period (6%)
  - Low birth weight (< 2.5 kg)
  - Prematurity (< 32 weeks)
  - Low Apgar score
  - Multiple births
  - Prenatal "TORCH" infections (toxoplasmosis, rubella, cytomegalovirus, and herpes)

- Maternal pathogenic factors
  - Breech presentation
  - Preeclampsia
  - Peripartum hemorrhage
  - Maternal hyperthyroidism
  - Fetal alcohol syndrome

**Acquired CP (20%) → develops during the first 2 years of life**
- Intracerebral hemorrhage
  - Viral encephalitis
  - Bacterial meningitis
  - Hyperbilirubinemia (kernicterus)
  - Head injury
  - Neonatal seizures

# COMPLICATIONS

Muscle weakness, muscle spasticity, and coordination problems may contribute to complications during childhood or adulthood
- **Contracture:** Muscle tissue shortening due to severe muscle tightening as a result of spasticity ➜ can inhibit bone growth, cause bones to bend, and result in joint deformities, dislocation, or partial dislocation (e.g., hip dislocation, scoliosis)
- **Malnutrition:** Swallowing or feeding problems limit the infant to get enough nutrition ➜ impaired growth and weakened bones
- **Mental health conditions:** Depression and behavioral problems
- **Cardiopulmonary disease**
  - Increased risk of aspiration pneumonitis and subsequent chronic lung scarring due to swallowing difficulties, esophageal dysmotility, abnormal lower esophageal sphincter tone, and spinal deformity ➜ gastroesophageal reflux disease (GERD)
  - Decreased immunity, poor nutrition, respiratory muscle hypotonia, and a weak cough in conjunction with GERD make patients more susceptible to recurrent chest infections, exacerbating the underlying chronic lung disease
  - Long-term truncal muscle spasticity can lead to scoliosis, restrictive lung defects, pulmonary hypertension, and ultimately cor pulmonale and respiratory failure
- **Osteoarthritis:** Pressure on joints or abnormal alignment of joints from muscle spasticity may lead to the early onset of osteoarthritis
- **Osteoporosis:** Fractures due to low bone density resulting from lack of mobility, inadequate nutrition, and anti-epileptic drug use
- **Other complications:** Sleep disorders, chronic pain, skin breakdown, intestinal problems, and issues with oral health

# PATHOPHYSIOLOGY

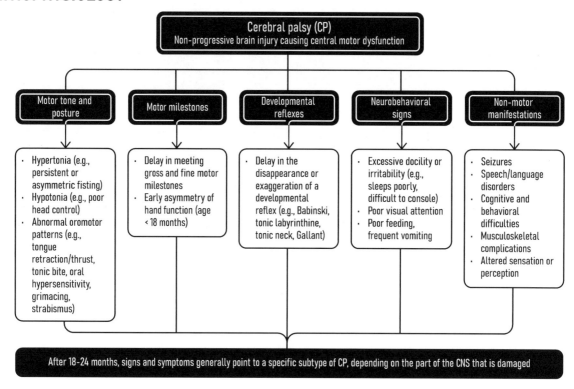

Cerebral palsy

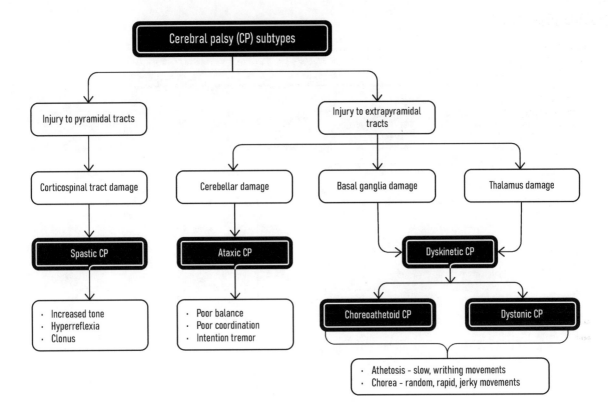

## TREATMENT

Treatment is focused on
- Improving posture and mobility by reducing spasticity, muscle spasms, and contractures
- Symptomatic relief of the associated medical problems (e.g., epilepsy, GERD, chest infections)

Combination therapies are more successful than single-treatment protocols: Physiotherapy, psychological counseling, occupational, speech, and behavioral therapy combined with
- Antispastic medications (e.g., baclofen)
- Neuromuscular denervation techniques (e.g., botulinum toxin injections, radiofrequency ablation of dorsal horn ganglia, and dorsal rhizotomy)
- Surgery (e.g., tenotomies, arthrodeses, osteotomies tendon transfer/lengthening, and multisegmental spinal fusion procedures)

# MANAGEMENT

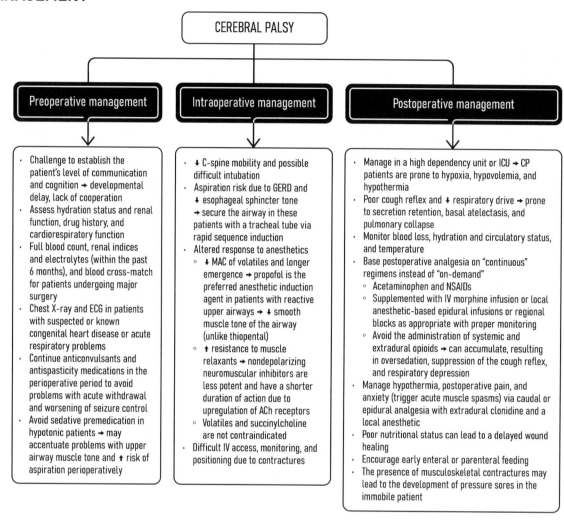

**CEREBRAL PALSY**

## Preoperative management

- Challenge to establish the patient's level of communication and cognition → developmental delay, lack of cooperation
- Assess hydration status and renal function, drug history, and cardiorespiratory function
- Full blood count, renal indices and electrolytes (within the past 6 months), and blood cross-match for patients undergoing major surgery
- Chest X-ray and ECG in patients with suspected or known congenital heart disease or acute respiratory problems
- Continue anticonvulsants and antispasticity medications in the perioperative period to avoid problems with acute withdrawal and worsening of seizure control
- Avoid sedative premedication in hypotonic patients → may accentuate problems with upper airway muscle tone and ↑ risk of aspiration perioperatively

## Intraoperative management

- ↓ C-spine mobility and possible difficult intubation
- Aspiration risk due to GERD and ↓ esophageal sphincter tone → secure the airway in these patients with a tracheal tube via rapid sequence induction
- Altered response to anesthetics
  ○ ↓ MAC of volatiles and longer emergence → propofol is the preferred anesthetic induction agent in patients with reactive upper airways → ↓ smooth muscle tone of the airway (unlike thiopental)
  ○ ↑ resistance to muscle relaxants → nondepolarizing neuromuscular inhibitors are less potent and have a shorter duration of action due to upregulation of ACh receptors
  ○ Volatiles and succinylcholine are not contraindicated
- Difficult IV access, monitoring, and positioning due to contractures

## Postoperative management

- Manage in a high dependency unit or ICU → CP patients are prone to hypoxia, hypovolemia, and hypothermia
- Poor cough reflex and ↓ respiratory drive → prone to secretion retention, basal atelectasis, and pulmonary collapse
- Monitor blood loss, hydration and circulatory status, and temperature
- Base postoperative analgesia on "continuous" regimens instead of "on-demand"
  ○ Acetaminophen and NSAIDs
  ○ Supplemented with IV morphine infusion or local anesthetic-based epidural infusions or regional blocks as appropriate with proper monitoring
  ○ Avoid the administration of systemic and extradural opioids → can accumulate, resulting in oversedation, suppression of the cough reflex, and respiratory depression
- Manage hypothermia, postoperative pain, and anxiety (trigger acute muscle spasms) via caudal or epidural analgesia with extradural clonidine and a local anesthetic
- Poor nutritional status can lead to a delayed wound healing
- Encourage early enteral or parenteral feeding
- The presence of musculoskeletal contractures may lead to the development of pressure sores in the immobile patient

GERD, gastroesophageal reflux disease; MAC, mean alveolar concentration; ACh, acetylcholine.

## KEEP IN MIND

- CP describes a spectrum of movement and posture disorders resulting from pathological injury to the developing fetal or infant brain
- Commonly associated comorbidities include dehydration, malnutrition, epilepsy, GERD, and impaired lung function
- Frequently encountered perioperative problems include difficulties with patient positioning and vascular access
- Regional analgesic techniques to reduce postoperative pain, muscle spasms, and respiratory complications are beneficial

## SUGGESTED READING

- GERD, gastroesophageal reflux disease; MAC, mean alveolar concentration; ACh, acetylcholine.
- Miller B, Rondeau B. Anesthetic Considerations In Patients With Cerebral Palsy. [Updated 2022 Jun 11]. In: StatPearls [Internet]. Treasure Island (FL): StatPearls Publishing; 2022 Jan. Available from: https://www.ncbi.nlm.nih.gov/books/NBK572057/
- Prosser DP, Sharma N. Cerebral palsy and anaesthesia. Continuing Education in Anaesthesia Critical Care & Pain. 2010;10(3):72-76.

Cerebral palsy

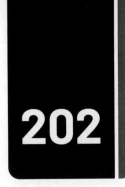

# CHARGE SYNDROME

## LEARNING OBJECTIVES

- Describe CHARGE syndrome
- Outline the major, minor, and occasional criteria to diagnose CHARGE syndrome
- Anesthetic management of a pediatric patient with CHARGE syndrome

## DEFINITION AND MECHANISM

- CHARGE syndrome is a rare genetic syndrome with a known pattern of features
  - **C: C**oloboma of the eye
  - **H: H**eart defects (e.g., most common tetralogy of Fallot, ventricular septal defect, atrioventricular canal defect, and aortic arch anomalies)
  - **A: A**tresia of the nasal choanae
  - **R: R**etardation of growth and development
  - **G: G**enital and/or urinary abnormalities (e.g., hypogonadism)
  - **E: E**ar abnormalities and deafness
- These features are no longer used in making the diagnosis

## DIAGNOSIS, SIGNS AND SYMPTOMS, AND COMPLICATIONS

- Individuals with all four major characteristics or three major and three minor characteristics are highly likely to have CHARGE syndrome

| Features of CHARGE syndrome | Later childhood/adolescent complications |
|---|---|
| **Major** | |
| Coloboma of the eye | Photophobia, retinal detachment, corneal abrasions |
| Choanal atresia/stenosis | Facial growth problems, recurrent closure and resurgeries, unilateral nasal discharge |
| Cranial nerve anomalies | Feeding/swallowing problems, gastroesophageal reflux, hiatus hernia |
| Abnormalities of the inner, middle, or external ear | Progressive hearing loss, chronic middle ear infections, vestibular problems affecting balance and/or motor skills |

| Minor | |
|---|---|
| Cardiovascular malformations: Tetralogy of Fallot, ventricular septal defect, atriventricular canal defect, and aortic arch anomalies | Arrhythmias, angina, further cardiac surgeries |
| Genital hypoplasia or delayed pubertal development: Micropenis and cryptorchidism (males), hypoplastic labia (females) | Pubertal delay, hormone replacement, fertility (unsure), hypogonadotrophic hypogonadism, osteoporosis |
| Cleft lip and/or palate | Cosmetic concerns, self-image |
| Tracheoesophageal defects: Tracheoesophageal fistula | Reflux esophagitis, feeding/swallowing problems |
| Distinctive CHARGE facies: Square face, broad forehead, arched eyebrows, large eyes, droopy eyelids, small mouth and chin, asymmetrical face) | Cosmetic concerns, self-image |
| Growth retardation: Short stature | Growth hormone replacement, obesity |
| Developmental delay: Delayed motor milestones, language delay, mental retardation | Educational, behavioral, social adjustment issues, autistic-like problems, obsessive compulsive disorders, ADHD |
| Occasional | |
| Renal anomalies: Duplex system, vesicoureteric reflux | Renal failure |
| Spinal anomalies: Scoliosis, osteoporosis | Scoliosis |
| Hand anomalies; Fifth finger clinodactyly, camptodactyly, and cutaneous syndactyly | Fine motor problems, cosmetic concern |
| Neck/shoulder anomalies: Sloping, Sprengel's deformity, kyphosis | Self-image problem |
| Immune system disorders | Recurrent infections |

## CAUSES

- A genetic mutation of the CHD7 gene on chromosome 8, autosomal dominant inheritance
- In rare cases, patients do not have a CHD7 mutation or have a mutation of another gene in their DNA

## TREATMENT

Treatment is unique per patient and focuses on improving symptoms
- Surgery to repair cleft lip or palate, cardiovascular problems, or atresia
- Occupational, physical, or speech therapy
- Feeding tube to help with swallowing
- Ventilator or CPAP to improve breathing difficulties or obstructive sleep apnea
- Hearing aids or implants to improve hearing loss
- Supportive education to improve cognitive development
- Medicine to treat specific symptoms

# MANAGEMENT

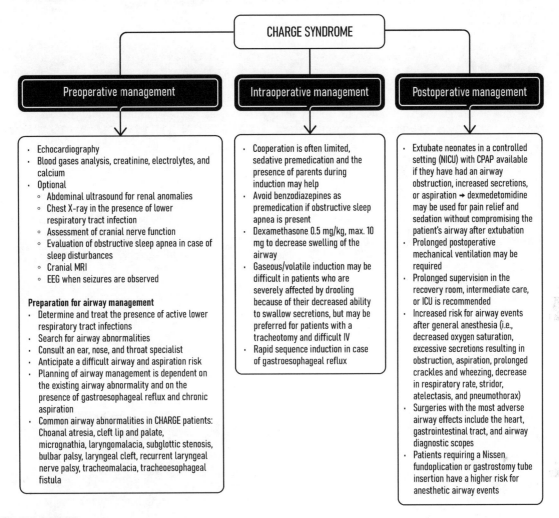

**CHARGE SYNDROME**

**Preoperative management**

- Echocardiography
- Blood gases analysis, creatinine, electrolytes, and calcium
- Optional
  - Abdominal ultrasound for renal anomalies
  - Chest X-ray in the presence of lower respiratory tract infection
  - Assessment of cranial nerve function
  - Evaluation of obstructive sleep apnea in case of sleep disturbances
  - Cranial MRI
  - EEG when seizures are observed

**Preparation for airway management**
- Determine and treat the presence of active lower respiratory tract infections
- Search for airway abnormalities
- Consult an ear, nose, and throat specialist
- Anticipate a difficult airway and aspiration risk
- Planning of airway management is dependent on the existing airway abnormality and on the presence of gastroesophageal reflux and chronic aspiration
- Common airway abnormalities in CHARGE patients: Choanal atresia, cleft lip and palate, micrognathia, laryngomalacia, subglottic stenosis, bulbar palsy, laryngeal cleft, recurrent laryngeal nerve palsy, tracheomalacia, tracheoesophageal fistula

**Intraoperative management**

- Cooperation is often limited, sedative premedication and the presence of parents during induction may help
- Avoid benzodiazepines as premedication if obstructive sleep apnea is present
- Dexamethasone 0.5 mg/kg, max. 10 mg to decrease swelling of the airway
- Gaseous/volatile induction may be difficult in patients who are severely affected by drooling because of their decreased ability to swallow secretions, but may be preferred for patients with a tracheotomy and difficult IV
- Rapid sequence induction in case of gastroesophageal reflux

**Postoperative management**

- Extubate neonates in a controlled setting (NICU) with CPAP available if they have had an airway obstruction, increased secretions, or aspiration → dexmedetomidine may be used for pain relief and sedation without compromising the patient's airway after extubation
- Prolonged postoperative mechanical ventilation may be required
- Prolonged supervision in the recovery room, intermediate care, or ICU is recommended
- Increased risk for airway events after general anesthesia (i.e., decreased oxygen saturation, excessive secretions resulting in obstruction, aspiration, prolonged crackles and wheezing, decrease in respiratory rate, stridor, atelectasis, and pneumothorax)
- Surgeries with the most adverse airway effects include the heart, gastrointestinal tract, and airway diagnostic scopes
- Patients requiring a Nissen fundoplication or gastrostomy tube insertion have a higher risk for anesthetic airway events

## KEEP IN MIND

- Have a formal cardiac evaluation for patients with choanal atresia
- The anesthetic management should ensure a calm, spontaneous breathing with a patent airway after the procedure
- Do not be surprised by difficult intubation and difficult mask ventilation

## SUGGESTED READING

- Blake KD, Prasad C. CHARGE syndrome. Orphanet J Rare Dis. 2006;1:34.
- Houck PJ. CHARGE SYNDROME. In: Houck PJ, Haché M, Sun LS. eds. Handbook of Pediatric Anesthesia. Mgraw Hill; 2015. Accessed February 03, 2023. https://accessanesthesiology.mhmedical.com/content.aspx?bookid=1189&sectionid=70364146

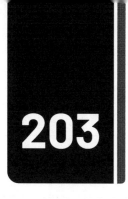

# CLEFT LIP AND PALATE

## LEARNING OBJECTIVES

- Describe cleft lip and palate
- Summarize the anticipated complications during the intraoperative and postoperative period among patients with cleft lip and palate
- Discuss the perioperative management of patients with orofacial clefts

## DEFINITION AND MECHANISM

- Orofacial clefts, encompassing cleft lip with or without cleft palate and cleft palate alone, are the most common craniofacial abnormalities
- They are birth defects and result from tissues of the face not joining properly during development
- These disorders affect the patient's feeding, speech, hearing, dental health, appearance, and psychological health
- **Cleft lip:** Fissure in the upper lip and may be incomplete or complete (through to the nasal cavity), unilateral, or bilateral
- **Cleft palate:** Gap in the soft palate that may or may not involve the hard palate, submucous (mildest form), incomplete or complete, unilateral or bilateral

| Chromosomal syndromes | Features |
|---|---|
| Velocardiofacial (DiGeorge) syndrome | Microcephaly and microstomia<br>Flat nasal bridge, small ears, short stature<br>Immune deficiency, congenital cardiac disease<br>Velopharyngeal incompetence with or without cleft palate<br>Laryngeal and tracheal anomalies<br>22q11 deletion (FISH test)<br>Cleft palate in 30% of cases |
| Trisomy 21 (Down syndrome) | Microstomia and relative macroglossia<br>Epicanthic folds, simian crease<br>Congenital cardiac disease<br>Atlantoaxial subluxation and instability |
| Monogenic syndromes | |
| Van der Woude syndrome | Lower lip pits<br>Hypodontia<br>Congenital cardiac disease<br>Musculoskeletal issues<br>Most common orofacial clefting syndrome |
| Treacher-Collins syndrome | Micrognathia and maxillary hypoplasia<br>Choanal atresia<br>Eye and ear malformations<br>Intubation may become more difficult with age<br>Cleft palate in 30% of cases |
| Hemifacial microsomia (Goldenhar syndrome) | Hemifacial and mandibular hypoplasia<br>Cervical spine abnormalities<br>Ear and eye abnormalities<br>Intubation may become more difficult with age |
| Stickler syndrome | Progressive connective tissue disorder (autosomal dominant)<br>Midface hypoplasia<br>Micrognathia/Pierre Robin sequence<br>Retinal detachment and early cataracts<br>Deafness<br>Hypermobility of joints |

Common syndromes associated with cleft lip and palate

| Sequence | |
|---|---|
| Pierre-Robin sequence (PRS) | Micrognathia<br>Glossoptosis<br>Underlying syndrome/anomalies<br>Usually easier to intubate with age<br>Cleft palate in 80% of cases |

## SIGNS AND SYMPTOMS

Opening in the upper lip that may extend into the nose or palate

**Cleft lip**
- Cleft does not affect the palate structure of the mouth
- Partial or incomplete cleft lip: Formed in the top of the lip as a small gap or indentation of the lip
- Complete cleft lip: Cleft continues into the nose
- Can occur as a one-sided (unilateral) or two-sided (bilateral) condition
- Due to failure of the fusion of the maxillary prominence and medial nasal processes (formation of the primary palate)

**Cleft palate**
- The two plates of the skull that form the roof of the mouth are not completely joined
- Cleft lip is also present in most cases
- Complete cleft palate: Soft and hard palate, possibly including a gap in the mandible
- Incomplete cleft palate: A hole in the roof of the mouth, usually as a cleft soft palate
- Submucous cleft palate: Mildest form with no visible cleft but a failure of the palatal muscles to unite
- The uvula is usually split
- Due to failure of the fusion of the lateral palatine processes, nasal septum, or median palatine processes (formation of the secondary palate)
- The hole in the roof of the mouth connects the mouth directly to the inside of the nose, resulting in velopharyngeal insufficiency (VPI) → hypernasal speech, nasal emission, and nasal turbulence

## CAUSES

- Most clefts are polygenic and multifactorial in origin with many genetic and environmental factors contributing
- Genetic factors cause clefts in 20% to 50% of the cases
- The remaining clefts are attributable to either environmental factors (e.g., teratogens) or gene-environment interactions

## RISK FACTORS

- Smoking during pregnancy
- Diabetes
- Obesity
- Advanced maternal age
- Certain medications (i.e., some used to treat seizures)

## COMPLICATIONS

- Feeding problems
- Speech problems
- Hearing problems
- Frequent ear infections

Cleft lip and palate

# PATHOPHYSIOLOGY

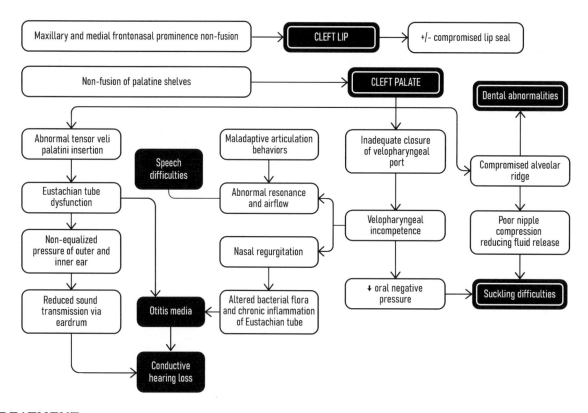

# TREATMENT

- Speech therapy: Improve velopharyngeal function and develop normal speech without compensatory articulations
- Dental care
- Corrective surgery
  - Cleft lip: 8-12 weeks
  - Cleft palate: 6-12 months (dependent upon the size of the cleft)

# MANAGEMENT

| Considerations for anesthesia for cleft lip and palate surgery | |
| --- | --- |
| Patient-related factors | Usually infants or young pediatric patients<br>Associated comorbidities and syndromes<br>Nutritional status<br>Airway obstruction<br>Potential difficult airway |
| Anesthetic factors | General anesthesia with tracheal tube<br>Shared airway |
| Surgical factors | Elective surgery (time to optimize) |

## CLEFT LIP AND PALATE

### Preoperative management

**PREOPERATIVE ASSESSMENT**
- Identify any signs of congenital heart disease (15% of patients), upper respiratory tract infection (URTI), obstructive sleep apnea (OSA), renal disorders, neuromuscular disorders, dehydration, or malnutrition
- Assess the airway → URTI increases the risk of airway complications and compromises wound healing
- Exclude other associated conditions
- Delay surgery in patients with multiple comorbities until their health is optimized
- Routine laboratory investigations are not required

**PREMEDICATION**
- Usually unnecessary; consider sedative premedication in patients with separation anxiety
- Avoid opiod or sedative premedication in children < 6 months or if airway is compromised
- Preoperative analgesia (e.g., 15-20 mg/kg acetaminophen PO) is recommended
- Give atropine 20 mcg/kg if a difficult airway is anticipated

**MONITORING**
- ECG - Noninvasive blood pressure
- $SpO_2$ - $EtCO_2$ and inhalational agent
- Nerve stimulator
- Core temperature
- Fluid balance
- Blood loss

### Postoperative management

- Monitor patients in the PACU with supplementary oxygen until fully awake and settled, often in the lateral or semi-prone position to allow drainage of secretions
- Extubate only when the patient is fully awake, breathing adequately and in tonsillar position → smooth pain-free emergence reduces crying and the risk of postoperative bleeding
- Main concerns during emergency are airway obstruction, bleeding, and disruption of the suture lines
- Postoperative airway complications
  - Laryngospasm
  - Edema/obstruction (surgery makes airway management more difficult)
- Postoperative analgesia
  - IV acetaminophen, NSAIDs (if not already given), and opiods (e.g., 20 mcg/kg morphine) with appropriate monitoring
  - Ketamine may be useful as a non-respiratory depressant analgesic in the early stages of postoperative management
- A nasopharyngeal airway or stent may be required in certain patients
- Close monitoring for the first 12-24 hours after palate surgery to identify potential airway obstruction, bleeding, or both
- Cleft lip patients may stay overnight and are disharged the next day, while cleft palate patients are usually discharged between day 1 and 3 after surgery
- Main determinant of discharge: Ensure patients are feeding well
- Oral medications for analgesia at home: Acetaminophen, ibuprofen, and morphine

## CLEFT LIP AND PALATE

### Intraoperative management

**INDUCTION OF ANESTHESIA**
- Inhalational or intravenous induction
  - Suspected airway problem: Sevoflurane in 100% oxygen
  - Use of CPAP will assist the maintenance of the airway
- Potential difficult airway (especially bag mask ventilation)
  - Careful airway plan required
  - Ensure direct laryngoscope does not enter the cleft
- Intubate deep with child breathing spontaneously or after a muscle relaxant once a safe airway is established
- Ideal airway device for cleft repair, allowing for optimal surgical access, is a preformed RAE tracheal tube, inserted orally and secured in the midline below the lower lip
  - Avoid endobronchial intubation by careful placement of the tip, visually at intubation and with auscultation of the chest
  - If the tube protrudes too far from the bottom lip, use padding (e.g., dental rolls of gauze) to build a platform that the tube can be secured to → reduce the risk of inadvertent advancement of the tip
  - Midline positioning → secure the tube so that it does not distort the tissues
- Throat pack

**MAINTENANCE OF ANESTHESIA**
- Controlled ventilation is appropriate, using volatile anesthetics or TIVA techniques
- IV fentanyl (1-2 mcg/kg) can supplement anesthesia but should be given with caution in neonates or in the presence of upper airway problems
- Addition of remifentanil reduces volatile and propofol anesthetic requirements → may allow controlled ventilation throughout, promoting a smooth, rapid emergence
- Use of muscle relaxation allows perfectly controlled ventilation, which may reduce blood loss secondary to tighter control of $PaCO_2$
- Local infiltration produces good analgesia, improved operating field, and reduced blood loss
- Regional anesthesia: Infraorbital nerve block for cleft lip repair or nasopalatine and palatine block for cleft palate surgery is effective

CPAP, continuous positive airway pressure; RAE, Ring, Adair & Elwyn; TIVA, total intravenous anesthesia.

Cleft lip and palate

## KEEP IN MIND

- Orofacial clefts are the most common craniofacial abnormality and patients with clefts require specialized multidisciplinary care from infancy through adulthood
- Assess patients appropriately in the preoperative period as cleft anomalies are associated with numerous congenital abnormalities
- Management of the airway may be challenging because of a difficult, shared airway, and postoperative airway obstruction
- Monitor patients for signs of airway obstruction throughout their recovery from anesthesia
- A multimodal approach to analgesia is important to provide optimal conditions for recovery

SUGGESTED READING

- Almeida-Chen GM. CLEFT LIP AND PALATE REPAIR. In: Houck PJ, Haché M, Sun LS. eds. Handbook of Pediatric Anesthesia. McGraw-Hill Education; 2015.
- Denning S, Ng E, Wong Riff KWY. Anaesthesia for cleft lip and palate surgery. BJA Education. 2021; 21(10): 384-389.

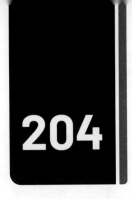

# CONGENITAL DIAPHRAGMATIC HERNIA

## LEARNING OBJECTIVES

- Describe congenital diaphragmatic hernia
- Understand the predictors for survival in congenital diaphragmatic hernia
- Management of congenital diaphragmatic hernia

## DEFINITION AND MECHANISM

- Congenital diaphragmatic hernia (CDH) is a birth defect characterized by the development of a hole in the diaphragm, leading to the protrusion of abdominal contents into the thoracic cavity affecting the normal development of the lungs
- 90% is left-sided
- Infants born with CDH experience respiratory failure due to pulmonary hypertension and pulmonary hypoplasia (decreased lung volume)
- Newborns born with CDH require immediate care at delivery → delivery should be as close to term as possible
- CDH is a life-threatening condition → death occurs due to:
  - Inadequate gas exchange surface
  - Fixed high pulmonary vascular resistance (decreased vascular cross-sectional area, normal cardiac output)
  - Reversible pulmonary hypertension
  - Pneumothorax
  - Additional anomalies (5%) and complications of intensive therapy

## DIAGNOSIS AND SURVIVAL

- CDH is usually discovered during a routine prenatal ultrasound
- The stomach, intestines, or liver may be present in the fetus' chest where the lungs should be; the fetus' heart may also be pushed to one side by the extra organs in the chest

**Antenatal ultrasound predictors of survival in CDH**
- Calculate the **lung-to-head ratio** (LHR) by dividing the fetal lung area (mm$^2$) by the fetal head circumference (mm)
  - LHR > 1.35: 100% survival
  - LHR 1.35 to 0.6: 61% survival
  - LHR < 0.6: No survival
- Calculate the **observed to expected LHR** (O/E LHR) by dividing the observed LHR by the expected ratio for gestational age
  - The fetal lung area increases 16-fold compared to a 4-fold increase in the head circumference between 12 and 32 weeks of gestation
  - O/E LHR < 25%: Severe CDH (survival 10% with liver up and 25% with liver down)
  - O/E LHR < 15% with liver up: No survival
- Position of the **liver** (or presence of liver herniation)
  - Liver herniation with LHR < 1.0: 40% survival
  - Liver in the thorax: 56% survival

## ANESTHETIC CONSIDERATIONS

- Emergency situation
- Critically ill neonate
- Hypoplastic lungs
  - Respiratory insufficiency (hypoxemia, hypercarbia, acidosis)
  - Permissive hypercarbia may be required
  - Consider HVO or ECMO
- Pulmonary hypertension
  - Potential for right ventricle failure, reduced cardiac output
  - Consider inhaled NO
- Transitional circulation
  - Potential for right-left and left-right shunting
  - Patent ductus arteriosus
- Delayed surgical repair, resuscitation is first priority
- NICU required

# MANAGEMENT

## *Resuscitation*

- Call NICU
- Indication for immediate tracheal intubation to facilitate intermittent positive pressure ventilation (IPPV)
- No bag-mask ventilation → distends herniated viscera, worsens mediastinal shift, and increases the risk of pneumothorax; while barotrauma further damages the hypoplastic lungs
- Nasal intubation helps with fixation and ventilator compliance
- Pass a nasogastric tube to deflate the gut and keep on free drainage
- Umbilical artery/vein lines
- Arterial blood gas, chest X-ray, echocardiogram
- Lung protective ventilation
  - Target $SaO_2$ > 85% and permissive hypercapnia ($PaCO_2$ < 65 mmHg, pH > 7.25)
  - PCV or PSV PIP < 25 cmH$_2$O
  - Inspiratory time 0.35 sec
  - PEEP 3-5 mmHg
  - RR < 65
  - Consider HVO, iNO, or ECMO
- Consider NO and inotropes for pulmonary hypertension
- Fluid: Target MAP 45-50 mmHg
- Sedation: Opioids and benzodiazepines, thoracic epidural
- Avoid neuromuscular blocking drugs

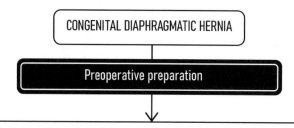

CONGENITAL DIAPHRAGMATIC HERNIA

Preoperative preparation

- Surgery worsens lung mechanics and is not an emergency
- Stabilize and improve gas exchange by medical management before surgery to avoid triggers for pulmonary vasoconstriction (hypoxia, hypercarbia, acidosis)
- Allow the normal physiological fall in pulmonary vascular resistance to occur

**Monitoring**
- Peripheral arterial cannulation for arterial pressure and blood gas monitoring with minimal disturbance
- Place pulse oximeters pre- and postductally to demonstrate the variability of shunting

**Ventilation**
- Risk of pneumothorax from high inflation pressures and asynchrony
- Muscle relaxants (e.g., atracurium or cisatracurium) by infusion give optimal control and decrease oxygen consumption → continue until weaning after surgery
- Gentle ventilation strategies (peak airway pressure < 25 mmHg) reduce barotrauma
- No firm evidence for benefits from individual treatment modalities (e.g., surfactant, HFOV, iNO, ECMO)

**Acid-base status**
- Correct metabolic acidosis with buffers
- Moderate alkalosis by systemic alkalinization (to pH 7.5-7.6) or hyperventilation (to $PaCO_2$ 30-35 mmHg) may enhance pulmonary circulation

**Pulmonary circulation**
- Echocardiography to estimate the severity of pulmonary hypertension
- Refractory hypoxemia may respond to pulmonary vasodilators (NO)

**Fluid balance**
- Preoperative restriction (6 mL/kg per 24 hours) avoids fluid retention
- Initial maintenance fluid should contain 5-10% glucose
- Switch to parenteral nutrition at 48 hours
- Maintain circulating blood volume with plasma or blood (maintain Hb > 14 g/dL)

**Sedation**
- A narcotic infusion (e.g., morphine) may help with lability in response to handling

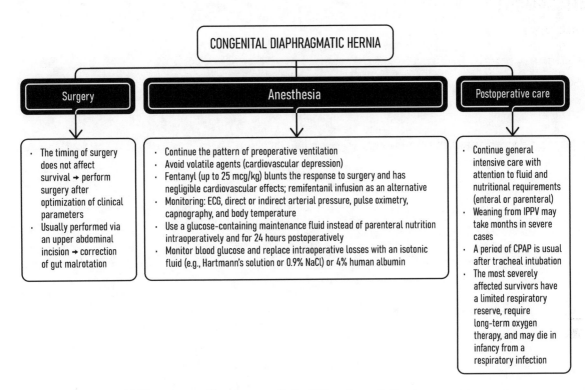

**CONGENITAL DIAPHRAGMATIC HERNIA**

**Surgery**

- The timing of surgery does not affect survival → perform surgery after optimization of clinical parameters
- Usually performed via an upper abdominal incision → correction of gut malrotation

**Anesthesia**

- Continue the pattern of preoperative ventilation
- Avoid volatile agents (cardiovascular depression)
- Fentanyl (up to 25 mcg/kg) blunts the response to surgery and has negligible cardiovascular effects; remifentanil infusion as an alternative
- Monitoring: ECG, direct or indirect arterial pressure, pulse oximetry, capnography, and body temperature
- Use a glucose-containing maintenance fluid instead of parenteral nutrition intraoperatively and for 24 hours postoperatively
- Monitor blood glucose and replace intraoperative losses with an isotonic fluid (e.g., Hartmann's solution or 0.9% NaCl) or 4% human albumin

**Postoperative care**

- Continue general intensive care with attention to fluid and nutritional requirements (enteral or parenteral)
- Weaning from IPPV may take months in severe cases
- A period of CPAP is usual after tracheal intubation
- The most severely affected survivors have a limited respiratory reserve, require long-term oxygen therapy, and may die in infancy from a respiratory infection

IPPV, Intermittent positive-pressure ventilation; CPAP, continuous positive airway pressure.

## KEEP IN MIND

- Immediate management at birth includes bowel decompression, avoidance of mask ventilation, and endotracheal tube placement if required
- The main focus of management includes gentle ventilation, hemodynamic monitoring, and treatment of pulmonary hypertension, followed by surgery

**SUGGESTED READING**

- Chandrasekharan PK, Rawat M, Madappa R, Rothstein DH, Lakshminrusimha S. Congenital Diaphragmatic hernia – a review. Matern Health Neonatol Perinatol. 2017;3:6.
- Leininger K, Chiu K. Anesthetic Considerations In Congenital Diaphragmatic Hernia. [Updated 2022 Nov 15]. In: StatPearls [Internet]. Treasure Island (FL): StatPearls Publishing; 2022 Jan. Available from: https://www.ncbi.nlm.nih.gov/books/NBK572077/
- Pollard BJ, Kitchen G. Handbook of Clinical Anaesthesia. 4th ed. Taylor & Francis group; 2018. Chapter 24 Paediatrics, Lomas B.

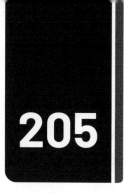

# CRANIOFACIAL DYSOSTOSIS

## 205

## LEARNING OBJECTIVES

- Definition and examples of craniofacial dysostosis
- Perioperative management of craniofacial dysostosis

## DEFINITION AND MECHANISM

- Craniofacial dysostosis or craniosynostosis is a condition in which premature fusion of one or more of the cranial sutures occurs, leading to abnormal skull development and head shape
- Abnormal premature fusion of one or several of these sutures results in restricted growth of the skull perpendicular to the affected suture
- Compensatory bone growth occurs parallel to the affected suture in order to allow for continued brain growth and results in distinct clinical skull characteristics
- Children may present with a broad range of conditions requiring correction, from otherwise well children with single suture craniosynostosis (80% of cases) to syndromic children with multiple synostoses with other cranial and extracranial anomalies
- Syndromes most frequently associated with craniosynostosis include:
  - Crouzon syndrome:
    - The most common craniofacial dysostosis syndrome
  - Apert syndrome:
    - Is similar to Crouzon syndrome but is more severe
    - Craniofacial characteristics of Crouzon syndrome and syndactyly (webbing of finger and toe) in addition
    - Intellectual disability is also more common in Apert syndrome
  - Pfeiffer syndrome:
    - Craniofacial characteristics and hand and feet abnormalities are also present (wide and deviated thumbs or big toes)
    - Mental and neurological problems are more likely
- Caused by an inherited or spontaneous autosomal dominant mutation in the fibroblast growth factor receptor 2 (FGFR2) located on chromosome 10
- Incidence is 1 in 2500 live births
- Correction may require extensive surgery that is commonly performed at a young age

## SIGNS AND SYMPTOMS

- Wide-set eyes (hypertelorism)
- Bulging eyeballs (proptosis)
- Crossed eyes (strabismus)
- Protruding forehead
- Small, beak-shaped nose
- Underdeveloped jaw
- Cleft lip and/or palate
- Abnormal head shape
- Insufficient growth of the midface

## COMPLICATIONS

- Vision problems
- Dental problems
- Hearing loss
- Breathing problems
- Hydrocephalus
- Rarely, intellectual disability

## DIAGNOSIS

- Physical appearance
- MRI/CT
- Genetic testing

## TREATMENT

- Surgical reconstruction (LeFort osteotomies) to prevent the closure of sutures of the skull from damaging the brain's development

# MANAGEMENT

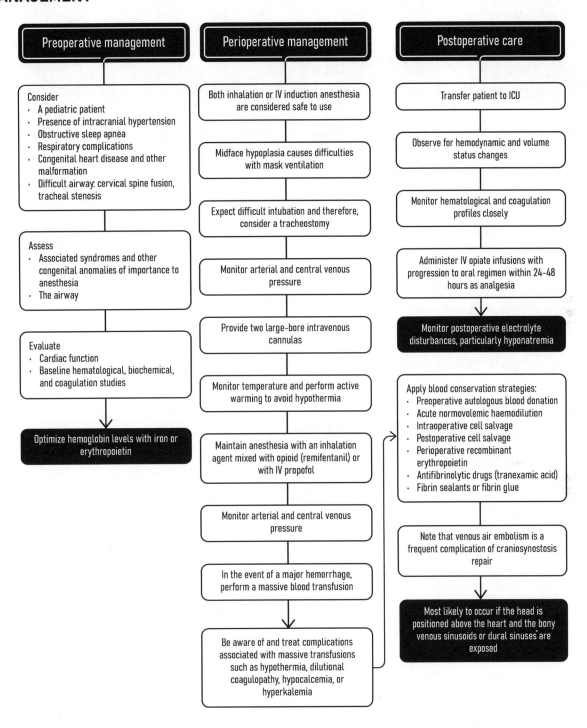

**Preoperative management**

Consider
- A pediatric patient
- Presence of intracranial hypertension
- Obstructive sleep apnea
- Respiratory complications
- Congenital heart disease and other malformation
- Difficult airway: cervical spine fusion, tracheal stenosis

Assess
- Associated syndromes and other congenital anomalies of importance to anesthesia
- The airway

Evaluate
- Cardiac function
- Baseline hematological, biochemical, and coagulation studies

Optimize hemoglobin levels with iron or erythropoietin

**Perioperative management**

Both inhalation or IV induction anesthesia are considered safe to use

Midface hypoplasia causes difficulties with mask ventilation

Expect difficult intubation and therefore, consider a tracheostomy

Monitor arterial and central venous pressure

Provide two large-bore intravenous cannulas

Monitor temperature and perform active warming to avoid hypothermia

Maintain anesthesia with an inhalation agent mixed with opioid (remifentanil) or with IV propofol

Monitor arterial and central venous pressure

In the event of a major hemorrhage, perform a massive blood transfusion

Be aware of and treat complications associated with massive transfusions such as hypothermia, dilutional coagulopathy, hypocalcemia, or hyperkalemia

**Postoperative care**

Transfer patient to ICU

Observe for hemodynamic and volume status changes

Monitor hematological and coagulation profiles closely

Administer IV opiate infusions with progression to oral regimen within 24-48 hours as analgesia

Monitor postoperative electrolyte disturbances, particularly hyponatremia

Apply blood conservation strategies:
- Preoperative autologous blood donation
- Acute normovolemic haemodilution
- Intraoperative cell salvage
- Postoperative cell salvage
- Perioperative recombinant erythropoietin
- Antifibrinolytic drugs (tranexamic acid)
- Fibrin sealants or fibrin glue

Note that venous air embolism is a frequent complication of craniosynostosis repair

Most likely to occur if the head is positioned above the heart and the bony venous sinusoids or dural sinuses are exposed

## SUGGESTED READING

- Pearson, A., Matava, C.T., 2016. Anaesthetic management for craniosynostosis repair in children. BJA Education 16, 410–416.
- Pollard BJ, Kitchen, G. Handbook of Clinical Anaesthesia. Fourth Edition. CRC Press. 2018. 978-1-4987-6289-2.
- Posnick JC, Ruiz RL. The craniofacial dysostosis syndromes: current surgical thinking and future directions. Cleft Palate Craniofac J. 2000;37(5):433.

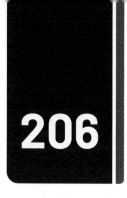

# CROUP/ LARYNGOTRACHEOBRONCHITIS

## LEARNING OBJECTIVES

- Describe the pathophysiology and symptoms of croup
- Diagnose croup and assess its severity
- Manage patients presenting with croup

## DEFINITION AND MECHANISM

- Laryngotracheobronchitis or croup refers to inflammation of the larynx, trachea, and bronchi
- Common cause of cough, stridor, and hoarseness in children with a fever
- Most children experiencing croup recover without complications
- Rarely, croup can be lethal to infants
- Most often caused by a viral infection (parainfluenza, RSV, rhinovirus, enterovirus, influenza, adenovirus)
- More common in boys compared to girls

## PATHOPHYSIOLOGY

- Inhalation of virus infecting nasal and pharyngeal mucosal epithelia, further spreading to the subglottic space
- In children, the subglottic space is the most narrow part of the airway
- The inability of the cricoid to expand causes significant narrowing of the subglottic region secondary to the inflamed mucosa
- When the patient cries or becomes agitated, further dynamic obstruction can occur

## SIGNS & SYMPTOMS

- Usually history of 1-3 days of rhinorrhea, nasal congestion, and fever
- Barking or seal-like cough
- Hoarse voice
- High-pitched inspiratory stridor
- Wheezing
- Crackles

- Air trapping
- Tachypnea
- Cyanosis
- Hypoxia requiring oxygenation
- Suprasternal, subcostal, and intercostal recessions

## DIAGNOSIS

- Mostly clinical diagnosis
- Abrupt onset of a barking cough, stridor, and hoarseness
- Often dyspnea and fever
- Overt inspiratory stridor in the neck on auscultation
- Steeple sign on radiography (usually not necessary)
- Laboratory studies are rarely needed

# DIFFERENTIAL DIAGNOSIS

| Condition | Typical age range | Clinical presentation | Diagnostic tests |
|---|---|---|---|
| Croup | 6 months to 3 years | Acute onset of barking cough, stridor, and hoarseness | None required |
| Bacterial tracheitis | < 6 years | High fever, barking cough, respiratory distress, and rapid deterioration | Neck radiography (irregular tracheal mucosa) and complete blood count |
| Epiglottitis | 3 to 12 years | Acute onset of dysphagia, odynophagia, drooling, high fever, anxiety, and muffled voice | Neck radiography (thickened epiglottis) and complete blood count |
| Foreign body aspiration | < 3 years | Acute onset of choking and/or drooling | Neck and chest radiography to see the location of foreign body and its impact |
| Hemangioma | < 6 months | Stridor worse with crying | Airway endoscopy |
| Large airway lesions (subglottic stenosis, laryngeal cleft, tracheomalacia, laryngomalacia) | < 6 months to 4.5 years | Recurrent episodes of barking cough and stridor | Airway endoscopy |
| Neoplasm | No age predilection | Progressive airway symptoms | Lateral neck radiography and CT |
| Peritonsillar abscess | 6 months to 3.5 years | Sore throat, fever, "hot potato" voice | Neck radiography, neck CT, and complete blood count |
| Retropharyngeal abscess | 2 to 4 years | Fever, drooling, dysphagia, odynophagia, and neck pain | Neck radiography (bulging posterior pharyngeal wall), neck CT, and complete blood count |
| Thermal injury/smoke inhalation | No age predilection | Exposure to heat, smoke, or chemical | Direct laryngoscopy |

## SEVERITY SCORING

- Westley Croup Score:

Total score:
- ≤ 2: Mild
- 3 – 7: Moderate
- 8 – 11: Severe
- ≥ 12: Impending respiratory failure

| Clinical sign | | Score |
|---|---|---|
| Level of consciousness | Normal (including sleep) | 0 |
| | Disoriented | 5 |
| Cyanosis | None | 0 |
| | With agitation | 4 |
| | At rest | 5 |
| Stridor | None | 0 |
| | When agitated | 1 |
| | At rest | 2 |
| Air entry | Normal | 0 |
| | Decreased | 1 |

# COMPLICATIONS

- Hospitalization
- Secondary bacterial infection
- Pneumothorax

- Otitis media
- Dehydration
- Lymphadenitis

# MANAGEMENT

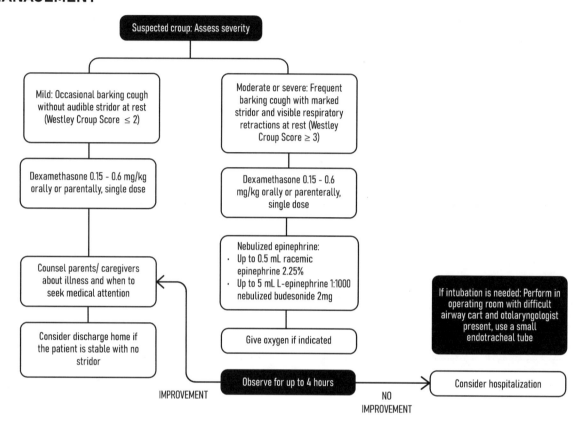

## SUGGESTED READING

- Ernest S, Khandhar PB. Laryngotracheobronchitis. [Updated 2022 Jun 27]. In: StatPearls [Internet]. Treasure Island (FL): StatPearls Publishing; 2022 Jan-. Available from: https://www.ncbi.nlm.nih.gov/books/NBK519531/
- Maloney E, Meakin GH. Acute stridor in children. Continuing Education in Anaesthesia Critical Care & Pain. 2007;7(6):183-6.
- Smith DK, McDermott AJ, Sullivan JF. Croup: Diagnosis and Management. Am Fam Physician. 2018;97(9):575-580.

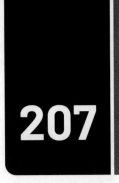

# DIGEORGE SYNDROME

## 207

## LEARNING OBJECTIVES

- Define DiGeorge syndrome
- Describe the signs, symptoms, and complications associated with DiGeorge syndrome
- Anesthetic management of a patient with DiGeorge syndrome

## DEFINITION AND MECHANISM

- DiGeorge syndrome, or 22q11.2 deletion syndrome, is a syndrome caused by a heterozygous microdeletion on the long arm of chromosome 22
- This deletion results in poor development of several body systems
- 90% of cases occur due to a new mutation during early development, while 10% are inherited (autosomal dominant)

- Memory aid: CATCH-22
- **C**yanotic congenital heart defect
- **A**bnormal facies
- **T**hymic aplasia or hypoplasia
- **C**ognitive impairment, cleft palate
- **H**ypoparathyroidism, hypocalcemia
- **22**q11.2 deletion

## SIGNS, SYMPTOMS, AND COMPLICATIONS

- Congenital heart disease (40%): Particularly conotruncal malformations (e.g., interrupted aortic arch, persistent truncus arteriosus, tetralogy of Fallot, and ventricular septal defect)
- Cyanosis
- Palatal abnormalities (50%): Velopharyngeal incompetence, submucosal cleft palate, and cleft palate with or without cleft lip
- Characteristic facial features (including hypertelorism): Underdeveloped chin (micrognathia and retrognathia), low-set ears, wide-set eyes, or a narrow groove in the upper lip
- Frequent infections due to thymic aplasia or hypoplasia
- Developmental delay
- Learning difficulties (90%) including cognitive deficits, attention deficit disorders
- Hypocalcemia (50%) due to hypoparathyroidism
- Significant feeding problems (30%), gastroesophageal reflux disease (GERD), and failure to thrive
- Renal anomalies (37%)
- Hearing loss
- Laryngotracheoesophageal anomalies
- Growth hormone deficiency
- Autoimmune disorders (e.g., rheumatoid arthritis or Graves disease)
- Immune disorders due to reduced T-cell numbers
- Seizures (with or without hypocalcemia)
- Skeletal abnormalities (e.g., scoliosis)
- Psychiatric disorders and behavioral problems (e.g., schizophrenia develops in 25-30% by adulthood, ADHD, autism spectrum disorder)

# PATHOPHYSIOLOGY

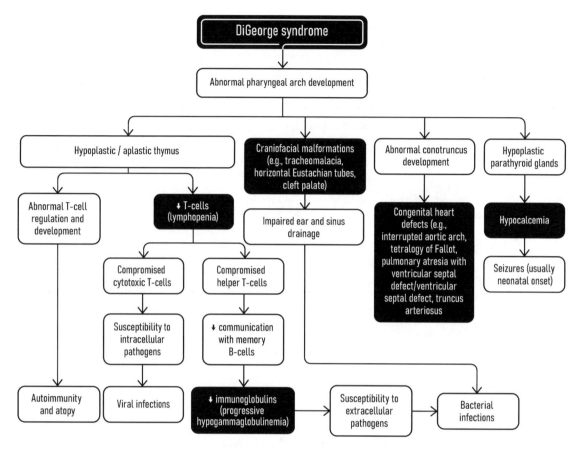

# TREATMENT

There is no cure for DiGeorge syndrome, but certain individual features are treatable using standard treatments
- **Hypoparathyroidism:** Calcium and vitamin D supplements
- **Congenital heart defects:** Surgical repair soon after birth to repair the defect and improve the supply of oxygen-rich blood
- **Limited thymus gland function:** Infections (e.g., colds and ear infections) are generally treated as they would be in any child; normal schedule of vaccines
- **Severe thymus gland function:** Transplant of thymus tissue, specialized bone marrow, or specialized disease-fighting blood cells
- **Cleft palate:** Surgical repair
- **Overall development:** Speech therapy, occupational therapy, and developmental therapy

# ANESTHESIA CONSIDERATIONS

- Airway
  - Difficult airway
    - Small mouth opening, retrognathia, micrognathia
    - Cleft palate, velopharyngeal insufficiency. Avoid nasal intubation
  - Aspiration risk
    - Pharyngeal insufficiency, GERD
- Breathing
  - Nasal obstruction
  - Obstructive sleep apnea (OSA)
- Circulation
  - Conotruncal anomalies
  - Long QT from hypocalcemia
- Disability
  - Developmental delay, behavioral issues
  - Tetany and seizures from hypocalcemia
- Genitourinary
  - Hypocalcemia from hypoparathyroidism (especially in newborns)
  - Renal anomalies
- Immunodeficiency
  - Thymic hypoplasia: Recurrent infections; aseptic technique needed
  - Thymic aplasia: Severe combined immunodeficiency (SCID)
- Musculoskeletal
  - Scoliosis

# MANAGEMENT

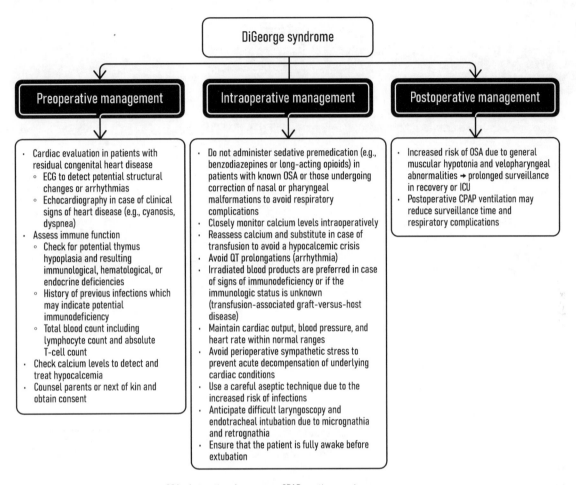

**DiGeorge syndrome**

**Preoperative management**

- Cardiac evaluation in patients with residual congenital heart disease
  - ECG to detect potential structural changes or arrhythmias
  - Echocardiography in case of clinical signs of heart disease (e.g., cyanosis, dyspnea)
- Assess immune function
  - Check for potential thymus hypoplasia and resulting immunological, hematological, or endocrine deficiencies
  - History of previous infections which may indicate potential immunodeficiency
  - Total blood count including lymphocyte count and absolute T-cell count
- Check calcium levels to detect and treat hypocalcemia
- Counsel parents or next of kin and obtain consent

**Intraoperative management**

- Do not administer sedative premedication (e.g., benzodiazepines or long-acting opioids) in patients with known OSA or those undergoing correction of nasal or pharyngeal malformations to avoid respiratory complications
- Closely monitor calcium levels intraoperatively
- Reassess calcium and substitute in case of transfusion to avoid a hypocalcemic crisis
- Avoid QT prolongations (arrhythmia)
- Irradiated blood products are preferred in case of signs of immunodeficiency or if the immunologic status is unknown (transfusion-associated graft-versus-host disease)
- Maintain cardiac output, blood pressure, and heart rate within normal ranges
- Avoid perioperative sympathetic stress to prevent acute decompensation of underlying cardiac conditions
- Use a careful aseptic technique due to the increased risk of infections
- Anticipate difficult laryngoscopy and endotracheal intubation due to micrognathia and retrognathia
- Ensure that the patient is fully awake before extubation

**Postoperative management**

- Increased risk of OSA due to general muscular hypotonia and velopharyngeal abnormalities → prolonged surveillance in recovery or ICU
- Postoperative CPAP ventilation may reduce surveillance time and respiratory complications

OSA, obstructive sleep apnea; CPAP, continuous airway pressure.

## KEEP IN MIND

- Perform a recent cardiac evaluation in patients with residual congenital heart disease
- Anticipate a difficult intubation
- Use a careful aseptic technique
- Check calcium levels

## SUGGESTED READING

- Haché M. DIGEORGE SYNDROME. In: Houck PJ, Haché M, Sun LS. eds. Handbook of Pediatric Anesthesia. Mgraw Hill; 2015. Accessed March 06, 2023. https://accessanesthesiology.mhmedical.com/content.aspx?bookid=1189&sectionid=70364073
- Sullivan KE. Chromosome 22q11.2 deletion syndrome and DiGeorge syndrome. Immunol Rev. 2019;287(1):186-201.
- Undergoing Cardiac Surgery. Journal of Cardiothoracic and Vascular Anesthesia. 2014;28(4):983-989.
- Yeng Yeoh T, Scavonetto F, Hamlin RJ, Burkhart HM, Sprung J, Weingarten TN. Perioperative Management of Patients With DiGeorge Syndrome

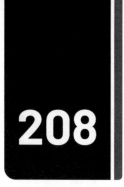

# DOWN SYNDROME

## LEARNING OBJECTIVES

- Anesthetic management of a patient with Down syndrome

## DEFINITION AND MECHANISM

- Down syndrome or trisomy 21 is a genetic disorder caused by an error in cell division
- Some or all body cells contain 47 chromosomes with the extra chromosome linked to chromosome 21
- Most frequent chromosomal abnormality

## PHYSIOLOGICAL CHANGES

| Physiological changes | |
|---|---|
| Neurological | Mental retardation |
| Airway/Respiratory | Microcephaly<br>Macroglossia<br>Subglottic stenosis<br>Obstructive sleep apnea<br>Airway obstruction<br>Small upper and lower airways<br>Pulmonary hypoplasia<br>Respiratory tract infections |
| Cardiovascular | Complete atrioventricular defect<br>Ventricular septal defect<br>Atrial septal defect (ASD)<br>Conduction disturbances<br>Pulmonary hypertension (PH) |
| Gastrointestinal | Gastroesophageal reflux disease<br>Duodenal atresia<br>Tracheoesophageal fistula<br>Hirschprung disease<br>Imperforate anus |
| Musculoskeletal | Atlantoaxial instability |
| Endocrine system | Hypothyroidism (in 50% of patients) |
| Hematology | Acute lymphoblastic leukemia<br>Acute myeloid leukemia (1.5%)<br>Polycythemia |
| Other | Difficult periperal venous access<br>Dental problems |

# MANAGEMENT

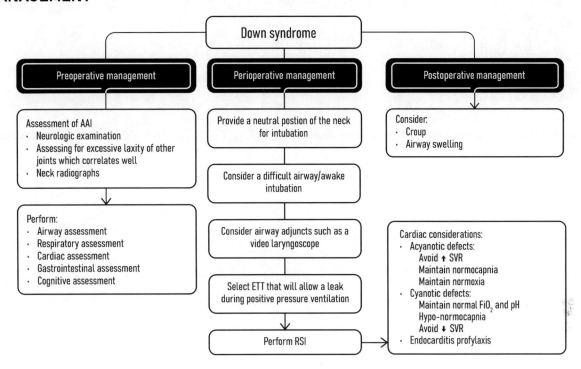

**Down syndrome**

**Preoperative management**

Assessment of AAI
- Neurologic examination
- Assessing for excessive laxity of other joints which correlates well
- Neck radiographs

Perform:
- Airway assessment
- Respiratory assessment
- Cardiac assessment
- Gastrointestinal assessment
- Cognitive assessment

**Perioperative management**

Provide a neutral postion of the neck for intubation

Consider a difficult airway/awake intubation

Consider airway adjuncts such as a video laryngoscope

Select ETT that will allow a leak during positive pressure ventilation

Perform RSI

**Postoperative management**

Consider:
- Croup
- Airway swelling

Cardiac considerations:
- Acyanotic defects:
  Avoid ↑ SVR
  Maintain normocapnia
  Maintain normoxia
- Cyanotic defects:
  Maintain normal $FiO_2$ and pH
  Hypo-normocapnia
  Avoid ↓ SVR
- Endocarditis profylaxis

AAI, atlantoaxial instability; ETT, endotracheal tube; RSI, rapid sequence intubation; SVR, systemic vascular resistance.

---

**SUGGESTED READING**

- Meitzner MC, Skurnowicz JA. Anesthetic considerations for patients with Down syndrome. AANA J. 2005;73(2):103-107.

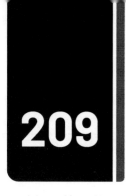

# DUCHENNE MUSCULAR DYSTROPHY

## LEARNING OBJECTIVES

- Signs and symptoms of Duchenne muscular dystrophy
- Anesthetic management of Duchenne muscular dystrophy

## DEFINITION AND MECHANISM

- Duchenne is an x-linked genetic disorder characterized by progressive muscle weakness and atrophy
- It is a multi-systemic condition and affects striated, smooth, and cardiac muscles
- Duchenne muscular dystrophy is the most common and severe form of muscular dystrophies, a group of genetically determined primary degenerative myopathies
- Duchenne is caused by a mutation in the gene that encodes for dystrophin, a protein that is essential to the proper functioning of our muscles
- Without dystrophin, muscles are not able to function or repair themselves properly
- Duchenne symptom onset is in early childhood (around the age of 4 years) and affects primarily males
- The prevalence is approximately 6 per 100,000 individuals
- Affected males are often wheelchair-bound before their teens and suffer from contractures, marked scoliosis, restrictive lung function, and cardiomyopathies
- The disease progresses differently for every person and the average life expectancy is 26-30 years
- Duchenne becomes eventually fatal due to respiratory or cardiac failure in the second or third decade

## SIGNS AND SYMPTOMS

- Muscle weakness
- Developmental delay
- Delayed speech and language development
- Enlargement of the calves
- Fatigue
- Difficulty climbing stairs
- Toe walking
- Frequent falls
- Lumbar lordosis
- Cardiomyopathy
- Shortness of breath
- Cognitive impairment
- Particular ECG pattern: Q-waves in the lateral leads, increased ST-segments, poor R-wave progression, resting tachycardia, and conduction defects
- Respiratory failure

## TREATMENT

- No cure available
- Manage symptoms with supportive therapy:
    - Corticosteroids
    - ACE inhibitors and/or beta-blockers to slow the progression of cardiomyopathy
    - Physical therapy
    - Braces
    - Surgery to treat scoliosis and contractures
    - Exercise
    - Tracheostomy and assisted ventilation for respiratory failure
    - Anticonvulsants to control seizures
    - Immunosuppressants to delay muscle damage

# MANAGEMENT

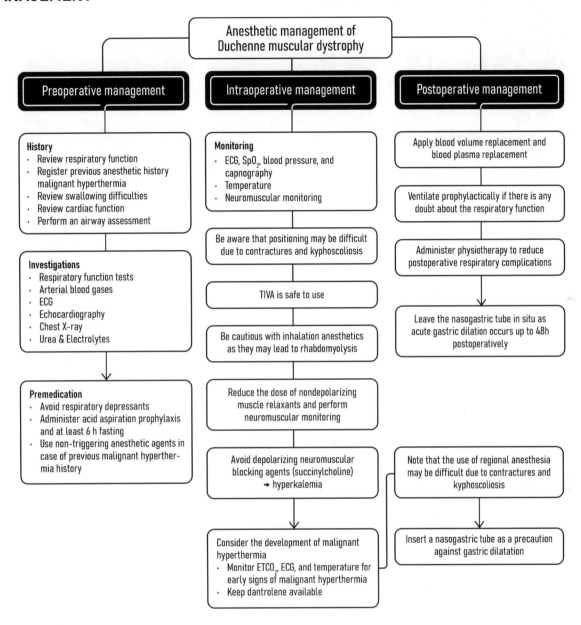

**Anesthetic management of Duchenne muscular dystrophy**

## Preoperative management

**History**
- Review respiratory function
- Register previous anesthetic history malignant hyperthermia
- Review swallowing difficulties
- Review cardiac function
- Perform an airway assessment

**Investigations**
- Respiratory function tests
- Arterial blood gases
- ECG
- Echocardiography
- Chest X-ray
- Urea & Electrolytes

**Premedication**
- Avoid respiratory depressants
- Administer acid aspiration prophylaxis and at least 6 h fasting
- Use non-triggering anesthetic agents in case of previous malignant hyperthermia history

## Intraoperative management

**Monitoring**
- ECG, SpO$_2$, blood pressure, and capnography
- Temperature
- Neuromuscular monitoring

Be aware that positioning may be difficult due to contractures and kyphoscoliosis

TIVA is safe to use

Be cautious with inhalation anesthetics as they may lead to rhabdomyolysis

Reduce the dose of nondepolarizing muscle relaxants and perform neuromuscular monitoring

Avoid depolarizing neuromuscular blocking agents (succinylcholine) → hyperkalemia

Consider the development of malignant hyperthermia
- Monitor ETCO$_2$, ECG, and temperature for early signs of malignant hyperthermia
- Keep dantrolene available

## Postoperative management

Apply blood volume replacement and blood plasma replacement

Ventilate prophylactically if there is any doubt about the respiratory function

Administer physiotherapy to reduce postoperative respiratory complications

Leave the nasogastric tube in situ as acute gastric dilation occurs up to 48h postoperatively

Note that the use of regional anesthesia may be difficult due to contractures and kyphoscoliosis

Insert a nasogastric tube as a precaution against gastric dilatation

## SUGGESTED READING

- Duan, D., Goemans, N., Takeda, S. et al. Duchenne muscular dystrophy. Nat Rev Dis Primers 7, 13 (2021).
- Lerman, J., 2011. Perioperative management of the paediatric patient with coexisting neuromuscular disease. British Journal of Anaesthesia 107, i79–i89.
- Marsh, S., Pittard, A., 2011. Neuromuscular disorders and anaesthesia. Part 2: specific neuromuscular disorders. Continuing Education in Anaesthesia Critical Care & Pain 11, 119–123.
- Pollard BJ, Kitchen, G. Handbook of Clinical Anaesthesia. Fourth Edition. CRC Press. 2018. 978-1-4987-6289-2.
- Ragoonanan, V., Russell, W., 2010. Anaesthesia for children with neuromuscular disease. Continuing Education in Anaesthesia Critical Care & Pain 10, 143–147.

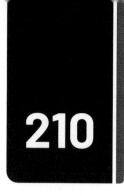

# EPIGLOTTITIS

## LEARNING OBJECTIVES

- Describe the pathophysiology and possible complications of epiglottitis
- Diagnose epiglottitis
- Manage patients with (suspected) epiglottitis

## DEFINITION AND MECHANISM

- Epiglottitis is a life-threatening inflammatory condition that causes swelling of the upper airways which can lead to asphyxia and respiratory arrest
- Usually caused by infection
- Noninfectious causes: Trauma from foreign objects, inhalation, and chemical burns
- Affects the epiglottis and nearby structures (arytenoids, aryepiglottic folds, vallecula)
- Symptoms can be exacerbated by patient discomfort or agitation

## PATHOPHYSIOLOGY

- The airway in the pediatric population differs from adults
- The epiglottis is located more superiorly and anteriorly
- More oblique angle with the trachea
- The narrowest part of the pediatric airway is the subglottis, in contrast to the glottis in adults
- The infant epiglottis is comprised of cartilage and is far more pliant
- Infectious processes that lead to edema and mass increase of the epiglottis are more likely to cause symptoms in children
- Each inspiration pulls the edematous epiglottis over the laryngeal airway, causing symptoms

## COMPLICATIONS

- Cellulitis
- Cervical adenitis
- Death
- Empyema
- Epiglottic abscess
- Hypoxia
- Meningitis
- Pneumonia
- Pneumothorax

- Prolonged ventilation
- Pulmonary edema
- Respiratory failure
- Sepsis
- Septic arthritis
- Septic shock
- Tracheostomy
- Vocal cord granuloma
- Ludwig angina-type submental infection

## SIGNS & SYMPTOMS

- Sudden onset
- Fever
- (Severe) sore throat
- Difficulty swallowing
- Hypersalivation
- Stridor
- "Tripod position"
- Inability to lie flat
- Voice changes
- Dysphagia
- Anxiety
- Tachypnea
- Cyanosis

Epiglottitis

## DIAGNOSIS

- Oropharyngeal exam may lead to loss of airway
- Lateral neck radiograph: Swelling of the epiglottis (only perform in stable, cooperative patients)
- When epiglottitis is suspected, transfer the patient to the operating room for airway assessment
- Differential diagnosis: laryngotracheobronchitis (croup), airway obstruction from a foreign object, acute angiedema, caustic ingestion, diphtheria, peritonsillar/retropharyngeal abscess

## MANAGEMENT

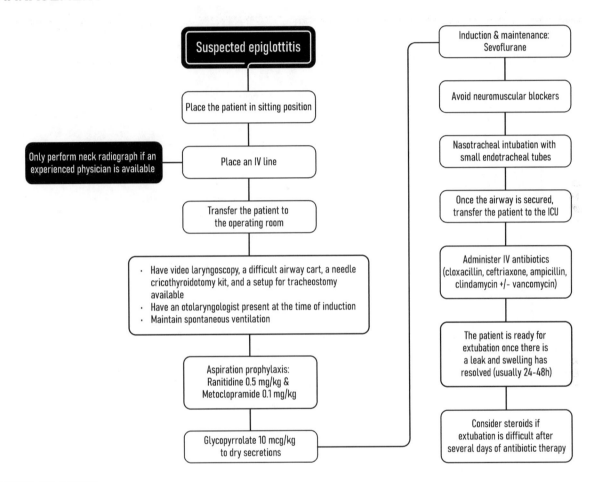

**Suspected epiglottitis**

Place the patient in sitting position

Only perform neck radiograph if an experienced physician is available

Place an IV line

Transfer the patient to the operating room

- Have video laryngoscopy, a difficult airway cart, a needle cricothyroidotomy kit, and a setup for tracheostomy available
- Have an otolaryngologist present at the time of induction
- Maintain spontaneous ventilation

Aspiration prophylaxis: Ranitidine 0.5 mg/kg & Metoclopramide 0.1 mg/kg

Glycopyrrolate 10 mcg/kg to dry secretions

Induction & maintenance: Sevoflurane

Avoid neuromuscular blockers

Nasotracheal intubation with small endotracheal tubes

Once the airway is secured, transfer the patient to the ICU

Administer IV antibiotics (cloxacillin, ceftriaxone, ampicillin, clindamycin +/- vancomycin)

The patient is ready for extubation once there is a leak and swelling has resolved (usually 24-48h)

Consider steroids if extubation is difficult after several days of antibiotic therapy

## KEEP IN MIND

- Do not agitate the patient
- Be prepared for sudden worsening of the clinical condition
- Oral exams may lead to loss of airway
- Always consider early intubation
- Awake intubation can be done in cooperative patient

## ═══ SUGGESTED READING ═══

- Guerra AM, Waseem M. Epiglottitis. [Updated 2022 Oct 17]. In: StatPearls [Internet]. Treasure Island (FL): StatPearls Publishing; 2022 Jan-. Available from: https://www.ncbi.nlm.nih.gov/books/NBK430960/
- Lichtor JL, Roche Rodriguez M, Aaronson NL, Spock T, Goodman TR, Baum ED. Epiglottitis: It Hasn't Gone Away. Anesthesiology. 2016;124(6):1404-7.

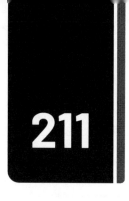

# FONTAN PHYSIOLOGY

## LEARNING OBJECTIVES

- Describe the Fontan procedure and its indications
- Manage patients with Fontan physiology

## DEFINITION AND MECHANISM

- In a normal biventricular heart, the systemic and pulmonary circulations are in series and each circulation is supported by a ventricle
- In patients with single-ventricle congenital heart disease, the two circulations are in parallel
- These patients only survive because the systemic and pulmonary venous blood mix
- The Fontan operation is a palliative procedure that connects the systemic and pulmonary circulations back in series
- Selected patients should be in sinus rhythm, have a good ventricular function, and adequately sized pulmonary arteries

## TECHNIQUE

- Contraindicated in the neonatal period due to high pulmonary vascular resistance
- Staged approach to facilitate the progressive adaptation of the heart and lungs
  - Stage 1: Systemic-pulmonary shunt
    - The placement of a restrictive synthetic conduit between a major systemic central vessel and a proximal pulmonary artery
    - Patients with hypoplastic left heart syndrome: Conduit placed between the right ventricle and the left pulmonary artery
  - Stage 2: Superior cavopulmonary connection
    - Bidirectional Glenn shunt or hemi-Fontan procedure
    - Usually performed as soon as the pulmonary arteries have grown sufficiently to allow a low pulmonary vascular resistance (2-6 months)
    - Cardiopulmonary bypass and ligation of the previous systemic-pulmonary shunt
  - Stage 3: Completion
    - Usually performed at 1-5 years of age
    - Blood in the inferior vena cava is directed into the pulmonary circuit via an extracardiac conduit or via an intra-atrial baffle

## COMPLICATIONS

- Decreased exercise tolerance
- Ventricular dysfunction
- Arrhythmias
- Shunts
- Protein-losing enteropathy
- Developmental deficits
- Thromboembolism

# MANAGEMENT

```
                    ┌──────────────────────────────────┐
                    │  FONTAN PHYSIOLOGY MANAGEMENT      │
                    └──────────────────────────────────┘
```

| Preoperative assessment | Intraoperative management | Postoperative management |

**Preoperative assessment**

- Detailed history & physical examination
- Baseline hematological & biochemical investigations
- 12-lead ECG
- Antibiotic prophylaxis with broad spectrum cover for all procedures likely to produce bacteremia
- Review and manage medications
- Consult cardiology
- Consider surgery at tertiary cardiac center

**Fenestrations**

- Patients with a fenestration are at high risk of air or fat emboli during major surgery
- Closing the fenestration preoperatively may be considered
- Have appropriate equipment and trained personnel available

**Monitoring**

- Oxygenation
- Gas analysis
- Cardiac rhythm
- Invasive arterial and central venous pressure
- Transesophageal echocardiography

**Anesthetic technique**

- Avoid induction agents that depress myocardial contractility (e.g., thiopental)
- Maintain normovolemia
- Avoid high concentrations (> 1.5 MAC) of volatile anesthetics
- Avoid hypercarbia, hypoxemia, acidosis, pain, stress, high intrathoracic pressures
- Low concentration of a volatile agent + short-acting opioid infusion
- Maintain peripheral oxygenation > 95%
- Guid fluid management by central venous pressure, transesophageal echocardiography or esophageal Doppler

**Ventilation**

- Maintain spontaneous breathing for short procedures, avoid hypercarbia
- Prevent atelectasis
- Avoid hyperventilation
- Maintain low respiratory rates, short inspiratory times, low positive end-expiratory pressure, tidal volumes of 5-6 mL/kg

**Postoperative management**

- ICU administration
- Monitor and maintain vascular volume status
- Maintain cardiac output (fluids, inotropes)
- Treat postoperative nausea and vomiting
- Patient-controlled IV or epidural opioid analgesia
- Monitor oxygen saturation for at least 24h after surgery and adjust inspired oxygen concentration to maintain saturation above preoperative levels
- Continue thromboprophylaxis
- Young healthy Fontan patients may have minor surgery as a day case

MAC, minimum alveolar concentration

## SUGGESTED READING

- Jolley M, Colan SD, Rhodes J, DiNardo J. Fontan Physiology Revisited. Anesthesia & Analgesia. 2015;121(1).
- Nayak S, Booker PD. The Fontan circulation. Continuing Education in Anaesthesia Critical Care & Pain. 2008;8(1):26-30.

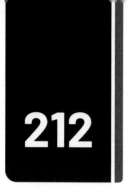

# FOREIGN BODY ASPIRATION

## LEARNING OBJECTIVES

- Diagnose an inhaled foreign body
- Manage patients with an inhaled foreign body

## DEFINITION AND MECHANISM

- Inhaled foreign bodies are a common emergency in young children
- Due to the high position of the larynx and epiglottis and narrow airways, there is a high risk of foreign body aspiration in this age group
- Distraction while eating like running or jumping, or while exploring metallic or plastic objects by mouthing, can lead to sudden onset difficulty in breathing
- It is the fourth leading cause of death in young children
- More often in boys compared to girls

## SIGNS & DIAGNOSIS

- Signs depend on the type of foreign body, time after aspiration, and exact location of the object, and can range from asymptomatic to severe respiratory distress
- Patients usually present with coughing, wheezing, dyspnea, and rarely with stridor, choking signs, and cyanosis
- The more proximal, the more severe the symptoms
- Many aspirated objects are not radiopaque, resulting in normal-appearing chest radiographs
- Pulmonary infectious or inflammatory infiltration, mediastinal shift, obstructive emphysema, atelectasis, air trapping, and very rarely pneumothorax or pneumomediastinum may be observed on chest x-ray
- Normal X-ray results are usually associated with upper airway obstruction, whereas emphysema and infiltration are seen more in distal airway obstruction
- Some organic materials may swell due to fluid absorption, resulting in increasing airway blockage with passage of time
- Sharp objects may perforate the airways
- History is crucial for making the correct diagnosis

## MANAGEMENT

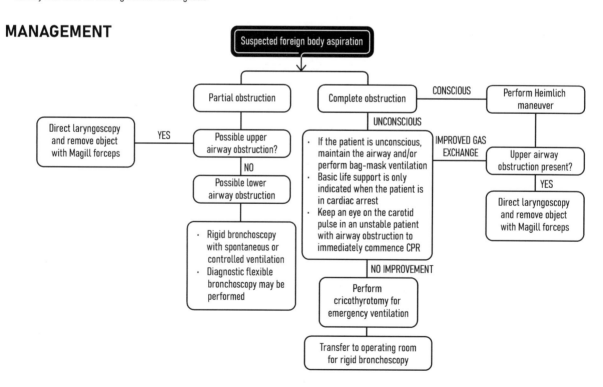

# RIGID BRONCHOSCOPY ANESTHETIC MANAGEMENT

## Preoperative assessment

- Ensure that anxiety is minimized
- Avoid sedative premedication
- Steroids like dexamethasone (0.4-1 mg/kg) can be used
- History: Allergies, medications, past medical/anesthesia history, last meal, events leading up to presentation
- Ask about family history of problems with anesthesia
- Neck and chest radiograph
- If not urgent ensure adequate fasting, else if urgent aspirate gastric contents using large bore NG tube

## Intraoperative management

### Airway
- Spontaneous breathing
- Positive pressure ventilation may push the foreign body further down the airway

### Induction
- Both IV and volatile agents can be used
- Sevoflurane in oxygen or IV fentanyl 0.5 μg/kg followed by incremental boluses of propofol (initial dose 1 mg/kg, then increments of 0.5 mg/kg or less)
- Alternative: Start with IV dexmedetomidine 1 μg/kg

### Maintenance
- Both volatile and IV agents can be used
- Ensure adequate depth of anesthesia
- Perform a direct laryngoscopy spray with lidocaine up to 4 mg/kg through the vocal cords
- For proximal obstruction-supported spontaneous ventilation and for deeper obstruction/longer procedures, use muscle relaxants with intermittent positive pressure ventilation

### Oxygenation
- If the surgeon has passed a ventilating bronchoscope through the vocal cords, attach a breathing circuit to the 22 mm connector on the bronchoscope
- If the surgeon is working at the level of the larynx, oxygen tubing can be attached to most surgical laryngoscopes or insufflate oxygen through a tracheal tube passed through the nares into the nasopharynx
- Perform manual jet ventilation during bronchoscopy in non-obstructed lung

## Postoperative management

- Many patients can breathe spontaneously with simple airway support until emergence
- Tracheal intubation may be necessary when there is significant swelling, trauma, or ongoing airway obstruction
- Treat postoperative croup with nebulized racemic epinephrine (1-5 mg) if it occurs

## SUGGESTED READING

- Bould MD. Essential notes: the anaesthetic management of an inhaled foreign body in a child. BJA Education. 2019;19(3):66-7.
- Kendigelen P. The anaesthetic consideration of tracheobronchial foreign body aspiration in children. J Thorac Dis. 2016;8(12):3803-3807.
- Moehrle NP, Jagannathan N. Management of foreign body aspiration in pediatric and adult patients. In: Berkow LC, Sakles JC, eds. Cases in Emergency Airway Management. Cambridge: Cambridge University Press; 2015:79-88.
- Rose D, Dubensky L. Airway Foreign Bodies. [Updated 2022 Aug 8]. In: StatPearls [Internet]. Treasure Island (FL): StatPearls Publishing; 2022 Jan-. Available from: https://www.ncbi.nlm.nih.gov/books/NBK539756/

Foreign body aspiration

# 213

# GENETIC SYNDROMES: GENERAL CONSIDERATIONS

## LEARNING OBJECTIVES

- Describe the general considerations for patients with genetic disorders

## DEFINITION AND MECHANISM

- Genetic syndromes are defined as the occurrence of more than one recognizable phenotypic trait in a specific association, caused by a specific genetic defect
- As molecular diagnosis is advancing rapidly, increasingly more syndromes are found to have a genetic cause
- Many children with genetic syndromes require anesthesia as part of their treatment

## ANESTHETIC CONSIDERATIONS

### AIRWAY

- Often abnormal and difficult airway
- Thorough history of airway problems
- Examination of previous anesthetic records or consulting the patient's previous anesthesiologist/surgeons
- Examination of the airway for mouth opening and visualization of the pharynx and soft palate, as well as the neck for range of motion
- Review imaging studies (chest, neck, facial radiographs, CT scans, MRI scans)
- Develop a management plan for the difficult airway
- Special attention is needed for syndromes with mandibular hypoplasia (e.g., Pierre Robin, Treacher Collins, Goldenhar) as well as patients with cleft lip/palate

### CARDIAC

- Thorough cardiac history and physical examination
- Cardiac anatomy and physiology must be understood
- Review recent diagnostic studies such as echocardiography
- Common syndromes with frequent cardiac involvement: VACTERL, CHARGE, trisomy 13, 18, and 21, and velocardiofacial syndromes
- Consult cardiology for severely affected patients

### ORTHOPEDIC

- Scoliosis, hip dysplasia, and limb contractures are common
- Carefully position the patient to not injure the affected areas
- Evaluate the respiratory and cardiac status of patients with severe scoliosis

### NEUROCOGNITIVE

- Malformations of the central/peripheral nervous system and developmental delays are common
- General intelligence lag, gross or fine motor problems, speech and language delay, behavioral problems
- Understanding neurodevelopmental status is important
- Patients may be very anxious and/or uncooperative
- Adjust the approach to preoperative preparation, communication, premedication, and parental presence accordingly

### VASCULAR ACCESS

- Limb abnormalities may complicate vascular access
- Provide external or internal jugular vein access if the limbs are not available
- Central veins may be thrombosed from previous catheters
- Additional studies (ultrasound, MRI, CT) may be necessary to plan for vascular access

### OTHER

- Consult a reference source with rare or unfamiliar disorders
- Consult parents and other caregivers about previous responses to interventions

## SUGGESTED READING

- Mann D, Garcia PJ, Andropoulos DB. Anesthesia for the Patient with a Genetic Syndrome. Gregory's Pediatric Anesthesia 2020. p. 1085-105.

# 214

# GOLDENHAR SYNDROME

## LEARNING OBJECTIVES

- Describe Goldenhar syndrome
- Understand how Goldenhar syndrome affects the airway
- Discuss the perioperative management of patients with Goldenhar syndrome

## DEFINITION AND MECHANISM

- Goldenhar syndrome (GS), also called oculo-auriculo-vertebral syndrome or hemifacial microsomia, is a rare disorder of craniofacial development
- Congenital malformation of the first and second branchial arches, resulting in the incomplete development of the ear, nose, soft palate, lip, and mandible (usually unilateral)
- It is characterized by the triad of mandibular hypoplasia resulting in facial asymmetry, ear and/or eye malformation, and vertebral anomalies
- Patients can also present with heart, kidney, and lung malformations, and central nervous system defects
- Male-to-female ratio 3:2
- Incidence - 1:5600

## SIGNS & DIAGNOSIS

- Mandibular hypoplasia (facial asymmetry)
- **Eye anomalies:** Microphthalmia, anophthalmia, epibulbar dermoids, and eyelid colobomas
- **Ear anomalies:** Preauricular tags, anotia (totally absent ear), and microtia (partially formed ear)
- **Vertebral anomalies:** Scoliosis, kyphosis, hemivertebrae, and cervical fusion
- Cleft lip and/or palate
- Wider than normal mouth
- Hydrocephalus
- Congenital heart defects in ⅓ of patients (most commonly septal and conotruncal defects, e.g., tetralogy of Fallot)
- Genitourinary malformations (e.g., ectopic or fused kidneys, renal agenesis, ureteropelvic junction obstruction, or vesicoureteral reflux)
- Partial or complete unilateral lung hypoplasia
- Developmental delay and autism spectrum disorder in some patients

## COMPLICATIONS

- Vision problems and/or loss
- Hearing loss
- Feeding difficulties
- Speech difficulties
- Obstructive sleep apnea (OSA)
- Strabismus
- Pulmonary hypoplasia might increase the risk for respiratory infections, pulmonary hypertension, and pneumothorax
- Severe spinal deformities might cause restrictive lung disease and lead to further decrease in pulmonary function

## TREATMENT

- Glasses or surgery to improve vision
- Hearing aids or bone-anchored auditory implants
- Feeding assistance with special bottles or nasogastric feedings
- Speech therapy to increase language and communication skills
- Reconstructive surgery
- Surgery to correct a congenital heart defect, cleft lip or palate, obstructive sleep apnea, microtia, or spinal defect

# MANAGEMENT

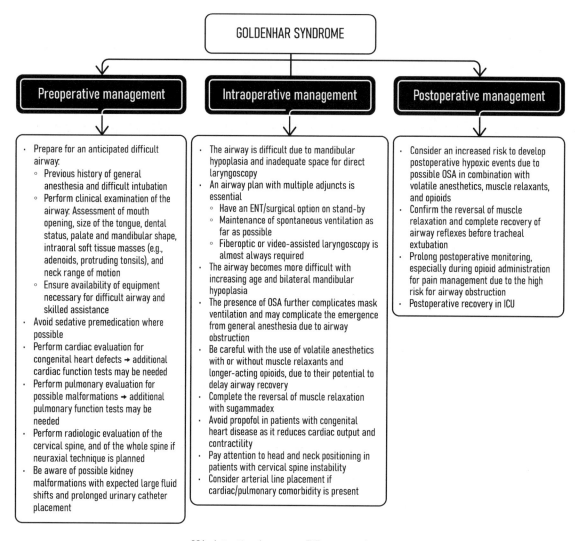

**GOLDENHAR SYNDROME**

**Preoperative management**

- Prepare for an anticipated difficult airway:
  - Previous history of general anesthesia and difficult intubation
  - Perform clinical examination of the airway: Assessment of mouth opening, size of the tongue, dental status, palate and mandibular shape, intraoral soft tissue masses (e.g., adenoids, protruding tonsils), and neck range of motion
  - Ensure availability of equipment necessary for difficult airway and skilled assistance
- Avoid sedative premedication where possible
- Perform cardiac evaluation for congenital heart defects → additional cardiac function tests may be needed
- Perform pulmonary evaluation for possible malformations → additional pulmonary function tests may be needed
- Perform radiologic evaluation of the cervical spine, and of the whole spine if neuraxial technique is planned
- Be aware of possible kidney malformations with expected large fluid shifts and prolonged urinary catheter placement

**Intraoperative management**

- The airway is difficult due to mandibular hypoplasia and inadequate space for direct laryngoscopy
- An airway plan with multiple adjuncts is essential
  - Have an ENT/surgical option on stand-by
  - Maintenance of spontaneous ventilation as far as possible
  - Fiberoptic or video-assisted laryngoscopy is almost always required
- The airway becomes more difficult with increasing age and bilateral mandibular hypoplasia
- The presence of OSA further complicates mask ventilation and may complicate the emergence from general anesthesia due to airway obstruction
- Be careful with the use of volatile anesthetics with or without muscle relaxants and longer-acting opioids, due to their potential to delay airway recovery
- Complete the reversal of muscle relaxation with sugammadex
- Avoid propofol in patients with congenital heart disease as it reduces cardiac output and contractility
- Pay attention to head and neck positioning in patients with cervical spine instability
- Consider arterial line placement if cardiac/pulmonary comorbidity is present

**Postoperative management**

- Consider an increased risk to develop postoperative hypoxic events due to possible OSA in combination with volatile anesthetics, muscle relaxants, and opioids
- Confirm the reversal of muscle relaxation and complete recovery of airway reflexes before tracheal extubation
- Prolong postoperative monitoring, especially during opioid administration for pain management due to the high risk for airway obstruction
- Postoperative recovery in ICU

OSA, obstructive sleep apnea; ENT, ear-nose-throat

## SUGGESTED READING

- Goldenhar Syndrome. In: Bissonnette B, Luginbuehl I, Marciniak B, Dalens BJ. eds. Syndromes: Rapid Recognition and Perioperative Implications. Mgraw Hill; 2006. Accessed February 09, 2023. https://accessanesthesiology.mhmedical.com/content.aspx?bookid=852&sectionid=49517623
- Kaymak C, Gulhan Y, Ozcan AO, Baltaci B, Unal N, Safak MA, Oguz H. Anaesthetic approach in a case of Goldenhar's syndrome. European Journal of Anaesthesiology. 2022; 19(11):836-838.
- Sun YH, Zhu B, Ji BY, Zhang XH. Airway Management in a Child with Goldenhar Syndrome. Chin Med J (Engl). 2017;130(23):2881-2882.

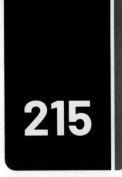

# MITOCHONDRIAL DISEASE

## LEARNING OBJECTIVES

- Describe the clinical features of mitochondrial disease
- Diagnose and treat mitochondrial disease
- Manage patients with mitochondrial disease presenting for surgery

## DEFINITION AND MECHANISM

- Mitochondrial disease refers to a group of genetic disorders affecting the mitochondria
- Results in a complex multisystem disease with varying degrees of severity
- Can present with a wide range of symptoms
- Organs and tissues that have a high ATP turnover are proportionally affected, e.g., the CNS, heart, GI tract and muscular system
- Associated with elevated lactate levels

## CLINICAL FEATURES

| System | Features |
|---|---|
| Neurological/myopathic | Developmental delay |
| | Regression |
| | Weakness |
| | Fatigability |
| | Hypotonia |
| | Spasticity |
| | Ataxia |
| | Seizure disorders |
| Respiratory | Respiratory failure |
| | Dysphagia |
| Cardiovascular | Cardiomyopathy |
| | Conduction abnormalities |

## DIAGNOSIS

| Diagnostic test | Signs of mitochondrial disease |
|---|---|
| Genetic testing | Genetic defects affecting the mitochondria |
| Muscle biopsy | Ragged-red fibers<br>cytochrome C-oxidase negative fibers |
| Biochemical analysis | Elevated lactate levels |
| Brain MRI | Stroke-like lesions in non-vascular distributions<br>Diffuse white matter disease<br>Bilateral<br>involvement of deep grey matter nuclei in the basal ganglia, mid-brain and/or brainstem<br>Lactate doublet |

# MANAGEMENT

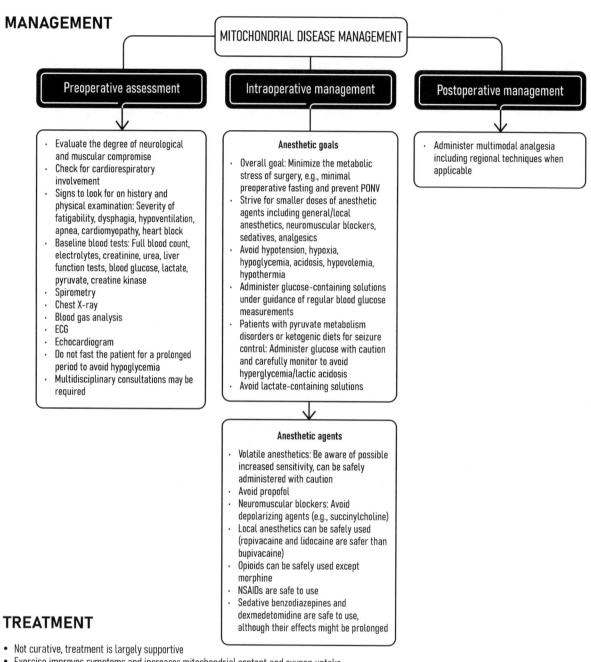

**MITOCHONDRIAL DISEASE MANAGEMENT**

## Preoperative assessment

- Evaluate the degree of neurological and muscular compromise
- Check for cardiorespiratory involvement
- Signs to look for on history and physical examination: Severity of fatigability, dysphagia, hypoventilation, apnea, cardiomyopathy, heart block
- Baseline blood tests: Full blood count, electrolytes, creatinine, urea, liver function tests, blood glucose, lactate, pyruvate, creatine kinase
- Spirometry
- Chest X-ray
- Blood gas analysis
- ECG
- Echocardiogram
- Do not fast the patient for a prolonged period to avoid hypoglycemia
- Multidisciplinary consultations may be required

## Intraoperative management

### Anesthetic goals

- Overall goal: Minimize the metabolic stress of surgery, e.g., minimal preoperative fasting and prevent PONV
- Strive for smaller doses of anesthetic agents including general/local anesthetics, neuromuscular blockers, sedatives, analgesics
- Avoid hypotension, hypoxia, hypoglycemia, acidosis, hypovolemia, hypothermia
- Administer glucose-containing solutions under guidance of regular blood glucose measurements
- Patients with pyruvate metabolism disorders or ketogenic diets for seizure control: Administer glucose with caution and carefully monitor to avoid hyperglycemia/lactic acidosis
- Avoid lactate-containing solutions

### Anesthetic agents

- Volatile anesthetics: Be aware of possible increased sensitivity, can be safely administered with caution
- Avoid propofol
- Neuromuscular blockers: Avoid depolarizing agents (e.g., succinylcholine)
- Local anesthetics can be safely used (ropivacaine and lidocaine are safer than bupivacaine)
- Opioids can be safely used except morphine
- NSAIDs are safe to use
- Sedative benzodiazepines and dexmedetomidine are safe to use, although their effects might be prolonged

## Postoperative management

- Administer multimodal analgesia including regional techniques when applicable

# TREATMENT

- Not curative, treatment is largely supportive
- Exercise improves symptoms and increases mitochondrial content and oxygen uptake
- Nutritional supplementation of multiple vitamins and cofactors including:
  - Coenzyme Q10
  - Alpha-lipoic acid
  - L-carnitine
  - Creatine
  - B-vitamins

# SUGGESTED READING

- Desai, V. (2021). Mitochondrial disease and anaesthesia : WFSA - resources. Mitochondrial Disease and Anaesthesia. Retrieved February 16, 2023, from https://resources.wfsahq.org/atotw/mitochondrial-disease-and-anaesthesia/.
- Hsieh VC, Krane EJ, Morgan PG. Mitochondrial Disease and Anesthesia. Journal of Inborn Errors of Metabolism and Screening. 2017;5:2326409817707770.
- Niezgoda J, Morgan PG. Anesthetic considerations in patients with mitochondrial defects. Paediatr Anaesth. 2013;23(9):785-793.

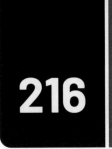

# MUCOPOLYSACCHARIDOSES

## LEARNING OBJECTIVES

- Describe mucopolysaccharidoses
- Understand the anesthetic risk factors and complications associated with mucopolysaccharidoses
- Anesthetic management of a patient with mucopolysaccharidosis

## DEFINITION AND MECHANISM

- Mucopolysaccharidoses (MPS) are rare, inherited, lysosomal storage diseases characterized by deficiencies in different lysosomal enzymes involved in the metabolism of glycosaminoglycans (mucopolysaccharides)
- MPS causes an accumulation of glycosaminoglycans in the brain, heart, liver, bone, cornea, and tracheobronchial tree
- Glycosaminoglycan accumulation in the upper airway results in hypertrophy of adenoids, tonsils, tongue (macroglossia), and laryngopharynx
- There are seven types and several subtypes of MPS, each with various clinical presentations → categorized in four broad categories
  - MPS I, II, and VII affect soft tissue storage and the skeleton with or without brain disease
  - MPS VI affects both soft tissues and the skeleton
  - MPS IV A and IV B are primarily associated with skeletal disorders
  - MPS III A-D are primarily associated with central nervous system disorders
- Autosomal recessive inheritance, except for MPS II, which is an inherited X-linked recessive disorder
- Patients with MPS often have a significantly shortened lifespan
- All types of MPS, except MPSIII, have facial and oral abnormalities posing a challenge for airway management

| MPS type | Accumulated product | Enzyme | Gene/locus | Clinical manifestations |
|---|---|---|---|---|
| MPS I H | Heparan sulfate, dermatan sulfate | α-L-iduronidase | IDUA/4p16.3 | Intellectual disability, facial dysmorphism, dwarfism, cardiomegaly, valvular disease, OSA, and hepatosplenomegaly |
| MPS I S  MPS I HS | | | | |
| MPS II | Heparan sulfate, dermatan sulfate | Iduronate-2-sulfatase | IDS/Xq28 | Macroglossia, vocal cord enlargement, hydrocephalus, narrow airway, spinal stenosis, cardiomegaly, valvular disease, OSA, and hepatosplenomegaly |
| MPS III A | Heparan sulfate | Heparan N-sulfatase | SGSH/17q25.3 | Dementia, seizures, language skills, deafness, blindness, enlarged tonsils, adenoids, and respiratory infections |
| MPS III B | | N-acetylglucosaminidase | NAGLU/17q21.2 | |
| MPS III C | | Heparan-α-glucosaminide N-acetyltransferase | HGSNAT/8p11.21 | |
| MPS III D | | N-acetylglucosamine 6-sulfatase | GNS/12q14.3 | |

| | | | | |
|---|---|---|---|---|
| MPS IV A | Keratan sulfate, chondroi-tin-6-sulfate | Galactose-6-sulfate sulfatase | GALNS/16q24.3 | Short stature, atlantoaxial instability, odontoid hypoplasia, pectus carinatum, spine deformities, hepatomegaly, and restrictive lung disease |
| MPS IV B | Keratan sulfate | β-galactosidase | GLB1/3p22.3 | |
| MPS VI | Dermatan sulfate | N-acetylgalactosamine-4-sulfatase | ARSB/5q14.1 | Short trunk, crouched stance, restricted joint movements, and heart disease |
| MPS VII | Heparan sulfate, dermatan sulfate, chondroitin-4,6-sulfate | β-glucuronidase | GUSB/7q11.21 | Skeletal dysplasia, short stature, nerve entrapment, developmental delay, and hepatomegaly |

## SIGNS & DIAGNOSIS

- Damage to neurons
- Pain and impaired motor function resulting from compressed nerves or nerve roots in the spinal cord or peripheral nervous system
- Coarse facial features (flat nasal bridge, thick lips, and enlarged mouth and tongue)
- Short stature with disproportionately short trunk/torso (dwarfism)
- Abnormal bone size and/or shape (dysplasia) and other skeletal abnormalities
- Thickened skin
- Hepatosplenomegaly
- Hernias
- Carpal tunnel syndrome restricting hand mobility and function
- Recurring respiratory infections, obstructive airway disease, and obstructive sleep apnea (OSA)
- Heart disease, often involving enlarged or diseased heart valves
- Hyperactivity
- Depression
- Speech difficulties
- Hearing impairment
- Hydrocephalus
- Corneal clouding, degeneration of the retina, and glaucoma → vision problems
- Intellectual disabilities, developmental delays, or behavioral problems

## TREATMENT

- Ventriculoperitoneal shunt
- Nerve decompression surgeries (spinal cord or skeletal nerves like median nerve)
- Herniorrhaphy or hernioplasty
- Corneal transplants to improve vision in patients with significant corneal clouding
- Adenotonsillectomy
- Enzyme replacement therapy (MPS I, II, IVA, VI, and VII) to reduce non-neurological symptoms and pain
- Orthopaedic surgery to correct deformities or skeletal defects, e.g., correction of kyphoscoliosis, varus and valgus deformities
- Heart valvular repair/replacement

## ANESTHESIA CHALLENGES

### Anesthetic risk factors

- Hypopharynx
  - Hyperplasia of adenoids, tonsils, swollen epiglottis and pharyngeal tissue
  - Narrow due to redundant tissue
  - High anterior larynx
- Neck pathology
  - Cervical cord compression
  - Short neck
  - Atlantoaxial instability (only for MPS IV)
  - Spinal cord injury and paralysis during intubation
- Oral cavity
  - Macroglossia (large tongue)
  - Limited mouth opening
- Cardiac
  - Coronary artery disease
  - Valvular heart disease
  - Heart failure
  - Significant arrhythmias
  - Pulmonary hypertension
  - Cardiomyopathy
- Respiratory

Mucopolysaccharidoses

- Restrictive lung disease
- Obstructive lung disease, OSA
- Breathing at closing capacity
- Recurrent pulmonary infections
- Pulmonary hypertension
- Cor pulmonale
- Respiratory failure
- Tracheobronchomalacia
- Neurological
  - Potential developmental delay, uncooperative behavior
  - Dural thickening can result in compressive myelopathy
  - Hydrocephalus
- Other
  - Hepatosplenomegaly
  - Hepatic dysfunction
  - Metabolic acidosis due to the inability to convert lactic acid to glycogen
  - Hemorrhagic diathesis due to platelet dysfunction

- Bone changes
  - Joint stiffness
  - Odontoid istability
  - Hypoplastic mandible
  - Kyphoscoliosis
  - Atlanto-axial instability

### Anesthetic complications that may occur during anesthesia in patients with MPS

- Inability to ventilate or intubate
- Temporary airway obstruction ➡ can cause negative pressure pulmonary edema
- Complete airway obstruction (mostly during induction or at extubation) ➡ can cause hypoxemia and cardiac arrest
- Post-extubation complications like inability to maintain airway
- Stridor
- Lower airway collapse/infection
- Need for reintubation or tracheostomy

## MANAGEMENT

MUCOPOLYSACCHARIDOSIS

### Preoperative management

- Review the patient's MPS type, age, and clinical features
- History of previous anesthesia and disease-targeting therapies
- Evaluate anesthetic risk factors (i.e., airway obstruction, OSA, cardiac disease, and pulmonary function)
- Preoperative examination for signs of airway obstruction using various techniques like flexible nasoendoscopy under local anaesthesia, CT thorax, multidetector CT of airway, dynamic CT study
- Identification of cardiac abnormalities and its optimisation
- X-rays of the chest and cervical spine if indicated
- Sedative premedication: Midazolam or diazepam orally in slightly reduced doses
- Anticholinergics: Atropine or glycopyrronium to reduce secretions and improve the view during fiberoptic bronchoscopy or intubation
- Monitor patients with a pulse oximeter after they have received sedative premedication

### Intraoperative management

- Difficult airway, both bag mask ventilation and laryngoscopy (with possibility of CICV), that worsens with time
- Safe establishment of the airway
  - Consider awake fiberoptic intubation
  - If uncooperative, spontaneous breathing fiberoptic intubation
  - Surgical backup for rigid bronchoscopy and tracheostomy should be immediately available
  - Use a 2-3 smaller ET tube than predicted
- Avoid/minimize the use of respiratory depressants if possible
- Consider using nitrous oxide instead of inhalational or intravenous agents for IV access placement
- Ketamine is better than midazolam or fentanyl for FOB as it maintains the airway better
- LMA or nasal airway may help in ventilation
- Induction in lateral position may be helpful
- Avoid muscle relaxants until airway is secured
- Perioperative monitoring of serum glucose, minimize fasting times when possible
- Use intraoperative steroids to prevent airway edema
- Most cases require general anesthesia as patients are mostly young children

### Postoperative management

- Continue airway management and monitoring until the patient regains full consciousness to detect airway obstruction and desaturation
- Only perform extubation when the patient is fully awake, coughing vigorously, breathing adequately, and moving deliberately
- Ensure full reversal of muscle relaxants
- Pace nasopharyngeal airway to avoid upper airway obstruction after extubation
- Consider using an airway exchange catheter to allow easy reintubation if needed
- FOB and ENT backup at all times should be available post-extubation
- Extubate patients early after surgery
  - Allows for early assessment of neurological status
  - Reduces airway swelling from intubation
- Possible need for postoperative ventilatory support

OSA, obstructive sleep apnea; FOB, fiberoptic bronchoscopy; LMA, laryngeal mask airway

## KEEP IN MIND

- MPS are a group of multisystem diseases, but the airway is the main concern (53% difficult intubation, 23% failed intubation)
- All MPS types, except for MPS III, have facial and airway characteristics which may challenge anesthetic airway management

## SUGGESTED READING

- Clark BM, Sprung J, Weingarten TN, Warner ME. Anesthesia for patients with mucopolysaccharidoses: Comprehensive review of the literature with emphasis on airway management. Bosn J Basic Med Sci. 2018;18(1):1-7.
- Walker R, Belani KG, Braunlin EA, et al. Anaesthesia and airway management in mucopolysaccharidosis. J Inherit Metab Dis. 2013;36(2):211-219.

# NECROTIZING ENTEROCOLITIS

## LEARNING OBJECTIVES

- Describe necrotizing enterocolitis
- Recognize signs and symptoms of necrotizing enterocolitis
- Anesthetic management of an infant with necrotizing enterocolitis

## DEFINITION AND MECHANISM

- Necrotizing enterocolitis (NEC) is a life-threatening intestinal disease that affects premature or very low birth-weight infants
- It is the most common gastrointestinal (GI) emergency in NICUs → leading cause of long-term disability in preterm infants
- Inflammation of the intestine leads to bacterial invasion causing cellular damage and cellular death, and necrosis of the colon and intenstines → as NEC progresses, it may lead to intestinal perforation, causing peritonitis, sepsis, and death
- Mortality up to 30%
- Usually presents within 2nd to 3rd week of life

## SIGNS AND SYMPTOMS

- Abdominal tenderness and distension
- Bradycardia, shock and respiratory distress
- Diarrhea with bloody stool
- Increased gastric residuals
- Vomiting of bile
- Lethargy

- Erythema of abdominal wall
- Intolerance to enteral feed
- Failure to thrive
- Temperature instability (hypothermia)
- In severe cases: Hypotension, disseminated intravascular coagulation (DIC) and metabolic acidosis

## DIAGNOSIS

Abdominal radiography with anterior-posterior and left lateral decubitus view—most important test for diagnosis and assessment of progression
Bell's stages of NEC

- **Stage I (suspected disease):** Mild systemic signs (apnea, bradycardia, temperature instability, lethargy), mild GI signs (abdominal distension, increased gastric residuals, bloody stools), non-specific or normal radiologic signs
- **Stage II (definite disease):** Mild systemic signs with additional GI signs (absent bowel sounds, abdominal tenderness), specific radiological signs (dilated loops of intestines, pneumatosis intestinalis or portal venous air), abnormal laboratory investigations (e.g., metabolic acidosis, thrombocytopenia)
- **Stage III (advanced disease):** Severe systemic illness (with hemodynamic instability), additional GI signs (gross abdominal distension, peritonitis), severe radiological signs (pneumoperitoneum), additional laboratory findings (e.g., metabolic and respiratory acidosis, disseminated intravascular coagulation) high C-reactive protein levels

## COMPLICATIONS

- Intestinal perforation: Peritonitis increases the risk of sepsis
- Intestinal strictures
- Short bowel (short-gut) syndrome: Results in malabsorption
- Growth failure, poor neurodevelopmental outcomes, and developmental delay: Mainly in infants requiring surgery

## RISK FACTORS

- Prematurity
- Low birth weight
- Birth asphyxia
- Hypoxemia
- Enteral formula feeding

- Cyanotic heart disease
- Patent ductus arteriosus
- Exchange transfusion
- Prolonged rupture of membranes

# PATHOPHYSIOLOGY

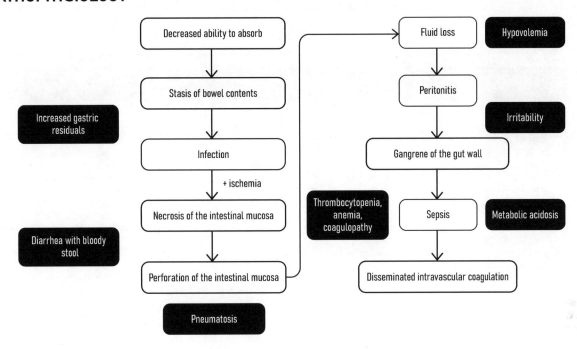

# TREATMENT

- Medical management will avoid surgery in 85% of cases
  - Fluid resuscitation and ionotropic support to maintain hemodynamics
  - Stop enteral nutrition
  - Decompress the stomach with a nasogastric tube
  - Broad spectrum antibitiotics
  - Packed red blood cells (PRBC) and platelet transfusions
- Surgery
  - Exploratory laparotomy for removal of the gangrenous bowel
  - Ileostomy
  - Peritoneal drain
- Indications for surgery
  - Perforation
  - Obstruction
  - Peritonitis
  - Worsening acidosis
  - Neonate becomes more septic
  - Bell's stage 3

# ANESTHETIC CONSIDERATIONS

- Premature infant considerations
- Increased risk of aspiration: Bowel obstruction, dilated bowel loops, pneumatosis intestinalis
- Associated multisystem derangements: Hypoxia, electrolyte imbalance, sepsis, hypovolemia, disseminated intravascular coagulation, thrombocytopenia, metabolic acidosis
- Associated conditions: Birth asphyxia, hypotension, respiratory distress syndrome, patent ductus arteriosus, recurrent apnea, intestinal ischemia, systemic infections

# MANAGEMENT

```
┌─────────────────────────────┐
│  NECROTIZING ENTEROCOLITIS  │
└─────────────────────────────┘
```

| Preoperative management | Intraoperative management | Postoperative management |

### Preoperative management

- Optimize the infant before surgery
- Investigations: Coagulation profile, serum electrolytes, arterial blood gas analysis, hematocrit, glycemic status
- Try to correct hypovolemia, metabolic acidosis, coagulopathy, hypocalcemia, and thrombocytopenia as much as possible
- Ensure adequate venous access for fluid replacement to replenish losses (third space and surgical losses)
- Crossmatch blood
- Have PRBC, fresh frozen plasma (FFP), and platelets available for transfusion

### Intraoperative management

- Continue resuscitation
- Large volumes of IV fluids along with appropriate maintenance fluids to maintain normoglycemia and euvolemia
- Inotropic support (i.e., dopamine, epinephrine, or vasopressin) to maintain adequate perfusion pressures
- Standard ASA monitoring (pulse oximeter, ECG, end-tidal $CO_2$, and noninvasive arterial pressure) plus peripheral arterial line
- Replace blood loss with appropriate blood products
- Prevent hypothermia: Increase ambient temperature, warmed fluids, radiant heat lamps, warming blanket, warming mattress, warmed and humidified gases
- Carefully titrate anesthetic medications (increased sensitivity)
- Most infants are already intubated, otherwise an awake intubation or rapid sequence intubation is preferred
- **Induction of anesthesia**
  - High dose of opioids (e.g., fentanyl 10 mcg/kg body weight or equivalent dose of remifentanil or sufentanil) with or without sevoflurane if hemodynamically tolerated
  - Succinylcholine or rocuronium
- **Maintenance of anesthesia**
  - Use opioids (e.g., fentanyl), muscle relaxants, and minimal concentrations of volatile anesthetics, if tolerated
  - Supplementation with ketamine
  - Use air/oxygen mixture to maintain $SpO_2$ around 90% ($PaO_2$ 50-70 mmHg)
- Ventilatory requirements increase during surgery as handling of the bowel reduces lung compliance
- Avoid nitrous oxide to prevent further bowel distension
- Better not to extubate

### Postoperative management

- Ventilation in the NICU
- Postoperative cardiovascular support
- Transport in warmed incubator with full monitoring
- Expect a prolonged ileus and consider central line for total parenteral nutrition and continued inotrope support until sepsis is controlled
- Intraoperative opioids usually make any further analgesia or sedation unnecessary for the first day
- Remove umbilical artery catheters if possible to improve mesenteric blood flow
- Acute complications include infections, disseminated intravascular coagulation, and further metabolic or respiratory compromise

# PROGNOSIS

Long-term survival depends on:
- Degree of prematurity
- Associated congenital anomalies
- Degree of surviving bowel
- Total length of affected bowel

# PREVENTION

- Breast milk
- Probiotics

# SUGGESTED READING

- Houck PJ. Chapter 175. Necrotizing Enterocolitis. In: Atchabahian A, Gupta R. eds. The Anesthesia Guide. Mgraw Hill; 2013. Accessed February 13, 2023. https://accessanesthesiology.mhmedical.com/content.aspx?bookid=572&sectionid=42543766
- Sodhi P, Fiset P. Necrotizing enterocolitis. Continuing Education in Anaesthesia Critical Care & Pain. 2012;12(1):1-4.

Necrotizing enterocolitis

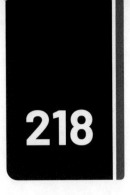

# OMPHALOCELE AND GASTROSCHISIS

**218**

## LEARNING OBJECTIVES

- Describe the difference between omphalocele and gastroschisis
- Anesthetic management of pediatric patients with abdominal wall defects

## DEFINITION AND MECHANISM

- Omphalocele and gastroschisis are congenital abdominal wall defects resulting in intestinal herniation from the abdominal cavity
- Resulting from major defects in the closure of the abdominal wall → exposure of abdominal viscera
- Main difference: There is no sac covering the intestines in gastroschisis
- Both can be detected antenatally using fetal ultrasound → allows timing, location, and mode of delivery to be planned in advance
  - Omphalocele: Delivery at term
  - Gastroschisis: Benefit from early delivery (37 weeks gestation) to limit bowel damage from exposure to amniotic fluid
- Both are associated with prematurity and low birth weight

### Omphalocele

- Herniation of abdominal contents through the middle of the abdominal wall at the umbilicus
  - The skin, muscle, and fibrous tissue are missing
  - The intestines herniate through the opening and are covered by a thin sac
  - The sac is formed from an outpouching of the peritoneum and protrudes in the midline, through the umbilicus
- Commonly occurs with other congenital defects (e.g., heart and kidney defects), chromosome abnormalities (e.g., Down syndrome, trisomy 18, trisomy 13), and genetic syndromes (e.g., Beckwith-Wiedemann syndrome)

### Gastroschisis

- Herniation of abdominal contents from a defect lateral to the umbilicus (usually right-sided), but not directly over it
- Protruding organs are not covered by a thin sac → damage due to direct contact with amniotic fluid in the uterus → inflammation
- Rarely have other congenital defects, seldom associated with chromosome abnormalities or genetic syndromes

## SIGNS AND SYMPTOMS

- External herniation of abdominal viscera

### Omphalocele

- Omphalocele minor: Minor herniation into the umbilical cord, small 5-8 cm defect
- Omphalocele major: Large defect, including the liver, with poorly developed abdominal and pulmonary hypoplasia
- Intestine looks normal

### Gastroschisis

- The intestine wall may be thickened, with a fibrin "peel" due to exposure to amniotic fluid
- May involve the stomach, bladder, uterus, and rarely liver

## COMPLICATIONS

- Intrauterine growth retardation
- Underdevelopment of the lungs → respiratory insufficiency may require mechanical ventilation
- Feeding difficulties
- Poor gut motility
- Malrotation
- Intestinal atresia
- Volvulus
- Stenosis
- Gastroesophageal reflux
- Short bowel syndrome → dehydration

- Sequelae of an open abdomen
  - Aspiration
  - Hypothermia
  - Fluid and electrolyte abnormalities
  - Sepsis

Omphalocele and gastroschisis

# TREATMENT

Initial post-delivery treatment
- Fluid resuscitation
- Care of herniated bowel/viscera and their blood supply: Cover exposed organs with a sterile dressing to keep them moist and protected
- Perform bowel decompression using a nasogastric tube
- Temperature regulation: Nurse in an incubator to reduce heat loss
- Omphalocele: Inspect the sac to check whether or not it is ruptured
- IV antibiotics to minimize the risk of infection

Single vs. staged surgery
- The surgery typically takes place shortly after birth
- Omphalocele: Semi-urgent surgery unless the sac is ruptured
- Gastroschisis: Urgent surgery
- Required to reinsert the intestines in the abdomen and to close the opening
- Single-stage surgery: Omphalocele minor
  - Intestines are moved back in the abdomen, and the opening is closed during the same surgery
- Staged-surgery: Omphalocele major and gastroschisis
  - Wrap intestines in a protective covering (i.e., silo)
  - Gradually move intestines back into the abdomen over several days or weeks
  - Surgically close the opening once all intestines are back in the abdomen

# KEEP IN MIND

- Neonates are highly susceptible to dehydration and heat loss before repair of the abdominal wall defect → Perform fluid resuscitation and temperature control
- Repair surgery may be primary or staged
- Improved survival is associated with optimal perioperative and postoperative care

Omphalocele and gastroschisis

# MANAGEMENT

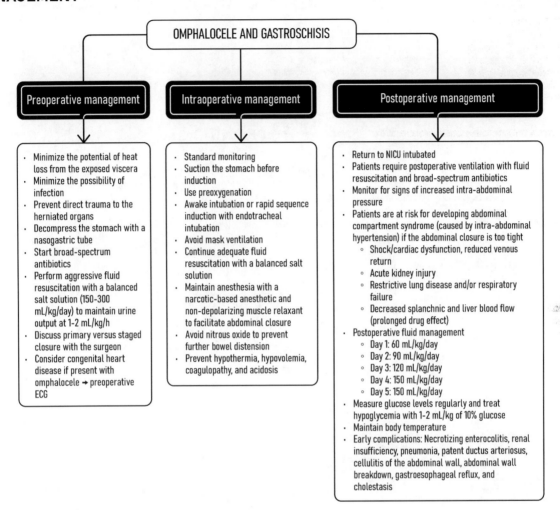

**OMPHALOCELE AND GASTROSCHISIS**

**Preoperative management**

- Minimize the potential of heat loss from the exposed viscera
- Minimize the possibility of infection
- Prevent direct trauma to the herniated organs
- Decompress the stomach with a nasogastric tube
- Start broad-spectrum antibiotics
- Perform aggressive fluid resuscitation with a balanced salt solution (150-300 mL/kg/day) to maintain urine output at 1-2 mL/kg/h
- Discuss primary versus staged closure with the surgeon
- Consider congenital heart disease if present with omphalocele ➜ preoperative ECG

**Intraoperative management**

- Standard monitoring
- Suction the stomach before induction
- Use preoxygenation
- Awake intubation or rapid sequence induction with endotracheal intubation
- Avoid mask ventilation
- Continue adequate fluid resuscitation with a balanced salt solution
- Maintain anesthesia with a narcotic-based anesthetic and non-depolarizing muscle relaxant to facilitate abdominal closure
- Avoid nitrous oxide to prevent further bowel distension
- Prevent hypothermia, hypovolemia, coagulopathy, and acidosis

**Postoperative management**

- Return to NICU intubated
- Patients require postoperative ventilation with fluid resuscitation and broad-spectrum antibiotics
- Monitor for signs of increased intra-abdominal pressure
- Patients are at risk for developing abdominal compartment syndrome (caused by intra-abdominal hypertension) if the abdominal closure is too tight
  - Shock/cardiac dysfunction, reduced venous return
  - Acute kidney injury
  - Restrictive lung disease and/or respiratory failure
  - Decreased splanchnic and liver blood flow (prolonged drug effect)
- Postoperative fluid management
  - Day 1: 60 mL/kg/day
  - Day 2: 90 mL/kg/day
  - Day 3: 120 mL/kg/day
  - Day 4: 150 mL/kg/day
  - Day 5: 150 mL/kg/day
- Measure glucose levels regularly and treat hypoglycemia with 1-2 mL/kg of 10% glucose
- Maintain body temperature
- Early complications: Necrotizing enterocolitis, renal insufficiency, pneumonia, patent ductus arteriosus, cellulitis of the abdominal wall, abdominal wall breakdown, gastroesophageal reflux, and cholestasis

## SUGGESTED READING

- Poddar R, Hartley L. Exomphalos and gastroschisis. Continuing Education in Anaesthesia Critical Care & Pain. 2009;9(2):48-51.
- Saraiya NR. GASTROSCHISIS AND OMPHALOCELE. In: Houck PJ, Haché M, Sun LS. eds. Handbook of Pediatric Anesthesia. Mgraw Hill; 2015. Accessed February 14, 2023. https://accessanesthesiology.mhmedical.com/content.aspx?bookid=1189&sectionid=70363342
- Wouters K, Walker I. Neonatal anaesthesia 2: Anaesthesia for neonates with abdominal wall defects. WFSA. August 28, 2008. Accessed February 14, 2023. https://resources.wfsahq.org/atotw/neonatal-anaesthesia-2-anaesthesia-for-neonates-with-abdominal-wall-defects/

# PATENT DUCTUS ARTERIOSUS

## LEARNING OBJECTIVES

- Define patent ductus arteriosus
- Describe the signs and symptoms of patent ductus arteriosus
- Anesthetic management of a patient with patent ductus arteriosus

## DEFINITION AND MECHANISM

- Patent ductus arteriosus (PDA) is a congenital heart defect in which there is a persistent opening between the aorta and pulmonary artery
- The ductus arteriosus is a blood vessel in the developing fetus that connects the trunk of the pulmonary artery to the proximal descending aorta, allowing most of the blood from the right ventricle to bypass the fetus's fluid-filled non-functioning lungs
- In PDA, the ductus arteriosus fails to close after birth
- PDA allows a portion of oxygenated blood from the left heart to flow back to the lungs by flowing from the aorta (higher pressure) to the pulmonary artery → left-to-right shunt

## SIGNS AND SYMPTOMS

- Rapid breathing
- Shortness of breath
- Sweating during feeding
- Fatigue or tiredness

- Feeding difficulties
- Failure to thrive
- Tachycardia
- Heart murmur

## COMPLICATIONS

- Pulmonary hypertension
- Pulmonary edema
- Heart failure
- Eisenmenger syndrome
- Endocarditis

- Necrotizing enterocolitis
- Bronchopulmonary dysplasia
- Intraventricular hemorrhage
- Neurodevelopmental delay
- Prolonged mechanical ventilation

## RISK FACTORS

- Premature birth
- Hypoxemia
- Congenital rubella syndrome
- Chromosomal abnormalities (e.g., Down syndrome)
- Family history and genetic conditions (e.g., CHARGE syndrome, Goldenhar syndrome, VACTERL)
- Female gender

## DIAGNOSIS

- Echocardiogram
- Chest X-ray
- ECG
- Cardiac catheterization (usually not needed to diagnose PDA, but might be used if PDA occurs with other heart problems)

# TREATMENT

- Nonsteroidal anti-inflammatory drugs (NSAIDs; e.g., ibuprofen, indomethacin) in premature babies
- NSAIDs will not close a PDA in full-term babies, children, or adults
- Surgery to close the PDA
  - Catheter procedure
  - Open-heart surgery (surgical closure)
  - Regular health checkups for life to check for complications, even after treatment to close the opening

# MANAGEMENT

## Preoperative management

- Hydration
- Avoid fluid overload
- Inotropic support, if required
- Crossmatch blood
- Premedication with midazolam 0.5 mg/kg PO or 0.05-0.2 mg/kg IV to reduce anxiety and smooth induction
- Pulse oximetry monitoring after giving premedication

## Intraoperative management

- Avoid hypothermia, hemodilution, hypoxia, and hyperoxia
- Anesthesia medications cause changes in systemic vascular resistance (SVR) and pulmonary vascular resistance (PVR), resulting in unbalancing of pulmonary blood flow (PBF)
  - High PBF leads to pulmonary edema and desaturation
  - Low PBF leads to desaturation and acidosis
- Monitoring: ECG, $SpO_2$, invasive blood pressure, $EtCO_2$, airway pressure, temperature, ABG, TEE, urine output
- Induction of anesthesia
  - Preoxygenation
  - Prolonged onset time of IV agents expected due to L → R shunt, no change in inhalational induction
  - IV agents: 1-2 mg/kg ketamine with 20 µg/kg glycopyrrolate
  - Neuromuscular blocking agent: 0.1 mg/kg rocuronium IV
  - If there is no IV line: Sevoflurane induction
  - Avoid succinylcholine (contracture of PDA)
  - Dexamethasone 0.2-0.5 mg/kg
  - Ondansetron 0.1 mg/kg to avoid nausea and vomiting

- Maintenance of anesthesia
  - Sevoflurane, air, and oxygen
  - Rocuronium
  - 1-2 µg/kg fentanyl (small doses) to blunt hemodynamic changes during stimuli
  - An increase in oxygen concentration decreases PVR
  - Avoid nitrous oxide (pulmonary hypertension)
- Ventilation
  - Controlled
  - Ventilatory goals: Tidal volume adjusted to keep PIP pressure between 15-25 cm $H_2O$
  - $FiO_2$ adjusted to keep $PaO_2$ between 50-70 mmHg
  - $SpO_2$ between 87-92%
  - $EtCO_2$ 30-35 cm $H_2O$
  - Hypoventilation can reverse shunt due to HPV
  - Hyperventilation can increase L → R shunt due to a reduction in PVR
- Hemodynamics
  - Maintenance fluid 4 mL/kg/h
  - IV tubing should be bubble-free to prevent embolization
  - Hematocrit is maintained as hemodilution leads to an increase in L → R shunt

## Postoperative management

- Paracetamol and local infiltration adequate for postprocedural analgesia
- Postoperative ventilation needed in premature babies

## SUGGESTED READING

- Kritzmire SM, Boyer TJ, Singh P. Anesthesia For Patients With Patent Ductus Arteriosus. [Updated 2022 Aug 9]. In: StatPearls [Internet]. Treasure Island (FL): StatPearls Publishing; 2022 Jan. Available from: https://www.ncbi.nlm.nih.gov/books/NBK572063/

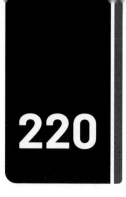

# PEDIATRIC ANXIETY

## LEARNING OBJECTIVES

- Understand the impact of preoperative anxiety in pediatric patients
- Management of preoperative anxiety in children with nonpharmacologic methods
- Describe the role of sedative premedication in managing preoperative anxiety in children
- Discuss the considerations for the selection of which premedication to use

## DEFINITION AND MECHANISM

- Hospitalization and surgery provoke stress and anxiety in pediatric patients
- Children experience the induction of anesthesia as the most stressful procedure during the entire perioperative period
- Intense levels of anxiety during anesthetic induction are associated with a higher risk of pain (i.e., increased opioid requirements), poor recovery, and emergence delirium
- Preoperative anxiety is also associated with psychological problems and negative behavioral changes in the two weeks after surgery, including apathy, separation anxiety, sleeping disturbances, enuresis, and aggression toward authority
- Predictors of anxiety are the age and temperament of the child → anesthetic plan must take these factors into account

## RISK FACTORS

- Age < 4 years
- Temperament: Shy, inhibited, dependent, withdrawn
- Limited time for preoperative preparation
- Anxious parents

- Previous negative experience with anesthesia or hospitalization
- Multiple previous hospital admissions
- Separation anxiety develops at 6-8 months old
- Age < 6 months can be soothed by a surrogate (i.e., nurse or physician)

## MANAGEMENT

- Use nonpharmacologic methods for all pediatric patients
- Use pharmacologic methods only in carefully selected pediatric patients
- Avoid pharmacologic methods in children with:
  - Potential difficult airway
  - OSA or central sleep apnea
  - Renal or hepatic impairment
  - Altered loss of consciousness (LOC)
  - Increased intracranial pressure
  - Acute systemic illness
  - Upper respiratory tract infection
  - New or unexplained oxygen desaturations
  - Allergies or adverse reactions to proposed medications
- When considering pharmacologic methods
  - Ensure patient monitoring
  - Have resuscitation equipment available
  - Transfer to OR or stretcher bed with portable suction and Ambu bag available, accompanied by a nurse or physician
  - Reduced LOC or respiratory depression → protect the airway, support ventilation, and consider naloxone (if opioid given) and flumazenil (if midazolam given)

### Nonpharmacologic methods

- Provide prehospital information and preparation (e.g., information leaflets, books, videos, OR tours)
- Play therapy (e.g., interaction with trained play therapists using visual aids and toys, and accompanying the patient to the OR)
- Distraction techniques (e.g., blowing bubbles, toys, videos, and games)
- Engagement with anesthetic equipment (e.g., holding the mask, "blowing up the balloon")
- Environment adjustments (e.g., lighting, music, minimal extraneous noise, limited healthcare staff)
- Actively involving parents/caregivers (e.g., parental presence for induction)
- Communication aids (e.g., info about the child's needs/routines)
- Relaxation techniques (e.g., breathing exercises, hypnosis)

*Pharmacologic methods – Sedative premedication*

| Drug | Route of administration | Dose | Remarks |
|---|---|---|---|
| Benzodiazepines | | | |
| Midazolam | PO | 0.5-0.75 mg/kg, max. 20 mg | Paradoxical agitation in some patients |
| | IN | 0.3 mg/kg | Causes stinging |
| Lorazepam | IV | 0.05-0.1 mg/kg | |
| Temazepam | PR | 0.05-0.1 mg/kg | Preferred in older children |
| | PO | 0.025-0.05 mg/kg, max. 4 mg | |
| | PO | 0.3-0.5 mg/kg, max. 20 mg | |
| Alpha-2 agonists | | | |
| Clonidine | PO | 3-4 mcg/kg | Added benefits of reduced need for rescue analgesia, reduced emergence agitation, PONV, and shivering<br><br>Caution in patients with grade 2 or 3 heart block, hypertension, cardiovascular disease, instability, on digoxin |
| | IN | 2-4 mcg/kg | |
| Dexmedetomidine | PR | 2.5-5 mcg/kg | |
| | IN | 1-2 mcg/kg | |
| NMDA antagonist | | | |
| Ketamine | PO | 5-8 mg/kg | Hallucinations and increased secretions can occur, as emergence delirium and PONV<br>IM ketamine is reserved for older uncooperative children with developmental problems |
| | IM | 4-6 mg/kg | |
| | IV | 0.5-1 mg/kg | |
| Opioids | | 0.2 mg/kg, max. 10 mg | Risk of respiratory depression |

PONV, postoperative nausea and vomiting; PO, per oral; PR, per rectal; IN, intranasal; IM, intramuscular; IV, intravenous.

## KEEP IN MIND

- Preoperative anxiety in pediatric patients is associated with adverse clinical and behavioral outcomes
- Multiple techniques may be valuable in managing preoperative anxiety
- Consider the need for sedative premedication during the preoperative assessment of every child
- Many factors influence the choice of premedication, including the pharmacological profile, possible adverse effects, and presence of comorbidities

### SUGGESTED READING

- Dave NM. Premedication and Induction of Anaesthesia in paediatric patients. Indian J Anaesth. 2019;63(9):713-720.
- Eijlers R, Staals LM, Legerstee JS, et al. Predicting Intense Levels of Child Anxiety During Anesthesia Induction at Hospital Arrival. J Clin Psychol Med Settings. 2021;28(2):313-322.
- Heikal S, Stuart G. Anxiolytic premedication for children. BJA Educ. 2020;20(7):220-225.

Pediatric anxiety

# PEDIATRIC PATIENT

## LEARNING OBJECTIVES

- Describe the differences in anatomy and physiology between pediatric patients and adults
- Understand how these differences impact anesthesia practice in pediatric patients

## DEFINITION AND MECHANISM

- Pediatric patients include the following groups
  - **Neonates:** A baby within 44 weeks of age from the date of conception
  - **Infants:** Up to 12 months of age
  - **Children:** 1-12 years
  - **Adolescents:** 13-16 years
- The differences between pediatric and adult anesthetic practice are reduced as patients become older

## ANATOMY AND PHYSIOLOGY

### Airway and respiratory system

- Large head, short neck, and prominent occiput
- The tongue is relatively large
- The larynx is high and anterior (C3-C4 level)
- The epiglottis is long, stiff, and U-shaped → flops anteriorly → the head needs to be in the neutral position to visualize the epiglottis
- Neonates breathe through their nose → narrow nasal passages are easily blocked by secretions and may be damaged by a nasogastric tube or nasally placed endotracheal tube (ETT)
- 50% of airway resistance comes from the nasal passages
- The airway is funnel-shaped and narrowest at the level of the cricoid cartilage
  - Trauma to the airway results in edema
  - Even 1 mm of edema can narrow a baby's airway by 60%
  - To prevent trauma that can cause subglottic edema and subsequent post-extubation stridor, it is important to ensure there is a leak around the endotracheal tube (ETT)
- ETT must be inserted to the correct length to sit at least 1 cm above the tracheal carina and should be securely taped to prevent tube dislodgement due to head movement
- Neonates and infants have a limited respiratory reserve
- Horizontal ribs prevent the "bucket handle" action seen in adult breathing and limit an increase in tidal volume (TV)
  - Ventilation is primarily diaphragmatic
  - Bulky abdominal organs or a stomach filled with gases from poor bag-mask ventilation can impinge on the contents of the chest and splint the diaphragm, reducing the ability to ventilate adequately
- The chest wall is more compliant → functional residual capacity (FRC) is relatively low
  - FRC decreases with apnea and anesthesia, causing lung collapse
- Minute ventilation is rate-dependent as there are little means to increase TV
- The closing volume is larger than the FRC until 6-8 years → increased tendency for airway closure at end-expiration → neonates and infants need intermittent positive-pressure ventilation (IPPV) during anesthesia and benefit from a higher respiratory rate (RR) and use of PEEP
- Continuous positive airway pressure (CPAP) during spontaneous ventilation improves oxygenation and decreases the work of breathing
- Work of respiration may be 15% of oxygen consumption
- Ventilation muscles are easily subject to fatigue due to the low percentage of type I muscle fibers in the diaphragm → number increases to the adult level over the first year of life
- Alveoli are thick-walled at birth → only 10% of the total number of alveoli found in adults → alveoli clusters develop over the first 8 years of life
- Postoperative apnea is common in premature infants → associated with desaturation and bradycardia
- RR = 24 – age/2
- Spontaneous ventilation TV = 6-8 mL/kg; IPPV TV = 7-10 mL/kg
- Physiological dead space = 30% and increased by anesthetic equipment

## Cardiovascular system

- The myocardium is less contractile in neonates, causing the ventricles to be less compliant and less able to generate tension during contraction → limits the size of the stroke volume → cardiac output is rate-dependent
- The infant behaves with a fixed cardiac output state
- The vagal parasympathetic tone is predominant, making neonates and infants more prone to bradycardia
- Bradycardia is associated with a reduced cardiac output
- Treat hypoxia-associated bradycardia with oxygen and ventilation
- External cardiac compression is required in neonates with a heart rate of ≤ 60 bpm or 60-80 bpm with adequate ventilation
- Cardiac output = 300-400 mL/kg/min at birth; 200 mL/kg/min within a few months
- Sinus arrhythmia is common in children, all other irregular rhythms are abnormal
- The patent ductus contracts in the first few days of life and will fibrose within 2-4 weeks
- Closure of the foramen ovale is pressure-dependent and closes in the first day of life but it may reopen within the next 5 years

## Normal heart rates (beats/min) and systolic blood pressure (mmHg)

| Age | Average HR (bpm) | Range HR (bpm) | Mean SBP (mmHg) |
|---|---|---|---|
| Preterm | 130 | 120-170 | 40-55 |
| Newborn | 120 | 100-170 | 50-90 |
| 1-11 months | 120 | 80-160 | 85-105 |
| 2 years | 110 | 80-130 | 95-105 |
| 4 years | 100 | 80-120 | 95-110 |
| 6 years | 110 | 75-115 | 95-110 |
| 8 years | 90 | 70-110 | 95-110 |
| 10 years | 90 | 70-110 | 100-120 |
| 14 years Boy | 80 | 60-100 | 110-130 |
| 14 years Girl | 85 | 65-105 | 110-130 |
| 16 years Boy | 75 | 55-95 | 110-130 |
| 16 years Girl | 80 | 60-100 | 110-130 |

## Normal blood volumes

| Age | Blood volume (mL/kg) |
|---|---|
| Newborns | 85-90 |
| 6 weeks to 2 years | 85 |
| 2 years to puberty | 80 |

## Renal system

- The renal blood flow and glomerular filtration are low in the first 2 years of life due to high renal vascular resistance
- The tubular function is immature until 8 months → infants are unable to excrete a large sodium load
- Dehydration is poorly tolerated
- Urine output = 1-2 mL/kg/h

## Hepatic system

- Immature liver function with decreased function of hepatic enzymes
- Barbiturates and opioids have a longer duration of action due to the slower metabolism

## Glucose metabolism

- Hypoglycemia is common in the stressed neonate
- Monitor glucose levels regularly
- Neurological damage may result from hypoglycemia → infusion of 10% glucose to prevent this
- Infants and older children maintain blood glucose better and rarely need glucose infusions
- Hyperglycemia is usually iatrogenic

## Hematology

- 70-90% of hemoglobin molecules are fetal hemoglobin (HbF)
- Within 3 months, the levels of HbF drop to 5%, and adult hemoglobin (HbA) predominates
- Vitamin K-dependent clotting factors (II, VII, IX, X) and platelet function are deficient in the first months → administer vitamin K at birth to prevent hemorrhagic disease
- Transfusion is recommended when 15% of the circulating blood volume has been lost

## Temperature control

- Babies and infants have a large surface area to weight ratio with minimal subcutaneous fat → poorly developed shivering, sweating, and vasoconstriction mechanisms
- Brown fat metabolism is required for non-shivering thermogenesis
- The optimal ambient temperature to prevent heat loss is 34°C for the premature infant, 32°C for neonates, and 28°C for adolescents and adults
- Hypothermia causes respiratory depression, acidosis, decreased cardiac output, increased duration of action of medications, decreased platelet function, and increased risk of infection

## Central nervous system

- Pain is associated with an increased heart rate, blood pressure, and neuroendocrine response
- Narcotics depress the ventilation response to a rise in $PaCO_2$
- The blood-brain barrier (BBB) is poorly formed → barbiturates, opioids, antibiotics, and bilirubin cross the BBB easily, causing a prolonged duration of action
- Cerebral vessels in the preterm infant are thin-walled and fragile → prone to intraventricular hemorrhages → risk is increased with hypoxia, hypercarbia, hypernatremia, low hematocrit, awake airway manipulations, rapid bicarbonate administration, fluctuations in blood pressure and cerebral blood flow
- Cerebral autoregulation is present and functional from birth

## Psychology

- Infants < 6 months are usually not upset by separation from their parents and will accept a stranger
- Children up to 4 years are upset by separation from their parents, as well as unfamiliar people and surroundings
- School-age children are more upset by the surgical procedure and the possibility of pain
- Adolescents fear narcosis and pain, loss of control, and the possibility of not being able to cope with the illness
- Parental anxiety is readily perceived and reacted to by the child

# ANESTHETIC CONSIDERATIONS

- Preoperative fasting
  - **Solids and milk > 12 months:** 6 hours
  - **Breast milk < 12 months:** 4 hours
  - **Formula feed < 12 months:** 6 hours
  - **Unlimited clear fluids:** 2 hours
  - Increased incidence of nausea and vomiting with long fasting periods
- Preoperative medical and anesthetic history
  - Previous problems with anesthetics, including family history
  - Allergies
  - Previous medical problems, including congenital anomalies

- □ Recent respiratory illness
- □ Current medications
- □ Recent immunizations
- □ Fasting times
- □ Presence of loose teeth
- Weigh the child → all medication doses are related to body weight
- Physical examination of the airway and cardiorespiratory systems
- Further investigations that may be necessary
  - □ **Hemoglobin:** Large expected blood loss, premature infants, systemic disease, congenital heart disease
  - □ **Electrolytes:** Renal or metabolic disease, intravenous fluids, dehydration
  - □ **Chest radiograph:** Active respiratory disease, scoliosis, congenital heart disease
- Uncooperative patient
- Altered airway anatomy
- Increased risk of laryngospasm
- **Inhalational induction:** Halothane and sevoflurane
- **Intravenous induction:** Propofol, thiopentone, or ketamine
- Rapid desaturation on induction
- Increased vagal tone and potential for bradycardia
- Rate-dependent cardiac output
- Altered pharmacokinetics and -dynamics
  - □ Increased minimum alveolar concentration (MAC)
  - □ Immature liver and kidney function
  - □ Increased total body water

## SUGGESTED READING

- Macfarlane F. Paediatric anatomy and physiology and the basics of paediatric anaesthesia. December 16, 2005. Accessed February 2, 2023. https://resources.wfsahq.org/atotw/paediatric-anatomy-and-physiology-and-the-basics-of-paediatric-anaesthesia/

# PIERRE-ROBIN SEQUENCE

## LEARNING OBJECTIVES

- Describe Pierre-Robin sequence
- Outline the anesthetic management considerations for patients with Pierre-Robin sequence
- Summarize the anticipated complications during the intraoperative and postoperative period among patients with Pierre-Robin sequence
- Describe the common intubation methods before administering general anesthesia among patients with (PRS)

## DEFINITION AND MECHANISM

- Pierre-Robin sequence (PRS), previously known as Pierre-Robin syndrome, is a rare congenital birth defect characterized by facial abnormalities
- The three main features are:
  - Micrognathia (mandibular hypoplasia), which causes glossoptosis (posterior displacement or retractation of the tongue), which in turn causes breathing problems due to upper airway obstruction
  - A wide, U-shaped cleft palate is commonly present in children with PRS
  - Airway obstruction and respiratory distress are clinical hallmarks of PRS
- At birth, neonates mainly show signs of respiratory distress (i.e., stridor, retractions, and cyanosis); some manifest with feeding difficulties, gastroesophageal reflux, aspiration, and failure to thrive
- PRS is more a sequence than a syndrome, because one initial malformation leads to a sequential chain of events causing the other anomalies
- PRS can occur as an isolated mandibular abnormality but is more often part of an underlying disorder or syndrome (e.g., fetal alcohol syndrome, Stickler syndrome, Treacher-Collins syndrome, and velocardiofacial syndrome)

| Associated syndrome | Associated anomalies | Anesthetic concerns |
|---|---|---|
| Fetal alcohol syndrome | Microcephaly, maxillary hypoplasia, micrognathia, short neck, ventricular septal defect, cognitive developmental delay, hyperactivity | May be difficult to ventilate and intubate<br>Preoperative echo indicated<br>Consider subacute bacterial endocarditis prophylaxis<br>May be uncooperative |
| Stickler syndrome | Marfanoid appearance, airway obstruction, micrognathia, joint laxity, mitral valve prolapse | May be difficult to ventilate and intubate<br>Care with positioning |
| Treacher-Collins syndrome | Craniofacial clefting, mandibular hypoplasia, may have obstructive sleep apnea, may have congenital heart disease | May be difficult or impossible to intubate<br>Preoperative echo indicated<br>Consider subacute bacterial endocarditis prophylaxis |
| Velocardiofacial (DiGeorge) syndrome | Microdeletion of chromosome 22, microcephaly, micrognathia, congenital heart disease, may have developmental delay, neonatal hypocalcemia, T-cell immune deficiency | May be difficult to intubate<br>Preoperative echo indicated<br>Consider subacute bacterial endocarditis prophylaxis<br>Blood products need to be irradiated |

## SIGNS AND SYMPTOMS

- Underdeveloped mandible and small chin
- Posterior displacement or retraction of the tongue due to the small mandible
- Obstructive sleep apnea (OSA) and upper airway obstruction due to tongue that falls toward the throat
- High-arched palate (roof of the mouth)
- Cleft palate (opening in the roof of the mouth)
- Natal teeth (teeth that are visible at birth)
- Dysphagia (difficulty swallowing)
- Repeated upper respiratory tract and ear infections
- Temporary hearing loss due to fluid buildup behind the ear (middle ear effusion), a common symptom of cleft palate
- Speech difficulty

## CAUSES

- Intrauterine compression of fetal mandible
- De-novo mutations on chromosomes 2 (possibly GAD1 gene), 4, 11 (possibly PVRL1 gene), or 17 (possibly SOX9 or KCNJ2 gene)

## COMPLICATIONS

Short-term complications are due to upper airway obstruction
- Breathing difficulties, respiratory distress
- Desaturations
- Choking episodes (asphyxia)
- Difficulty feeding, malnutrition
- Aspiration risk
- Hypoxemia

Long-term complications are due to hypoxic injury and inability to feed well
- Cerebral impairment
- Pulmonary hypertension
- Cor pulmonale
- Failure to thrive
- Gastroesophageal reflux

## PROGNOSIS

- Left untreated, PRS can be fatal
- Children usually reach full development and size
- General prognosis is good once the initial breathing and feeding difficulties are overcome in infancy

## TREATMENT

- **Mild airway obstruction:** Manage conservatively with nasopharyngeal airways (NPAs), prone positioning, and mechanical feeders
- **Moderate or severe obstruction:** Requires invasive interventions such as gastrostomy tube placement, tongue-lip adhesion (TLA), mandibular distraction osteogenesis (MDO), and tracheostomy

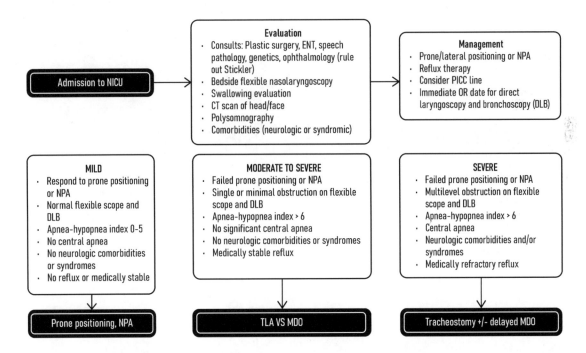

ENT, ear, nose and throat; DLB, direct laryngoscopy and bronchoscopy; NPA, nasopharyngeal airway; PICC line, peripherally inserted central catheter; TLA, tongue-lip adhesion; MDO, mandibular distraction osteogenesis

Pierre-Robin sequence

# ANESTHESIA CHALLENGES

- Airway is challenging to ventilate and intubate due to craniofacial dysmorphology
  - Maintaining a seal for ventilation (facemask) can be challenging due to facial deformities
  - Direct laryngoscopy and tracheal intubation are difficult during infancy but become more manageable with age and (mandibular) growth
- Postoperatively, patients can spontaneously develop airway collapse
  - Occurs due to preexisting airway obstruction, possible OSA, chronic hypoxia, and increased opioid sensitivity
  - Diagnosed with paradoxical breathing patterns, intercostal indrawing, subcostal & sternal recession, and tracheal tug
- Neonates are increasingly sensitive to opioids
  - Infants who develop OSA due to glossoptosis have increased opioid sensitivity due to the upregulation of opioid receptors in the brainstem
  - Patients with severe obstruction have reduced opioid requirements and require careful dose adjustments
- Feeding difficulties, swallowing disorders, and co-existing gastroesophageal reflux are frequently complicated by bronchial microaspirations and pulmonary infections → implement aspiration precautions before elective procedures
- Malnutrition and associated failure to thrive due to difficulties with feeding and airway

# MANAGEMENT

## Preoperative management

- History includes micrognathia, glossoptosis, and airway obstruction; additionally, a cleft palate may be present but this is not a required feature of PRS
- PRS can be seen as an isolated anomaly or as part of other syndromes
- Perform induction with a pediatric otolaryngology present in the OR with emergency bronchoscopy and tracheostomy equipment

## Anesthetic management

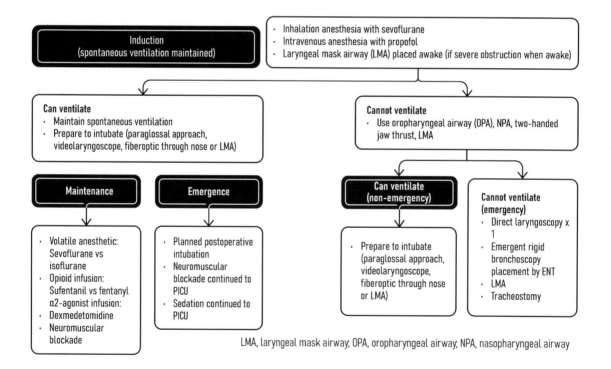

LMA, laryngeal mask airway; OPA, oropharyngeal airway; NPA, nasopharyngeal airway

### *Postoperative management*

- Acute postoperative airway obstruction may result in hypoxia, negative pressure pulmonary edema, and death
- Patients are prone to postoperative respiratory complications (i.e., airway obstruction, oxygen desaturation, and an escalation of postoperative respiratory care) from airway obstructions due to previous airway obstruction, opioid sensitivity (associated with OSA), and surgically induced airway edema (release the mouth retractor periodically to minimize the risk of postoperative tongue edema)
- Maximize nonopioid analgesics including local anesthetic (regional blocks or local infiltration), acetaminophen, and ketorolac
- Reduce opioid doses
- Observe patients in a monitored setting with pulse oximetry

## KEEP IN MIND

- The primary concern in PRS is upper airway obstruction with subsequent respiratory distress and feeding difficulty
- Feeding difficulty may manifest as gastroesophageal reflux and failure to thrive

## SUGGESTED READING

- Cladis F, Kumar A, Grunwaldt L, Otteson T, Ford M, Losee JE. Pierre Robin Sequence: a perioperative review. Anesth Analg. 2014;119(2):400-412.
- Hegde N, Singh A. Anesthetic Consideration In Pierre-Robin Sequence. [Updated 2022 Jul 26]. In: StatPearls [Internet]. Treasure Island (FL): StatPearls Publishing; 2022 Jan. Available from: https://www.ncbi.nlm.nih.gov/books/NBK576442/

# PREMATURE INFANT

## LEARNING OBJECTIVES

- Define prematurity and describe its classification
- Describe the specific anatomical, physiological, and pharmacological difficulties in premature infants
- Understand how these difficulties impact anesthesia in premature infants

## DEFINITION AND MECHANISM

- Prematurity is defined as a live birth before 37 weeks of gestational age
  - Moderate to late preterm: 32-37 weeks
  - Very preterm: 28-32 weeks
  - Extremely preterm: < 28 weeks
- Preterm infants can also be categorized based on their birth weight
  - Low birth weight: < 2500 g
  - Very low birth weight: < 1500 g
  - Extremely low birth weight: < 1000 g
- Approximately 10% of infants are born prematurely
- The earlier the baby is born, the higher the risk of complications
- Important growth occurs in the final months and weeks of pregnancy (e.g., the brain, lungs, and liver need the final weeks of pregnancy to develop fully)

### Known risk factors of premature delivery

- Previous premature birth
- Pregnancy with twins, triplets, or other multiples
- Interval of < 6 months between pregnancies
- Conceiving through in vitro fertilization
- Problems with the uterus, cervix, or placenta
- Smoking and drug use
- Infections (of the amniotic fluid and lower genital tract)
- Chronic conditions (e.g., hypertension and diabetes)
- Being underweight or overweight before pregnancy
- Stressful life events
- Multiple miscarriages or abortions
- Physical injury or trauma
- Many women who have a premature birth have no known risk factors

## ANATOMICAL AND PHYSIOLOGICAL CONSIDERATIONS

- Altered airway anatomy
- Respiratory derangements
  - Development of conducting airways, alveoli, and pulmonary vasculature is interrupted
  - Surfactant is produced in insufficient quantities until 35 weeks
  - Respiratory distress syndrome
  - Bronchopulmonary dysplasia
  - Rapid desaturation
  - Postoperative apnea
  - Persistent pulmonary hypertension
- Cardiovascular derangements
  - Heart rate/preload-dependent cardiac output
  - Transitional circulation/patent ductus arteriosus (PDA)
  - Bradycardia
  - Congenital heart disease
- CNS derangements
  - Intraventricular hemorrhage
  - Seizures
  - Cerebral palsy
  - Retinopathy of prematurity
  - Apnea

- Gastrointestinal derangements
  - Gastroesophageal reflux disease
  - Necrotizing enterocolitis
- Metabolic derangements
  - Impaired temperature and glucose regulation
    - Prone to hypothermia
    - Hyperglycemia is caused by incomplete suppression of hepatic glucose production and defective insulin secretion
    - Hypoglycemia results from minimal glycogen reserves and limited ketogenesis and lipolysis
- Hematologic derangements
  - Anemia
  - Thrombocytopenia
  - Coagulopathy

## PHARMACOLOGICAL CONSIDERATIONS

- Altered pharmacology
- Increased volume of distribution
- Opioid sensitivity
- Decreased clearance, protein binding, metabolism, and minimum alveolar concentration
- Drugs will accumulate with repeated doses or infusions
- Immature renal and hepatic function

## TREATMENT

- Admission to NICU
  - Supportive care
  - Incubator: To maintain normothermia
  - Monitoring vital signs: Blood pressure, heart rate, breathing, and temperature
  - Ventilator may be used to help with breathing
  - Placement of a nasogastric tube
  - Fluid therapy
  - Bilirubin lights: To treat infant jaundice
  - Blood transfusion if needed
- Medications: To promote maturing and stimulation of normal functioning of the lungs, heart, and circulation
  - Surfactant to treat respiratory distress syndrome
  - Aerosolized or IV medication to strengthen breathing and heart rate
  - Antibiotics to treat infections
  - Diuretics to increase urine output and manage excess fluid
  - Medicine to close PDA
- Surgery (e.g., PDA closure)

## MANAGEMENT

### Preoperative management

- Manage premature infants in specialized pediatric centers
- Risk stratification
  - Five times higher in-hospital mortality for non-cardiac surgery than term neonates
  - Discuss proposed interventions with the surgical and NICU multidisciplinary teams and family
- Some surgical procedures can be performed in the NICU (e.g., PDA closure), especially if the patient is unstable or difficult to transport
- Preoperatively optimize respiratory, cardiovascular, hepatic, renal, and hematological derangements
- Preoperatively optimize fluid, electrolyte, and glucose derangements
- Airway and ventilation
  - Assess the presence of subglottic stenosis, tracheal or laryngomalacia, frequency and severity of apneas, history of difficult intubation or ventilation
  - Administer methylxanthine medications to prevent apneas and facilitate extubation
- Cardiovascular system
  - Inotropic support
  - Perform echocardiography to assess ventricular function and the presence of shunts or other congenital defects
- Neurological system
  - Administer morphine (10-40 µg/kg/h) to sedate patients to tolerate tracheal tube
  - Perform neurological assessment in case of preexisting neurological concerns
- Difficult IV access

*Intraoperative management*

## PREMATURE INFANT: INTRAOPERATIVE MANAGEMENT

**INDUCTION OF ANESTHESIA**

- Balanced anesthetic including a narcotic (e.g., 1-5 mcg/kg fentanyl), IV anesthetic agent (e.g., 3-5 mg/kg propofol or 1-2 mg/kg ketamine) and a nondepolarizing muscle relaxant
- Perform inhalational induction if spontaneous ventilation has to be preserved in case of a difficult airway
- Premedication with 20 mcg/kg atropine or 10 mcg/kg glycopyrrolate IV can attenuate the vagal response to intubation

**MAINTENANCE OF ANESTHESIA**

- With volatile anesthetics (e.g., sevoflurane)

**VENTILATION**

- Continue with NICU ventilation parameters
- Volume-targeted or pressure-limited mode targeting tidal volumes of 5 mL/kg
- Ventilatory frequency: 30-60 bpm
- PEEP: 6-8 cm $H_2O$
- Titrate above to maintain normocapnia or mild hypercapnia
- Titrate $FiO_2$ to achieve $SpO_2$ 90-95%

**FLUIDS**

- Balanced isotonic electrolyte solution with 1-2.5% glucose for maintenance at a rate of 10 mL/kg/h → reduces hyperglycemia and hyponatremia
- Manage hypoglycemia with a bolus of 2 mL/kg 10% glucose
- Maintain urine output at 1-2 mL/kg/h
- Regular intraoperative glucose checks

**TEMPERATURE**

- Ensure continuous temperature monitoring and maintain normothermia

**ANALGESIA**

- Paracetamol unless contraindicated
- Avoid opioids

**AIRWAY MANAGEMENT**

- Tracheal intubation to secure the airway
- Securely tape the tracheal tube to prevent dislodgement
- Use uncuffed tubes as the smallest cuffed tube is not recommended for neonates < 3 kg
- Increased risk for difficult airway if the neonate < 32 weeks or < 1500 g

| Gestation (weeks) | Weight (kg) | Blade size | Tube size (uncuffed) | Oral depth (cm) | Nasal depth (cm) |
|---|---|---|---|---|---|
| ≤ 29 | <1 | 00 | 2.5 | 5.5-6.5 | 7.0-7.5 |
| 30-35 | 1-2 | 0 | 3.0 | 7.0-7.5 | 8.0-8.5 |
| < 35 | >2 | 1 | 3.5 | 8.0-9.0 | 9.0-10 |

*Postoperative management*

- The majority of premature infants remain intubated after surgery
- Awake extubation after full reversal of neuromuscular block and adequate ventilation
- Postoperative apnea monitoring for 24-48 hours after surgery (unless if the infant is >50-60 weeks postmenstrual age and has no other risk factors for apnea)

# KEEP IN MIND

- Premature infants are a high-risk group and present with unique anatomical, physiological, and pharmacological challenges
- Anesthetic considerations are based on the physiological immaturity of various body systems, associated congenital disorders, and poor tolerance of anesthetic medications
- The benefits of adequate anesthesia and analgesia must outweigh the risk of cardiorespiratory depression
- The main goal of anesthesia in this pediatric patient population is to titrate anesthetics to the desired effect while carefully monitoring the cardiorespiratory status

## SUGGESTED READING

- Macrae J, Ng E, Whyte H. Anaesthesia for premature infants. BJa Education. 2021;21(9):355-363.
- Taneja B, Srivastava V, Saxena KN. Physiological and anaesthetic considerations for the preterm neonate undergoing surgery. J Neonatal Surg. 2012;1(1):14.

Premature infant

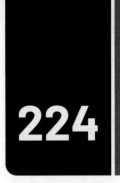

# 224

# PYLORIC STENOSIS

## LEARNING OBJECTIVES

- Describe the electrolyte and acid-base abnormalities associated with pyloric stenosis
- Explain why these electrolyte and acid-base abnormalities need to be corrected preoperatively
- Anesthetic management of a pediatric patient with pyloric stenosis

## DEFINITION AND MECHANISM

- Pyloric stenosis, or infantile hypertrophic pyloric stenosis, is an uncommon condition in infants characterized by abnormal thickening of the pylorus muscles in the stomach, leading to gastric outlet obstruction
- Typically seen between 2 and 12 weeks of age, patients present with projectile vomiting after feedings, dehydration, and failure to thrive
- The danger of pyloric stenosis comes from the dehydration and electrolyte disturbance rather than the underlying problem itself → infant has to be stabilized by correcting the dehydration and hypochloremic alkalosis with IV fluids

## SIGNS AND SYMPTOMS

- Symptoms usually appear within 3-5 weeks after birth
- Bile-free projectile vomiting after every feeding
- Persistent hunger
- Stomach contractions (visible peristalsis in the left upper quadrant from left to right)
- Changes in bowel movements
- Weight problems

## COMPLICATIONS

- Failure to grow and develop, failure to thrive
- Dehydration, hypovolemia
- Metabolic alkalosis
- Electrolyte abnormalities (hypochloremia, hyponatremia, hypokalemia)
- Stomach irritation
- Jaundice

## RISK FACTORS

- First-born male children
- Preterm birth
- Cesarean section
- Family history
- Smoking during pregnancy
- Bottle feeding
- Early antibiotic use (e.g., erythromycin to treat whooping cough)
- White and Hispanic children

## PATHOPHYSIOLOGY

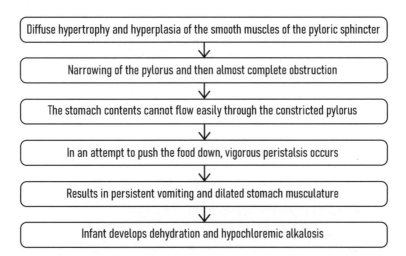

Diffuse hypertrophy and hyperplasia of the smooth muscles of the pyloric sphincter

↓

Narrowing of the pylorus and then almost complete obstruction

↓

The stomach contents cannot flow easily through the constricted pylorus

↓

In an attempt to push the food down, vigorous peristalsis occurs

↓

Results in persistent vomiting and dilated stomach musculature

↓

Infant develops dehydration and hypochloremic alkalosis

# TREATMENT

- Correction of dehydration and hypochloremic alkalosis before surgery with IV fluids ➔ accomplished within 24-48 hours
- Surgery: Pyloromyotomy

# MANAGEMENT

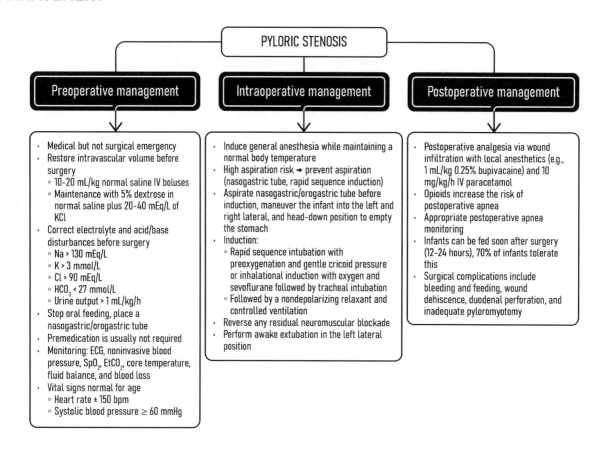

**PYLORIC STENOSIS**

**Preoperative management**

- Medical but not surgical emergency
- Restore intravascular volume before surgery
  - 10-20 mL/kg normal saline IV boluses
  - Maintenance with 5% dextrose in normal saline plus 20-40 mEq/L of KCl
- Correct electrolyte and acid/base disturbances before surgery
  - Na > 130 mEq/L
  - K > 3 mmol/L
  - Cl > 90 mEq/L
  - $HCO_3$ < 27 mmol/L
  - Urine output > 1 mL/kg/h
- Stop oral feeding, place a nasogastric/orogastric tube
- Premedication is usually not required
- Monitoring: ECG, noninvasive blood pressure, $SpO_2$, $EtCO_2$, core temperature, fluid balance, and blood loss
- Vital signs normal for age
  - Heart rate ± 150 bpm
  - Systolic blood pressure ≥ 60 mmHg

**Intraoperative management**

- Induce general anesthesia while maintaining a normal body temperature
- High aspiration risk ➔ prevent aspiration (nasogastric tube, rapid sequence induction)
- Aspirate nasogastric/orogastric tube before induction, maneuver the infant into the left and right lateral, and head-down position to empty the stomach
- Induction:
  - Rapid sequence intubation with preoxygenation and gentle cricoid pressure or inhalational induction with oxygen and sevoflurane followed by tracheal intubation
  - Followed by a nondepolarizing relaxant and controlled ventilation
- Reverse any residual neuromuscular blockade
- Perform awake extubation in the left lateral position

**Postoperative management**

- Postoperative analgesia via wound infiltration with local anesthetics (e.g., 1 mL/kg 0.25% bupivacaine) and 10 mg/kg/h IV paracetamol
- Opioids increase the risk of postoperative apnea
- Appropriate postoperative apnea monitoring
- Infants can be fed soon after surgery (12-24 hours), 70% of infants tolerate this
- Surgical complications include bleeding and feeding, wound dehiscence, duodenal perforation, and inadequate pyloromyotomy

# KEEP IN MIND

- Vomiting associated with pyloric stenosis results in hypochloremia, hyponatremia, hypokalemia, metabolic alkalosis, and dehydration, all of which have to be corrected before general anesthesia and surgery
- Empty the stomach using a nasogastric or orogastric tube before induction of anesthesia
- Ensure an adequate depth of anesthesia with a complete neuromuscular block before laryngoscopy to minimize the risk of regurgitation and pulmonary aspiration

---

## SUGGESTED READING

- Craig R, Deeley A. Anaesthesia for pyloromyotomy. BJA Educ. 2018;18(6):173-177.
- Houck PJ. PYLORIC STENOSIS. In: Houck PJ, Haché M, Sun LS. eds. Handbook of Pediatric Anesthesia. Mgraw Hill; 2015. Accessed February 14, 2023. https://accessanesthesiology.mhmedical.com/content.aspx?bookid=1189&sectionid=70363285
- Pollard BJ, Kitchen G. Handbook of Clinical Anaesthesia. 4th ed. Taylor & Francis group; 2018. Chapter 24 Paediatrics, Lomas B.

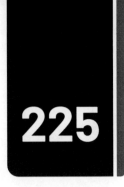

# SCOLIOSIS

**225**

## LEARNING OBJECTIVES

- Definition and types of scoliosis
- Non-operative treatment options
- Pre-operative evaluation

## DEFINITION AND MECHANISM

- Scoliosis refers to lateral curvature of the spine, vertebral body rotation, and angulation of the rib
- These are classified as structural or non-structural (e.g., length discrepancy)
- Men and women are equally affected, with women often requiring more surgical intervention
- Congenital scoliosis:
  - May present at any age and is a result of either failure of vertebral segmentation (a bar) or failure of formation (a hemivertebra)
  - Congenital scoliosis is often part of a generalized condition, such as Goldenhar syndrome or spina bifida
  - It may be associated with abnormalities in renal, cardiac, respiratory, or neurological systems
- Acquired scoliosis:
  - Mainly idiopathic
  - Infantile onset idiopathic scoliosis (scoliosis before the age of 8 years) carries the most serious prognosis and if left unchecked is likely to result in cardiopulmonary failure in middle age

## TYPES OF SCOLIOSIS

| Idiopathic scoliosis is the most common with a wide range of causes | Collagen abnormalities, hormones, genetics, and growth abnormalities |
|---|---|
| Neuromuscular | Neuropathic<br>Upper motor neuron (e.g., cerebral palsy, spinal cord injury)<br>Lower motor neuron (e.g., poliomyelitis, myelomeningocele, spinal muscular atrophy)<br>Familial dysautonomia |
| Myopathic | Muscular dystrophy<br>Myotonic dystrophy |
| Congenital | Hemivertebrae<br>Congenitally fused ribs |
| Neurofibromatosis | Marfan's syndrome<br>Osteogenesis imperfecta<br>Arthrogryposis |
| Trauma | Vertebral fracture or surgery<br>Post thoracoplasty<br>Post radiation |

Neuromuscular scoliosis has been associated with increased intraoperative blood loss compared with idiopathic scoliosis

## DIAGNOSIS

- X-ray
- Clinical examinations

## CLASSIFICATION OF SEVERITY

- Cobb Angle:
  - Measured from a standing anteroposterior radiograph of the spine
  - The surgical treatment is recommended if the Cobb angle is greater than 45° – 50°
  - The degre e of Cobb Angle is associated with pulmonary and cardiovascular dysfunction

Scoliosis

# CONDITIONS ASSOCIATED WITH SCOLIOSIS

- Decreased overall lung function (restrictive) with a significantly reduced vital capacity and respiratory muscle function can be impaired as well
- An increased pulmonary vascular resistance and pulmonary hypertension, possibly leading to right ventricular hypertrophy and failure
- An increased risk of mitral valve prolapse
- An increased risk for malignant hyperthermia if scoliosis results from muscular dystrophies
- A potentially difficult airway

# NON-OPERATIVE TREATMENT

- Rigid bracing (thoracolumbosacral orthosis)
  - Indicated for a progressive curve greater than 25°
  - Results depend on compliance (social stigma and discomfort)
- Serial full-body casting
  - Indicated for infantile scoliosis
  - General anesthesia is required every 2-3 months

# MANAGEMENT

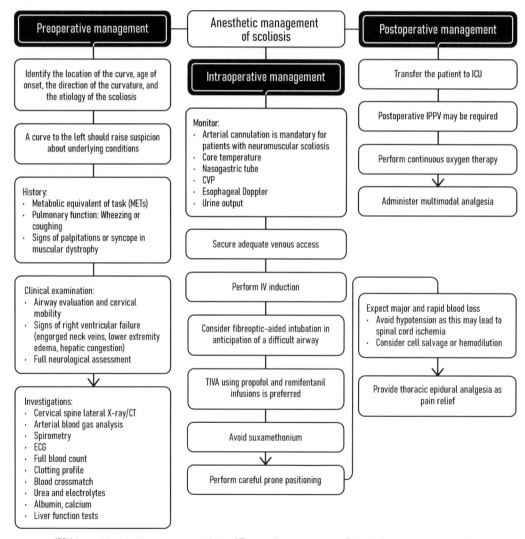

IPPV, intermittent positive pressure ventilation; VP, central venous pressure; TIVA, total intravenous anesthesia
See also spine surgery

Scoliosis

■ **SUGGESTED READING** ■

- Gadsden, J., & Jones, D. (2011). Anesthesiology Oral Board Flash Cards. Mgraw-Hill Education.
- Gambrall MA. Anesthetic implications for surgical correction of scoliosis. AANA J. 2007;75(4):277-285.
- Pollard BJ, Kitchen, G. Handbook of Clinical Anaesthesia. Fourth Edition. CRC Press. 2018. 978-1-4987-6289-2.
- Yao FS, Hemmings HC, Malhotra V, Fong J. 2021. Yao & Artusio's Anesthesiology: Problem-Oriented Patient Management. Chapter 58 – scoliosis (9th edition). Wolters Kluwer Health/ Lippincott Williams & Wilkins.

Scoliosis

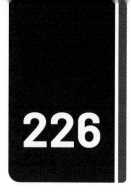

# 226

# STATUS EPILEPTICUS IN PEDIATRIC PATIENTS

## LEARNING OBJECTIVES

- Describe the overall mechanisms and etiology of status epilepticus in pediatric patients
- Manage status epilepticus in pediatric patients

## DEFINITION AND MECHANISM

- Status epilepticus is defined as more than 30 minutes of either 1) continuous seizure activity or 2) two or more sequential seizures without full recovery of consciousness between seizures
- Epilepsy is twice as common in children compared to adults
- Cerebral damage is more likely if the seizure is prolonged
- There are many different types of seizures and not all of them involve obvious convulsive activity
- Epilepsy can occur at any age but is commonly diagnosed in those aged below 20 or over 65 years
- First stage is characterized by an increase in:
  - Cerebral metabolism
  - Blood flow
  - Glucose and lactate concentration

- Compensatory mechanisms:
  - Massive catecholamine release
  - Raised cardiac output
  - Hypertension
  - Increased central venous pressure
- After 30-60 min, compensatory mechanisms fail:
  - Hypoxia
  - Hypoglycemia
  - Increased intracranial pressure
  - Cerebral edema
  - Hyponatremia
  - Potassium imbalance
  - Evolving metabolic acidosis
  - Consumptive coagulopathy
  - Rhabdomyolysis
  - Multi-organ failure

## ETIOLOGY

- Acute
  - Stroke
  - Metabolic abnormalities
  - Hypoxia
  - Systemic infection
  - Anoxia
  - Trauma
  - Traumatic brain injury
  - Drug overdose
  - CNS infection
  - CNS hemorrhage

- Chronic
  - Inheritance tendency
  - Low concentration of anti-epileptic drugs
  - Structural changes to the brain (trauma) or space occypying lesions (tumor, stroke)
  - Idiopathic

## SIGNS AND SYMPTOMS

Status epilepticus can present in several forms:
- Convulsive: unresponsiveness and tonic, clonic, or tonic-clonic movements of the extremities
- Non-convulsive: prolonged seizure activity evidenced by epileptiform discharges on EEG, change in behavior or cognition in some patients
- Electrographic: commonly used for comatose patients who show electrographic evidence of prolonged seizure activity

## DIAGNOSIS

- Based on history and clinical examination
- Often present either actively convulsing or minimal time between clustered seizures

## PREVENTION

- Seizure detection based on EEG and immediate treatment
- In patients with a history of well-controlled epilepsy, avoid disruption of antiepileptic medication perioperatively

# MANAGEMENT

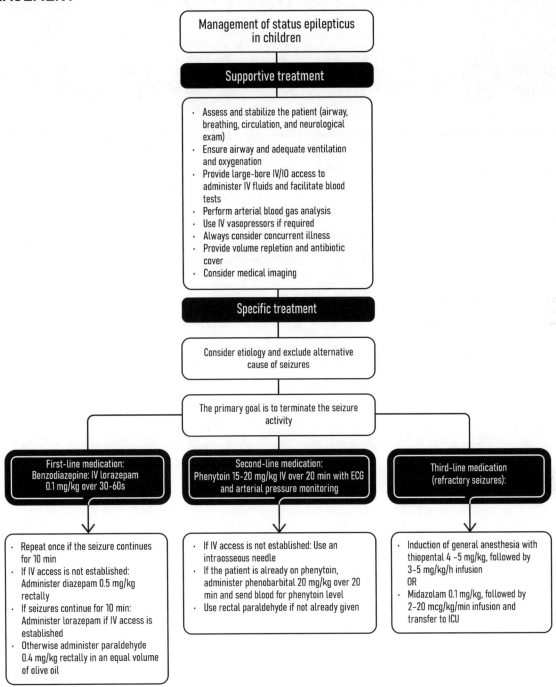

**Management of status epilepticus in children**

**Supportive treatment**

- Assess and stabilize the patient (airway, breathing, circulation, and neurological exam)
- Ensure airway and adequate ventilation and oxygenation
- Provide large-bore IV/IO access to administer IV fluids and facilitate blood tests
- Perform arterial blood gas analysis
- Use IV vasopressors if required
- Always consider concurrent illness
- Provide volume repletion and antibiotic cover
- Consider medical imaging

**Specific treatment**

Consider etiology and exclude alternative cause of seizures

The primary goal is to terminate the seizure activity

**First-line medication:** Benzodiazepine: IV lorazepam 0.1 mg/kg over 30-60s

- Repeat once if the seizure continues for 10 min
- If IV access is not established: Administer diazepam 0.5 mg/kg rectally
- If seizures continue for 10 min: Administer lorazepam if IV access is established
- Otherwise administer paraldehyde 0.4 mg/kg rectally in an equal volume of olive oil

**Second-line medication:** Phenytoin 15-20 mg/kg IV over 20 min with ECG and arterial pressure monitoring

- If IV access is not established: Use an intraosseous needle
- If the patient is already on phenytoin, administer phenobarbital 20 mg/kg over 20 min and send blood for phenytoin level
- Use rectal paraldehyde if not already given

**Third-line medication** (refractory seizures):

- Induction of general anesthesia with thiopental 4 –5 mg/kg, followed by 3-5 mg/kg/h infusion
  OR
- Midazolam 0.1 mg/kg, followed by 2–20 mcg/kg/min infusion and transfer to ICU

## SUGGESTED READING

- Barakat, A.R., Mallory, S., 2011. Anaesthesia and childhood epilepsy. Continuing Education in Anaesthesia Critical Care & Pain 11, 93–98.
- Betjemann JP, Lowenstein DH. Status epilepticus in adults. Lancet Neurol. 2015;14(6):615-624.
- Glauser T, Shinnar S, Gloss D, et al. Evidence-Based Guideline: Treatment of Convulsive Status Epilepticus in Children and Adults: Report of the Guideline Committee of the American Epilepsy Society. Epilepsy Curr. 2016;16(1):48-61.
- Perks A, Cheema S, Mohanraj R. Anaesthesia and epilepsy. BJA: British Journal of Anaesthesia. 2012;108(4):562-71.

Status epilepticus in pediatric patients

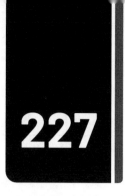

# STRABISMUS SURGERY

## LEARNING OBJECTIVES

- Recognize the signs and symptoms of strabismus
- Describe the risk factors of strabismus
- Anesthetic management for patients undergoing strabismus surgery

## DEFINITION AND MECHANISM

- Strabismus surgery is surgery of the extraocular muscles (tightening, lengthening, transposing, or shortening the eye muscles) to correct strabismus, the misalignment of the eyes
- It is the most common ophthalmic surgery in pediatric patients
- Strabismus occurs in 3-5% of children worldwide
- Strabismus results from an imbalance in extraocular muscle function → two different images (one from each eye) are transmitted to the brain, resulting in loss of visual depth → in children, the brain may suppress the image from the weaker eye, impairing visual development and leading to amblyopia (decreased vision in a normal healthy eye; lazy eye)
- The prognosis is good if the correction is performed as early as possible (before the child reaches the age of 8 years)

## SIGNS AND SYMPTOMS

- Strabismus may involve one or both eyes
- The affected eye can deviate outward (exotropia), inward (esotropia), upward (hypertropia), or downward (hypotropia)
- The deviation may be intermittent or constant, large magnitude (large angle) or small magnitude (small angle)
- Diplopia (double vision)
- Loss of stereopsis
- Headache
- Inability to read comfortably
- Fatigue when reading
- Amblyopia (loss of visual acuity)
- Psychosocial issues (interferes with normal eye contact with others)

## RISK FACTORS

- Premature birth
- Low birth weight
- Smoking during pregnancy
- Family history
- Down syndrome (29%)
- Cerebral palsy (53%)
- Syndromes with craniofacial dysostosis (up to 90%)

## PATIENT CHARACTERISTICS

- Infantile strabismus needs early surgery (6-12 months) for the best visual outcome
- Rare association with primary muscle diseases and malignant hyperthermia
- Associated syndromes: Apert syndrome, Cri du chat syndrome, Crouzon syndrome, Down syndrome, Goldenhar syndrome, Marfan syndrome, Moebius syndrome, Stickler syndrome, Turner syndrome

# PROBLEMS

- Airway not accessible because of the microscope's position
- Avoid suxamethonium
- Can trigger malignant hyperthermia in susceptible patients
- Can cause tonic contracture of extraocular muscles, interferes with forced duction test
- Oculocardiac reflex
- Topical adrenaline is often used to reduce bleeding and may be absorbed systemically, watch dose in small children
- High incidence of postoperative nausea and vomiting (PONV)

# MANAGEMENT

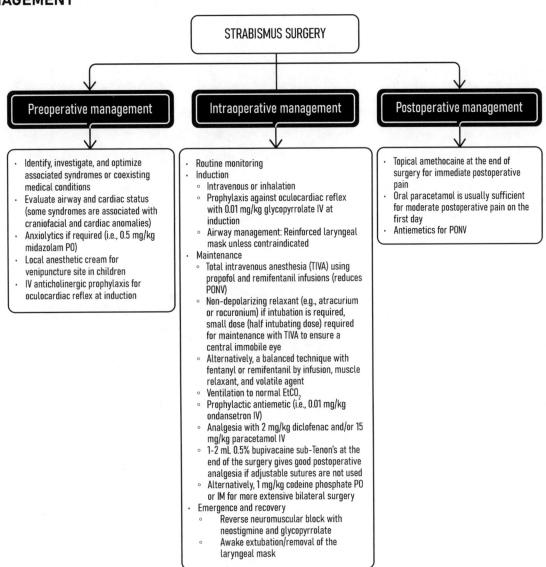

STRABISMUS SURGERY

**Preoperative management**

- Identify, investigate, and optimize associated syndromes or coexisting medical conditions
- Evaluate airway and cardiac status (some syndromes are associated with craniofacial and cardiac anomalies)
- Anxiolytics if required (i.e., 0.5 mg/kg midazolam PO)
- Local anesthetic cream for venipuncture site in children
- IV anticholinergic prophylaxis for oculocardiac reflex at induction

**Intraoperative management**

- Routine monitoring
- Induction
  - Intravenous or inhalation
  - Prophylaxis against oculocardiac reflex with 0.01 mg/kg glycopyrrolate IV at induction
  - Airway management: Reinforced laryngeal mask unless contraindicated
- Maintenance
  - Total intravenous anesthesia (TIVA) using propofol and remifentanil infusions (reduces PONV)
  - Non-depolarizing relaxant (e.g., atracurium or rocuronium) if intubation is required, small dose (half intubating dose) required for maintenance with TIVA to ensure a central immobile eye
  - Alternatively, a balanced technique with fentanyl or remifentanil by infusion, muscle relaxant, and volatile agent
  - Ventilation to normal $EtCO_2$
  - Prophylactic antiemetic (i.e., 0.01 mg/kg ondansetron IV)
  - Analgesia with 2 mg/kg diclofenac and/or 15 mg/kg paracetamol IV
  - 1–2 mL 0.5% bupivacaine sub-Tenon's at the end of the surgery gives good postoperative analgesia if adjustable sutures are not used
  - Alternatively, 1 mg/kg codeine phosphate PO or IM for more extensive bilateral surgery
- Emergence and recovery
  - Reverse neuromuscular block with neostigmine and glycopyrrolate
  - Awake extubation/removal of the laryngeal mask

**Postoperative management**

- Topical amethocaine at the end of surgery for immediate postoperative pain
- Oral paracetamol is usually sufficient for moderate postoperative pain on the first day
- Antiemetics for PONV

# SUGGESTED READING

- Chua AW, Chua MJ, Leung H, Kam PC. Anaesthetic considerations for strabismus surgery in children and adults. Anaesthesia and Intensive Care. 2020;48(4):277-288.
- Lewis H, James I. Update on anaesthesia for paediatric ophthalmic surgery. BJA Educ. 2021;21(1):32-38.
- Pollard BJ, Kitchen G. Handbook of Clinical Anaesthesia. 4th ed. Taylor & Francis group; 2018. Chapter 18 Ophthalmic surgery, Slater RM.

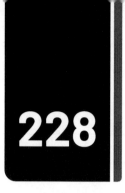

# TETRALOGY OF FALLOT

## LEARNING OBJECTIVES

- Define tetralogy of Fallot
- Describe the signs and symptoms of tetralogy of Fallot
- Understand the pathophysiology of tetralogy of Fallot
- Anesthetic management of a patient with tetralogy of Fallot

## DEFINITION AND MECHANISM

- Tetralogy of Fallot (TOF) is one of the most common congenital heart defects (10%), resulting in a right-to-left shunt characterized by:
  - Large non-restrictive ventricular septal defect (VSD)
  - Valvular, subvalvular, or supravalvular pulmonary stenosis, causing right ventricular outflow tract obstruction (RVOTO)
  - Right ventricular hypertrophy
  - Overriding aorta
- Cyanotic heart disease
- TOF often presents with low birth weight and prematurity
- TOF may present with other anatomical anomalies
  - Stenosis of the left pulmonary artery (40%)
  - Bicuspid pulmonary valve (60%)
  - Right-sided aortic arch (25%)
  - Coronary artery anomalies (10%)
  - Patent foramen ovale or atrial septal defect → pentalogy of Fallot
  - Atrioventricular septal defect
  - Partially or totally anomalous pulmonary venous return

## SIGNS AND SYMPTOMS

- Right-to-left shunt
- Cyanosis (bluish coloration of the skin caused by hypoxemia)
- Hypoxia/low $SpO_2$ (60-90%) with little or no response to oxygen therapy
- Shortness of breath and rapid breathing, especially during feeding or exercise
- Heart murmurs (pansystolic and ejection systolic)
- Abnormal, rounded shape of the nail bed in the fingers and toes (clubbing)
- Poor weight gain
- Tiring easily during feeding or exercise
- Irritability
- Prolonged crying
- Polycythemia
- Baby may turn blue with breastfeeding or crying

### Tet spells

- Infants and children with unrepaired TOF may develop tet spells → acute hypoxia spells, characterized by shortness of breath, cyanosis, agitation, and loss of consciousness (syncope)
- Initiated by any event (i.e., crying, bowel movements, anxiety, pain, dehydration, or fever) that leads to decreased oxygen saturation or that causes decreased systemic vascular resistance (SVR) → increased shunting through the VSD (increased right-to-left shunt)
- Decrease in frequency after the first four years of life
- Older children will squat to increase the SVR → temporary reversal of shunt

## COMPLICATIONS

- Endocarditis
- Arrhythmias (particularly supraventricular or ventricular)
- Pulmonary regurgitation
- Dizziness, fainting, or seizures due to hypoxemia
- Delayed growth and development

Tetralogy of Fallot

## RISK FACTORS

- Viral illness during pregnancy (rubella)
- Maternal alcohol consumption
- Maternal smoking
- Maternal diabetes mellitus or gestational diabetes
- Maternal age > 40

- Family history of TOF
- Down syndrome or DiGeorge syndrome
- Tracheoesophageal fistula or VACTERL association
- Male gender

## PATHOPHYSIOLOGY

- Anatomy of TOF allows mixing of blood between the pulmonary and systemic circulations (usually at VSD) → right-to-left shunt adding deoxygenated blood to the systemic circulation → cyanosis

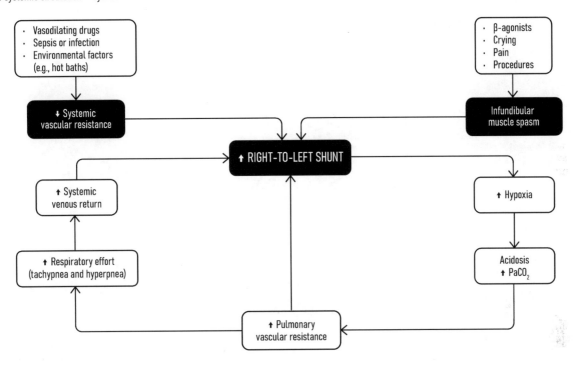

## DIAGNOSIS

- Many patients are diagnosed prenatally
- **Chest radiography:** Abnormal "coeur-en-sabot" (boot-like) appearance of the heart
- **Electrocardiogram:** Right ventricular hypertrophy (tall R-waves in lead V1 and deep S-waves in lead V5-V6) along with right-axis deviation
- **Echocardiogram:** Presence of VSD, right ventricular hypertrophy, and aortic override; color Doppler to measure the degree of pulmonary stenosis

## TREATMENT

- Surgical repair
  - Patch closure of the VSD to separate the pulmonary and systemic circulation
  - Enlargement of the RVOT (increase the size of the pulmonary valve and pulmonary arteries) to relieve RVOTO
- Usually takes place in the first year following birth, at age 3-6 months
- Intraoperative transesophageal echocardiography to evaluate the VSD closure and RVOT

### *Long-term complications after TOF surgery*

- Chronic pulmonary valve regurgitation
- Tricuspid valve regurgitation
- VSD that may continue to leak after repair or may need re-repair
- Hypertrophic right or left ventricle and dysfunction
- Arrhythmias
- Coronary artery disease
- Aortic root and valve dilation
- Sudden cardiac death

# MANGEMENT

```
┌─────────────────────────────────┐
│       TETRALOGY OF FALLOT        │
└─────────────────────────────────┘
```

| Preoperative management | Intraoperative management | Postoperative management |

**Preoperative management**

- Full and thorough history and review of investigations
- Proceed cautiously in children with uncorrected TOF
- Subacute bacterial endocarditis prophylaxis
- Awareness, early detection of, and management of tet spells are crucial
- Premedication with 0.5 mg/kg midazolam 30 min preoperatively in children with a history of tet spells

**Intraoperative management**

- Goal: Prevent significant right-to-left shunt
  - Avoid an increase in pulmonary vascular resistance
  - Avoid a decrease in SVR
  - Avoid myocardial depression
  - Keep full preload
- Avoid prolonged fasting and dehydration
- Avoid hypercarbia, hypoxemia, and acidosis
- Avoid hypothermia
- Pulse oximetry monitoring
- Full invasive monitoring including central venous and arterial access
- Induction of anesthesia
  - Inhalation: Sevoflurane, then place IV, then paralyze, then endotracheal tube
  - Intravenous: Ketamine (2 mg/kg), then paralyze, then endotracheal tube
  - Avoid propofol/remifentanil to prevent reduced SVR/contractility

**Postoperative management**

- Admission to pediatric ICU
- Continue invasive monitoring with careful IV filling to minimize the effect of residual RVOTO
- Inotropic support following bypass (e.g., phosphodiesterase inhibitor such as enoximone or milrinone)
- Addition of norepinephrine may be required to counteract the reduction in SVR
- Continue ventilation until the child is warm with minimal bleeding and adequate peripheral perfusion
- Maintain potassium levels at 4.5-5.0 mmol/L and magnesium levels at 1.5-2.0 mmol/L to reduce the risk of cardiac arrhythmias
- Treat junctional escape tachycardias with cooling to 34°C, maintenance of serum electrolytes, and amiodarone loading

SVR, systemic vascular resistance; RVOTO, right ventricular outflow tract obstruction.

### Management of tet spells during anesthesia

- Goal: Increase oxygenation, improve cardiac output, and reduce infundibular spasm and right-to-left shunt
- Give 100% oxygen and check the endotracheal tube position
- Deepen anesthesia and give an opiate bolus (e.g., 0.1 mg/kg morphine)
- Fluid bolus
- Vasopressor therapy (e.g., 5 μg/kg phenylephrine)
- β-blockers (e.g., 0.1-0.3 mg/kg propranolol)
- Knee-to-chest flexion position

## KEEP IN MIND

- TOF is characterized by the presence of a VSD, RVOTO, right ventricular hypertrophy, and overriding aorta
- TOF is one of the most common cyanotic heart defects
- Prevention of tet spells is the key for safe anesthesia

## SUGGESTED READING

- Pollard BJ, Kitchen G. Handbook of Clinical Anaesthesia. 4th ed. Taylor & Francis group; 2018. Chapter 2 Cardiovascular system, Tully RP and Turner R.
- Wilson R, Ross O, Griksaitis MJ. Tetralogy of Fallot. BJA Educ. 2019;19(11):362-369.

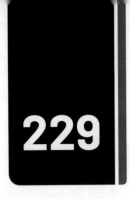

# TONSILLECTOMY

## LEARNING OBJECTIVES

- Understand the indications and contraindications for tonsillectomy
- Anesthetic management for patients undergoing tonsillectomy
- Discuss the management of post-tonsillectomy bleeding

## DEFINITION AND MECHANISM

- Tonsillectomy is a surgical procedure to remove the palatine tonsils, which are lymphoid tissue covered in the respiratory epithelium and invaginated to create crypts
- It is a common procedure in children to treat recurrent acute sore throat
- Adenotonsillar hypertrophy can present with nasal obstruction, recurrent infections, secretory otitis media, deafness (secondary to Eustachian tube dysfunction), and obstructive sleep apnea (OSA)
- The surgery is performed through the mouth using a Boyle-Davis gag ➜ difficulties may be encountered due to a poorly placed gag, obstructing the tracheal tube or laryngeal mask airway

## PATIENT CHARACTERISTICS

- Chronic/recurrent throat infections
- Comorbidities
- OSA
  - Congenital abnormalities (e.g., Down syndrome)
  - May have malignancy
  - Other incidental medical conditions
  - Cor pulmonale due to long-term hypoxia

## INDICATIONS AND CONTRAINDICATIONS FOR SURGERY

### Absolute indications

- Upper airway obstruction, dysphagia, and OSA
- Peritonsillar abscess, which is unresponsive to adequate medical management and surgical drainage
- Recurrent tonsillitis with associated febrile convulsions
- Requirement for biopsy to confirm tissue pathology

### Relative indications

- Recurrent tonsillitis, which is unresponsive to medical treatment
  - Sore throat secondary to tonsilitis
  - > 5 episodes of tonsillitis in one year
  - Symptoms > 1 year
  - Episodes of sore throats are disabling
- Persistent bad breath and taste in the mouth due to chronic tonsillitis
- Persistent tonsillitis in streptococcus carrier, which is unresponsive to beta-lactamase-resistant antibiotics
- Pathology thought to be neoplastic

### Contraindications

- Bleeding diathesis
- Acute infection
- Anemia
- Significant anesthetic risk

Tonsillectomy

# MANAGEMENT

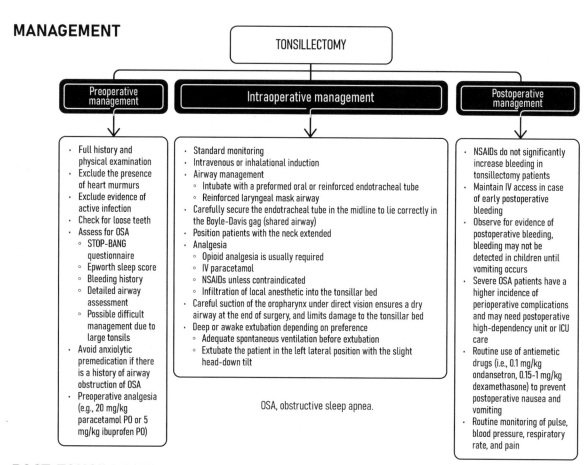

**TONSILLECTOMY**

**Preoperative management**

- Full history and physical examination
- Exclude the presence of heart murmurs
- Exclude evidence of active infection
- Check for loose teeth
- Assess for OSA
  - STOP-BANG questionnaire
  - Epworth sleep score
  - Bleeding history
  - Detailed airway assessment
  - Possible difficult management due to large tonsils
- Avoid anxiolytic premedication if there is a history of airway obstruction of OSA
- Preoperative analgesia (e.g., 20 mg/kg paracetamol PO or 5 mg/kg ibuprofen PO)

**Intraoperative management**

- Standard monitoring
- Intravenous or inhalational induction
- Airway management
  - Intubate with a preformed oral or reinforced endotracheal tube
  - Reinforced laryngeal mask airway
- Carefully secure the endotracheal tube in the midline to lie correctly in the Boyle-Davis gag (shared airway)
- Position patients with the neck extended
- Analgesia
  - Opioid analgesia is usually required
  - IV paracetamol
  - NSAIDs unless contraindicated
  - Infiltration of local anesthetic into the tonsillar bed
- Careful suction of the oropharynx under direct vision ensures a dry airway at the end of surgery, and limits damage to the tonsillar bed
- Deep or awake extubation depending on preference
  - Adequate spontaneous ventilation before extubation
  - Extubate the patient in the left lateral position with the slight head-down tilt

OSA, obstructive sleep apnea.

**Postoperative management**

- NSAIDs do not significantly increase bleeding in tonsillectomy patients
- Maintain IV access in case of early postoperative bleeding
- Observe for evidence of postoperative bleeding, bleeding may not be detected in children until vomiting occurs
- Severe OSA patients have a higher incidence of perioperative complications and may need postoperative high-dependency unit or ICU care
- Routine use of antiemetic drugs (i.e., 0.1 mg/kg ondansetron, 0.15-1 mg/kg dexamethasone) to prevent postoperative nausea and vomiting
- Routine monitoring of pulse, blood pressure, respiratory rate, and pain

# POST-TONSILLECTOMY BLEEDING

- Serious complication of tonsillectomy that can occur in the recovery room or hours later
- Emergency with limited time to optimize
- Persistent swallowing can be an early indicator of bleeding from the tonsillar bed
- Patient may be hypovolemic and require fluid resuscitation before induction → assess patient's fluid status and cardiovascular parameters
- Risk of aspiration due to potential full stomach with blood
- Potential difficult airway due to blood in the airway and edema from recent intubation

## Intraoperative management

- Resuscitate patients and apply full monitoring
- Assess previous anesthetic record
- Suction must be immediately available
- Head-down tilt helps to drain blood away from the larynx
- Rapid sequence induction ensures quick intubation and protects the airway during induction
- Intubation may require a smaller sized endotracheal tube than originally inserted
- Continue fluid resuscitation throughout surgery
- Empty the stomach with a wide-bore naso- or orogastric tube, and ensure that the stomach is empty before extubation
- Extubate patients only when fully awake, in the head-down, left lateral position

## Postoperative management

- Patients have to stay in the recovery for an extended period to ensure that the bleeding has stopped
- Check the hemoglobin and coagulation, and transfuse blood if necessary
- Closely monitor patients for further bleeding

# SUGGESTED READING

- Davies K. Anaesthesia for tonsillectomy. WFSA. April 2, 2007. Accessed February 10, 2023. https://resources.wfsahq.org/atotw/anaesthesia-for-tonsillectomy/.
- Pollard BJ, Kitchen G. Handbook of Clinical Anaesthesia. 4th ed. Taylor & Francis group; 2018. Chapter 19 ENT Surgery, MacNab R, Bexon K, Clegg S, Hutchinson A.

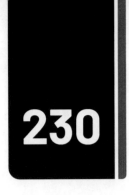

# TRACHEOESOPHAGEAL FISTULA

## 230

### LEARNING OBJECTIVES

- Describe tracheoesophageal fistula and esophageal atresia, and their classification
- Define the associated congenital anomalies of tracheoesophageal fistulas
- Anesthetic management of pediatric patients with a tracheoesophageal fistula and/or esophageal atresia

## DEFINITION AND MECHANISM

- A tracheoesophageal fistula (TEF) is one of the most common congenital anomalies and is an abnormal connection (fistula) between the esophagus and trachea
- TEF commonly occurs with esophageal atresia (EA), a related congenital malformation with a similar presentation to TEF
- EA is an abnormal connection between the esophagus and stomach, the esophagus ends in a blind-ended pouch rather than connecting normally to the stomach, can occur with or without the presence of a fistula

| Classification | | |
|---|---|---|
| Type A | No TEF, only EA → isolated EA<br>The esophagus is divided into two parts with both portions ending in blind pouches | 8% of all cases |
| Type B | Proximal TEF and distal EA<br>The lower portion of the esophagus ends in a blind pouch and the upper portion is connected to the trachea by a TEF | 2% of all cases |
| Type C | Proximal EA and distal TEF<br>The upper portion of the esophagus ends in a blind pouch and the lower portion is connected to the trachea by a TEF | Most common,<br>85% of all cases |
| Type D | Both proximal and distal TEF<br>TEF connects both the upper and lower portions of the esophagus and trachea | Rarest form, <1%<br>of all cases |
| Type E<br>(H-type) | Isolated TEF<br>The esophagus connects to the stomach normally and is fully intact, a TEF connects the esophagus and trachea | 4% of all cases |

## SIGNS AND SYMPTOMS

- Excessive oral secretions, salivation
- Breathing difficulties, respiratory distress
- Coughing or choking when feeding
- Vomiting
- Cyanosis, especially during feeding

- Feeding difficulties
- Frequent lung infections
- Risk of aspiration
- EA and the inability to swallow may cause polyhydramnios in utero

## ASSOCIATED CONGENITAL ANOMALIES

50% of babies with TEF/EA also have associated congenital anomalies
- Prematurity (30%)
- Congenital heart disease (30%): Ventricular septal defect, tetralogy of Fallot, patent ductus arteriosus, atrial septal defect, right-sided aortic arch
- Gastrointestinal anomalies (14%): Diaphragmatic hernia, duodenal atresia, pyloric stenosis, imperforate anus, malrotation, omphalocele
- Genitourinary anomalies (14%): Renal agenesis, hypospadias, horseshoe/polycystic kidney, ureteric/urethral abnormalities
- Musculoskeletal anomalies (10%): Radial limb abnormalities, polydactyly, lower limb defects, hemivertebrae, rib defects, scoliosis
- VACTERL syndrome (10%)
- Respiratory anomalies (6%): Tracheobronchomalacia, pulmonary hypoplasia, tracheal agenesis/stenosis, tracheal upper pouch
- Chromosome abnormalities (4%): Trisomy 13, 18, or Down syndrome

# TREATMENT

- Surgical correction with resection of any fistula and anastomosis of any discontinuous segments
- Usually repaired within 24 hours of birth to minimize the risk and complications of aspiration
- Complications after surgery
  - Anastomotic leaks
  - Esophageal strictures (abnormal tightening)
  - Damage to the laryngeal nerve
  - Recurrence of the fistula
  - Gastroesophageal reflux disease
  - Dysphagia
  - Asthma-like symptoms: Persistent coughing or wheezing
  - Recurrent chest infections
  - Tracheomalacia

# MANAGEMENT

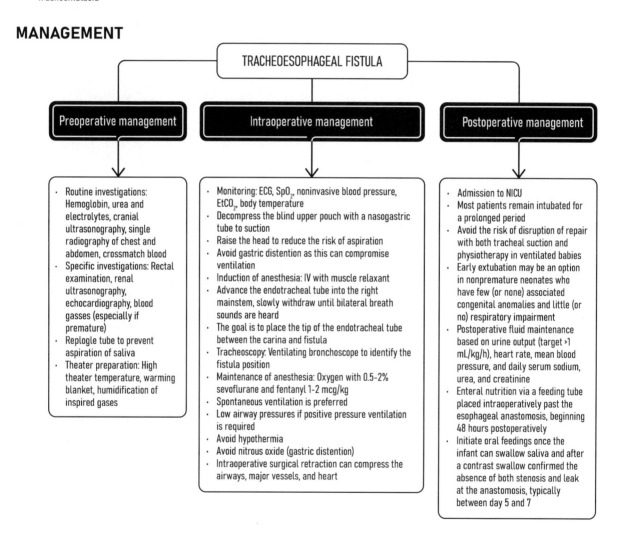

**TRACHEOESOPHAGEAL FISTULA**

**Preoperative management**

- Routine investigations: Hemoglobin, urea and electrolytes, cranial ultrasonography, single radiography of chest and abdomen, crossmatch blood
- Specific investigations: Rectal examination, renal ultrasonography, echocardiography, blood gasses (especially if premature)
- Replogle tube to prevent aspiration of saliva
- Theater preparation: High theater temperature, warming blanket, humidification of inspired gases

**Intraoperative management**

- Monitoring: ECG, $SpO_2$, noninvasive blood pressure, $EtCO_2$, body temperature
- Decompress the blind upper pouch with a nasogastric tube to suction
- Raise the head to reduce the risk of aspiration
- Avoid gastric distention as this can compromise ventilation
- Induction of anesthesia: IV with muscle relaxant
- Advance the endotracheal tube into the right mainstem, slowly withdraw until bilateral breath sounds are heard
- The goal is to place the tip of the endotracheal tube between the carina and fistula
- Tracheoscopy: Ventilating bronchoscope to identify the fistula position
- Maintenance of anesthesia: Oxygen with 0.5-2% sevoflurane and fentanyl 1-2 mcg/kg
- Spontaneous ventilation is preferred
- Low airway pressures if positive pressure ventilation is required
- Avoid hypothermia
- Avoid nitrous oxide (gastric distention)
- Intraoperative surgical retraction can compress the airways, major vessels, and heart

**Postoperative management**

- Admission to NICU
- Most patients remain intubated for a prolonged period
- Avoid the risk of disruption of repair with both tracheal suction and physiotherapy in ventilated babies
- Early extubation may be an option in nonpremature neonates who have few (or none) associated congenital anomalies and little (or no) respiratory impairment
- Postoperative fluid maintenance based on urine output (target >1 mL/kg/h), heart rate, mean blood pressure, and daily serum sodium, urea, and creatinine
- Enteral nutrition via a feeding tube placed intraoperatively past the esophageal anastomosis, beginning 48 hours postoperatively
- Initiate oral feedings once the infant can swallow saliva and after a contrast swallow confirmed the absence of both stenosis and leak at the anastomosis, typically between day 5 and 7

# SUGGESTED READING

- Choumanovai I, Sanusii A, Evansii F. Anaesthetic management of tracheo-oesophageal fistula/ oesophageal atresia. WFSA. October 17, 2017. Accessed February 16, 2023. https://resources.wfsahq.org/atotw/anaesthetic-management-of-tracheo-oesophageal-fistula-oesophageal-atresia/
- Pollard BJ, Kitchen G. Handbook of Clinical Anaesthesia. 4th ed. Taylor & Francis group; 2018. Chapter 24 Paediatrics, Lomas B.
- Saraiya NR. TRACHEOESOPHAGEAL FISTULA. In: Houck PJ, Haché M, Sun LS. eds. Handbook of Pediatric Anesthesia. Mgraw Hill; 2015. Accessed February 16, 2023. https://accessanesthesiology.mhmedical.com/content.aspx?bookid=1189&sectionid=70363324

Tracheoesophageal fistula

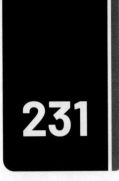

# TREACHER COLLINS SYNDROME

## LEARNING OBJECTIVES

**231**

- Describe Treacher Collins syndrome
- Understand how Treacher Collins syndrome affects the airway
- Discuss the perioperative management of patients with Treacher Collins syndrome

---

## DEFINITION AND MECHANISM

- Treacher Collins syndrome (TCS) or mandibulofacial dysostosis is a rare autosomal dominant disorder of craniofacial development
- Congenital malformation of the first and second branchial arches, which may affect the size, shape, and position of the ears, eyelids, zygomatic (cheek) bones, and maxilla and mandible (jaws)
- TCS is characterized by hypoplasia of the facial bones, especially the zygoma and mandible
- It is bilateral, symmetrical, and restricted to the head and neck region

## SIGNS AND SYMPTOMS

Main features of TCS
- Malar hypoplasia and a cleft in the zygoma
- Eyes have an antimongoloid slant with colobomas (eyelid notch) along the lateral ⅓ of the lower lid
- Lashes are absent from the medial ⅔ of the lower eyelid
- Face has a convex profile with a retrusive chin and jaw, associated with an overbite
- External ear abnormalities are common
- A cleft lip and/or palate is present in up to 35% of patients

| System affected | Features seen |
|---|---|
| Facial bones | Hypoplasia of the malar bones<br>Underdeveloped zygoma<br>Hypoplastic orbits<br>Hypoplasia of maxilla, mandible, and temporomandibular joint |
| Eyes | Antimongoloid slant of palpebrae<br>Coloboma of the lower eyelid<br>Hypoplasia of lower eyelids with partial absence of cilia<br>Hypoplasia of lateral canthi<br>Hypertelorism |
| Ears | Abnormality of the external ear<br>Abnormality of the auditory canal<br>Malformed middle ear ossicles<br>Conductive hearing loss |
| Facial features | External nose deformity<br>Deviated nasal septum<br>Macrostomia with typical "fish-mouth" appearance<br>"Bird-face" appearance<br>Tongue-shaped hair process in the preauricular region |
| Intraoral features | Cleft palate<br>Anterior open bite<br>Steep occlusal plane<br>Supernumerary teeth<br>T-shaped teeth<br>Enamel opacity/hypoplasia<br>Microdontia, tooth agenesis<br>Ectopic eruption/rotation of teeth |
| Other features | Choanal stenosis/atresia<br>Occlusion of oropharynx and hypopharynx by the tongue<br>Constricted nasal passages<br>Obstructive sleep apnea |

## CAUSES

- De novo mutation (60%) or inherited (40%)
- Mutations in TCOF1, POLR1B, POLR1C, or POLR1D genes

## COMPLICATIONS

- Facial abnormalities can result in airway narrowing and respiratory compromise
- Feeding difficulties
- Vision problems
- Hearing loss
- Obstructive sleep apnea (OSA)

## TREATMENT

- Patients may require prone positioning or surgery to maintain a patent airway (e.g., tracheostomy)
- Patients may require a gastrostomy to ensure adequate food intake while protecting the airway
- Reconstructive surgery
- Hearing aids
- Speech therapy

## MANAGEMENT

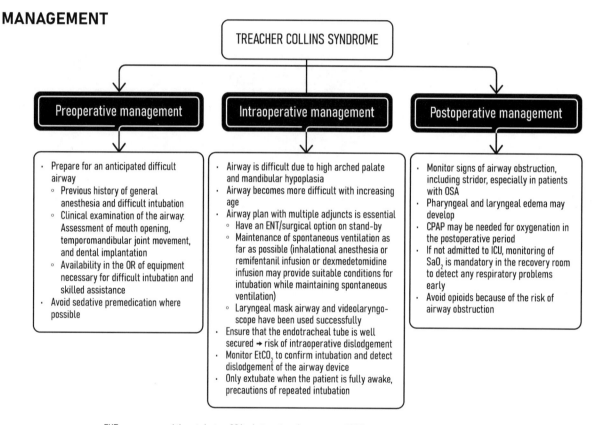

ENT, ear, nose, and throat doctor; OSA, obstructive sleep apnea; CPAP, continuous positive airway pressure.

## KEEP IN MIND

- Prepare for an anticipated difficult airway in all children with TCS
- Direct laryngoscopy may become more difficult with increasing age

## SUGGESTED READING

- Goel L, Bennur SK, Jambhale S. Treacher-collins syndrome-a challenge for anaesthesiologists. Indian J Anaesth. 2009;53(4):496-500.
- Hosking J, Zoanetti D, Carlyle A, Anderson P, Costi D. Anesthesia for Treacher Collins syndrome: a review of airway management in 240 pediatric cases. Paediatr Anaesth. 2012;22(8):752-758.

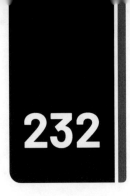

# 232

# UPPER RESPIRATORY TRACT INFECTION

## LEARNING OBJECTIVES

- Recognize the signs and symptoms of an upper respiratory tract infection
- Decide whether or not surgery should be postponed in children with an acute upper respiratory tract infection
- Anesthetic management of pediatric patients with upper respiratory tract infections

## DEFINITION AND MECHANISM

- An upper respiratory tract infection (URTI) is an illness caused by an acute infection, which involves the upper respiratory tract, including the nose, sinuses, pharynx, larynx, or trachea
- URTIs are characterized by cough, nasal congestion and discharge, sore throat, and sneezing
- URTIs include the common cold, epiglottitis, tonsillitis, rhinitis, pharyngitis, laryngitis, sinusitis, and otitis media
- Children experience 6 to 8 URTIs per year
- Risk of perioperative adverse respiratory complications (i.e., coughing, breath holding, laryngospasm, bronchospasm, airway obstruction, oxygen desaturation < 90%, atelectasis, post-extubation stridor, pneumonia, and unanticipated tracheal intubation or reintubation) is greatest during acute infection but remains increased for 2-6 weeks after an URTI
- Independent risk factors for adverse respiratory events in children with active URTI include intubation, prematurity (< 37 weeks), child < 1 year, history of asthma or atopy, passive smoking, airway surgery, presence of copious secretions, nasal congestion, parental confirmation "my child has a cold", snoring, and use of an endotracheal tube (ETT)
- Airway hyperreactivity is present for up to 6-8 weeks following a URTI

## SIGNS AND SYMPTOMS

- Cough
- Runny nose
- Nasal congestion
- Sore throat
- Headache
- Low-grade fever
- Facial pressure
- Sneezing
- Malaise
- Hoarse voice
- Fatigue and lack of energy
- Red eyes
- Swollen lymph nodes

## CAUSES

- 95% of URTIs are secondary to viral causes, with rhinoviruses accounting for 30-40% of infections

## PATHOPHYSIOLOGY

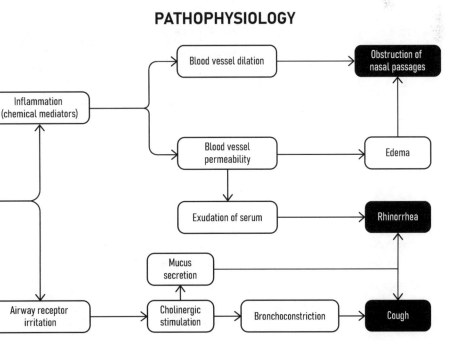

Upper respiratory tract infection

# TREATMENT

- Rest
- Fluids to stay hydrated
- Over-the-counter pain medications
- Antibiotics in case of bacterial origin (i.e., Beta-lactam antibiotics)

# MANAGEMENT

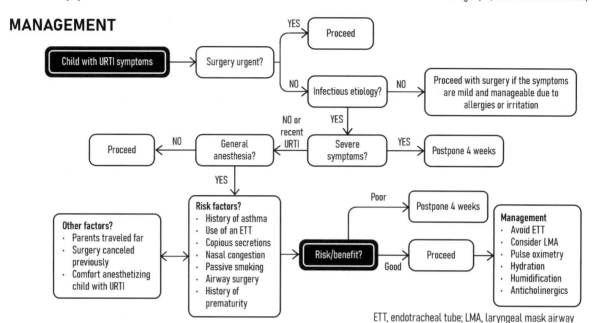

ETT, endotracheal tube; LMA, laryngeal mask airway

## Preoperative assessment

- Parents statement
- Check for the presence of respiratory and cardiovascular comorbidities
- Monitor vital signs and baseline saturation
- Anticipate perioperative adverse respiratory events
- Chest X-ray if physical examination suggests signs of lower respiratory tract involvement
- Categorize URTI based on medical history and physical examination
  - **Mild URTIs:** Clear runny nose, dry cough, appear healthy otherwise, clear lungs to auscultation, no fever
  - **Moderate URTIs:** Green runny nose, mild moist cough, no wheezing or involvement of lower respiratory tract, no fever or irritability for 1-2 days
  - **Severe URTIs:** Green runny nose, productive cough, mucopurulent secretion, nasal congestion, fever > 38°C, severe sore or scratchy throat, pulmonary involvement (lower respiratory tract), wheezing, and lethargy

## Anesthetic management

- **Goal:** Minimize secretions and avoid or limit stimulation of a potentially irritable airway
- Experienced pediatric anesthesia team
- Preoperative bronchodilators 10-30 min before surgery to reduce bronchoconstriction and perioperative respiratory events
- Humidifiers may help to clear secretions and prevent bronchial mucus plugging
- Combining β2-agonist (e.g., salbutamol) with inhaled corticosteroids is more effective in minimizing bronchoconstriction due to intubation compared to inhaled β2-agonist alone
- Avoid tracheal intubation, particularly in children < 5 years
- A laryngeal mask airway or facemask is preferred
- IV lidocaine may be helpful in reducing the laryngospasm reflex
- Less adverse respiratory events with propofol than sevoflurane as induction agent
- Maintenance of anesthesia: Intravenous or inhalation techniques, anesthesia should be deep enough
- Suction airway only under deep anesthesia

# KEEP IN MIND

- Children with active and recent URTI are at increased risk of perioperative respiratory complications
- Assessment of suitability of any child with URTI symptoms for surgery includes the child's age and presenting symptoms, frequency of URTIs, urgency and type of procedure, and presence of comorbidities
- The decision to postpone or proceed with surgery for children with URTI should be made on an individual basis by considering the presence of identified risk factors and the anesthesiologist's experience

# SUGGESTED READING

- Lema GF, Berhe YW, Gebrezgi AH, Getu AA. Evidence-based perioperative management of a child with upper respiratory tract infections (URTIs) undergoing elective surgery: A systematic review. International Journal of Surgery Open. 2018;12:17-24.
- Regli A, Becke K, von Ungern-Sternberg BS. An update on the perioperative management of children with upper respiratory tract infections. Curr Opin Anaesthesiol. 2017;30(3):362-367.
- Tait AR, Malviya S. Anesthesia for the child with an upper respiratory tract infection: still a dilemma?. Anesth Analg. 2005;100(1):59-65.

Upper respiratory tract infection

# VACTERL

## LEARNING OBJECTIVES

- Define VACTERL
- Anesthetic management of a pediatric patient with VACTERL

## DEFINITION AND MECHANISM

- VACTERL association (VATER association, VACTERL syndrome) refers to a group of congenital defects that tend to co-occur
  - **V:** Vertebral anomalies
  - **A:** Anorectal malformations
  - **C:** Cardiovascular anomalies
  - **T:** Tracheoesophageal fistula (TEF)
  - **E:** Esophageal atresia (EA)
  - **R:** Renal anomalies
  - **L:** Limb defects, including radial anomalies
- Refers to abnormalities in structures derived from the embryonic mesoderm
- Patients may also have other congenital anomalies
- Most patients are developmentally normal and have normal intelligence

## SIGNS AND SYMPTOMS, AND COMPLICATIONS

| VACTERL | Congenital malformations |
|---|---|
| V: Vertebral anomalies (70%) | Small hypoplastic, dysplastic, missing, or supernumery vertebrae<br>Hemivertebrae<br>Wedge vertebrae<br>Vertebral clefts and fusion<br>Caudal regression<br>Tethered cord<br>Branchial arch/cleft abnormalities<br>Rib anomalies<br>Sacral agenesis<br>Dysplastic sacral vertebrae<br>Scoliosis or kyphoscoliosis secondary to costovertebral anomalies<br>C5-C6 dislocation and severe stenosis with spinal cord impingement (rare)<br>Single umbilical artery (20%) |
| A: Anorectal malformations (55%, up to 90%) | Anal atresia/imperforate anus |
| C: Cardiovascular anomalies (75%) | Most common defects: Ventricular septal defect, atrial septal defect, tetralogy of Fallot<br>Less common defects: Truncus arteriosus, transposition of great arteries, patent ductus arteriosus, coarctation of aorta |
| T: TEF / E: EA (32%) | TEF<br>EA can occur as an isolated effect (8%) |
| R: Renal anomalies (50-80%) | Urological problems (e.g., severe reflux or obstruction of outflow of urine from both kidneys)<br>Horseshoe kidneys<br>Cystic, aplastic, dysplastic, or ectopic kidneys<br>Hydronephrosis<br>Unilateral/bilateral agenesis<br>Pyelonephritis<br>Nephrolithiasis |

| | |
|---|---|
| L: Limb defects, including radial anomalies (up to 70%) | Displaced, absent, or hypoplastic thumbs<br>Polydactyly<br>Syndactyly<br>Radial aplasia, dysplasia, or hypoplasia<br>Radial ray deformities<br>Radioulnar synostosis<br>Club foot<br>Hypoplasia of great toe/tibia<br>Lower limb tibial deformities<br>Bilateral limb defects usually have kidney/urological problems on both sides while unilateral limb defects have kidney/urological problems on the same side |
| Other | Growth deficiencies<br>Failure to thrive |

## DIAGNOSIS

- VACTERL association is a diagnosis of exclusion
- Not all malformations are always present
- At least three of the malformations (including TEF) have to be present and there must be no clinical or laboratory-based evidence for the presence of one of the many similar overlapping conditions to make the diagnosis

## TREATMENT

- Surgical correction of the specific congenital anomalies (e.g., TEF, certain types of severe cardiac malformations, and imperforate anus/anal atresia in the immediate postnatal/neonatal period)
- Long-term medical management of sequelae of congenital malformations (e.g., renal and vertebral anomalies)

VACTERL

# MANAGEMENT

```
                              ┌─────────────────────┐
                              │       VACTERL        │
                              └─────────────────────┘
        ┌──────────────────────────────┼──────────────────────────────┐
        ▼                               ▼                               ▼
┌──────────────────┐          ┌──────────────────────┐        ┌──────────────────────┐
│  Preoperative    │          │   Intraoperative     │        │   Postoperative      │
│   management     │          │     management       │        │     management       │
└──────────────────┘          └──────────────────────┘        └──────────────────────┘
        │                               │                               │
        ▼                               ▼                               ▼
```

**Preoperative management**

- Baseline investigations to rule out or determine the severity of the condition
  - **V:** X-ray, ultrasound, and/or CT/MRI of the spine
  - **A:** Physical examination/observation, abdominal ultrasound +/- additional testing for genitourinary anomalies
  - **C:** ECG (arrhythmias), echocardiogram +/- cardiac CT/MRI/angiogram (exclude cardiac or vascular abnormalities; evaluate structure and function of the heart), chest X-ray (cardiomegaly)
  - **TE:** Physical examination/observation, chest X-ray, CT/MRI (tracheoesophageal cleft) + chest X-ray (aspiration evidence) and endoscopy, abdominal X-ray (diaphragmatic hernia)
  - **R:** Renal ultrasound +/- voiding cystourethrogram, CT urogram multislice, abdominal CT, urine M/C/S
  - **L:** Physical examination, X-rays (skeletal survey, limbs, hips, rib), angiography (radial artery hypoplasia)
- Other investigations
  - **Blood work:** Full blood count, hemoglobin, hematocrit, electrolytes, renal function, liver and bone profiles, vitamin D, glucose, crossmatch, coagulation/bleeding time, chromosome analysis
  - **Post dialysis:** Blood urea, electrolytes, weight
  - **Pulmonary workup:** Chest X-ray +/- respiratory function tests

**Intraoperative management**

- Potential difficult airway due to craniofacial-vertebral deformities
- TEF/EA considerations
- Perform rigid bronchoscopy in patients with TEF to help endotracheal tube positioning
- Avoid succinylcholine in patients with chronic renal failure due to hyperkalemic arrhythmias and arrest
- Use intravenous or inhalational anesthetics
- Spontaneous ventilation in a non-intubated patient would increase the aspiration risk
- Avoid hypothermia
- History of an increased aspiration risk (e.g., cleft lip/palate, TEF) excludes early extubation
- Consider difficult IV access in patients with limb abnormalities
- Insert arterial and central venous lines in patients undergoing surgeries involving hemodynamic instability or major fluid shifts (e.g., cardiac and TEF/EA repairs)

**Postoperative management**

- Postoperative monitoring depends on type of surgery and preoperative medical condition
- ICU admission for: Continued ventilation and/or paralysis, hemodynamic monitoring, appropriate fluid management, observation for the development of potential complications resulting from surgery, feeding including parenteral nutrition, antibiotics, and analgesia for patients who underwent major surgeries (e.g., TEF/EA repair, laryngeal cleft, cardiac surgery)

---

**SUGGESTED READING**

- Aycan IO. Turgut H, Yildirim ZB, Kavak GO. Anesthetic management in VACTERL syndrome. J Clin Exp Invest. 2014;5(1):103-105.

# PSYCHIATRIC DISORDERS

# ELECTROCONVULSIVE THERAPY (ECT)

## LEARNING OBJECTIVES

- Understand the effects of Electroconvulsive therapy (ECT)
- Anesthetic management of ECT

## DEFINITION AND MECHANISM

- Electroconvulsive therapy (ECT) is a procedure in which small electric currents are passed through the brain to intentionally trigger a brief tonic-clonic epileptic seizure
- Is a safe and effective treatment for severe medication-resistant depression
- Can also be beneficial in:
  - Severe mania
  - Catatonia
  - Agitation and aggression in people with dementia
  - Schizophrenia
- Performed under general anesthesia
- Modern ECT devices deliver brief electrical stimuli via two electrodes and are equipped with controls to adjust the duration and frequency of the stimulus
- The electrodes can either be attached on both sides of the head, typically bitemporal, for bilateral ECT or on the dominant hemisphere for unilateral ECT

| Effects | |
|---|---|
| Cardiovascular effects | Bradycardia<br>Hypotension<br>Possibly asystole<br>Systolic arterial pressure may increase by 30-40%<br>Heart rate may increase by 20% or peak at 3-5 min<br>Myocardial oxygen consumption increases while myocardial oxygen supply may be reduced<br>Myocardial ischemia and infarction may occur<br>Left ventricular systolic and diastolic function can remain decreased up to 6 h after ECT |
| Cerebral effects | Increase in:<br>Cerebral oxygen consumption<br>Blood flow<br>Intracranial pressure<br>Reports of:<br>Transient ischemic deficits<br>Intracranial hemorrhage<br>Cortical blindness<br>Prolonged seizures<br>Status epilepticus<br>Postictal:<br>Disorientation<br>Impaired attention<br>Memory problems<br>Short-term memory impairment lasting several weeks<br>Permanent memory loss<br>Retrograde and aterograde amnesia |
| Other physiological effects | Increased intraocular pressure<br>Increased intragastric pressure |
| General physical effects | Headaches<br>Myalgia<br>Drowsiness<br>Weakness<br>Nausea<br>Anorexia<br>Increased salivation<br>Dental damage<br>Oral cavity lacerations |

# MANAGEMENT

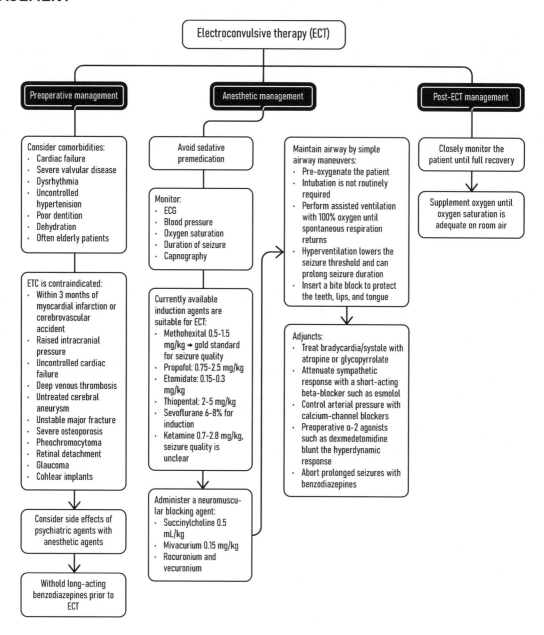

**Electroconvulsive therapy (ECT)**

**Preoperative management**

Consider comorbidities:
- Cardiac failure
- Severe valvular disease
- Dysrhythmia
- Uncontrolled hypertenision
- Poor dentition
- Dehydration
- Often elderly patients

ETC is contraindicated:
- Within 3 months of myocardial infarction or cerebrovascular accident
- Raised intracranial pressure
- Uncontrolled cardiac failure
- Deep venous thrombosis
- Untreated cerebral aneurysm
- Unstable major fracture
- Severe osteoporosis
- Pheochromocytoma
- Retinal detachment
- Glaucoma
- Cohlear implants

Consider side effects of psychiatric agents with anesthetic agents

Withold long-acting benzodiazepines prior to ECT

**Anesthetic management**

Avoid sedative premedication

Monitor:
- ECG
- Blood pressure
- Oxygen saturation
- Duration of seizure
- Capnography

Currently available induction agents are suitable for ECT:
- Methohexital 0.5-1.5 mg/kg → gold standard for seizure quality
- Propofol: 0.75-2.5 mg/kg
- Etomidate: 0.15-0.3 mg/kg
- Thiopental: 2-5 mg/kg
- Sevoflurane 6-8% for induction
- Ketamine 0.7-2.8 mg/kg, seizure quality is unclear

Administer a neuromuscular blocking agent:
- Succinylcholine 0.5 mL/kg
- Mivacurium 0.15 mg/kg
- Rocuronium and vecuronium

Maintain airway by simple airway maneuvers:
- Pre-oxygenate the patient
- Intubation is not routinely required
- Perform assisted ventilation with 100% oxygen until spontaneous respiration returns
- Hyperventilation lowers the seizure threshold and can prolong seizure duration
- Insert a bite block to protect the teeth, lips, and tongue

Adjuncts:
- Treat bradycardia/systole with atropine or glycopyrrolate
- Attenuate sympathetic response with a short-acting beta-blocker such as esmolol
- Control arterial pressure with calcium-channel blockers
- Preoperative α-2 agonists such as dexmedetomidine blunt the hyperdynamic response
- Abort prolonged seizures with benzodiazepines

**Post-ECT management**

Closely monitor the patient until full recovery

Supplement oxygen until oxygen saturation is adequate on room air

## SUGGESTED READING

- Pollard BJ, Kitchen, G. Handbook of Clinical Anaesthesia. Fourth Edition. CRC Press. 2018. 978-1-4987-6289-2.
- Uppa Vl, Dourish J, Macfarlane A. Anaesthesia for electroconvulsive therapy. Continuing Education in Anaesthesia Critical Care & Pain. 2010. 10;(6); 192-196.

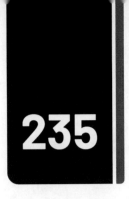

# 235

# MONOAMINE OXIDASE INHIBITORS (MAOI)

## LEARNING OBJECTIVES

- Describe the side effects and anesthetic consequences of patients on monoamine oxidase inhibitors (MAOI)

## DEFINITION AND MECHANISM

- Monoamine oxidase inhibitors (MAOI) inhibit the activity of one or both monoamine oxidase enzymes A and B, thus preventing the breakdown of monoamine neurotransmitters serotonin and norepinephrine and thereby increasing their availability
  - MAO type A has a preference for norepinephrine and serotonin
  - MAO type B deaminates tyramine and phenylethylamine
- Risk of hypertensive crisis with norepinephrine release
- MAOIs are effective antidepressants and are used in the treatment of:
  - Panic disorder
  - Atypical depression
  - Anxiety disorder
  - Depression
  - Bulimia
  - Post-traumatic stress disorder
  - Borderline personality disorder
  - Obsessive compulsive disorder
  - Bipolar depression
- Be cautious of withdrawal symptoms and recurrence of the psychiatric illness if the psychoactive drug is stopped
- MAOIs interact severely with commonly used anesthetic agents
  - MAOIs inhibit the metabolism of indirectly acting sympathomimetics resulting in the potentiation of their action
  - Where necessary, direct sympathomimetics are preferable

## SIDE EFFECTS

- Dry mouth
- Nausea, diarrhea, or constipation
- Headache
- Drowsiness
- Insomnia
- Dizziness or lightheadedness
- Skin reaction at the patch site
- Involuntary muscle jerks
- Low blood pressure
- Reduced sexual desire or difficulty reaching orgasm
- Weight gain
- Difficulty starting a urine flow
- Muscle cramps
- Prickling or tingling sensation in the skin (paresthesia)

# MANAGEMENT

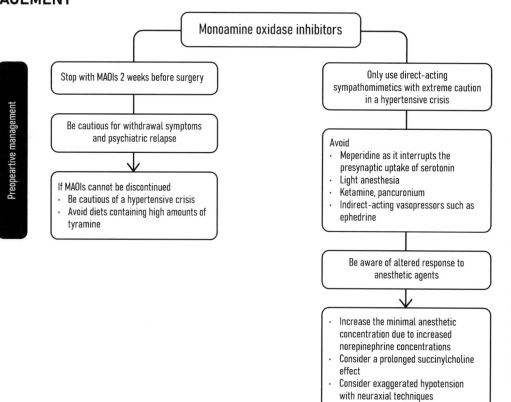

Monoamine oxidase inhibitors

**Preopeartive management**

Stop with MAOIs 2 weeks before surgery

Be cautious for withdrawal symptoms and psychiatric relapse

If MAOIs cannot be discontinued
- Be cautious of a hypertensive crisis
- Avoid diets containing high amounts of tyramine

**Perioperative management**

Only use direct-acting sympathomimetics with extreme caution in a hypertensive crisis

Avoid
- Meperidine as it interrupts the presynaptic uptake of serotonin
- Light anesthesia
- Ketamine, pancuronium
- Indirect-acting vasopressors such as ephedrine

Be aware of altered response to anesthetic agents

- Increase the minimal anesthetic concentration due to increased norepinephrine concentrations
- Consider a prolonged succinylcholine effect
- Consider exaggerated hypotension with neuraxial techniques
- Use direct-acting vasopressors only, consider reduced doses

**SUGGESTED READING**

- Peck T, Wong A, Norman E. 2010. Anaesthetic implications of psychoactive drugs. Continuing Education in Anaesthesia Critical Care & Pain.10;(6); 177-181.

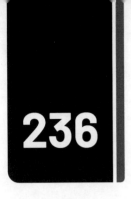

# NEUROLEPTIC MALIGNANT SYNDROME

**236**

## LEARNING OBJECTIVES

- Recognize neuroleptic malignant syndrome (NMS)
- Management of NMS

## DEFINITION AND MECHANISM

- Neuroleptic malignant syndrome (NMS) is a rare, potentially fatal neurological condition caused by an adverse reaction to neuroleptic (haloperidol) or antipsychotic agents
- Caused by either treatment with dopamine receptor antagonists or by the withdrawal of dopamine receptor agonists
- This leads to an acute blockade of dopaminergic transmission in the:
  - Nigrostriatum – which produces rigidity
  - Hypothalamus – which produces hyperthermia
  - Corticolimbic system – which produces an altered mental state
- Usually develops within the first 2 weeks of treatment with the agent but can occur at any time
- The mortality risk is 10%

- Clinical manifestations: remember the mnemonic FEVERS:
  - **F**ever
  - **E**ncephalopathy
  - **V**ital signs unstable
  - **E**levated labs
  - **R**igidity (vs myoclonus in serotonin syndrome)
  - **S**weating

## SIGNS AND SYMPTOMS

Autonomic signs and symptoms
- Fever
- Sweating
- Unstable blood pressure
- Tachycardia
- Autonomic dysfunction

Neuromuscular/behavioral signs and symptoms
- Muscle cramps/rigidity
- Tremor
- Stupor
- Confusion
- Delirium
- Agitation

## RISK FACTORS

- Dehydration
- Agitation
- Catatonia
- Typical neuroleptics: e.g., haloperidol, chlorpromazine
- Atypical neuroleptics: e.g., olanzapine, clozapine, risperidone

- Anti-dopaminergic antiemetics: e.g., droperidol
- Withdrawal of dopaminergic agents: levodopa, amantadine

## CRITERIA FOR DIAGNOSIS

| Major criteria | Minor criteria |
|---|---|
| High fever | Tachycardia |
| Muscular rigidity | Raised blood pressure |
| Elevated serum creatine kinase | Tachypnea |
| | Altered consciousness level |
| | Sweating |

# MANAGEMENT

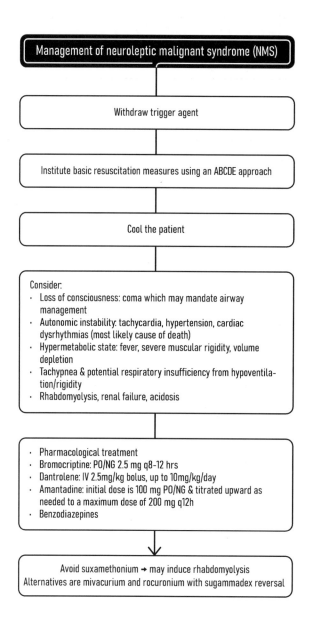

**Management of neuroleptic malignant syndrome (NMS)**

Withdraw trigger agent

Institute basic resuscitation measures using an ABCDE approach

Cool the patient

Consider:
- Loss of consciousness: coma which may mandate airway management
- Autonomic instability: tachycardia, hypertension, cardiac dysrhythmias (most likely cause of death)
- Hypermetabolic state: fever, severe muscular rigidity, volume depletion
- Tachypnea & potential respiratory insufficiency from hypoventilation/rigidity
- Rhabdomyolysis, renal failure, acidosis

- Pharmacological treatment
- Bromocriptine: PO/NG 2.5 mg q8-12 hrs
- Dantrolene: IV 2.5mg/kg bolus, up to 10mg/kg/day
- Amantadine: initial dose is 100 mg PO/NG & titrated upward as needed to a maximum dose of 200 mg q12h
- Benzodiazepines

Avoid suxamethonium → may induce rhabdomyolysis
Alternatives are mivacurium and rocuronium with sugammadex reversal

## SUGGESTED READING

- Adnet, P., Lestavel, P., Krivosic-Horber, R., 2000. Neuroleptic malignant syndrome. British Journal of Anaesthesia 85, 129–135.
- Bartakke, A., Corredor, C., Van Rensburg, A., 2020. Serotonin syndrome in the perioperative period. BJA Education 20, 10–17.
- Pollard BJ, Kitchen, G. Handbook of Clinical Anaesthesia. Fourth Edition. CRC Press. 2018. 978-1-4987-6289-2.

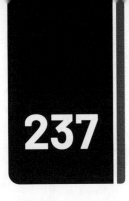

# SEROTONIN SYNDROME

## LEARNING OBJECTIVES

- Describe the wide variety of signs and symptoms of serotonin syndrome (SS)
- Management of a patient with SS

## DEFINITION AND MECHANISM

- Serotonin syndrome (SS) is a potentially life-threatening drug interaction caused by excessive serotoninergic activity in the central nervous system (CNS)
- Can arise from therapeutic drug use, drug interactions, or intentional overdose of medications that affect the serotonergic system, use the mnemonic MAD HOT:
  - **M**yoclonus
  - **A**utonomic instability
  - **D**elirium, Diarrhea
  - **H**ot (fever)
- Central nervous system (CNS): seizure, altered level of consciousness (LOC)
- Cardiovascular system (CVS): tachycardia & hypertension, autonomic instability, arrhythmia
- Musculoskeletal system (MSK): rigidity, rhabdomyolysis, hyperkalemia & renal failure
- Hyperthermia
- Disseminated intravascular coagulation
- Onset of SS typically occurs all of a sudden within 24-48h of exposure to the triggering agents and usually resolves quickly after the triggering agent is discontinued
- Note that the washout period after discontinuation is highly variable between psychotropic drugs

## SIGNS AND SYMPTOMS

| Signs and symptoms | |
|---|---|
| Mild | Sweating |
| | Fever |
| | Agitation |
| | Confusion |
| | Anxiety |
| | Tachycardia |
| | Diarrhea |
| | Tremors |
| | Poor coordination |
| Full-blown | Hyperthermia |
| | Shivering |
| | Diaphoresis |
| | Hypomania |
| | Hypervigilance |
| | Hypertension |
| | Hyperreflexia |
| | Clonus |
| | Myoclonus |
| Severe | Hyperthermia > 40°C |
| | Seizures |
| | Coma |
| | Rigidity |

## DIFFERENTIAL DIAGNOSIS

| Disease | Medication exposure | Shared clinical features | Distinguishing clinical features |
|---|---|---|---|
| Serotonin Syndrome | Serotonergic medications | Hypertension | Clonus<br>Hyperreflexia<br>Hyperactive bowel sounds |
| Neuroleptic malignant syndrome | Dopamine antagonists | Tachycardia | Bradykinesia<br>Normal reflexes (no clonus or hyperreflexia)<br>*Pertinent positive first, then pertinent negative |
| Anticholinergic toxicity | Acetylcholine antagonist | Hyperthermia | Dry skin<br>Absent bowel sounds<br>Normal reflexes (no clonus or hyperreflexia)<br>*Pertinent positive first, then pertinent negative |
| Malignant hyperthermia | Halogenated anesthetics<br>Succinylcholine | Altered mental status | Extreme muscular rigidity<br>Normal reflexes (no clonus or hyperreflexia)<br>*Pertinent positive first, then pertinent negative |

# MANAGEMENT

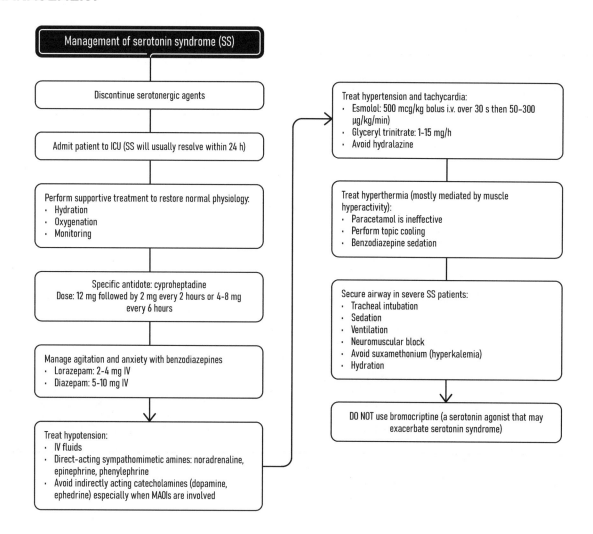

**Management of serotonin syndrome (SS)**

Discontinue serotonergic agents

Admit patient to ICU (SS will usually resolve within 24 h)

Perform supportive treatment to restore normal physiology:
- Hydration
- Oxygenation
- Monitoring

Specific antidote: cyproheptadine
Dose: 12 mg followed by 2 mg every 2 hours or 4-8 mg every 6 hours

Manage agitation and anxiety with benzodiazepines
- Lorazepam: 2-4 mg IV
- Diazepam: 5-10 mg IV

Treat hypotension:
- IV fluids
- Direct-acting sympathomimetic amines: noradrenaline, epinephrine, phenylephrine
- Avoid indirectly acting catecholamines (dopamine, ephedrine) especially when MAOIs are involved

Treat hypertension and tachycardia:
- Esmolol: 500 mcg/kg bolus i.v. over 30 s then 50–300 µg/kg/min)
- Glyceryl trinitrate: 1-15 mg/h
- Avoid hydralazine

Treat hyperthermia (mostly mediated by muscle hyperactivity):
- Paracetamol is ineffective
- Perform topic cooling
- Benzodiazepine sedation

Secure airway in severe SS patients:
- Tracheal intubation
- Sedation
- Ventilation
- Neuromuscular block
- Avoid suxamethonium (hyperkalemia)
- Hydration

DO NOT use bromocriptine (a serotonin agonist that may exacerbate serotonin syndrome)

## SUGGESTED READING

- Bartakke, A., Corredor, C., Van Rensburg, A., 2020. Serotonin syndrome in the perioperative period. BJA Education 20, 10–17.
- Chinniah, S., French, J.L.H., Levy, D.M., 2008. Serotonin and anaesthesia. Continuing Education in Anaesthesia Critical Care & Pain 8, 43–45.
- Francescangeli, J., Karamchandani, K., Powell, M., Bonavia, A., 2019. The Serotonin Syndrome: From Molecular Mechanisms to Clinical Practice. International Journal of Molecular Sciences 20, 2288.

Serotonin syndrome

# RARE CO-EXISTING DISEASES

# AMYLOIDOSIS

## LEARNING OBJECTIVES

- Involved systems in and classification of amyloidosis
- Anesthetic management of amyloidosis

## DEFINITION AND MECHANISM

- Amyloidosis constitutes a group of diseases characterized by the extracellular deposition of insoluble protein aggregates
- Precursor proteins, produced by various mechanisms, are deposited extracellularly as insoluble fibrils resulting in disruption of tissue architecture and organ dysfunction
- The disease spectrum may be inherited or acquired and localized or systemic
- May occur as its own entity or in association with dialysis-dependent renal failure, chronic infection, or inflammation
- Diagnosed based on histological demonstration of amyloid deposits in affected tissues

## CLASSIFICATION OF AMYLOID SUBTYPES

| Abbreviation | Protein type | Major anesthetic considerations | Treatment |
|---|---|---|---|
| AL | Light chain (plasma cell-derived) | Airway difficulties, cardiomyopathy, arrhythmias, renal failure, hepatic failure, bleeding, autonomic/peripheral neuropathy, endocrine organ dysfunction, treatment-related complications | Symptomatic, chemotherapy, immunosuppression, endocrine supplementation, stem cell/organ transplantation |
| AA | Serum amyloid A (acute phase protein) | Features of underlying cause: Infection: Tuberculosis, leprosy, Bronchiectasis Inflammation Autoimmune disease Malignancy: Hodgkin's lymphoma Respiratory tract lesions Hepatic failure Renal failure Treatment-related complications | Treat underlying cause, surgical (localized disease) |
| Ab | b-Amyloid | Consent issues (Alzheimer's dementia) | Supportive |
| Ab2M | b2-Microglobulin | Dialysis-dependent renal failure, difficult positioning (arthropathy) | Symptomatic, renal transplant |
| ATTR | Transthyretin Wild type ('Senile') Mutant type (Hereditary) | Heart failure (males, slow progressive) Autonomic/peripheral neuropathy, cardiomyopathy, gastrointestinal dysfunction | Symptomatic Symptomatic, liver transplant |

# SYSTEMS INVOLVED

| Associated complications | |
|---|---|
| Airway and the respiratory system | Failed intubation<br>Hemorrhage<br>Obstruction<br>Macroglossia predisposes to difficult intubation<br>Laryngeal amyloid presents with hoarseness, dyspnea, cough, stridor, and odynophagia<br>Tracheobronchial involvement is relatively uncommon<br>Parenchymal amyloid may be unilateral or bilateral, diffuse or nodular |
| Cardiovascular system | Restrictive cardiomyopathy<br>Diastolic heart failure<br>Conduction disorders<br>Ischaemic heart disease<br>Arrhythmias<br>Orthostatic hypotension<br>Congestive heart failure |
| Hematological system | Microvascular fragility<br>Platelet dysfunction<br>Impaired fibrin formation<br>Clotting factor deficiencies: factor X is most common, factors II, VI, VII, and IX also reported<br>Impaired vasoconstriction<br>Increased risk of hemorrhage |
| Neurological system | Autonomic and peripheral neuropathy |
| Other systems | Renal dysfunction: nephrotic syndrome & renal failure<br>Visceral organomegaly<br>Early satiety<br>Malabsorption<br>Protein-losing enteropathy<br>Ascites<br>Dysmotility<br>Gastrointestinal hemorrhage<br>Deranged liver function<br>Thyroid, adrenals, and testes infiltration |

# ANESTHETIC DRUGS IN AMYLOIDOSIS

| Class of drug | Caution |
|---|---|
| Anticholinergics | Blunted, or absent response |
| Anticoagulants | Use is contentious if bleeding risk evident |
| Benzylisoquinoliniums | Effect antagonized by anticholinesterase inhibitors |
| b-Blockers, Ca-channel blockers | Negative inotropic effects risk cardiac decompensation |
| Cardiac glycosides | Drug binding to protein fibrils risks toxicity at therapeutic levels |
| Depolarizing neuromuscular blocking agents | Potential for hyperkalaemic response in neurological dysfunction<br>Prolonged action with anticholinesterase inhibitors |
| Halogenated volatile agents | Exposure increases in b-amyloid deposition in animal models |
| IV sedatives | Predictable haemodynamic depressant effects (except ketamine)<br>Increased b-amyloid deposition not demonstrated with propofol, barbiturates and benzodiazepines |

# MANAGEMENT

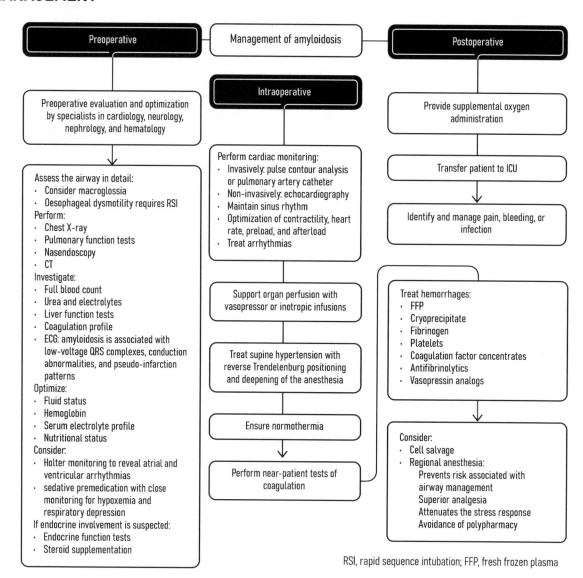

**Management of amyloidosis**

**Preoperative**

Preoperative evaluation and optimization by specialists in cardiology, neurology, nephrology, and hematology

Assess the airway in detail:
- Consider macroglossia
- Oesophageal dysmotility requires RSI

Perform:
- Chest X-ray
- Pulmonary function tests
- Nasendoscopy
- CT

Investigate:
- Full blood count
- Urea and electrolytes
- Liver function tests
- Coagulation profile
- ECG: amyloidosis is associated with low-voltage QRS complexes, conduction abnormalities, and pseudo-infarction patterns

Optimize:
- Fluid status
- Hemoglobin
- Serum electrolyte profile
- Nutritional status

Consider:
- Holter monitoring to reveal atrial and ventricular arrhythmias
- sedative premedication with close monitoring for hypoxemia and respiratory depression

If endocrine involvement is suspected:
- Endocrine function tests
- Steroid supplementation

**Intraoperative**

Perform cardiac monitoring:
- Invasively: pulse contour analysis or pulmonary artery catheter
- Non-invasively: echocardiography
- Maintain sinus rhythm
- Optimization of contractility, heart rate, preload, and afterload
- Treat arrhythmias

Support organ perfusion with vasopressor or inotropic infusions

Treat supine hypertension with reverse Trendelenburg positioning and deepening of the anesthesia

Ensure normothermia

Perform near-patient tests of coagulation

**Postoperative**

Provide supplemental oxygen administration

Transfer patient to ICU

Identify and manage pain, bleeding, or infection

Treat hemorrhages:
- FFP
- Cryoprecipitate
- Fibrinogen
- Platelets
- Coagulation factor concentrates
- Antifibrinolytics
- Vasopressin analogs

Consider:
- Cell salvage
- Regional anesthesia:
  Prevents risk associated with airway management
  Superior analgesia
  Attenuates the stress response
  Avoidance of polypharmacy

RSI, rapid sequence intubation; FFP, fresh frozen plasma

## SUGGESTED READING

- Wani Z, Harkawat DK, Sharma M. Amyloidosis and Anesthesia. Anesth Essays Res. 2017;11(1):233-237.
- Fleming I, Dubrey S, Williams B. 2012. Amyloidosis and anaesthesia, Continuing Education in Anaesthesia Critical Care & Pain.12;(2);72-77.

# 239

# GLYCOGEN STORAGE DISORDERS

## LEARNING OBJECTIVES

- Understanding of glycogen storage disorders (GSD)
- Pre- and perioperative management of GSD

## DEFINITION AND MECHANISM

- Glycogen storage disorders (GSD) are metabolic disorders caused by an enzyme deficiency affecting glycogen synthesis, glycogen breakdown, or glucose breakdown, typically in muscles and/or liver cells
- Glycogen in skeletal muscles provides a ready source of fuel during exercise, and hepatic glycogen helps maintain plasma glucose levels during fasting
- Attempts to maintain glucose homeostasis can result in muscle degradation as amino acids are used as an alternative substrate
- Patients are at risk of hypoglycemia
- GSD is hereditary and occurs in about 1/20 000 babies
- There are 14 types of GS, with type I being the most common

## TYPES OF GSD

| Disease and eponym | Inheritance and incidence | Organs affected | Clinical features |
|---|---|---|---|
| Type I (von Gierke disease) | Autosomal recessive, 1:100 000–200 000 | Liver (and renal) | Hypoglycemia, lactic acidosis, ketosis, hepatomegaly, truncal obesity, short stature, hypertriglyceridemia, hyperuricemia and gout, platelet dysfunction, renal dysfunction<br>Good prognosis with supportive treatment |
| Type II (Pompe disease) | Autosomal recessive, 1:50 000 | Cardiac, muscle, liver | Hypotonia and skeletal muscle weakness, hypertrophic cardiomyopathy. Death from cardiorespiratory failure by 2 yr in severe infantile form |
| Type III (Cori disease) | Autosomal recessive, 1:100 000–150 000 | Liver, muscles | Hypoglycemia, ketonuria, hepatomegaly, muscle fatigue<br>Good prognosis |
| Type IV (Andersen disease) | Autosomal recessive, 1:500 000 | Liver | Failure to thrive, hypotonia, hepatosplenomegaly<br>Hepatic cirrhosis leading to death by 5 yr |
| Type V (McArdle disease) | Autosomal recessive, 1:500 000 | Muscles | Exercise intolerance, muscle cramps, fatigability<br>Good prognosis |
| Type VI (Hers disease) | 1:200 000 | Liver | Hepatomegaly, mild hypoglycemia, hyperlipidemia, ketosis<br>Good prognosis |
| Type VII (Tarui disease) | Autosomal recessive, 1:500 000 | Muscles | Similar to GSD type V |
| Type VIII/IX (phosphorylase kinase deficiency) | Autosomal and X-linked | Liver | Similar to GSD type III, but no myopathy |

## SIGNS AND SYMPTOMS

General symptoms of GSD may include:
- Poor growth
- Heat intolerance
- Bruising too easily
- Hypoglycemia
- An enlarged liver
- A swollen abdomen
- Low muscle tone
- Muscle pain and cramping during exercise
- Fatigue
- Obesity
- Kidney problems
- Low resistance to infections
- Mouth sores
- Heart problems
- Gout

Symptoms for babies may include:
- Too much acid in the blood (acidosis)
- High blood cholesterol levels (hyperlipidemia)

## DIAGNOSIS

- A low blood glucose level
- Abdominal ultrasound to detect an enlarged liver
- Tissue biopsy
- Abnormal blood tests
- Gene testing

# MANAGEMENT

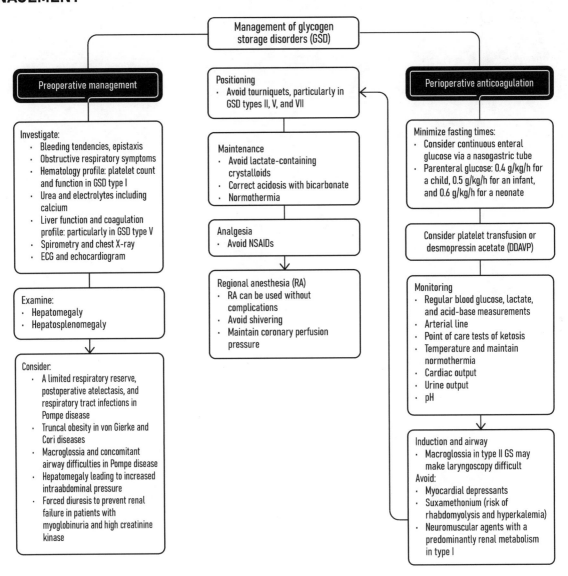

**Management of glycogen storage disorders (GSD)**

## Preoperative management

**Investigate:**
- Bleeding tendencies, epistaxis
- Obstructive respiratory symptoms
- Hematology profile: platelet count and function in GSD type I
- Urea and electrolytes including calcium
- Liver function and coagulation profile: particularly in GSD type V
- Spirometry and chest X-ray
- ECG and echocardiogram

**Examine:**
- Hepatomegaly
- Hepatosplenomegaly

**Consider:**
- A limited respiratory reserve, postoperative atelectasis, and respiratory tract infections in Pompe disease
- Truncal obesity in von Gierke and Cori diseases
- Macroglossia and concomitant airway difficulties in Pompe disease
- Hepatomegaly leading to increased intraabdominal pressure
- Forced diuresis to prevent renal failure in patients with myoglobinuria and high creatinine kinase

## Positioning
- Avoid tourniquets, particularly in GSD types II, V, and VII

## Maintenance
- Avoid lactate-containing crystalloids
- Correct acidosis with bicarbonate
- Normothermia

## Analgesia
- Avoid NSAIDs

## Regional anesthesia (RA)
- RA can be used without complications
- Avoid shivering
- Maintain coronary perfusion pressure

## Perioperative anticoagulation

**Minimize fasting times:**
- Consider continuous enteral glucose via a nasogastric tube
- Parenteral glucose: 0.4 g/kg/h for a child, 0.5 g/kg/h for an infant, and 0.6 g/kg/h for a neonate

Consider platelet transfusion or desmopressin acetate (DDAVP)

**Monitoring**
- Regular blood glucose, lactate, and acid-base measurements
- Arterial line
- Point of care tests of ketosis
- Temperature and maintain normothermia
- Cardiac output
- Urine output
- pH

**Induction and airway**
- Macroglossia in type II GS may make laryngoscopy difficult

Avoid:
- Myocardial depressants
- Suxamethonium (risk of rhabdomyolysis and hyperkalemia)
- Neuromuscular agents with a predominantly renal metabolism in type I

## SUGGESTED READING

- Grant S, Nargis A. 2011. Perioperative care of children with inherited metabolic disorders. Continuing Education in Anaesthesia Critical Care & Pain.11:2;62-68.
- Pollard BJ, Kitchen, G. Handbook of Clinical Anaesthesia. Fourth Edition. CRC Press. 2018. 978-1-4987-6289-2.
- Yeoh C, Teng H, Jackson J, et al. Metabolic Disorders and Anesthesia. Curr Anesthesiol Rep. 2019;9(3):340-359.

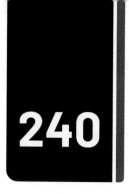

# 240

# HEREDITARY ANGIEDEMA (C1 ESTERASE DEFICIENCY)

## LEARNING OBJECTIVES

- Describe hereditary angiedema
- Anesthetic management of hereditary angiedema

## DEFINITION AND MECHANISM

### *Angiedema:*

- Angiedema is painless swelling of subcutaneous or submucosal tissues in any part of the body due to increased vascular permeability
- It can cause symptoms secondary to a pressure effect on neighboring structures
- It can lead to life-threatening complications when occurring in the airway
- C1 esterase inhibitor deficiency can be hereditary or acquired, and these two entities are indistinguishable

### *Hereditary C1 esterase inhibitor deficiency (HAE):*

- The prevalence of HAE is 1:50000
- Either due to:
  - Impaired production of C1 esterase inhibitor (type 1, 85% of cases)
  - Poor function of the protein (type 2, 15% of cases)
- C1 esterase inhibitor (C1-INH) prevents the autoactivation of C1, the first factor of the classical pathway in the complement system
- The lack of C1-INH leads to uncontrolled complement activation with the release of vasoactive and chemotactic peptides
- Thereby causing increased vascular permeability, vasodilatation, and contraction of the vascular smooth muscle
- And resulting in acute, localized, non-pitting, nonpruritic, non-erythematous, and demarcated angiedema
- Swelling typically lasts for 2–5 days before resolving spontaneously
- The first attack occurs often before the age of 15 and the condition lasts lifelong but symptoms tend to decrease with increasing age
- Attacks can be precipitated by a variety of triggers:
  - Dental treatment
  - Surgery
  - Trauma
  - Stress (mental or physical)
  - Exercise
  - Infection
  - Alcohol consumption
  - Anesthesia
  - Menstruation
  - Certain agents: angiotensin-converting enzyme (ACE)- inhibitors and estrogens

## SYMPTOMS

- Potential airway compromise
- Symptoms of acute bowel obstruction: vomiting, anorexia, and severe abdominal pain
- Swollen lips, eyelids, tongue, extremities, and genitals

# MANAGEMENT

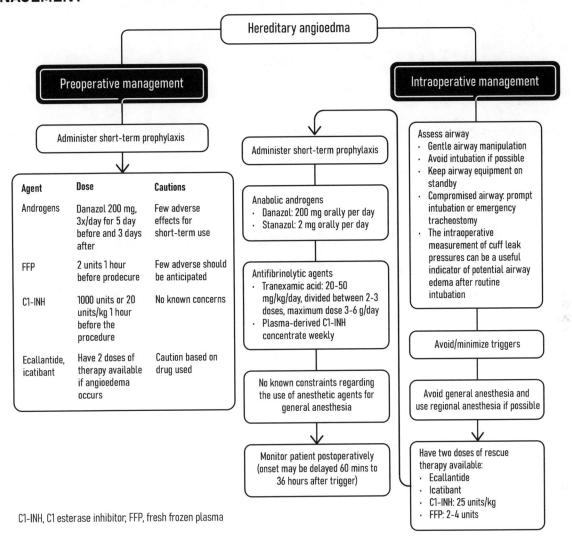

**Hereditary angioedema**

## Preoperative management

### Administer short-term prophylaxis

| Agent | Dose | Cautions |
|---|---|---|
| Androgens | Danazol 200 mg, 3x/day for 5 day before and 3 days after | Few adverse effects for short-term use |
| FFP | 2 units 1 hour before prodecure | Few adverse should be anticipated |
| C1-INH | 1000 units or 20 units/kg 1 hour before the procedure | No known concerns |
| Ecallantide, icatibant | Have 2 doses of therapy available if angioedema occurs | Caution based on drug used |

C1-INH, C1 esterase inhibitor; FFP, fresh frozen plasma

### Administer short-term prophylaxis

**Anabolic androgens**
- Danazol: 200 mg orally per day
- Stanazol: 2 mg orally per day

**Antifibrinolytic agents**
- Tranexamic acid: 20-50 mg/kg/day, divided between 2-3 doses, maximum dose 3-6 g/day
- Plasma-derived C1-INH concentrate weekly

No known constraints regarding the use of anesthetic agents for general anesthesia

Monitor patient postoperatively (onset may be delayed 60 mins to 36 hours after trigger)

## Intraoperative management

**Assess airway**
- Gentle airway manipulation
- Avoid intubation if possible
- Keep airway equipment on standby
- Compromised airway: prompt intubation or emergency tracheostomy
- The intraoperative measurement of cuff leak pressures can be a useful indicator of potential airway edema after routine intubation

Avoid/minimize triggers

Avoid general anesthesia and use regional anesthesia if possible

**Have two doses of rescue therapy available:**
- Ecallantide
- Icatibant
- C1-INH: 25 units/kg
- FFP: 2-4 units

## SUGGESTED READING

- Hoyer C, Hill MR, Kaminski ER. 2012. An overview of differential diagnosis and clinical management. Continuing Education in Anaesthesia Critical Care & Pain. 1:6;307–311.
- Williams AH, Craig TJ. Perioperative management for patients with hereditary angiedema. Allergy Rhinol (Providence). 2015;6(1):50-55.

# 241

# HEREDITARY HEMORRHAGIC TELANGIECTASIAS

## LEARNING OBJECTIVES

- Signs and symptoms, complications and management of hereditary hemorrhagic telangiectasias (HHT)

## DEFINITION AND MECHANISM

- Hereditary hemorrhagic telangiectasias (HHT) causes abnormal connections, called arteriovenous malformations (AVMs), to develop between arteries and veins
- The most common locations affected are the nose, lungs, brain, and liver
- These AVMs may enlarge over time and are more prone to hemorrhage
- Telangiectasias refers to malformations of small vessels and can be described as dilated arterioles in communication with dilated post-capillary venules
- HHT is an autosomal dominant genetic disorder and is also known as **Osler-Weber-Rendu disease**

## SIGNS AND SYMPTOMS

- Nosebleeds, sometimes daily and often starting in childhood
- Abnormal blood vessels (telangiectasia) may appear just underneath the skin, which show as red or purple spots
- Red or purple spots usually form on the fingertip pads, the lips, and the lining of the nose or the gut
- Iron deficiency anemia
- Shortness of breath
- Headaches
- Seizures
- Abnormal artery-vein connections within the brain, lungs, and liver
- Iron deficiency anemia

## COMPLICATIONS

- Hemorrhage
- Embolism
- Stroke

## DIAGNOSIS

The diagnosis can be made depending on the presence of four criteria, known as the "Curaçao criteria":
- Spontaneous recurrent epistaxis
- Multiple telangiectasias in typical locations
- Proven visceral AVM (lung, liver, brain, spine)
- First-degree family member with HHT

# MANAGEMENT

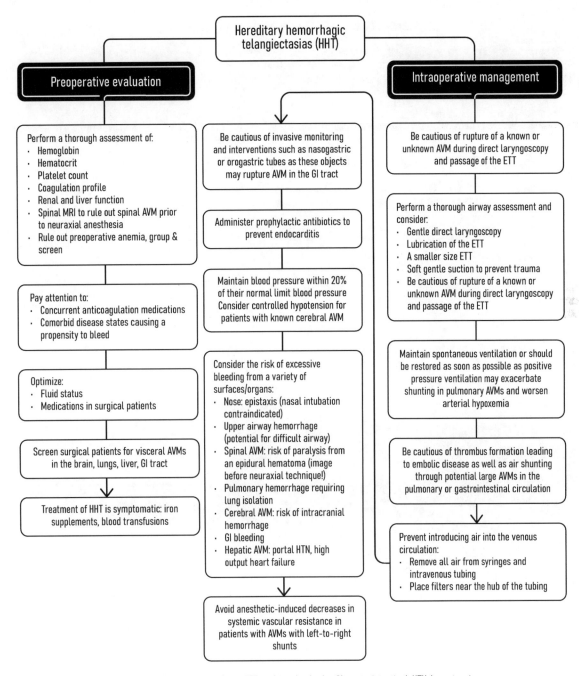

**Hereditary hemorrhagic telangiectasias (HHT)**

## Preoperative evaluation

Perform a thorough assessment of:
- Hemoglobin
- Hematocrit
- Platelet count
- Coagulation profile
- Renal and liver function
- Spinal MRI to rule out spinal AVM prior to neuraxial anesthesia
- Rule out preoperative anemia, group & screen

Pay attention to:
- Concurrent anticoagulation medications
- Comorbid disease states causing a propensity to bleed

Optimize:
- Fluid status
- Medications in surgical patients

Screen surgical patients for visceral AVMs in the brain, lungs, liver, GI tract

Treatment of HHT is symptomatic: iron supplements, blood transfusions

Be cautious of invasive monitoring and interventions such as nasogastric or orogastric tubes as these objects may rupture AVM in the GI tract

Administer prophylactic antibiotics to prevent endocarditis

Maintain blood pressure within 20% of their normal limit blood pressure Consider controlled hypotension for patients with known cerebral AVM

Consider the risk of excessive bleeding from a variety of surfaces/organs:
- Nose: epistaxis (nasal intubation contraindicated)
- Upper airway hemorrhage (potential for difficult airway)
- Spinal AVM: risk of paralysis from an epidural hematoma (image before neuraxial technique!)
- Pulmonary hemorrhage requiring lung isolation
- Cerebral AVM: risk of intracranial hemorrhage
- GI bleeding
- Hepatic AVM: portal HTN, high output heart failure

Avoid anesthetic-induced decreases in systemic vascular resistance in patients with AVMs with left-to-right shunts

## Intraoperative management

Be cautious of rupture of a known or unknown AVM during direct laryngoscopy and passage of the ETT

Perform a thorough airway assessment and consider:
- Gentle direct laryngoscopy
- Lubrication of the ETT
- A smaller size ETT
- Soft gentle suction to prevent trauma
- Be cautious of rupture of a known or unknown AVM during direct laryngoscopy and passage of the ETT

Maintain spontaneous ventilation or should be restored as soon as possible as positive pressure ventilation may exacerbate shunting in pulmonary AVMs and worsen arterial hypoxemia

Be cautious of thrombus formation leading to embolic disease as well as air shunting through potential large AVMs in the pulmonary or gastrointestinal circulation

Prevent introducing air into the venous circulation:
- Remove all air from syringes and intravenous tubing
- Place filters near the hub of the tubing

AVM, arteriovenous malformations; ETT, endotracheal tube; GI, gastrointestinal; HTN, hypertension

## SUGGESTED READING

- Robinson, D., Rogers, B., Kapoor, R., Swan, J., Speas, G., Gutmann, R., 2014. Anesthetic Considerations for a Patient With Hereditary Hemorrhagic Telangiectasia (Osler-Weber-Rendu Syndrome) Undergoing a Five-Box Thoracoscopic Maze Procedure for Atrial Fibrillation. Journal of Investigative Medicine High Impact Case Reports 2, 232470961455366.

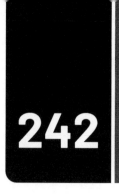

# HIV AND AIDS

## LEARNING OBJECTIVES

- Stages of HIV (human immunodeficiency virus)
- Progression to AIDS (acquired immunodeficiency syndrome)
- Anesthetic management of HIV and AIDS

## DEFINITION AND MECHANISM

- HIV is a virus that attacks the body's immune system, making a person more vulnerable to other infections and diseases
- If HIV is not treated, it can lead to AIDS
- Effective treatment with antiretroviral therapy to reduce the viral load is available, however, no cure exists
- AIDS is the late stage of HIV infection that occurs when the body's immune system is badly damaged because of the virus

## SIGNS AND SYMPTOMS

- Flu-like symptoms within 2-4 weeks after infection
- Fever
- Headache
- Diarrhea
- Weight loss
- Cough
- Sore throat
- Swollen lymph nodes
- Rash
- Muscle aches
- Night sweats
- Mouth ulcers
- Fatigue

## STAGES OF HIV

| Stage 1: acute HIV infection | Stage 2: chronic or clinically latent HIV infection | Stage 3: AIDS |
|---|---|---|
| 2-4 weeks after infection, the body responds with flu like symptoms, a highly contagious stage | Asymptomatic HIV infection or clinical latency. HIV is still active and continues to replicate. Patients may not have any symptoms but can still transmit HIV. Intake of HIV treatment can prevent the development of stage 3 (AIDS). At the end of this stage, the HIV viral load increases, and the patient moves into stage 3 (AIDS) | The most advanced stage of HIV infection. High viral load and can easily transmit HIV to other people. Opportunistic infections or other serious illnesses are common in this stage. People with AIDS typically survive about three years without HIV treatment |
| | | A person with HIV is considered to have progressed to AIDS when: The number of th eir CD4 cells falls below 200 cells per cubic millimeter of blood (200 cells/mm$^3$) OR If they develop one or more opportunistic infections regardless of their CD4 count |

| Major opportunistic pathogens in HIV/AIDS | |
|---|---|
| Protozoa | Pnemocystis carinii |
| | Toxoplasma gondii |
| | Cryptosporidium parvum |
| | Microsporidia spp. |
| | Isospora belli |
| Fungi and yeasts | Candida spp. |
| | Cryptococcus neoformans |
| | Histoplasma capsulatum |
| | Coccidioides immitis |
| Viruses | Cytomegalovirus |
| | Herpes simplex |
| | Varicella zoster |
| Bacteria | Mycobacterium avium intracellulare |
| | Mycobacterium tuberculosis |
| | Streptococcus pneumoniae |
| | Haemophillus influenzae |
| | Salmonella spp. |
| | Nocardia |
| | Moraxella catarrhalis |

## TREATMENT

- Highly active antiretroviral therapy (HAART) to slow the progression of the disease
- Combination or cocktail of antiretroviral agents to prevent resistance to the virus, typically:
  - A non-nucleoside reverse transcriptase inhibitor (NNRTI)
  - Two nucleoside reverse transcriptase inhibitors (NRTIs)
- Consider side effects of antiretrovirals:
  - Bone marrow suppression
  - Renal failure
  - Peripheral neuropathy
  - p450 activation
  - Lactic acidosis
  - Insulin resistance
  - Dyslipidemia

# MANAGEMENT

## *Preoperative management*

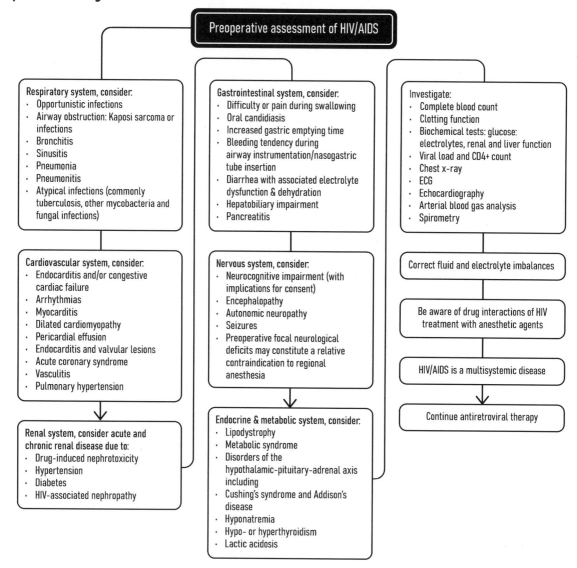

**Preoperative assessment of HIV/AIDS**

**Respiratory system, consider:**
- Opportunistic infections
- Airway obstruction: Kaposi sarcoma or infections
- Bronchitis
- Sinusitis
- Pneumonia
- Pneumonitis
- Atypical infections (commonly tuberculosis, other mycobacteria and fungal infections)

**Gastrointestinal system, consider:**
- Difficulty or pain during swallowing
- Oral candidiasis
- Increased gastric emptying time
- Bleeding tendency during airway instrumentation/nasogastric tube insertion
- Diarrhea with associated electrolyte dysfunction & dehydration
- Hepatobiliary impairment
- Pancreatitis

**Investigate:**
- Complete blood count
- Clotting function
- Biochemical tests: glucose: electrolytes, renal and liver function
- Viral load and CD4+ count
- Chest x-ray
- ECG
- Echocardiography
- Arterial blood gas analysis
- Spirometry

**Cardiovascular system, consider:**
- Endocarditis and/or congestive cardiac failure
- Arrhythmias
- Myocarditis
- Dilated cardiomyopathy
- Pericardial effusion
- Endocarditis and valvular lesions
- Acute coronary syndrome
- Vasculitis
- Pulmonary hypertension

**Nervous system, consider:**
- Neurocognitive impairment (with implications for consent)
- Encephalopathy
- Autonomic neuropathy
- Seizures
- Preoperative focal neurological deficits may constitute a relative contraindication to regional anesthesia

**Correct fluid and electrolyte imbalances**

**Be aware of drug interactions of HIV treatment with anesthetic agents**

**HIV/AIDS is a multisystemic disease**

**Continue antiretroviral therapy**

**Renal system, consider acute and chronic renal disease due to:**
- Drug-induced nephrotoxicity
- Hypertension
- Diabetes
- HIV-associated nephropathy

**Endocrine & metabolic system, consider:**
- Lipodystrophy
- Metabolic syndrome
- Disorders of the hypothalamic-pituitary-adrenal axis including
- Cushing's syndrome and Addison's disease
- Hyponatremia
- Hypo- or hyperthyroidism
- Lactic acidosis

## *Intraoperative management*

- Reduce the risk of cross infection
  - Vigilance in the use of universal precautions
  - Administer post-exposure prophylaxis (PEP) to healthcare workers as soon as possible after the injury, ideally within 1–2 hours

- Obstetric anesthesia
  - Cesarean section reduces the incidence of mother-to-child transmission
  - Administer antiretroviral therapy (ART)
  - RA is not contraindicated
  - Epidural blood patch for post dural puncture headache (PDPH) is safe
- Pain management
- Multidisciplinary pain management

# SUGGESTED READING

- Leelanukrom R. Anaesthetic considerations of the HIV-infected patients. Curr Opin Anaesthesiol. 2009;22(3):412-418.
- Prout J, Agarwal B. 2005. Anaesthesia and critical care for patients with HIV infection. Continuing Education in Anaesthesia Critical Care & Pain. 5;5:153-156.
- Wilson, S. 2009 HIV and anaesthesia. Updtae in anaesthesia.

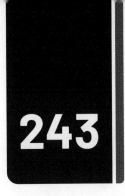

# HUNTINGTON'S DISEASE

## LEARNING OBJECTIVES

- Describe Huntington's Disease (HD)
- Management of HD

## DEFINITION AND MECHANISM

- Huntington's disease (HD) is an autosomal dominant genetic disease that causes the progressive degeneration of nerve cells in the brain
- HD results in an increased production of a mutant protein, Huntington
- This protein initially leads to cell loss and atrophy
- The disease attacks areas of the brain that help to control voluntary (intentional) movement, as well as other areas
- People living with HD develop uncontrollable dance-like movements (chorea) and abnormal body postures, as well as problems with behavior, emotion, thinking, and personality
- Adult-onset Huntington's disease is the most common form of Huntington's disease
  - People typically develop the symptoms in their mid-30s and 40s
- Early-onset Huntington's disease is developed in rare instances by children or adolescents

## SIGNS AND SYMPTOMS

The symptoms usually start at 30 to 50 years of age, but can begin much earlier or later:
- Difficulty concentrating and memory lapses
- Depression
- Stumbling and clumsiness
- Involuntary jerking or fidgety movements of the limbs and body (chorea)
- Mood swings and personality changes
- Irritability
- Hallucinations, paranoia, and psychosis
- Problems swallowing (dysphagia), speaking, and breathing
- Muscle problems, such as rigidity or muscle contracture (dystonia)
- Slow or unusual eye movements
- Impaired gait, posture, and balance
- Full-time nursing care is needed in the later stages of the condition

In children, the symptoms often include Parkinson disease-like features such as:
- Slow movements
- Rigidity
- Tremors

## DIAGNOSIS

- Neurological examination
- Family history
- CT, MRI, or PET

# MANAGEMENT

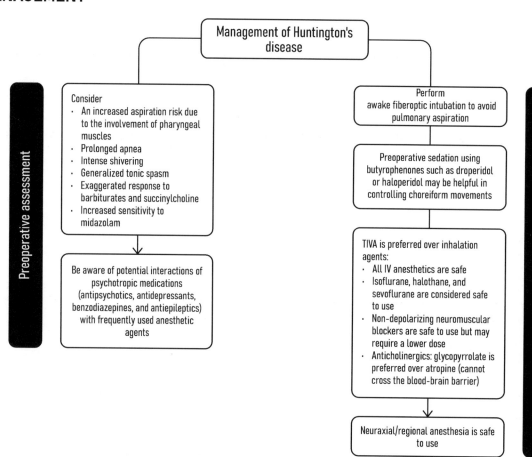

**Management of Huntington's disease**

**Preoperative assessment**

Consider
- An increased aspiration risk due to the involvement of pharyngeal muscles
- Prolonged apnea
- Intense shivering
- Generalized tonic spasm
- Exaggerated response to barbiturates and succinylcholine
- Increased sensitivity to midazolam

Be aware of potential interactions of psychotropic medications (antipsychotics, antidepressants, benzodiazepines, and antiepileptics) with frequently used anesthetic agents

**Perioperative management**

Perform awake fiberoptic intubation to avoid pulmonary aspiration

Preoperative sedation using butyrophenones such as droperidol or haloperidol may be helpful in controlling choreiform movements

TIVA is preferred over inhalation agents:
- All IV anesthetics are safe
- Isoflurane, halothane, and sevoflurane are considered safe to use
- Non-depolarizing neuromuscular blockers are safe to use but may require a lower dose
- Anticholinergics: glycopyrrolate is preferred over atropine (cannot cross the blood-brain barrier)

Neuraxial/regional anesthesia is safe to use

## SUGGESTED READING

- Batra A, Sahni N, Mete UK. Anesthetic management of a patient with Huntington's chorea undergoing robot-assisted nephron-sparing surgery. Indian J Anaesth. 2016;60(11):866-867.
- Kang JM, Chung JY, Han JH, Kim YS, Lee BJ, Yi JW. Anesthetic management of a patient with Huntington's chorea -A case report-. Korean J Anesthesiol. 2013;64(3):262-264.

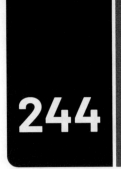

# NEUROFIBROMATOSIS

## LEARNING OBJECTIVES

- Signs and symptoms and management of neurofibromatosis

## DEFINITION AND MECHANISM

- Neurofibromatoses are a group of genetic disorders that cause tumors to form on nerve tissue
- Tumors can develop in the brain, spinal cord, or nerves
- An autosomal dominant disorder caused by a genetic mutation in oncogenes
- Three types of neurofibromatosis:
  - Neurofibromatosis 1: usually diagnosed in childhood
  - Neurofibromatosis 2: usually diagnosed in early adulthood
  - Schwannomatosis: usually diagnosed in early adulthood
- Tumors are usually benign but can sometimes become malignant

## SIGNS AND SYMPTOMS

| Neurofibromatosis 1 (NF1) | Neurofibromatosis 2 (NF2) | Schwannomatosis |
|---|---|---|
| Flat, light brown spots on the skin (cafe au lait spots) Freckling in the armpits or groin area Tiny bumps on the iris of the eye (Lisch nodules) Soft, pea-sized bumps on or under the skin (neurofibromas) Bone deformities Tumor on the optic nerve (optic glioma) Learning disabilities Larger than average head size Short stature | Signs and symptoms of NF2 usually result from the development of benign, slow-growing acoustic neuromas Gradual hearing loss Ringing in the ears Poor balance Headaches | Causes tumors to develop on the cranial, spinal, and peripheral nerves Chronic pain, which can occur anywhere in the body and can be disabling Numbness or weakness in various parts of the body Loss of muscle |
| | Sometimes NF2 can lead to the growth of schwannomas in other nerves, including the cranial, spinal, visual (optic), and peripheral nerves Numbness and weakness in the arms or legs Pain Imbalance or unstable gait Facial drop Vision problems or cataracts Seizures Headache | |

## TREATMENT

- Surgical removal
- Chemotherapy
- Radiotherapy

# MANAGEMENT

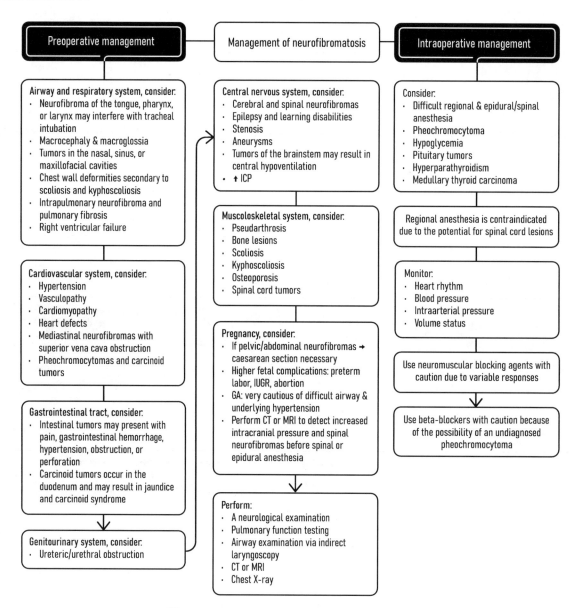

**Preoperative management** — **Management of neurofibromatosis** — **Intraoperative management**

**Airway and respiratory system, consider:**
- Neurofibroma of the tongue, pharynx, or larynx may interfere with tracheal intubation
- Macrocephaly & macroglossia
- Tumors in the nasal, sinus, or maxillofacial cavities
- Chest wall deformities secondary to scoliosis and kyphoscoliosis
- Intrapulmonary neurofibroma and pulmonary fibrosis
- Right ventricular failure

**Cardiovascular system, consider:**
- Hypertension
- Vasculopathy
- Cardiomyopathy
- Heart defects
- Mediastinal neurofibromas with superior vena cava obstruction
- Pheochromocytomas and carcinoid tumors

**Gastrointestinal tract, consider:**
- Intestinal tumors may present with pain, gastrointestinal hemorrhage, hypertension, obstruction, or perforation
- Carcinoid tumors occur in the duodenum and may result in jaundice and carcinoid syndrome

**Genitourinary system, consider:**
- Ureteric/urethral obstruction

**Central nervous system, consider:**
- Cerebral and spinal neurofibromas
- Epilepsy and learning disabilities
- Stenosis
- Aneurysms
- Tumors of the brainstem may result in central hypoventilation
- ↑ ICP

**Muscoloskeletal system, consider:**
- Pseudarthrosis
- Bone lesions
- Scoliosis
- Kyphoscoliosis
- Osteoporosis
- Spinal cord tumors

**Pregnancy, consider:**
- If pelvic/abdominal neurofibromas → caesarean section necessary
- Higher fetal complications: preterm labor, IUGR, abortion
- GA: very cautious of difficult airway & underlying hypertension
- Perform CT or MRI to detect increased intracranial pressure and spinal neurofibromas before spinal or epidural anesthesia

**Perform:**
- A neurological examination
- Pulmonary function testing
- Airway examination via indirect laryngoscopy
- CT or MRI
- Chest X-ray

**Consider:**
- Difficult regional & epidural/spinal anesthesia
- Pheochromocytoma
- Hypoglycemia
- Pituitary tumors
- Hyperparathyroidism
- Medullary thyroid carcinoma

Regional anesthesia is contraindicated due to the potential for spinal cord lesions

**Monitor:**
- Heart rhythm
- Blood pressure
- Intraarterial pressure
- Volume status

Use neuromuscular blocking agents with caution due to variable responses

Use beta-blockers with caution because of the possibility of an undiagnosed pheochromocytoma

ICP, intracranial pressure; IUGR, intrauterine growth restriction

# SUGGESTED READING

- Fox CJ, Tomajian S, Kaye AJ, Russo S, Abadie JV, Kaye AD. Perioperative management of neurofibromatosis type 1. Ochsner J. 2012;12(2):111-121.
- Griffiths, S., Durbridge, J.A., 2011. Anaesthetic implications of neurological disease in pregnancy. Continuing Education in Anaesthesia Critical Care & Pain 11, 157–161.
- Hirsch NP, Murphy A, Radcliffe JJ. Neurofibromatosis: clinical presentations and anaesthetic implications. Br J Anaesth. 2001;86(4):555-564.

# PERIODIC PARALYSIS

## LEARNING OBJECTIVES

- Distinguish the four forms of periodic paralysis (PP)
- Anesthetic management of PP

## DEFINITION AND MECHANISM

- Periodic paralysis (PP) is a group of rare genetic diseases that lead to weakness or paralysis
- The underlying mechanisms of these diseases are malfunctions in the ion channels in skeletal muscle cell membranes that allow electrically charged ions to leak in or out of the muscle cell
- Thereby causing the cell to depolarize and become unable to move
- It causes sudden attacks of short-term muscle weakness, stiffness, or paralysis
- These attacks may affect the whole body or just 1 or 2 limbs
- Four forms of PP exist and most forms affect the skeletal muscles

## MAIN FORMS

| Hypokalemic PP | Hyperkalemic PP | Thyrotoxic PP | Andersen-Tawil syndrome |
|---|---|---|---|
| Potassium leaks into the muscle cells from the bloodstream | Potassium leaks out of the cells into the bloodstream | High levels of thyroid hormone | Swings in potassium blood levels |
| Often starts in the late childhood or teenage years | Often starts by age 10 | It tends to start between 20 and 40 years of age | Usually starts before age 18 |
| Attacks of skeletal muscle weakness may last from a couple of hours to a day | Attacks of skeletal muscle weakness last an average of 30 minutes to 4 hours | Attacks happen anywhere from a few times per year to a few times per week. Attacks can last from hours to days | The attacks last from 1 to 36 hours |
| Paralysis usually affects the limbs and trunk but spares the diaphragm. Chronic muscle weakness occurs in most patients as they age | Acute attacks can be fatal because of cardiac dysrhythmias or respiratory failure. A chronic myopathy frequently develops in older patients | The patient may also have thyroid-related symptoms such as anxiety, sweating, weight loss, and an abnormal sensation of the heartbeat (palpitations) | Includes significant heart rhythm problems, fainting, and risk of sudden death |
| The genetic defect is a rare autosomal dominant condition that results in defective calcium channels | The underlying abnormality is a dysfunctional sodium channel | It appears mostly in men, especially in those of Asian background | Set of facial features: a broad forehead, widely spaced eyes, low-set ears, and a small chin |
| Caused by: Strenuous exercise High carbohydrate meals Licorice Stress Cold temperatures Infusion of glucose and insulin | Caused by: Strenuous exercise Fasting Stress Cold Infusion of potassium Metabolic acidosis Hypothermia | Caused by: Exercise High carbohydrate meals Stress | Caused by: Exercise Stress Certain medicines |

Periodic paralysis

## SIGNS AND SYMPTOMS

- Attacks of muscle weakness that may last for minutes to days
- Muscle pain in muscles after exercise
- Muscle cramping
- Feeling tingles
- Permanent weakness, more likely later in life

## TREATMENT

- Carbonic anhydrase inhibitors: acetazolamide, methazolamide or dichlorphenamide
- Hypokalemia:
  - Supplemental oral potassium chloride
  - Potassium-sparing diuretics
- Hyperkalemia:
  - Avoid potassium
  - Thiazide diuretics to increase the renal excretion of potassium

## MANAGEMENT

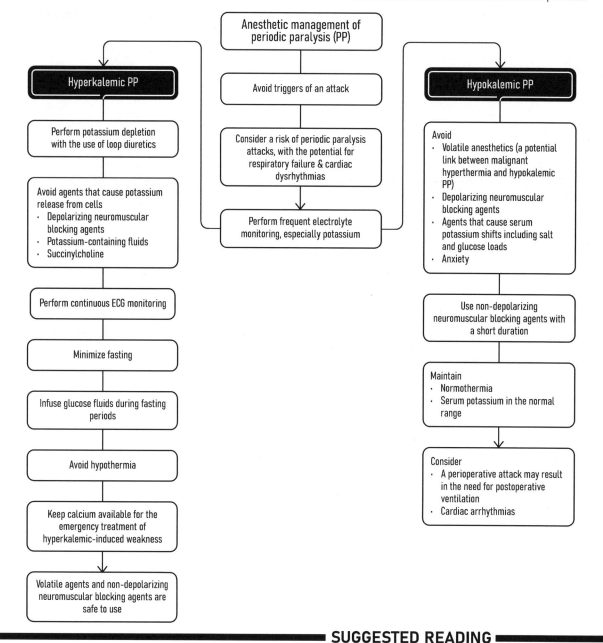

**Anesthetic management of periodic paralysis (PP)**
↓
Avoid triggers of an attack
↓
Consider a risk of periodic paralysis attacks, with the potential for respiratory failure & cardiac dysrhythmias
↓
Perform frequent electrolyte monitoring, especially potassium

**Hyperkalemic PP**
↓
Perform potassium depletion with the use of loop diuretics
↓
Avoid agents that cause potassium release from cells
- Depolarizing neuromuscular blocking agents
- Potassium-containing fluids
- Succinylcholine
↓
Perform continuous ECG monitoring
↓
Minimize fasting
↓
Infuse glucose fluids during fasting periods
↓
Avoid hypothermia
↓
Keep calcium available for the emergency treatment of hyperkalemic-induced weakness
↓
Volatile agents and non-depolarizing neuromuscular blocking agents are safe to use

**Hypokalemic PP**
↓
Avoid
- Volatile anesthetics (a potential link between malignant hyperthermia and hypokalemic PP)
- Depolarizing neuromuscular blocking agents
- Agents that cause serum potassium shifts including salt and glucose loads
- Anxiety
↓
Use non-depolarizing neuromuscular blocking agents with a short duration
↓
Maintain
- Normothermia
- Serum potassium in the normal range
↓
Consider
- A perioperative attack may result in the need for postoperative ventilation
- Cardiac arrhythmias

## SUGGESTED READING

- Marsh, S., Pittard, A., 2011. Neuromuscular disorders and anaesthesia. Part 2: specific neuromuscular disorders. Continuing Education in Anaesthesia Critical Care & Pain 11, 119–123.

# SARCOIDOSIS

## LEARNING OBJECTIVES

- Describe sarcoidosis
- Anesthetic management of sarcoidosis

## DEFINITION AND MECHANISM

- Sarcoidosis is a disease characterized by the growth of tiny collections of inflammatory cells (granulomas) in any part of the body
- Most commonly the lungs and hilar lymph nodes
- Less commonly affected are the eyes, skin, liver, and brain
- An uncommon side effect of sarcoidosis is vocal cord paralysis
  - Sarcoidosis can impact the function of the vocal cord by directly impacting it
  - Or by involving the neuronal routes that lead to it, such as the superior and recurrent laryngeal nerves, the nucleus ambiguus, and the 10th cranial nerves
- The supraglottic region is commonly a site of sarcoid infiltration
- Cardiac involvement is less common but potentially fatal
- Unknown etiology
  - Thought to be an immune reaction to a trigger such as infection or chemicals
- Diagnosed by biopsy

## SIGNS AND SYMPTOMS

| Signs and symptoms | |
| --- | --- |
| General symptoms | Sarcoidosis can begin with these signs and symptoms:<br>Fatigue<br>Enlarged lymph nodes<br>Weight loss<br>Pain and swelling in joints, such as the ankles |
| Lung symptoms | Persistent dry cough<br>Shortness of breath<br>Wheezing<br>Chest pain |
| Skin symptoms | A red rash or reddish-purple bumps<br>Disfiguring sores (lesions) on the nose, cheeks, and ears<br>Areas of skin that are darker or lighter in color<br>Growths under the skin (nodules), particularly around scars or tattoos |
| Eye symptoms | Blurred vision<br>Eye pain<br>Burning, itching, or dry eyes<br>Severe redness<br>Sensitivity to light |
| Heart symptoms | Chest pain<br>Dyspnea<br>Syncope<br>Fatigue<br>Arrhythmias<br>Palpitations<br>Edema |

Sarcoidosis

# MANAGEMENT

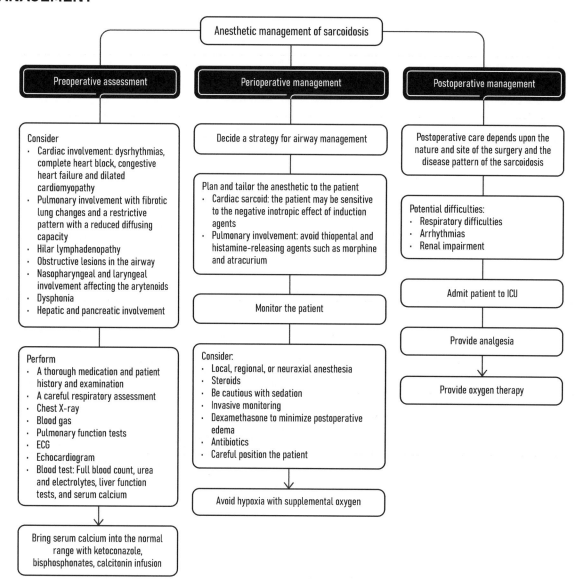

**Anesthetic management of sarcoidosis**

## Preoperative assessment

**Consider**
- Cardiac involvement: dysrhythmias, complete heart block, congestive heart failure and dilated cardiomyopathy
- Pulmonary involvement with fibrotic lung changes and a restrictive pattern with a reduced diffusing capacity
- Hilar lymphadenopathy
- Obstructive lesions in the airway
- Nasopharyngeal and laryngeal involvement affecting the arytenoids
- Dysphonia
- Hepatic and pancreatic involvement

**Perform**
- A thorough medication and patient history and examination
- A careful respiratory assessment
- Chest X-ray
- Blood gas
- Pulmonary function tests
- ECG
- Echocardiogram
- Blood test: Full blood count, urea and electrolytes, liver function tests, and serum calcium

Bring serum calcium into the normal range with ketoconazole, bisphosphonates, calcitonin infusion

## Perioperative management

Decide a strategy for airway management

Plan and tailor the anesthetic to the patient
- Cardiac sarcoid: the patient may be sensitive to the negative inotropic effect of induction agents
- Pulmonary involvement: avoid thiopental and histamine-releasing agents such as morphine and atracurium

Monitor the patient

**Consider:**
- Local, regional, or neuraxial anesthesia
- Steroids
- Be cautious with sedation
- Invasive monitoring
- Dexamethasone to minimize postoperative edema
- Antibiotics
- Careful position the patient

Avoid hypoxia with supplemental oxygen

## Postoperative management

Postoperative care depends upon the nature and site of the surgery and the disease pattern of the sarcoidosis

**Potential difficulties:**
- Respiratory difficulties
- Arrhythmias
- Renal impairment

Admit patient to ICU

Provide analgesia

Provide oxygen therapy

---

**SUGGESTED READING**

- Pollard BJ, Kitchen, G. Handbook of Clinical Anaesthesia. Fourth Edition. CRC Press. 2018. 978-1-4987-6289-2.
- Sanders, D., Rowland, R., Howell, T., 2016. Sarcoidosis and anaesthesia. BJA Education 16, 173–177.

Sarcoidosis

# RENAL DISEASES

# ACUTE KIDNEY INJURY (AKI)

**247**

## LEARNING OBJECTIVES

- Definition of AKI
- Pre- and perioperative management of AKI

## DEFINITION AND MECHANISM

- Acute kidney injury (AKI) is an acute decline (hours to days) in renal function leading to the retention of plasma urea and creatinine
- AKI leads to dysregulation of volume status, metabolic acidosis, and electrolytes
- Perioperative AKI:
  - Occurs in approximately 1% of patients undergoing general surgery
  - Is associated with an increased risk of sepsis, anemia, coagulopathy, and mechanical ventilation

## SIGNS AND SYMPTOMS

- ↑ Serum creatinine concentration
- ↑ Blood urea nitrogen concentration
- Patients are not necessarily oliguric

## CLASSIFICATION AND CAUSES OF AKI

- Pre-renal - inadequate perfusion - 40%-70%
- Renal - intrinsic renal disease - 10%-50%
- Post-renal - Obstructive uropathy - 10%

| Hemodynamic prerenal | Instrinsic renal disease | Postrenal |
|---|---|---|
| Hypovolemia: Bleeding Dehydration Extravasation | Acute tubular injury: Systemic inflammation Sepsis Major surgery Prolonged or total ischemia | Obstruction: Prostatic hypertrophy Nephrolithiasis Retroperitoneal fibrosis (kidney stones) Pelvic masses Bladder tumors |
| Vasodilatory hypotension: Sepsis | Exogenous nephrotoxins: Aminoglycosides Radiological contrast | |
| Low cardiac output states | Pigment nephropathy: Rhabdomyolysis Hemolysis including cardiopulmonary bypass | |
| Acute and chronic heart failure | Metabolic syndromes: Hypercalcemia Hyperuricemia | |
| Locally impaired renal circulation: Medication (ACEI, ARB, NSAIDs) Renovascular disease Chronic kidney disease Chronic liver disease Abdominal compartment syndrome | Autoimmune/inflammatory: Glomerulonephritis Vasculitis Thrombotic microangiopathies Interstitial nephritis | |

ACEI, angiotensin-converting enzyme inhibitors; ARB, angiotensin II receptor blockers; NSAIDs, non-steroidal anti-inflammatory drugs.

# MANAGEMENT

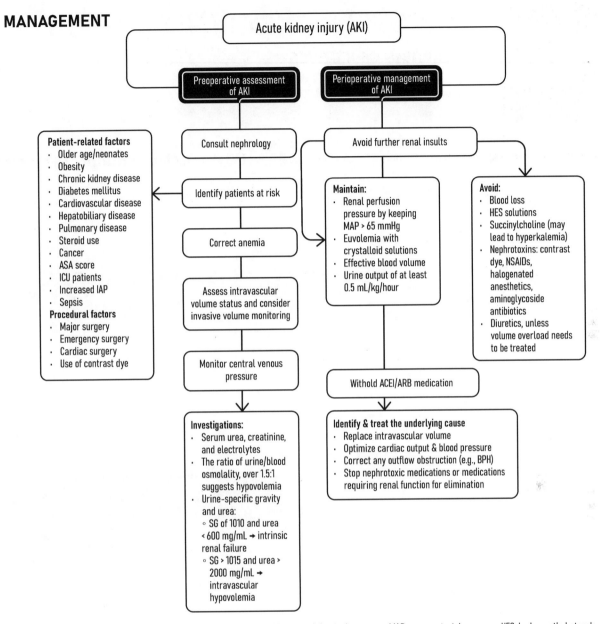

**Acute kidney injury (AKI)**

**Preoperative assessment of AKI**

**Perioperative management of AKI**

**Patient-related factors**
- Older age/neonates
- Obesity
- Chronic kidney disease
- Diabetes mellitus
- Cardiovascular disease
- Hepatobiliary disease
- Pulmonary disease
- Steroid use
- Cancer
- ASA score
- ICU patients
- Increased IAP
- Sepsis

**Procedural factors**
- Major surgery
- Emergency surgery
- Cardiac surgery
- Use of contrast dye

Consult nephrology

Identify patients at risk

Correct anemia

Assess intravascular volume status and consider invasive volume monitoring

Monitor central venous pressure

**Investigations:**
- Serum urea, creatinine, and electrolytes
- The ratio of urine/blood osmolality, over 1.5:1 suggests hypovolemia
- Urine-specific gravity and urea:
  ○ SG of 1010 and urea < 600 mg/mL → intrinsic renal failure
  ○ SG > 1015 and urea > 2000 mg/mL → intravascular hypovolemia

Avoid further renal insults

**Maintain:**
- Renal perfusion pressure by keeping MAP > 65 mmHg
- Euvolemia with crystalloid solutions
- Effective blood volume
- Urine output of at least 0.5 mL/kg/hour

**Avoid:**
- Blood loss
- HES solutions
- Succinylcholine (may lead to hyperkalemia)
- Nephrotoxins: contrast dye, NSAIDs, halogenated anesthetics, aminoglycoside antibiotics
- Diuretics, unless volume overload needs to be treated

Withold ACEI/ARB medication

**Identify & treat the underlying cause**
- Replace intravascular volume
- Optimize cardiac output & blood pressure
- Correct any outflow obstruction (e.g., BPH)
- Stop nephrotoxic medications or medications requiring renal function for elimination

ASA, American society of anesthesiologists; ICU, intensive care unit; IAP, intra-abdominal pressure; MAP, mean arterial pressure; HES, hydroxyethyl starch; NSAIDs, non-steroidal anti-inflammatory drugs; ACEI, angiotensin-converting enzyme inhibitors; ARB, angiotensin II receptor blockers; BPH, benign prostatic hyperplasia.

## KEEP IN MIND

- Patients in whom chronic diuretic therapy has caused hypo- or hyperkalemia may have:
  □ Potentiation of the effects of muscle relaxants
  □ A predisposition to cardiac arrhythmias and AKI

## SUGGESTED READING

- Goren O, Matot I. Perioperative acute kidney injury. Br J Anaesth. 2015;115 Suppl 2:ii3-ii14.
- Gross JL, Prowle JR. Perioperative acute kidney injury, BJA Education, Volume 15, Issue 4, 2015, Pages 213-218.
- Gumbert SD, Kork F, Jackson ML, et al. Perioperative Acute Kidney Injury. Anesthesiology. 2020;132(1):180-204.
- Pollard BJ, Kitchen, G. Handbook of Clinical Anaesthesia. Fourth Edition. CRC Press. 2018. 978-1-4987-6289-2.

# 248

# CHRONIC KIDNEY DISEASE (CKD)

## LEARNING OBJECTIVES

- Recognize CKD
- Management of CKD

## DEFINITION AND MECHANISM

- A slow and gradual loss of kidney function over a period of months to years
- Retention of fluid and waste products
- Can get worse over time and may lead to kidney failure

## SIGNS AND SYMPTOMS

Few symptoms in the early stages
- Nausea
- Vomiting
- Loss of appetite
- Fatigue
- Sleep problems
- Increased or decreased urination
- Headaches
- Muscle cramps
- Swelling of feet and ankles
- Dry, itchy skin
- Hypertension
- Shortness of breath
- Chest pain
- Weight loss
- Blood in urine

## CAUSES

- Hypertension
- Diabetes
- High cholesterol
- Kidney infection
- Glomerulonephritis
- Polycystic kidney disease
- Heart disease/failure
- Longterm regular use of lithium or NSAIDs

## COMPLICATIONS

## STAGES OF CKD

| CKD Stage | eGFR (mL/ min/ 1.73 m³) | Description |
|---|---|---|
| 1 | > 90 | Kidney damage with normal GFR |
| 2 | 60-89 | Kidney damage with mildly decreased GFR |
| 3 | 30-59 | Moderately decreased GFR |
| 4 | 15-29 | Severely decreased GFR |
| 5 | < 15 | Kidney failure |

CKD, chronic kidney disease; eGFR, estimated glomerular filtration rate; GFR, glomerular filtration rate.

| System | Effects |
|---|---|
| Cardiovascular system | Hypertension<br>Ischemic heart disease<br>Pericarditis<br>Heart failure |
| Respiratory system | Pulmonary edema<br>Pleural effusion<br>Respiratory infection |
| Central nervous system | Autonomic neuropathy<br>Coma |
| Hematological | Perioperative anemia<br>Bleeding tendency |
| Gastrointestinal | Stress ulcertion<br>Delayed gastric emptying |
| Renal and metabolic | Fluid retention<br>Hyperkalemia<br>Metabolic acidosis |
| Immunological aspects | Immunosuppressant |

Chronic kidney disease

# MANAGEMENT

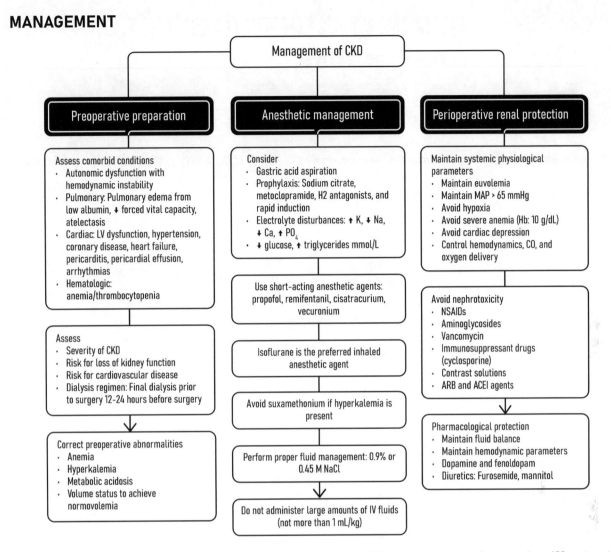

**Management of CKD**

**Preoperative preparation**

Assess comorbid conditions
- Autonomic dysfunction with hemodynamic instability
- Pulmonary: Pulmonary edema from low albumin, ↓ forced vital capacity, atelectasis
- Cardiac: LV dysfunction, hypertension, coronary disease, heart failure, pericarditis, pericardial effusion, arrhythmias
- Hematologic: anemia/thrombocytopenia

Assess
- Severity of CKD
- Risk for loss of kidney function
- Risk for cardiovascular disease
- Dialysis regimen: Final dialysis prior to surgery 12-24 hours before surgery

Correct preoperative abnormalities
- Anemia
- Hyperkalemia
- Metabolic acidosis
- Volume status to achieve normovolemia

**Anesthetic management**

Consider
- Gastric acid aspiration
- Prophylaxis: Sodium citrate, metoclopramide, H2 antagonists, and rapid induction
- Electrolyte disturbances: ↑ K, ↓ Na, ↓ Ca, ↑ $PO_4$
- ↓ glucose, ↑ triglycerides mmol/L

Use short-acting anesthetic agents: propofol, remifentanil, cisatracurium, vecuronium

Isoflurane is the preferred inhaled anesthetic agent

Avoid suxamethonium if hyperkalemia is present

Perform proper fluid management: 0.9% or 0.45 M NaCl

Do not administer large amounts of IV fluids (not more than 1 mL/kg)

**Perioperative renal protection**

Maintain systemic physiological parameters
- Maintain euvolemia
- Maintain MAP > 65 mmHg
- Avoid hypoxia
- Avoid severe anemia (Hb: 10 g/dL)
- Avoid cardiac depression
- Control hemodynamics, CO, and oxygen delivery

Avoid nephrotoxicity
- NSAIDs
- Aminoglycosides
- Vancomycin
- Immunosuppressant drugs (cyclosporine)
- Contrast solutions
- ARB and ACEI agents

Pharmacological protection
- Maintain fluid balance
- Maintain hemodynamic parameters
- Dopamine and fenoldopam
- Diuretics: Furosemide, mannitol

CKD, chronic kidney disease; LV, left ventricle; MAP, mean arterial pressure; Hb, hemoglobin; NSAIDs, non-steroidal anti-inflammatory drugs; ARB, angiotensin II receptor blockers; ACEI, angiotensin-converting enzyme inhibitors.

## KEEP IN MIND

- Decreased renal function can prolong anesthetic drug effects by decreased elimination of these agents

## SUGGESTED READING

- Domi R, Huti G, Sula H, et al. From Pre-Existing Renal Failure to Perioperative Renal Protection: The Anesthesiologist's Dilemmas. Anesth Pain Med. 2016;6(3):e32386. Published 2016 May 14.
- Sladen RN. Chronic kidney disease: the silent enemy?. Anesth Analg. 2011;112(6):1277-1279.

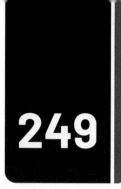

# HEMOLYTIC UREMIC SYNDROME

## LEARNING OBJECTIVES

- Describe the etiology of hemolytic uremic syndrome
- Management of hemolytic uremic syndrome

## DEFINITION AND MECHANISM

- Hemolytic uremic syndrome (HUS) is a triad of renal failure, hemolytic anemia, and thrombocytopenia and is the most common cause of renal failure in infancy and childhood
- HUS can lead to widespread inflammation and thrombotic microangiopathy, the formation of platelet microthrombi in the walls of small blood vessels
- Most cases occur after infectious diarrhea due to a specific type of E. coli
- Other causes include S. pneumoniae, Shigella, Salmonella, and certain medications
- Two predominant types:
  - Typical HUS
    - Preceded by 4-6 days of diarrhea
    - Most commonly caused by infection with Shiga toxin-producing E. coli (O157:H7)
    - The mortality rate is 3%-5%
    - Approximately two-thirds of children require dialysis although 85% regain normal renal function
  - Atypical HUS
    - 60-50% can be attributed to dysregulation of the alternative complement pathway
    - Involves mutations in factor H, factor I, CD46/MCP, factor B, and C3 components
    - A mortality rate of up to 25% in the acute phase
    - 50% of patients require renal replacement therapy at some point
- The first symptoms of infection can emerge between 1 to 10 days later, but usually after 3 to 4 days
- Affects about 1.5 per 100,000 people each year
- A multisystemic disease affecting:

| | |
|---|---|
| Cardiovascular system | Myocarditis<br>Congestive heart failure<br>Severe hypertension |
| Respiratory system | Severe respiratory insufficiency<br>Pulmonary edema<br>Congestive heart failure |
| CNS | Drowsiness<br>Seizures<br>Hemiparesis<br>Coma |
| Biochemical | Evidence of acute kidney injury<br>Acid-base and electrolyte disturbances<br>Abnormal liver function tests associated with hepatitis |
| Hematological | Hemolysis rapidly appears<br>Hemoglobin falls to as low as 4 g/L<br>Thrombocytopenia<br>Hepatosplenomegaly |
| Renal system | Proteinuria, hematuria, and oliguria leading to anuria |
| Gastrointestinal tract | Hemorrhagic gastritis |
| Immunological | Severe infections: peritonitis, meningitis, osteomyelitis |

## SIGNS AND SYMPTOMS

- Abdominal pain, cramping, or bloating
- Bloody diarrhea
- Fever
- Vomiting
- Pale coloring, including loss of pink color in cheeks and inside the lower eyelids
- Extreme fatigue
- Shortness of breath
- Easy bruising or unexplained bruises
- Unusual bleeding
- Decreased urination or blood in the urine
- Edema
- Confusion, seizures, or stroke
- High blood pressure
- Low platelets

## COMPLICATIONS

- Kidney failure
- Hypertension
- Stroke or seizures
- Coma
- Clotting problems
- Heart problems
- Digestive tract problems

## TREATMENT

- Fluid resuscitation
- Treat hyperkalemia
- Dialysis
- Control hypertension with standard antihypertensive agents
- Steroids
- Blood transfusion
- Plasmapheresis

## DIAGNOSIS

- Travel and dietary history
- Complete blood count: anemia (Hb < 10 g/dL) and thrombocytopenia
- Comprehensive metabolic panel (elevated creatinine, elevated indirect bilirubin, and elevated lactate dehydrogenase)
- Urinalysis
- Peripheral smear

## MANAGEMENT

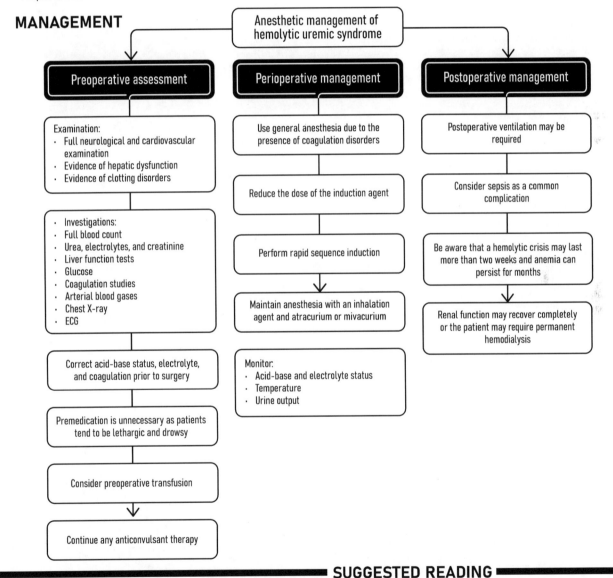

Anesthetic management of hemolytic uremic syndrome

**Preoperative assessment**

Examination:
- Full neurological and cardiovascular examination
- Evidence of hepatic dysfunction
- Evidence of clotting disorders

- Investigations:
- Full blood count
- Urea, electrolytes, and creatinine
- Liver function tests
- Glucose
- Coagulation studies
- Arterial blood gases
- Chest X-ray
- ECG

Correct acid-base status, electrolyte, and coagulation prior to surgery

Premedication is unnecessary as patients tend to be lethargic and drowsy

Consider preoperative transfusion

Continue any anticonvulsant therapy

**Perioperative management**

Use general anesthesia due to the presence of coagulation disorders

Reduce the dose of the induction agent

Perform rapid sequence induction

Maintain anesthesia with an inhalation agent and atracurium or mivacurium

Monitor:
- Acid-base and electrolyte status
- Temperature
- Urine output

**Postoperative management**

Postoperative ventilation may be required

Consider sepsis as a common complication

Be aware that a hemolytic crisis may last more than two weeks and anemia can persist for months

Renal function may recover completely or the patient may require permanent hemodialysis

## SUGGESTED READING

- Noris M, Remuzzi G. Hemolytic uremic syndrome. J Am Soc Nephrol. 2005;16(4):1035-1050.
- Pollard BJ, Kitchen, G. Handbook of Clinical Anaesthesia. Fourth Edition. CRC Press. 2018. 978-1-4987-6289-2.

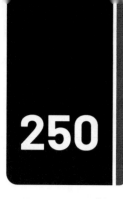

# NEPHRECTOMY

## LEARNING OBJECTIVES

- Definition of a nephrectomy
- Management of a nephrectomy

## DEFINITION AND MECHANISM

- A nephrectomy involves the removal of a kidney with or without part of the ureter and may be open, laparoscopic, or robot-assisted
- Often performed in the treatment of renal cell carcinoma but may also be performed for hydronephrosis, trauma, shrunken kidney, hypertension, or chronic infection
- Nephrectomy is also performed to remove a healthy kidney from a donor (either living or deceased) for transplantation
- In partial nephrectomy or kidney-sparing (nephron-sparing) surgery, only the diseased or injured portion of the kidney is removed
- Radical (complete) nephrectomy involves removing the entire kidney, part of the ureter, the renal fascia, the adrenal gland, the regional lymph nodes
- The open surgery is carried out via a dorsal, anterior subcostal, flank, midline, or thoracoabdominal incision
- The laparoscopic approach is associated with less pain and quicker recovery times and may be performed transperitoneal or retroperitoneal

## COMPLICATIONS

- Hemorrhage
- Urinary fistula
- Urethral obstruction
- Infection
- Pneumothorax
- Postoperative pneumonia
- Vascular injury
- Splenic injury
- Bowel injury
- Acute renal failure
- Bowel obstruction
- Peritonitis
- Deep venous thrombosis and pulmonary embolism
- Chronic renal failure

# MANAGEMENT

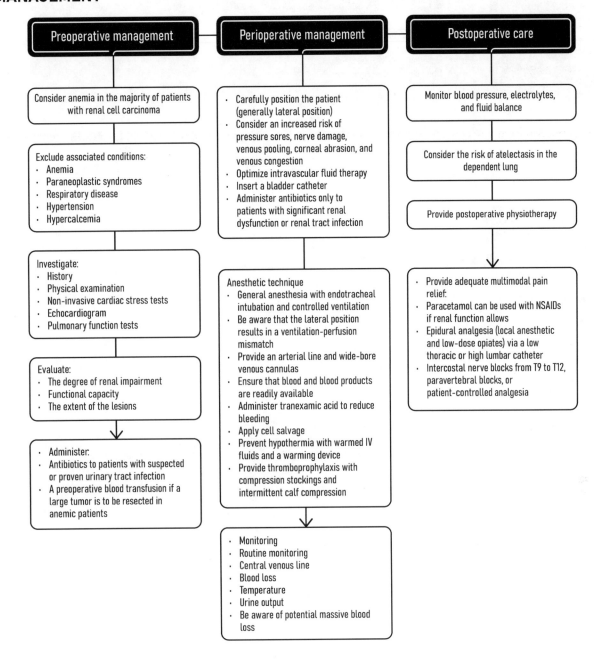

**Preoperative management**

Consider anemia in the majority of patients with renal cell carcinoma

Exclude associated conditions:
- Anemia
- Paraneoplastic syndromes
- Respiratory disease
- Hypertension
- Hypercalcemia

Investigate:
- History
- Physical examination
- Non-invasive cardiac stress tests
- Echocardiogram
- Pulmonary function tests

Evaluate:
- The degree of renal impairment
- Functional capacity
- The extent of the lesions

- Administer:
- Antibiotics to patients with suspected or proven urinary tract infection
- A preoperative blood transfusion if a large tumor is to be resected in anemic patients

**Perioperative management**

- Carefully position the patient (generally lateral position)
- Consider an increased risk of pressure sores, nerve damage, venous pooling, corneal abrasion, and venous congestion
- Optimize intravascular fluid therapy
- Insert a bladder catheter
- Administer antibiotics only to patients with significant renal dysfunction or renal tract infection

Anesthetic technique
- General anesthesia with endotracheal intubation and controlled ventilation
- Be aware that the lateral position results in a ventilation-perfusion mismatch
- Provide an arterial line and wide-bore venous cannulas
- Ensure that blood and blood products are readily available
- Administer tranexamic acid to reduce bleeding
- Apply cell salvage
- Prevent hypothermia with warmed IV fluids and a warming device
- Provide thromboprophylaxis with compression stockings and intermittent calf compression

- Monitoring
- Routine monitoring
- Central venous line
- Blood loss
- Temperature
- Urine output
- Be aware of potential massive blood loss

**Postoperative care**

Monitor blood pressure, electrolytes, and fluid balance

Consider the risk of atelectasis in the dependent lung

Provide postoperative physiotherapy

- Provide adequate multimodal pain relief:
- Paracetamol can be used with NSAIDs if renal function allows
- Epidural analgesia (local anesthetic and low-dose opiates) via a low thoracic or high lumbar catheter
- Intercostal nerve blocks from T9 to T12, paravertebral blocks, or patient-controlled analgesia

---

### SUGGESTED READING

- Chapman, E., Pichel, A., 2016. Anaesthesia for nephrectomy. BJA Education 16, 98–101.
- Pollard BJ, Kitchen, G. Handbook of Clinical Anaesthesia. Fourth Edition. CRC Press. 2018. 978-1-4987-6289-2.

# NEPHROTIC SYNDROME

## LEARNING OBJECTIVES

- Definition of nephrotic syndrome
- Management of nephrotic syndrome

## DEFINITION AND MECHANISM

- Nephrotic syndrome is a collection of symptoms due to kidney damage including protein in the urine, low blood albumin levels, high blood lipids, and edema
- Characterized by glomerular injury
- Can be primary, being a disease specific to the kidneys, or secondary to a systemic condition
- Primary causes:
  - Minimal-change disease (nephropathy)
  - Focal segmental glomerulosclerosis
  - Membranous glomerulonephritis
  - Membranoproliferative glomerulonephritis
  - Hereditary nephropathies
- Secondary causes:
  - Diabetes mellitus
  - Systemic lupus erythematosus
  - Sarcoidosis
  - Amyloidosis and paraproteinemias
  - Viral infections (e.g., hepatitis B, hepatitis C, HIV)
  - Preeclampsia
  - Sjögren's syndrome
  - Multiple myeloma
  - Vasculitis
  - Cancer
  - Medications: penicillin, captopril
- A defect in the glomerular barrier leads to an increased glomerular permeability resulting in proteinuria/albuminuria
- Leading to a decrease in plasma oncotic pressure, retention of sodium and water, peripheral edema, ascites, pleural effusions, and hypovolemia
- Most cases spontaneously remit without treatment, hypertension occurs commonly, and renal failure is rare
- Patients may develop renal failure as well as secondary complications including arterial and venous thromboembolism and infection

## SIGNS AND SYMPTOMS

- Proteinuria (> 3 g/24 h) and foamy urine
- Hypoalbuminemia (< 3.5 g/dL)
- Hypercholesterolemia and hyperlipidemia
- Thromboembolic episodes
- Puffy eyelids and swelling in the legs, ankles, feet, or lower abdomen
- Weight gain
- Fatigue
- Loss of appetite

## RISK FACTORS

- Nephrotoxic medication
- Diabetes mellitus
- Systemic lupus erythematosus
- Amyloidosis
- Reflux nephropathy
- Infections: HIV, hepatitis B, hepatitis C, malaria

# COMPLICATIONS

- Arterial and venous thrombosis
- Infections
- Hypertension
- High blood cholesterol and elevated blood triglycerides
- Acute kidney injury
- Chronic kidney disease
- Pulmonary edema
- Hypothyroidism
- Vitamin D deficiency
- Hypocalcemia
- Microcytic hypochromic anemia
- Protein malnutrition
- Growth retardation
- Cushing's syndrome

# DIAGNOSIS

- Urine dipstick test to check for albuminuria
- 24-hour urine collection
- Urine albumin-to-creatinine ratio
- Blood tests: serum albumin level, creatinine concentrations
- Kidney ultrasound
- Kidney biopsy

# TREATMENT

- Diuretics
- Angiotensin-converting enzyme (ACE) inhibitors and angiotensin-receptor blockers are used alone or in combination
- Prednisolone
- Cyclophosphamide
- Mycophenolate
- Cyclosporin
- Low salt diet and limited fluid intake
- Specific treatment depending on etiology:
  - Statins to lower cholesterol
  - Glucocorticosteroids for minimal-change nephropathy
  - Prednisone and cyclophosphamide are useful in some forms of lupus nephritis
  - Secondary amyloidosis with nephrotic syndrome may respond to anti-inflammatory treatment of the primary disease

# MANAGEMENT

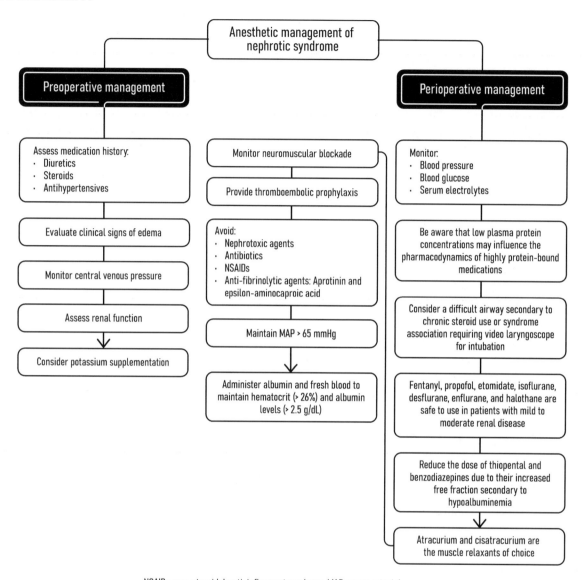

**Anesthetic management of nephrotic syndrome**

**Preoperative management**

- Assess medication history:
  - Diuretics
  - Steroids
  - Antihypertensives
- Evaluate clinical signs of edema
- Monitor central venous pressure
- Assess renal function
- Consider potassium supplementation

- Monitor neuromuscular blockade
- Provide thromboembolic prophylaxis
- Avoid:
  - Nephrotoxic agents
  - Antibiotics
  - NSAIDs
  - Anti-fibrinolytic agents: Aprotinin and epsilon-aminocaproic acid
- Maintain MAP > 65 mmHg
- Administer albumin and fresh blood to maintain hematocrit (> 26%) and albumin levels (> 2.5 g/dL)

**Perioperative management**

- Monitor:
  - Blood pressure
  - Blood glucose
  - Serum electrolytes
- Be aware that low plasma protein concentrations may influence the pharmacodynamics of highly protein-bound medications
- Consider a difficult airway secondary to chronic steroid use or syndrome association requiring video laryngoscope for intubation
- Fentanyl, propofol, etomidate, isoflurane, desflurane, enflurane, and halothane are safe to use in patients with mild to moderate renal disease
- Reduce the dose of thiopental and benzodiazepines due to their increased free fraction secondary to hypoalbuminemia
- Atracurium and cisatracurium are the muscle relaxants of choice

NSAIDs, non-steroidal anti-inflammatory drugs; MAP, mean arterial pressure.

## SUGGESTED READING

- Pollard BJ, Kitchen, G. Handbook of Clinical Anaesthesia. Fourth Edition. CRC Press. 2018. 978-1-4987-6289-2.
- Vishnu D, Tempe D, Arora K, Virmani S, Chander J, Agarwal S.(2012). Anesthetic management of a child with nephrotic syndrome undergoing open heart surgery. Report of a rare case. Annals of cardiac anaesthesia. 15. 305-8.

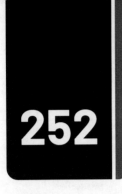

# RENAL TRANSPLANT

## LEARNING OBJECTIVES

- Definition of a renal transplant
- Management of a living donor during a nephrectomy
- Management of a renal transplant recipient

## DEFINITION AND MECHANISM

- A renal transplant is the organ transplant of a kidney into a patient with end-stage renal disease (ESRD)
- Classified as deceased-donor nephrectomy (formerly known as cadaveric) or living-donor nephrectomy (LDN)
- Improves both length and quality of life for patients with ESRD
- ESRD is defined as chronic kidney disease (CKD) with a glomerular filtration rate (GFR) < 15 mL/min/1.73 m² or where renal replacement therapy is needed
- Diabetes is the most common cause of ESRD followed by glomerulonephritis, polycystic kidney disease, pyelonephritis, hypertension, and autoimmune disorders
- Two-year graft survival is > 80% for cadaveric and 90% for living-donor grafts, and overall patient survival is > 95%

## SIGNS AND SYMPTOMS

Few symptoms in the early stages of CKD

- Nausea
- Vomiting
- Loss of appetite
- Fatigue
- Sleep problems
- Increased or decreased urination
- Headaches
- Muscle cramps
- Swelling of feet and ankles
- Dry, itchy skin
- Hypertension
- Shortness of breath
- Chest pain
- Weight loss
- Blood in urine

## COMPLICATIONS

- Bleeding
- Vascular thrombosis and stenosis
- Transplant rejection (hyperacute, acute, or chronic)
- Ureteral obstruction
- Urinary leakage
- Infections and sepsis due to immunosuppression
- Post-transplant lymphoproliferative disorder
- Electrolyte imbalance (particularly calcium and phosphate)
- Proteinuria
- Hypertension

Renal transplant

# MANAGEMENT OF THE LIVING DONOR DURING NEPHRECTOMY

### SELECTION OF DONOR

- ASA I or II patients
- Age > 18 years
- Hypertension is not a contraindication as long as kidney function and urine protein are normal
- Relative contraindications
    - Obesity
- Absolute contraindications
    - Diabetes mellitus
    - Malignancy
    - Hypertension with evidence of end-stage organ damage
    - Albumin/creatinine ratio > 30 mg/mmol
    - Protein/creatinine ratio > 50 mg/mmol
    - 24-hour total protein > 300 mg/day

### ASSESSMENT OF THE DONOR

- Systematic history
- Blood tests
- Infection screening
- Malignancy screening
- Cardiorespiratory assessment
- Psychological assessment
- Renal anatomy assessment with CT/MRI
- Usually the left kidney is chosen because it has a longer renal vein
- Assessment of kidney function: GFR has to be 37.5 mL/min/1.73m² prior to donation

### PERIOPERATIVE MANAGEMENT

- Perform adequate preoperative hydration (overnight fluid preloading)
- Provide:
    - An adequate wide-bore IV access
    - An arterial line in patients with preexisting hypertension and in case of a left nephrectomy (potential damage to the spleen)
    - Noninvasive monitoring
- Use general anesthesia with endotracheal intubation
- Consider:
    - Combining general anesthesia with TAP, paravertebral, or rectus sheath blocks
    - LA catheter in wound
    - Local infiltration
- Maintain:
    - Normoxia
    - Normocarbia
    - Normothermia
    - Normotension (keep renal perfusion pressures/MAP at preoperative values)
    - Urine output of 1.5-2 mL/kg/h
- Administer:
    - Adequate perioperative hydration Hartmann's solution (10-15 mL/kg/h)
    - Heparin (5000 IU) before application of the arterial clamp
    - Protamin (50 mg) after kidney isolation
- Avoid:
    - NSAIDs
    - Vasoconstrictors
- Provide comprehensive thromboembolism prophylaxis:
    - Low molecular weight heparin
    - Graduated stockings
    - Pneumatic compression devices

GFR, glomerular filtration rate; IV, intravenous; TAP, transversus abdominis plane; LA, local anesthetic; MAP, mean arterial pressure; NSAIDs, non-steroidal anti-inflammatory drugs.

# POSTOPERATIVE CARE OF THE LIVING DONOR

- Provide postoperative analgesia via a fentanyl patient-controlled analgesia (PCA)
- Consider a paravertebral or transversus abdominis plane (TAP) block to complement analgesia
- Avoid NSAIDs
- Apply early mobilization along with breathing exercises and incentive spirometry
- Consider postoperative complications:
    - Pulmonary embolism
    - Hepatitis
    - Myocardial infarction
    - Arrhythmias
    - Pneumonia
    - Atelectasis
    - Urinary tract infection
    - Wound infections
    - Splenic lacerations

Renal transplant

# MANAGEMENT OF THE RECIPIENT

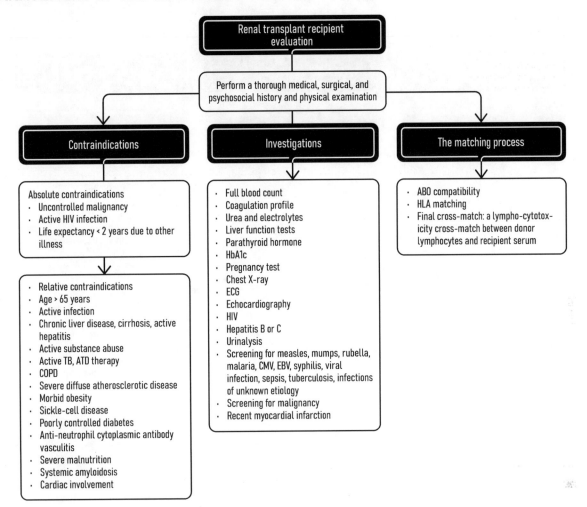

```
                    ┌─────────────────────────────┐
                    │  Renal transplant recipient  │
                    │         evaluation           │
                    └─────────────────────────────┘
                                  │
                    ┌─────────────────────────────────────┐
                    │ Perform a thorough medical, surgical, │
                    │ and psychosocial history and physical │
                    │            examination               │
                    └─────────────────────────────────────┘
```

## Contraindications

**Absolute contraindications**
- Uncontrolled malignancy
- Active HIV infection
- Life expectancy < 2 years due to other illness

- Relative contraindications
- Age > 65 years
- Active infection
- Chronic liver disease, cirrhosis, active hepatitis
- Active substance abuse
- Active TB, ATD therapy
- COPD
- Severe diffuse atherosclerotic disease
- Morbid obesity
- Sickle-cell disease
- Poorly controlled diabetes
- Anti-neutrophil cytoplasmic antibody vasculitis
- Severe malnutrition
- Systemic amyloidosis
- Cardiac involvement

## Investigations

- Full blood count
- Coagulation profile
- Urea and electrolytes
- Liver function tests
- Parathyroid hormone
- HbA1c
- Pregnancy test
- Chest X-ray
- ECG
- Echocardiography
- HIV
- Hepatitis B or C
- Urinalysis
- Screening for measles, mumps, rubella, malaria, CMV, EBV, syphilis, viral infection, sepsis, tuberculosis, infections of unknown etiology
- Screening for malignancy
- Recent myocardial infarction

## The matching process

- ABO compatibility
- HLA matching
- Final cross-match: a lympho-cytotoxicity cross-match between donor lymphocytes and recipient serum

HIV, human immunodeficiency virus; TB, tuberculosis; ATD, anti-tuberculosis drug; COPD, chronic obstructive pulmonary disease; HbA1c, hemoglobin A1c; CMV, cytomegalovirus; EBV, Epstein-Barr virus; HLA, human leukocyte antigen.

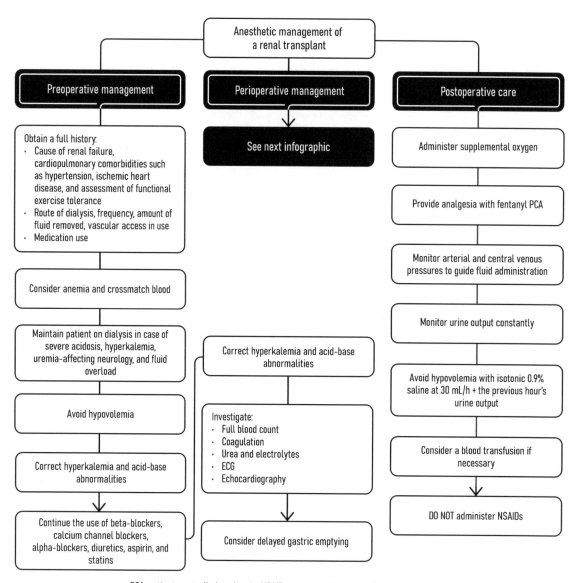

**Anesthetic management of a renal transplant**

**Preoperative management**

Obtain a full history:
- Cause of renal failure, cardiopulmonary comorbidities such as hypertension, ischemic heart disease, and assessment of functional exercise tolerance
- Route of dialysis, frequency, amount of fluid removed, vascular access in use
- Medication use

Consider anemia and crossmatch blood

Maintain patient on dialysis in case of severe acidosis, hyperkalemia, uremia-affecting neurology, and fluid overload

Avoid hypovolemia

Correct hyperkalemia and acid-base abnormalities

Continue the use of beta-blockers, calcium channel blockers, alpha-blockers, diuretics, aspirin, and statins

**Perioperative management**

See next infographic

Correct hyperkalemia and acid-base abnormalities

Investigate:
- Full blood count
- Coagulation
- Urea and electrolytes
- ECG
- Echocardiography

Consider delayed gastric emptying

**Postoperative care**

Administer supplemental oxygen

Provide analgesia with fentanyl PCA

Monitor arterial and central venous pressures to guide fluid administration

Monitor urine output constantly

Avoid hypovolemia with isotonic 0.9% saline at 30 mL/h + the previous hour's urine output

Consider a blood transfusion if necessary

DO NOT administer NSAIDs

PCA, patient-controlled analgesia; NSAIDs, non-steroidal anti-inflammatory drugs.

Renal transplant

## Perioperative management of a renal transplant patient

### ANESTHESIA
- General anesthesia is preferred
- Combined spinal-epidural is acceptable for patients with an increased risk of respiratory complications

### INDUCTION
- Protect the airway with an endotracheal tube
- Propofol and thiopental are safe to use but titrate to minimize the risk of hypotension
- Fentanyl and remifentanil (opioids) are safe to use
- Cisatracurium and atracurium (muscle relaxants) are safe to use
- Note that succinylcholine leads to hyperkalemia and can only be used if a rapid sequence induction when serum potassium is < 5.5 mmol/L
- TIVA with propofol and remifentanil is safe to use

### MONITORING
- Routine AAGBI monitoring
- Neuromuscular block
- Temperature
- Central venous pressure
- Arterial lines are not necessary unless there is LV dysfunction or valvular heart disease

### MAINTENANCE
- Isoflurane, desflurane, and sevoflurane are all safe to use
- Analgesia: IV paracetamol, incremental fentanyl are safe to use
- Consider a TAP block or wound infiltration catheter
- Keep MAP > 80 mmHg when administering central neuraxial blocks
- DO NOT administer NSAIDs!

### FLUID THERAPY
- Administer a balanced salt solution (Hartmann's)
  Consider albumin and gelatins as alternative colloids
  Avoid hydroxyethyl starch
  Avoid 0.9% saline → hyperchloremia and hyperkalemia
- Keep MAP at 80-90 mmHg
- Maintain a low CVP (5 mmHg) until vessels are clamped followed by high CVP (15 mmHg) when clams are released to promote graft function
- Decrease vasopressors and diuretics as required
- A blood transfusion is required if hemoglobin < 7 g/dL
- Treat hyperkalemia with sodium bicarbonate, calcium chloride, or insulin dextrose solution (see also "hyperkalemia")

### IMMUNOSUPPRESSION
- Administer methylprednisolone
- Administer basiliximab 20 mg to reduce the risk of acute injection
- Consider anti-thymocyte globulin (ATG), alemtuzumab, and rituximab in patients with ABO/HLA incompatibility

TIVA, total intravenous anesthesia; LV, left ventricle; IV, intravenous; TAP, transversus abdominis plane; MAP, mean arterial pressure; NSAIDs, non-steroidal anti-inflammatory drugs; CVP, central venous pressure; HLA, human leukocyte antigen.

## SUGGESTED READING

- Mayhew D, Ridgway d, Hunter JM. 2016. Update on the intraoperative management of adult cadaveric renal transplantation. BJA education. 16;2:53-57.
- O'Brien, B., Koertzen, M., 2012. Anaesthesia for living donor renal transplant nephrectomy. Continuing Education in Anaesthesia Critical Care & Pain 12, 317-321.
- Pollard BJ, Kitchen, G. Handbook of Clinical Anaesthesia. Fourth Edition. CRC Press. 2018. 978-1-4987-6289-2.
- Rabey P. 2001. Anesthesia for renal transplantation. BJA CEPD Reviews. 1;1:24-17.

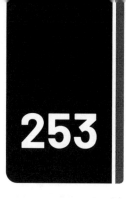

# TURP AND TURP SYNDROME

## LEARNING OBJECTIVES

- Definition of transurethral resection of the prostate (TURP) syndrome
- Management of TURP

## DEFINITION AND MECHANISM

- Benign prostatic hyperplasia (BPH) occurs in over 40% of men aged over 60 years and prostate resection is the second-line treatment if BPH symptoms are resistant to medical management
- Transurethral resection of the prostate (TURP) syndrome is a rare but potentially life-threatening complication of the TURP procedure
- The prostate at the bladder neck is shaved away during the procedure
- As the body of the prostate is removed, veins are exposed, but the capsule is maintained
- The exposed veins can bleed, causing significant blood loss, and can also absorb large amounts of irrigation fluid (1.5% glycine solution) resulting in TURP syndrome
- Treatment is largely supportive and relies on the removal of the underlying cause, and organ and physiological support
- Mortality is 0.2-0.8%
- Preoperative prevention strategies are extremely important

## SIGNS AND SYMPTOMS

- Signs and symptoms are often vague and non-specific as there is no classical TURP presentation
- Symptoms result from fluid overload, and disturbed electrolyte balance, and hyponatremia

## COMPLICATIONS OF TURP PROCEDURE

- Retrograde ejaculation
- Urinary incontinence
- Erectile dysfunction
- Urethral strictures (narrowing of the urethra)
- Bleeding
- Urinary tract infection
- Urinary retention

## RISK FACTORS

- The size of the opened venous sinuses
- The amount of irrigation fluid used
- The use of excess amounts of hypotonic intravenous fluids
- Duration of the resection (> 1 hour)
- Perforation of the bladder

## DIAGNOSIS

- Acutely unwell, confused patient with a reduced Glasgow Coma Scale score
- Hyponatremia: Na < 120 mmol/L
- Hyperkalemia: K > 6.0 mmol/L
- Glycine toxicity
- Intravascular hemolysis
- Disseminated intravascular coagulation

| Signs and symptoms | |
|---|---|
| Central nervous system | Restlessness<br>Headache<br>Nausea and vomiting<br>Confusion<br>Visual disturbances<br>Cerebral edema<br>Seizures<br>Coma |
| Cardio-respiratory | Bradycardia<br>Hypotension or hypertension<br>Tachypnea<br>Hypoxia<br>Cyanosis<br>Pulmonary edema |
| Systemic | Hypothermia<br>Abdominal pain and distension |

# PREVENTION

- Regional anesthesia is preferred over general anesthesia
- Avoid large amounts of glycine-containing fluids
- Keep the length of surgery under 1 hour
- Keep the patient horizontal and avoid the Trendelenburg position
- Resect large prostates in staged procedures to avoid prolonged operative times
- The optimal height of the irrigation fluid bag above the patient is 60 cm

# MANAGEMENT

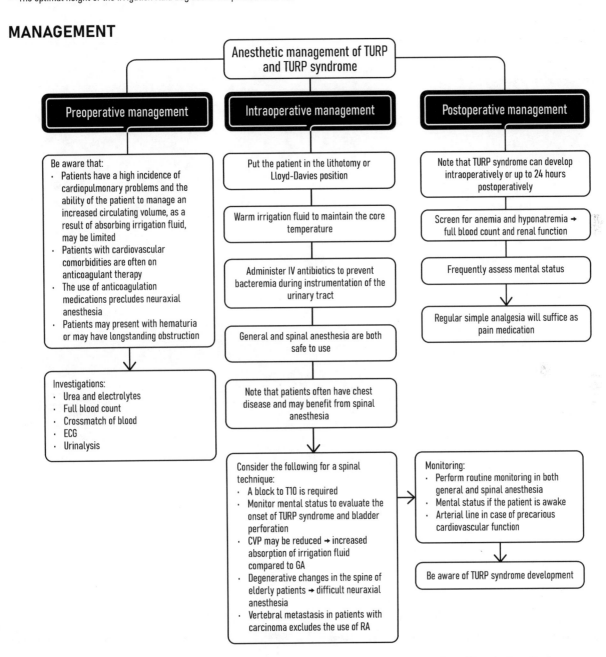

TURP, transurethral resection of the prostate; CVP, central venous pressure; GA, general anesthesia; RA, regional anesthesia.

# TREATMENT OF TURP SYNDROME

- Stop the procedure as soon as possible
- Provide oxygenation (intubation) and circulatory support (inotropes)
- Perform invasive monitoring if hemodynamically unstable
- Treat hypotension
- Correct hyponatremia
- Treat fluid overload with diuretics
- Manage disseminated intravascular coagulation
- Perform regular blood tests to monitor improvement in the clotting status
- Control seizures with benzodiazepines
- Treat nausea and vomiting with antiemetics

## SUGGESTED READING

- Demirel I, Ozer AB, Bayar MK, Erhan OL. TURP syndrome and severe hyponatremia under general anaesthesia. BMJ Case Rep. 2012;2012:bcr-2012-006899.
- Nakahira, J., Sawai, T., Fujiwara, A., Minami, T., 2014. Transurethral resection syndrome in elderly patients: a retrospective observational study. BMC Anesthesiology 14, 30.
- O'Donnell AM, Foo I. 2009. Anaesthesia for transurethral resection of the prostate. Continuing Education in Anaesthesia Critical Care & Pain. 9;3:92-96.
- Pollard BJ, Kitchen, G. Handbook of Clinical Anaesthesia. Fourth Edition. CRC Press. 2018. 978-1-4987-6289-2.

TURP and TURP syndrome

# RESPIRATORY & THORACICS

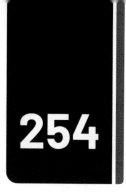

# ANTERIOR MEDIASTINAL MASS

## LEARNING OBJECTIVES

- Describe the common causes and symptoms of anterior mediastinal masses
- Manage patients with anterior mediastinal masses

## DEFINITION AND MECHANISM

- Mediastinal masses constitute a heterogeneous group of benign and malignant tumors
- Most common masses in the anterior mediastinum:
  - Thymoma
  - Teratoma
  - Thyroid goiter
  - Lymphoma
  - Germ cell tumor
  - Thymic cyst
  - Parathyroid adenoma

## SIGNS AND SYMPTOMS

- Anterior mediastinal masses can manifest as systemic syndromes (e.g., myasthenia gravis and thyroid disease) or symptoms stemming from localized pathology

| Pathology | |
|---|---|
| Tracheobronchial obstruction | Dyspnea<br>Noisy breathing<br>Nonspecific cough<br>Chest discomfort<br>Tachypnea<br>Stridor<br>Rhonchi<br>Decreased breath sounds |
| Superior vena cava syndrome | Dyspnea<br>Headache<br>Visual disturbance<br>Altered mentation<br>Dilated collateral veins in the upper body<br>Edema of the face, neck, and arms |
| Right heart and pulmonary vascular compression | Dyspnea<br>Syncope during a forced Valsalva maneuver<br>Arrhythmias<br>Cardiac murmur |

# MANAGEMENT

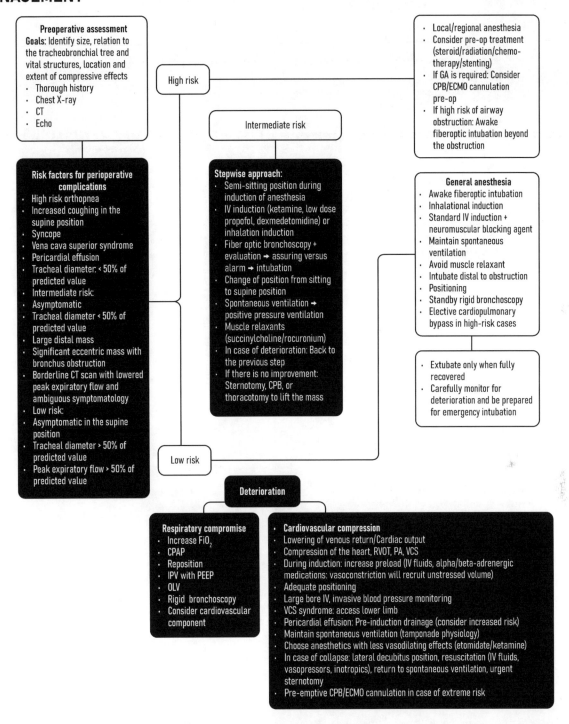

**Preoperative assessment**
**Goals:** Identify size, relation to the tracheobronchial tree and vital structures, location and extent of compressive effects
- Thorough history
- Chest X-ray
- CT
- Echo

**High risk**

**Intermediate risk**

**Low risk**

**Risk factors for perioperative complications**
- High risk orthopnea
- Increased coughing in the supine position
- Syncope
- Vena cava superior syndrome
- Pericardial effusion
- Tracheal diameter: < 50% of predicted value
- Intermediate risk:
- Asymptomatic
- Tracheal diameter < 50% of predicted value
- Large distal mass
- Significant eccentric mass with bronchus obstruction
- Borderline CT scan with lowered peak expiratory flow and ambiguous symptomatology
- Low risk:
- Asymptomatic in the supine position
- Tracheal diameter > 50% of predicted value
- Peak expiratory flow > 50% of predicted value

**Stepwise approach:**
- Semi-sitting position during induction of anesthesia
- IV induction (ketamine, low dose propofol, dexmedetomidine) or inhalation induction
- Fiber optic bronchoscopy + evaluation → assuring versus alarm → intubation
- Change of position from sitting to supine position
- Spontaneous ventilation → positive pressure ventilation
- Muscle relaxants (succinylcholine/rocuronium)
- In case of deterioration: Back to the previous step
- If there is no improvement: Sternotomy, CPB, or thoracotomy to lift the mass

- Local/regional anesthesia
- Consider pre-op treatment (steroid/radiation/chemo-therapy/stenting)
- If GA is required: Consider CPB/ECMO cannulation pre-op
- If high risk of airway obstruction: Awake fiberoptic intubation beyond the obstruction

**General anesthesia**
- Awake fiberoptic intubation
- Inhalational induction
- Standard IV induction + neuromuscular blocking agent
- Maintain spontaneous ventilation
- Avoid muscle relaxant
- Intubate distal to obstruction
- Positioning
- Standby rigid bronchoscopy
- Elective cardiopulmonary bypass in high-risk cases

- Extubate only when fully recovered
- Carefully monitor for deterioration and be prepared for emergency intubation

**Deterioration**

**Respiratory compromise**
- Increase $FiO_2$
- CPAP
- Reposition
- IPV with PEEP
- OLV
- Rigid bronchoscopy
- Consider cardiovascular component

- **Cardiovascular compression**
- Lowering of venous return/Cardiac output
- Compression of the heart, RVOT, PA, VCS
- During induction: increase preload (IV fluids, alpha/beta-adrenergic medications: vasoconstriction will recruit unstressed volume)
- Adequate positioning
- Large bore IV, invasive blood pressure monitoring
- VCS syndrome: access lower limb
- Pericardial effusion: Pre-induction drainage (consider increased risk)
- Maintain spontaneous ventilation (tamponade physiology)
- Choose anesthetics with less vasodilating effects (etomidate/ketamine)
- In case of collapse: lateral decubitus position, resuscitation (IV fluids, vasopressors, inotropics), return to spontaneous ventilation, urgent sternotomy
- Pre-emptive CPB/ECMO cannulation in case of extreme risk

## SUGGESTED READING

- Almeida PT, Heller D. Anterior Mediastinal Mass. [Updated 2022 Sep 26]. In: StatPearls [Internet]. Treasure Island (FL): StatPearls Publishing; 2022 Jan-. Available from: https://www.ncbi.nlm.nih.gov/books/NBK546608/
- Ku, Chih Min. "Anesthesia for patients with mediastinal masses." Principles and Practice of Anesthesia for Thoracic Surgery. Springer New York, 2011. 201-210.
- McLeod M, Dobbie M. Anterior mediastinal masses in children. BJA Education. 2019;19(1):21-6.

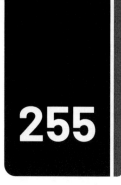

# ASTHMA

## LEARNING OBJECTIVES

- Manage patients with asthma in the pre-, and perioperative period

## DEFINITION AND MECHANISM

- Asthma is an airway condition characterized by variable respiratory symptoms and variable airflow limitation, typically, but not always, associated with airway inflammation and airway remodeling
- In between asthma attacks, a patient might be asymptomatic, and lung function tests might be normal

### ABOUT

- Episodic recurrent lower airway obstruction affecting 3-5% of the population
- 65% of people become symptomatic before 5 years
- **Peak expiratory flow (PEF) rate**
  - Measurement of severity of asthma → PEF rates < 50% of the predicted value (corrected for age/gender/height) indicate severe asthma
  - PEF ↑ > 15% after bronchodilator administration suggests inadequate treatment

### CLINICAL PRESENTATION

- Inflammation of the airways → inflamed airway is hyperresponsive to irritant stimuli → bronchospasm and mucous secretions
- **Bronchospastic stimuli:** Allergens, dust, cold air, instrumentation of the airways, and medications (i.e., aspirin or histamine-releasing drugs)
- Life-threatening bronchospasm during anesthesia if improperly managed, particularly during or recently after a respiratory tract infection → delay elective surgery at least 6 weeks after a respiratory infection

| Normal airway | Asthma |
|---|---|
| · Thin airway walls | · Thick airway walls |
| · Muscles around airways are relaxed | · Muscles around airways contract |
| · No mucus | · Mucus present |

### STEPWISE THERAPY FOR TREATMENT

1. Inhaled short-acting β2-agonists (e.g., salbutamol 100-200 µg prn)
2. Inhaled short-acting β2-agonists and inhaled steroids at up to 400 µg/day
3. Step 2 and additional long-acting β2-agonist (LABA)
4. Inhaled steroids up to 800 µg/day and LABA/leukotriene receptor antagonist
5. Oral steroids/additional therapy as required ↓ steroid use
! Take caution when anesthetizing patients after step 3

### MANAGEMENT OF ANESTHESIA

- Assess adequacy of asthma control during preoperative evaluation
- Exclude symptoms uncharacteristic of asthma
- Perioperative management
- Usual inhalers per normal on day of surgery → inhaled β2-agonists prior to anesthesia
- Avoid lower airway manipulation (e.g., endotracheal intubation) → use regional anesthesia or laryngeal mask airway for general anesthesia
- Avoid medications that release histamine (e.g., thiopental, morphine, atracurium)
- Use anesthetic drugs that promote bronchodilation (e.g., propofol, ketamine, sevoflurane)
- If instrumentation of the lower airway is necessary, use a deep level of general anesthesia to ↓ airway reflexes

## SYMPTOMS

- Symptoms are nonspecific and include wheezing, shortness of breath, chest tightness, and cough
- The most characteristic features relate to the pattern of symptoms, including symptom nature, timing, triggers, and response to treatment
- Childhood-onset allergic asthma is commonly associated with atopy
- Late-onset asthma ( > 12 years) is often non-atopic
- Exercise-induced bronchoconstriction might be the only symptom of asthma

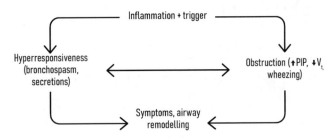

Pathophysiology of asthma and bronchospasm. PIP, peak inspiratory pressure; $V_t$, tidal volume. Adopted from Expert Panel Report 3 (EPR-3), from Elsevier.

# EXACERBATION TREATMENT

- Exacerbations are characterized by progressively increasing shortness of breath, cough, wheezing or chest tightness, and decreasing lung function
- Onset is usually rapid in children but can develop over a week or more in adults

## Acute exacerbation treatment

1. Give **short-acting β2-agonists (SABAs)** to resolve acute symptoms, they can be used every 15 to 20 minutes for the first hour
2. Add **ipratropium bromide** to decrease hospitalization rate and shorten emergency department (ED) stay for patients with severe or moderate asthma exacerbations
3. Give **systemic corticosteroids** as these decrease the rate of hospital admission, there is no difference between oral or IV corticosteroids

## Preventative measures

4. A 5-day course of oral corticosteroids after ED treatment reduces the rate of relapse
5. A single dose of benralizumab, an anti-IL-5 receptor monoclonal antibody, reduces the rate and severity of subsequent exacerbations when given at the time of an initial exacerbation

# ANESTHESIOLOGICAL MANAGEMENT

- Poorly controlled asthma poses a high additional risk for perioperative complications, well-controlled asthma confers almost no additional risk
- Question the patient on exacerbations, recent respiratory infections, and hospital visits
- Commence strict smoking cessation as soon as possible
- Signs of acute bronchospasm or active lung infection should defer elective surgery
- Optimize medications and therapy compliance, consider a short course of oral methylprednisolone 40 mg for 5 days before surgery, as it has been shown to decrease post-intubation wheezing in newly diagnosed or poorly compliant patients with reversible airway obstruction
- Consider locoregional anesthesia where possible
- Give a short-acting bronchodilator prophylactically before surgery, ideally the patient's own metered dose inhaler (MDI)
  - Avoid bronchospasm
    - Ensure adequate depth of anesthesia when manipulating the airway to avoid bronchospasm
    - Consider using ketamine and/or sevoflurane which have a protective bronchodilating effect
    - Don't stimulate the airway (e.g., when suctioning) during emergence
    - Practice good pain control
    - Give preventive bronchodilator therapy
- Treatment of acute intraoperative bronchospasm

# SUGGESTED READING

- Papi A, Brightling C, Pedersen SE, Reddel HK. Asthma. Lancet. 2018;391(10122):783-800.
- Castillo JR, Peters SP, Busse WW. Asthma Exacerbations: Pathogenesis, Prevention, and Treatment. J Allergy Clin Immunol Pract. 2017;5(4):918-927.
- Woods BD, Sladen RN. Perioperative considerations for the patient with asthma and bronchospasm. BJA. 2009;103(1):i57-i65.

# BRONCHIECTASIS

## LEARNING OBJECTIVES

- Describe the pathology, common causes, and symptoms of bronchiectasis
- Manage patients with bronchiectasis

## DEFINITION AND MECHANISM

- Bronchiectasis is characterized by prolonged abnormal dilatation of bronchi with chronic inflammation
- Patients are extremely productive of sputum with a predisposition to either chronic infection or colonization with intermittent acute episodes of infection

## CAUSES

- Cystic fibrosis
- Tuberculosis
- Smoking
- Chronic obstructive pulmonary disease (COPD)
- Asthma
- Childhood pneumonia or recurrent adult infections
- Bronchial cartilage deficiency
- Abnormal ciliary motility (Kartageners)
- Hypogammaglobulinemia
- Immunodeficiency
- Inhaled foreign body
- Tumor

## SIGNS & SYMPTOMS

- High sputum production: Severe bronchiectasis patients can produce up to 500 mL of purulent sputum per day, which gets dramatically worse during an acute exacerbation
- Hemoptysis from areas of severe inflammation
- Pulmonary hypertension and cor pulmonale may develop in long-standing disease
- Metastatic abscess formation can occur
- Amyloidosis (rare)

## TREATMENT

- Chest physiotherapy with percussion and postural drainage
- Early intervention with antibiotics to prevent acute exacerbations

## MANAGEMENT

### BRONCHIECTASIS ANESTHETIC MANAGEMENT

**Preoperative assessment**

- Blood gas analysis
- ECG: Assess for signs of ventricular strain or cor pulmonale
- Echocardiography: Assess right ventricular hypertrophy, myocardial function and raised pulmonary pressures

- Extensive physiotherapy
- Ensure that the patient is exacerbation free prior to surgery
- Determine appropriate preoperative antibiotic use

**Intraoperative management**

- Regional anesthesia is preferred
- Routine monitoring + low threshold for arterial line
- No particular anesthetic agents are contraindicated
- Optimize ventilation to avoid barotrauma, dynamic hyperinflation, pulmonary tamponade
- Keep oxygen saturation high ( > 90%)
- Humidify all gases and persist with tracheal suction
- Bronchoscopy may be necessary to remove aspirated secretions and sputum
- Bronchial blocker may be feasible to isolate a part of the lung with localized severe bronchiectasis
- Avoid nasal tubes
- Pay attention to sterile technique

**Postoperative management**

- Arrange early postoperative therapy in advance
- High dependency unit care may be helpful
- Analgesia: Patient-controlled, epidural or NSAIDs
- Avoid postoperative ventilation

## SUGGESTED READING

- Chalmers, J.D., Chang, A.B., Chotirmall, S.H. et al. Bronchiectasis. Nat Rev Dis Primers 4, 45 (2018).
- Pollard BJ, Kitchen, G. Handbook of Clinical Anaesthesia. Fourth Edition. CRC Press. 2018. 978-1-4987-6289-2.

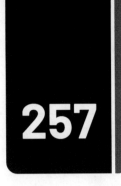

# BRONCHOPLEURAL FISTULA

## LEARNING OBJECTIVES

- Describe bronchopleural fistula, its causes, symptoms, and diagnosis
- Manage patients with a bronchopleural fistula

## DEFINITION AND MECHANISM

- A bronchopleural fistula (BPF) is a pathologic connection between the bronchus and the pleural space
- Potentially serious complication following pneumonectomy or other pulmonary resection
- Can be classified as acute, subacute, and chronic
  - Acute: Caused by surgical dehiscence, potentially life-threatening, requires prompt surgical intervention
  - Subacute & chronic: Mainly associated with infection, subacute is more severe

## CAUSES

- Breakdown of suture/staple line following lung resection
- Rupture of a cavity (cyst, abscess, bulla, bleb)
- Erosion of the bronchial wall by infection (empyema, pneumonia, tuberculosis)
- Erosion of the bronchial wall by neoplasm
- Penetrating trauma
- Pulmonary infarction
- Persistent spontaneous pneumothorax
- Chemotherapy or radiotherapy
- Iatrogenic

### Diagnosis

- Instillation of methylene blue into the pleural space
- Bronchography
- Bronchoscopy
- CT
- Capnography

| Signs and symptoms | |
|---|---|
| Acute BPF | Dyspnea<br>Hypotension<br>Subcutaneous emphysema<br>Cough with expectoration of purulent fluid<br>Tracheal or mediastinal shift<br>Persistent air leak<br>Reduction or disappearance of pleural effusion on chest radiograph |
| Subacute BPF | Wasting<br>Malaise<br>Fever |
| Chronic BPF | Infectious processes<br>Fibrosis of the pleural space |

Bronchopleural fistula

# MANAGEMENT

## *Bronchopleural fistula (BPF) Anesthetic Management*

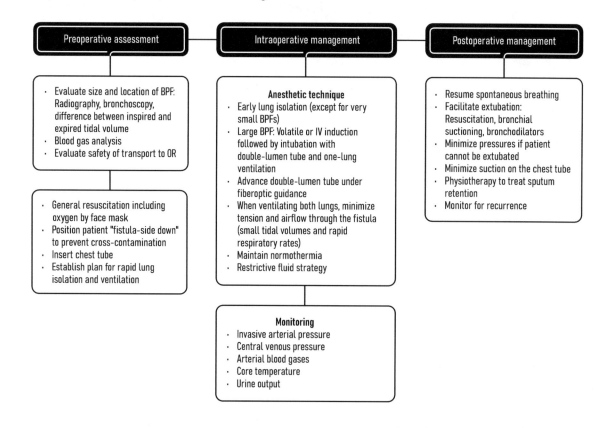

**Preoperative assessment**

- Evaluate size and location of BPF: Radiography, bronchoscopy, difference between inspired and expired tidal volume
- Blood gas analysis
- Evaluate safety of transport to OR

- General resuscitation including oxygen by face mask
- Position patient "fistula-side down" to prevent cross-contamination
- Insert chest tube
- Establish plan for rapid lung isolation and ventilation

**Intraoperative management**

**Anesthetic technique**
- Early lung isolation (except for very small BPFs)
- Large BPF: Volatile or IV induction followed by intubation with double-lumen tube and one-lung ventilation
- Advance double-lumen tube under fiberoptic guidance
- When ventilating both lungs, minimize tension and airflow through the fistula (small tidal volumes and rapid respiratory rates)
- Maintain normothermia
- Restrictive fluid strategy

**Monitoring**
- Invasive arterial pressure
- Central venous pressure
- Arterial blood gases
- Core temperature
- Urine output

**Postoperative management**

- Resume spontaneous breathing
- Facilitate extubation: Resuscitation, bronchial suctioning, bronchodilators
- Minimize pressures if patient cannot be extubated
- Minimize suction on the chest tube
- Physiotherapy to treat sputum retention
- Monitor for recurrence

## SUGGESTED READING

- Kiyota Y, Topulos GP, Hartigan PM. Bronchopleural fistula. In: Aglio LS, Lekowski RW, Urman RD, eds. Essential Clinical Anesthesia Review: Keywords, Questions and Answers for the Boards. Cambridge: Cambridge University Press; 2015:518-519.
- Pollard BJ, Kitchen, G. Handbook of Clinical Anaesthesia. Fourth Edition. CRC Press. 2018. 978-1-4987-6289-2.
- Salik I, Vashisht R, Abramowicz AE. Bronchopleural Fistula. [Updated 2022 May 8]. In: StatPearls [Internet]. Treasure Island (FL): StatPearls Publishing; 2022 Jan-. Available from: https://www.ncbi.nlm.nih.gov/books/NBK534765/

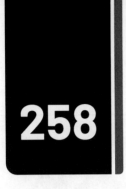

# BULLOUS LUNG DISEASE

## LEARNING OBJECTIVES

- Definition of bullous lung disease
- Anesthetic management of bullous lung disease

## DEFINITION AND MECHANISM

- Bullous lung disease is an uncommon cause of respiratory distress
- Characterized by the development of bullae within the lung parenchyma
- A bulla is a permanent, air-filled space within the lung parenchyma that is at least 1 cm in size and has a thin or poorly defined wall
- The term giant bulla is used for bullae that occupy at least 30 percent of a hemithorax
- Bullae do not take part in gas exchange and cause hypoxia and dyspnea
- Bullae are to be distinguished from other air-filled spaces within the lung:
  - Blebs are air-filled collections within the layers of the visceral pleura and are < 1 cm in diameter
  - Cysts are round, well-circumscribed collections that have an epithelial or fibrous lining
  - Cavities are usually thick-walled collections formed by focal necrosis within a consolidation, mass, or nodule
  - Pneumatoceles are temporary tents in the lung parenchyma that usually arise from blunt trauma or over-distension of the lung
- Bullae grow in size over time
- If positive pressure is used, the intra-bulla pressure will rise in relation to surrounding lung regions with a concomitant risk of hyperinflation and rupture
- Bulla rupture could be life-threatening due to hemodynamic collapse from a tension pneumothorax or inadequate ventilation due to a resultant bronchopleural fistula

## SIGNS AND SYMPTOMS

- Shortness of breath or chest tightness, particularly with exertion
- Cough
- Sputum production
- Abdominal fullness or bloating, usually associated with severe obstruction and prominent air-trapping on pulmonary function testing

## ETIOLOGY

- A consequence of cigarette or marijuana smoking
- HIV infection
- Intravenous drug users
- Alpha-1 antitrypsin deficiency
- Marfan syndrome
- Loeys-Dietz syndrome
- Ehlers-Danlos syndrome
- Sjögren syndrome
- Sarcoidosis
- Idiopathic

## DIAGNOSIS

- Chest X-ray
- CT
- Arterial blood gas
- Pulmonary function test

## TREATMENT

- If symptoms are absent, bullae do not require intervention
- Perform surgical extraction when the patient has incapacitating dyspnea or for patients who have complications related to bullous diseases, such as infection or pneumothorax

# MANAGEMENT

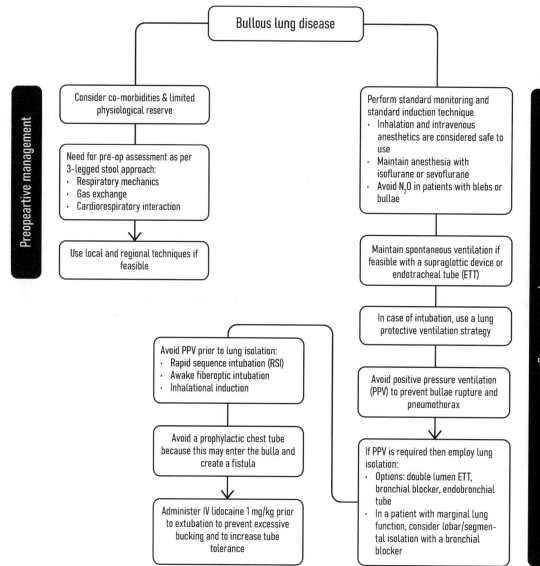

Bullous lung disease

**Preopeartive management**

Consider co-morbidities & limited physiological reserve

Need for pre-op assessment as per 3-legged stool approach:
- Respiratory mechanics
- Gas exchange
- Cardiorespiratory interaction

Use local and regional techniques if feasible

**Perioperative management**

Perform standard monitoring and standard induction technique
- Inhalation and intravenous anesthetics are considered safe to use
- Maintain anesthesia with isoflurane or sevoflurane
- Avoid $N_2O$ in patients with blebs or bullae

Maintain spontaneous ventilation if feasible with a supraglottic device or endotracheal tube (ETT)

In case of intubation, use a lung protective ventilation strategy

Avoid positive pressure ventilation (PPV) to prevent bullae rupture and pneumothorax

If PPV is required then employ lung isolation:
- Options: double lumen ETT, bronchial blocker, endobronchial tube
- In a patient with marginal lung function, consider lobar/segmental isolation with a bronchial blocker

Avoid PPV prior to lung isolation:
- Rapid sequence intubation (RSI)
- Awake fiberoptic intubation
- Inhalational induction

Avoid a prophylactic chest tube because this may enter the bulla and create a fistula

Administer IV lidocaine 1 mg/kg prior to extubation to prevent excessive bucking and to increase tube tolerance

## SUGGESTED READING

- Goldberg, C., Carey, K., 2013. Bullous Lung Disease. Western Journal of Emergency Medicine 14, 450–451.
- Johnson MK, Smith RP, Morrison D, et alLarge lung bullae in marijuana smokersThorax 2000;55:340-342.
- Saini V, Assu SM, Bhatia N, Sethi S. Abdominal surgery in a patient with bullous emphysema: Anesthetic concerns. J Anaesthesiol Clin Pharmacol. 2019;35(3):414-415.

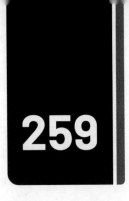

# 259

# CHRONIC OBSTRUCTIVE PULMONARY DISEASE

## LEARNING OBJECTIVES

- Manage patients with chronic obstructive pulmonary disease (COPD) in the pre-, and perioperative period

---

## DEFINITION AND MECHANISM

- COPD is an inflammatory lung disease characterized by abnormalities of the airways (bronchitis, bronchiolitis) and alveoli (emphysema), causing chronic dyspnea, cough, excessive sputum production, and progressive airway obstruction

### ABOUT
- Progressive lung disease characterized by long-term respiratory symptoms and airflow limitation
- **Symptoms:** Shortness of breath and a cough (with or without mucus)
- **Incorporates three disorders:** Emphysema, peripheral airway disease, and chronic bronchitis
- FEV1/FVC ratio < 70% - RV ↑

- Different stages based on FEV1
  - **Stage I:** > 50% predicted FEV1
  - **Stage II:** 35-50%
  - **Stage III:** < 35%

### COMPLICATIONS OF COPD
#### Carbon dioxide retention
- Many stage II or III patients have an ↑ $PaCO_2$ (> 45 mmHg) at rest
- When these patients are given supplemental oxygen $PaCO_2$ ↑ because ↑ inspired oxygen concentrations cause an ↑ in alveolar dead space owing to a ↓ in regional hypoxic pulmonary vasoconstriction and the Haldane effect
- ↑ $CO_2$ concentrations above baseline lead to respiratory acidosis → cardiovascular changes (tachycardia, hypotension, and pulmonary vasoconstriction)
- $PaCO_2$ levels > 80 mmHg can cause a ↓ level of consciousness
#### Right ventricular dysfunction
- In up to 50% of patients with severe COPD
- Cor pulmonale occurs in 70% of COPD patients with an FEV1 < 0.6 L
- Chronic recurrent hypoxemia is the cause of right ventricular dysfunction and subsequent progression to cor pulmonale
#### Bullae
- Many patients with moderate to severe COPD develop cystic air spaces in the lung parenchyma (= bullae)
- Localized loss of structural support tissue in the lung with elastic recoil of surrounding parenchyma
#### Flow limitation
- Occurs when any ↑ in expiratory effort will not produce an ↑ in flow at that given lung volume

### PERIOPERATIVE MANAGEMENT
- Manage and treat these 4 complications at the time of preoperative assessment: Atelectasis, bronchospasm, respiratory tract infections, and congestive heart failure
- Atelectasis impairs local lung lymphocyte and macrophage function predisposing to infection
- Wheezing may be a symptom both of airway obstruction and congestive heart failure
- All patients should receive bronchodilator therapy as guided by their symptoms
- Start corticosteroid therapy if sympathomimetic and anticholinergic bronchodilators provide inadequate therapy
- COPD patients have fewer postoperative pulmonary complications when intensive chest physiotherapy is initiated preoperatively → those with excessive sputum benefit the most from physiotherapy

FEV1, forced expiratory volume; RV, residual volume

## BACKGROUND INFORMATION

- In 2017, 300 million people worldwide were living with COPD

## RISK FACTORS

COPD is caused by a complicated interaction between chronic exposure to noxious stimuli, individual risk factors, and socioeconomic risk factors

### Noxious stimuli
- Tobacco smoke
- Air pollution caused by burning carbon-based fuels or biomass

- Occupational exposure such as chemical fumes or other fine particulate matter

### Individual risk factors

- History of previous lung infections, including tuberculosis
- Genetics
- Maternal and prenatal exposure
- Asthma
- Premature birth

### Socio-economic risk factors

- Access to healthcare
- Diet

## PATHOPHYSIOLOGY

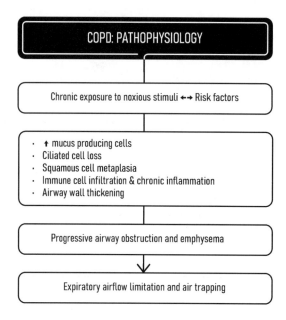

## EXACERBATION TREATMENT

### 1. Assess severity

- Use ABCDE approach – take arterial blood gas, perform chest X-ray, apply full ASA-monitoring

### 2. Treat symptoms

- Give supplemental $O_2$ – titrate to achieve $SaO_2$ of 88-92%
- Bronchodilators
  - ↑ dose and/or frequency of short-acting bronchodilators
  - Combine short-acting beta-2-agonists and anticholinergics
  - Give long-acting beta-2-agonists when stable
- Give corticosteroids
- Give antibiotics if signs of bacterial infection
- If necessary, start noninvasive ventilation (NIV)

### 3. Identify and treat associated conditions

- e.g., Heart failure, pulmonary embolism, arrhythmia

# ANESTHETIC IMPLICATIONS

## *Preoperative assessment*

- Assess maximal level of exertion attainable
- Perform
  - Routine preoperative blood tests
  - Electrocardiogram – to exclude concomitant heart disease
  - Chest X-ray – if evidence of current infection or recent worsening of symptoms
  - Spirometry – to confirm the diagnosis and to assess the severity of COPD
- Treat symptoms aggressively
- If signs of active respiratory infection, postpone non-emergency surgery
- Strict smoking cessation
- Preoperative physiotherapy may help reduce the incidence of intraoperative bronchial plugging or pneumonitis
- Optimize nutritional status
  - Obesity and underweight both increase perioperative risk
  - Serum albumin level < 35 mg/L is a strong predictor of postoperative pulmonary complications, give preoperative nutritional supplementation

## *Anesthetic regimen*

- Regional anesthesia (RA) decreases postoperative pulmonary complications
- Light sedation, flexible positioning, or NIV might comfort patients who find it uncomfortable lying supine
- General anesthesia in COPD carries higher risk for laryngospasm, bronchospasm, cardiovascular instability, barotraumas, and hypoxemia
- To reduce the harmful effects of air trapping when mechanically ventilating
  - Reduce the respiratory rate or the I:E ratio (to 1:3–1:5) to lengthen expiration
  - Give PEEP to help keep small airways open during late exhalation
  - Promptly treat bronchospasm
- Fully reverse the neuromuscular blocking agent before extubation
- Consider periextubation bronchodilator treatment
- NIV postextubation reduces the work of breathing and air trapping and has been shown to reduce the need for reintubation in the postoperative period after major surgery

## SUGGESTED READING

- Christenson SA, Smith BM, Bafadhel M, Putcha N. Chronic obstructive pulmonary disease. Lancet. 2022;399(10342):2227-2242.
- Lumb AB, Biercamp C. Chronic obstructive pulmonary disease and anaesthesia. Continuing Education in Anaesthesia, Critical Care & Pain. 2014;14:1-5.
- National Institute for Health and Care Excellence. (2018) Chronic Obstructive Pulmonary Disease in over 16s: diagnosis and management (NICE guideline 115) available at https://www.nice.org.uk/guidance/ng115.

# CYSTIC FIBROSIS

## LEARNING OBJECTIVES

- Describe the pathophysiology and clinical manifestations of cystic fibrosis
- Diagnose cystic fibrosis
- Manage patients with cystic fibrosis

## DEFINITION AND MECHANISM

- Cystic fibrosis is a multisystem autosomal recessive disease
- Most common lethal genetic disease in Caucasians
- Best considered as a disease spectrum rather than a distinct single clinical entity

## PATHOPHYSIOLOGY AND CLINICAL MANIFESTATIONS

| Site | Pathology | Clinical manifestations |
|------|-----------|-------------------------|
| Lower respiratory tract | Viscid mucous secretions, hypertrophy of goblet cells, decreased mucociliary clearance | Frequent lower respiratory tract infection (LRTI), chronic hypoxemia, cor pulmonale |
| Upper respiratory tract | Abnormal viscid nasal secretions | Sinusitis, nasal polyposis |
| Hepatobiliary system | Obstruction of bile ductules | Focal biliary cirrhosis, portal hypertension, multinodular biliary cirrhosis |
| Gastrointestinal tract | Abnormally viscid intestinal secretions at the level of the terminal ileum in the neonate | Meconium ileus, recurrent abdominal pain (distal intestinal obstruction syndrome) |
| Pancreas | Obstructed pancreatic ducts, fibrosis | Pancreatic exocrine insufficiency, CF-related diabetes (CFRD) |
| Reproductive system | Congenital absence of vas deferens, viscid cervical secretions | Infertility in men (98%), decreased fertility in women |
| Bone | Impaired calcium, vitamin D absorption, increased catabolism | Osteoporosis |
| Skin | Increased chloride levels | Abnormal 'sweat test', diminished thermoregulation |

# DIAGNOSIS

- Based on the presence of:
  - One or more characteristic clinical features

Or
  - History of cystic fibrosis in a sibling

Or
  - Positive newborn screening (NBS) test
- PLUS laboratory evidence of an abnormality in the CF transmembrane conductance regulator (CFTR) gene or protein:
  - Sweat testing: Transdermal administration of pilocarpine by iontophoresis to stimulate sweating and analysis of electrolyte concentrations
  - Genetic testing

# TREATMENT

- No curative treatment is available
- Treatment is supportive and aims to
  - Minimize pulmonary infection
  - Optimize nutritional status
  - Slow disease progress
  - Ease symptoms

| | |
|---|---|
| Respiratory | Physical therapy |
| | Inhaled bronchodilators and mucolytics |
| | Oscillatory devices, positive expiratory pressure devices, and high-frequency chest compression devices |
| | Oxygen therapy |
| Pharmacologic | Mucolytics: DNA-ase, inhaled hypertonic saline |
| | Anti-inflammatories: Oral corticosteroids, ibuprofen, azithromycin |
| | Antibiotics |
| Nutrition | Enteral supplementation or parenteral nutrition |
| | Subcutaneous insulin when needed |
| Gene therapy | Under investigation |

Cystic fibrosis

# MANGEMENT

CYSTIC FIBROSIS ANESTHETIC MANAGEMENT

## Preoperative assessment

- Thorough history
- Medication review
- More intense daily physiotherapy
- Nebulized medications as late as possible
- Chest radiograph
- Arterial blood gas analysis
- Bedside spirometry
- Microbiological infection
- Volume and purulence of sputum
- Full blood count
- Blood glucose
- Urea and electrolytes
- Coagulation study
- Liver function tests

**Surgical factors that increase the risk of pulmonary complications**
- Duration of surgery/anesthesia
- Surgical site: upper abdominal and thoracic incisions carry the highest risk
- Nasogastric tube insertion
- Emergency surgery

## Intraoperative management

**Anesthetic goals**
- Maintain baseline blood gas levels
- Facilitate rapid emergence
- Avoid hypothermia
- Careful positioning and padding
- Balance of analgesia against respiratory depression: Minimize opioid use (e.g., local and/or regional anesthesia)

**Monitoring**
- Arterial line for blood gas analysis
- Cardiac output monitoring for patients with cor pulmonale or presenting for major surgery

**Airway management**
- For short or non-abdominal or thoracic procedures: Laryngeal mask with spontaneous breathing
- Endotracheal tube facilitates tracheal suctioning of secretions and allows improved control of gas exchange
- Avoid nasal intubation
- Keep airway pressures as low as possible
- Humidify gases
- Volatile anesthetics (e.g., sevoflurane) facilitate bronchodilation

## Postoperative management

**Goals**
- Minimize the development of postoperative respiratory tract infection
- Early extubation
- Fully reverse neuromuscular block
- Have patient's own ventilation equipment available
- Resume chest physiotherapy as soon as possible
- Monitored postoperative care for patients with advanced respiratory disease or non-respiratory manifestations
- Consider postoperative ventilation for patients with advanced respiratory disease

## SUGGESTED READING

- Fitzgerald M, Ryan D. Cystic fibrosis and anaesthesia. Continuing Education in Anaesthesia Critical Care & Pain. 2011;11(6):204-9.
- Huffmyer JL, Littlewood KE, Nemergut EC. Perioperative Management of the Adult with Cystic Fibrosis. Anesthesia & Analgesia. 2009;109(6).

Cystic fibrosis

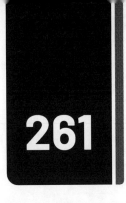

# 261

# ESOPHAGECTOMY

## LEARNING OBJECTIVES

- Describe the indications for esophagectomy
- Manage patients presenting for esophagectomy

## DEFINITION AND MECHANISM

- Esophageal cancer is the eighth most common malignancy worldwide
- Curative therapy for many patients involves surgery (esophagectomy), often with preoperative chemotherapy
- Esophagectomy remains high-risk with substantial associated morbidity and mortality

## RISK FACTORS FOR ESOPHAGEAL MALIGNANCY

| Risk factor | Adenocarcinoma | Squamos cell carcinoma |
|---|---|---|
| Lifestyle | Smoking | Alcohol, smoking (may show synergism), poor oral hygiene |
| Racial origin | Caucasian more common than Asian or African | Sub-Saharan African Heritage three times higher than Caucasians<br>Far East Asian Heritage |
| Age and gender | Increasing age, male greater than female | Male > female |
| Dietary | Low dietary intake of fruit and vegetables | Salted vegetables, preserved fish |
| Disease | Gastro-oesophageal reflux, Barrett's oesophagus, obesity, family history (rare) | Mutations of alcohol metabolic pathways, achalasia, caustic injury, nutritional deficiencies, non-epidermolytic palmoplantar keratoderma |
| Economic | Developed world → High income countries<br>Developing world → Low & middle income countries | Low socioeconomic status<br>Developing world |
| Medical/industrial | Thoracic radiation, medications that relax the lower oesophageal sphincter | Thoracic radiation |

## RISK FACTORS FOR PERIOPERATIVE MORBIDITY AND MORTALITY

- Poor cardiac and/or pulmonary function
- Advanced age
- Tumor stage
- Diabetes mellitus
- Impaired general health

- Hepatic dysfunction
- Peripheral vascular disease
- Smoker
- Chronic use of steroids

Esophagectomy

# MANAGEMENT

**Preoperative assessment & prehabilitation**
- Evaluation of cardiopulmonary exercise
- Pre-optimization of comorbid disease management
- Encouragement of smoking cessation
- Management of preoperative anemia
- Careful nutritional support with fortified drinks and/or nasogastric or jejunostomy feeding
- Physiotherapy and exercise training (requires further research)

**Surgical approaches**
- Excision of the esophagus and relocation of the stomach in the mediastinum to form gastric conduit
- Revision esophagectomy: Colonic interposition using a section of colon on a pedicle
- Ivor Lewis approach: Laparotomy to assess tumor extent and mobilize the stomach, followed by a right thoracotomy for the resection and anastomosis
- Tri-incisional or McKeown technique: Cervical incision for the upper anastomosis
- Transdiaphragmatic approach: Incision from the thoracotomy site to the umbilicus, dividing the diaphragm surgically
- Transhiatal esophagectomy: Laparotomy and dissection of the lower esophagus through an enlarged diaphragmatic hiatus, followed by removal of the esophagus and re-anastomosis via a left cervical incision
- Minimally invasive esophagectomy: Thoracoscopic and laparoscopic surgical techniques in place of open incisions
- Many surgeons perform hybrid techniques

**Analgesia**
- Pre-emptive thoracic epidural
- Paravertebral block or catheter when epidural is strongly contraindicated or difficult
- Patient-controlled analgesia for step-down analgesia or if regional anesthesia failed

**One-lung ventilation**
- Lung isolation is necessary for the open thoracic or thoracoscopic phase of surgery
- Most frequently achieved with a left-sided double-lumen tube
- Prevent, detect, and correct tube migration, especially if the prone position is used

**Protective lung ventilation**
- Low tidal volumes and lung-protective strategies to prevent atelectasis and minimize shunt

**Fluid management**
- Excess fluid administration: Risk of pulmonary edema and venous congestion of the anastomosis
- Insufficient fluid: Excess vasopressor use, increased myocardial strain, and vasoconstriction, risking ischemia of the anastomosis and systemic effects including acute kidney injury
- Suboptimal anastomotic perfusion: Risk of leak development

# POSTOPERATIVE COMPLICATIONS

| Postoperative complications | |
| --- | --- |
| Respiratory | Pneumonia <br> Atelectasis <br> Acute respiratory stress syndrome <br> Recurrent laryngeal nerve palsy |
| Surgical | Anastomotic leak |
| Cardiac | Supraventricular arrhythmias (e.g., atrial fibrillation) |

- The risk of respiratory complications can be minimized by adequate analgesia, reversal of muscular block, normothermia, chest physiotherapy and hemodynamic stability
- Major anastomotic leaks require surgical exploration and revision surgery
- Smaller leaks are managed by keeping the patient nil by mouth, giving high protein enteral feed or total parenteral nutrition, antibiotics, chest physiotherapy, radiologically guided drainage collection and performing serial contrast studies

## SUGGESTED READING

- Howells P, Bieker M, Yeung J. Oesophageal cancer and the anaesthetist. BJA Education. 2017;17(2):68-73.
- Veelo DP, Geerts BF. Anaesthesia during oesophagectomy. J Thorac Dis. 2017;9(Suppl 8):S705-S712. doi:10.21037/jtd.2017.03.153

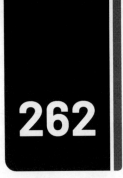

# 262

# LUNG CANCER

## LEARNING OBJECTIVES

- Anesthetic management of lung cancer

## DEFINITION AND MECHANISM

- Lung cancer is the most common cause of cancer mortality worldwide for men and women
- Lung cancer or lung carcinoma is a malignant tumor characterized by uncontrolled cell growth in lung tissue
- Lung carcinomas derive from transformed, malignant cells that originate as epithelial cells, or from tissues composed of epithelial cells
- Sarcomas are generated by the malignant transformation of connective tissues, which arise from mesenchymal cells
- Lung cancer often starts in the bronchi, bronchioles, or alveoli

- Two types:
  □ Non-small-cell lung cancer
    ▪ The most common form, accounting for around 80% of lung cancer cases
    ▪ Common types include: squamous cell carcinoma, adenocarcinoma, or large-cell carcinoma
  □ Small-cell lung cancer
    ▪ Less common
    ▪ Spreads faster and harder to treat than non-small-cell lung cancer
- Other tumors including large cell, neuroendocrine (carcinoid), bronchioloalveolar and rarer forms can all present as lung malignancies
- The presentation includes airway obstruction, lung collapse, and distal infection or through spread via the peribronchial tissues with subsequent invasion of the mediastinum
- Spreads by both lymphatic and hematological routes and distal metastasis is common in the liver, adrenals, bone, and brain

## SIGNS AND SYMPTOMS

- A persistent cough
- Shortness of breath
- Chest pain
- Wheezing
- Hemoptysis
- Fatigue
- Hoarseness
- Weight loss
- Bone pain
- Headache
- Swelling in the face, neck, arms, or upper chest (superior vena cava (SVC) syndrome)

## RISK FACTORS

- Smoking
- Older age
- Genetic mutations
- Exposure to harmful substances such as air pollution, radon, asbestos, uranium, silica, coal products
- Previous radiation treatment to the thorax
- Family history of lung cancer

## DIAGNOSIS

- Physical exam
- Blood test
- Chest X-ray
- CT/PET
- Biopsy

## MANAGEMENT

- Anesthetic involvement is mainly for lung resection (e.g., lobectomy, pneumonectomy)
- Consider:
  □ Potentially compromised respiratory function with risk of perioperative respiratory complications
  □ Mass effects: obstructive pneumonia, lung abscess, SVC syndrome, tracheobronchial distortion, Pancoast's syndrome, recurrent laryngeal nerve or phrenic nerve paresis, chest wall or mediastinal extension

  □ Metabolic effects: Lambert–Eaton syndrome, hypercalcemia, hyponatremia, Cushing's syndrome
  □ Metastases: particularly to the brain, bone, liver, & adrenal
  □ Medications: chemotherapy agents, pulmonary toxicity (bleomycin, mitomycin), cardiac toxicity (doxorubicin), renal toxicity (cisplatin)
  □ Comorbidities including smoking, chronic obstructive lung disease, coronary artery disease, hypertension

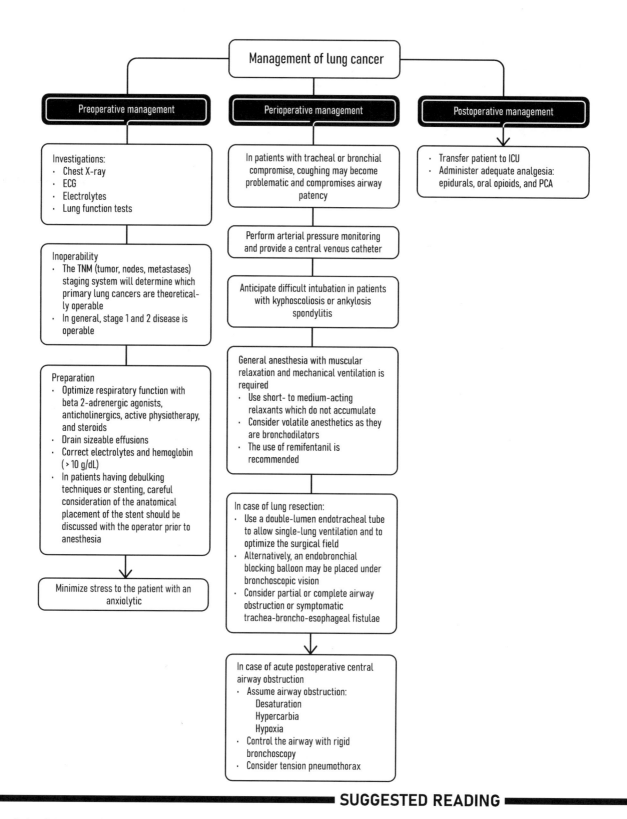

## Management of lung cancer

### Preoperative management

Investigations:
- Chest X-ray
- ECG
- Electrolytes
- Lung function tests

Inoperability
- The TNM (tumor, nodes, metastases) staging system will determine which primary lung cancers are theoretically operable
- In general, stage 1 and 2 disease is operable

Preparation
- Optimize respiratory function with beta 2-adrenergic agonists, anticholinergics, active physiotherapy, and steroids
- Drain sizeable effusions
- Correct electrolytes and hemoglobin ( > 10 g/dL)
- In patients having debulking techniques or stenting, careful consideration of the anatomical placement of the stent should be discussed with the operator prior to anesthesia

Minimize stress to the patient with an anxiolytic

### Perioperative management

In patients with tracheal or bronchial compromise, coughing may become problematic and compromises airway patency

Perform arterial pressure monitoring and provide a central venous catheter

Anticipate difficult intubation in patients with kyphoscoliosis or ankylosis spondylitis

General anesthesia with muscular relaxation and mechanical ventilation is required
- Use short- to medium-acting relaxants which do not accumulate
- Consider volatile anesthetics as they are bronchodilators
- The use of remifentanil is recommended

In case of lung resection:
- Use a double-lumen endotracheal tube to allow single-lung ventilation and to optimize the surgical field
- Alternatively, an endobronchial blocking balloon may be placed under bronchoscopic vision
- Consider partial or complete airway obstruction or symptomatic trachea-broncho-esophageal fistulae

In case of acute postoperative central airway obstruction
- Assume airway obstruction:
  Desaturation
  Hypercarbia
  Hypoxia
- Control the airway with rigid bronchoscopy
- Consider tension pneumothorax

### Postoperative management

- Transfer patient to ICU
- Administer adequate analgesia: epidurals, oral opioids, and PCA

---

**SUGGESTED READING**

- Hackett, S., Jones, R., Kapila, R., 2019. Anaesthesia for pneumonectomy. BJA Education 19, 297–304.
- Pollard BJ, Kitchen, G. Handbook of Clinical Anaesthesia. Fourth Edition. CRC Press. 2018. 978-1-4987-6289-2.

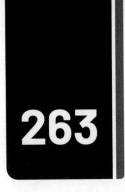

# MASSIVE HEMOPTYSIS

## LEARNING OBJECTIVES

- Describe the definition and possible causes of massive hemoptysis
- Diagnose massive hemoptysis
- Manage massive hemoptysis occurrence

## DEFINITION AND MECHANISM

- Hemoptysis is defined as the expectoration of blood originating from the lower respiratory tract
- There is no agreed definition of massive hemoptysis, with volumes ranging from 100 mL to 1000 mL within 24 hours
- In practice, life-threatening hemoptysis occurs with any volume of blood that could obstruct the airway or cause significant hemodynamic compromise
- Emergency that requires prompt management

## PATHOPHYSIOLOGY

- In 90% of cases, the source is the bronchial circulation

| Causes | |
|---|---|
| Infectious | Mycobacteria<br>Fungal infections (mycetomas)<br>Necrotizing pneumonia and lung abscess (Klebsiella, Pseudomonas, Streptococcus, Actinomyces)<br>Bacterial endocarditis with septic emboli<br>Parasitic (paragonimiasis, hydatid cyst) |
| Parasitic (paragonimiasis, hydatid cyst) | Bronchogenic carcinoma<br>Endobronchial tumors (carcinoid, adenoid cystic carcinoma)<br>Pulmonary metastases<br>Sarcoma |
| Pulmonary | Bronchiectasis (including cystic fibrosis)<br>Chronic bronchitis<br>Alveolar hemorrhage and underlying causes<br>Diffuse alveolar damage |
| Cardiac/pulmonary vascular | Pulmonary artery aneurysm (Rasmussen aneurysm, mycotic, arteritis)<br>Bronchial artery aneurysm<br>Pulmonary infarct (embolism)<br>Pulmonary hypertension<br>Congenital cardiac or pulmonary malformations<br>Airway-vascular fistulae<br>Arteriovenous malformations<br>Mitral stenosis<br>Left-ventricular failure<br>Pulmonary veno-occlusive disease |
| Vasculitis/collagen vascular disease | Granulomatosis with polyangiitis<br>Goodpasture's syndrome<br>Behçet's disease<br>Systemic lupus erythematosus<br>Essential mixed cryoglobulinemia<br>Henoch-Schonlein purpura<br>Mixed connective tissue disease<br>Progressive systemic sclerosis<br>Rheumatoid arthritis<br>Systemic necrotizing vasculitis<br>Immune complex associated glomerulonephritis<br>Pauci-immune glomerulonephritis |

| Causes | |
|---|---|
| Hematologic | Coagulopathy (congenital, acquired or iatrogenic)<br>Platelet disorders<br>Thrombotic thrombocytopenic purpura |
| Drugs and toxins | Penicillamine<br>Solvents<br>Crack cocaine<br>Trimellitic anhydride<br>Bevacizumab<br>Isocyanates<br>Nitrofurantoin |
| Trauma | Catheter-induced pulmonary artery rupture<br>Blunt or penetrating chest injury<br>Transtracheal procedures<br>Iatrogenic secondary to interventional pulmonology procedures<br>Bronchoscopic biopsy |
| Miscellaneous | Cryptogenic<br>Endometriosis<br>Lymphangiolyomyomatosis<br>Broncholithiasis<br>Foreign body aspiration<br>Lung transplantation<br>Tuberous sclerosis<br>Idiopathic pulmonary hemosiderosis |

## DIAGNOSIS

- The main goals are identifying the site of bleeding and revealing the underlying cause
- Diagnostic tools:
  - Chest radiography
  - Computed tomography
  - Fiberoptic bronchoscopy

## MANAGEMENT

- Hemoptysis ABCs:
  - Bleeding side down (if known bleeding site)
  - Intubation
    1. Rigid intubation
    2. Single-lumen endotracheal intubation
  - Contralateral isolation and single-lung ventilation
  - Volume resuscitation (crystalloids/colloids)
  - Multidisciplinary call/page
    - Interventional radiology
    - ICU
    - Interventional pulmonology
    - Anesthesiology
- Surgery: Lung resection

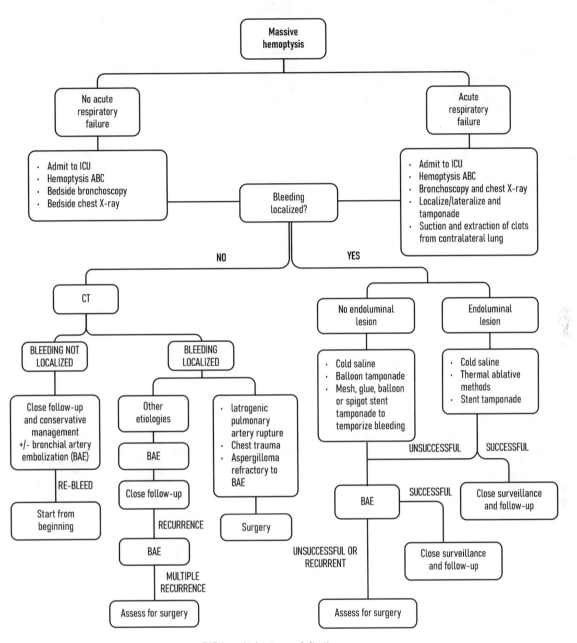

**Massive hemoptysis**

**No acute respiratory failure**
- Admit to ICU
- Hemoptysis ABC
- Bedside bronchoscopy
- Bedside chest X-ray

**Acute respiratory failure**
- Admit to ICU
- Hemoptysis ABC
- Bronchoscopy and chest X-ray
- Localize/lateralize and tamponade
- Suction and extraction of clots from contralateral lung

**Bleeding localized?**

**NO**

CT

BLEEDING NOT LOCALIZED

Close follow-up and conservative management +/- bronchial artery embolization (BAE)

RE-BLEED

Start from beginning

BLEEDING LOCALIZED

Other etiologies

BAE

Close follow-up

RECURRENCE

BAE

MULTIPLE RECURRENCE

Assess for surgery

- Iatrogenic pulmonary artery rupture
- Chest trauma
- Aspergilloma refractory to BAE

Surgery

**YES**

No endoluminal lesion
- Cold saline
- Balloon tamponade
- Mesh, glue, balloon or spigot stent tamponade to temporize bleeding

Endoluminal lesion
- Cold saline
- Thermal ablative methods
- Stent tamponade

UNSUCCESSFUL

SUCCESSFUL

Close surveillance and follow-up

BAE

SUCCESSFUL

Close surveillance and follow-up

UNSUCCESSFUL OR RECURRENT

Assess for surgery

BAE, bronchial-artery embolisation

**SUGGESTED READING**

- Radchenko C, Alraiyes AH, Shojaee S. A systematic approach to the management of massive hemoptysis. J Thorac Dis. 2017;9(Suppl 10):S1069-S1086.
- Thomas, A. and Lynch, G. (2011) Management Of Massive Haemoptysis, WFSA. Available at: https://resources.wfsahq.org/atotw/management-of-massive-haemoptysis/ (Accessed: January 23, 2023).

Massive hemoptysis

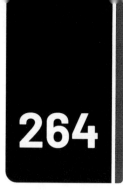

# MEDIASTINOSCOPY

## LEARNING OBJECTIVES

- Describe the indications and contraindications for mediastinoscopy
- Describe the possible complications of mediastinoscopy
- Manage patients presenting for mediastinoscopy

**DEFINITION AND MECHANISM**

- Mediastinoscopy is a diagnostic procedure with high sensitivity and specificity for lung cancer staging
- Also used for biopsy of mediastinal masses and diagnosis in diseases presenting with mediastinal lymphadenopathy
- The majority of mediastinoscopies are performed via the cervical approach:
  - Entering the mediastinum through a 3 cm incision in the suprasternal notch
  - A dissection is made between the left innominate vein and the sternum creating a tunnel in the fascial layers
  - The mediastinoscope is then inserted anterior to the aortic arch

## INDICATION & CONTRAINDICATIONS

- Indications
  - Evaluation of lymph node involvement in patients with carcinoma of the lung
  - Tissue biopsy of mediastinal masses
  - Removal of mediastinal masses and enlarged lymph nodes
    - Conditions presenting as a mediastinal mass:

| Tumors | |
|---|---|
| Anterior mediastinum | Thymic tumors<br>Thyroid and parathyroid tumors<br>Lymphoma<br>Germ cell tumors |
| Middle mediastinum | Lymphoma<br>Mesenchymal tumors |
| Posterior mediastinum | Esophageal cancer<br>Neurogenic tumors |
| **Benign conditions** | |
| Developmental cysts | Pericardial cyst<br>Esophageal cyst |
| Granulomatous lymphadenopathy | Tuberculosis<br>Sarcoidosis |
| Vascular | Aneurysms (e.g., thoracic aorta, innominate vein)<br>Aberrant vessels (e.g., persistent left superior vena cava, anomalous left pulmonary artery) |

| Contraindications | |
|---|---|
| Absolute | Anterior mediastinal mass<br>Inoperable tumor<br>Previous recurrent laryngeal nerve injury<br>Extremely debilitated patients<br>Ascending aortic aneurysm<br>Previous mediastinoscopy |
| Relative | Thoracic inlet obstruction<br>Superior vena cava (SVC) syndrome<br>Severe tracheal deviation<br>History of radiation therapy to the chest<br>Cerebrovascular disease<br>Severe cervical spine disease with limited neck extension<br>Thoracic aortic aneurysm |

## POSSIBLE COMPLICATIONS

- Major hemorrhage
- Stroke
- Air embolism
- Pneumothorax
- Reflex arrhythmias
- Phrenic nerve paralysis
- Recurrent laryngeal nerve palsy
- Esophageal tear
- Tracheobronchial laceration
- Thoracic duct injury
- Minor bleeding

## MANAGEMENT

### MEDIASTINOSCOPY ANESTHETIC MANAGEMENT

#### Preoperative assessment

**Investigations**
- Routine hematology and biochemistry
- ECG
- Chest X-ray
- CT scan to evaluate location of the tumor/mass and the degree of tracheal compression
- Pulmonary function tests
- Flow-volume curves in upright and supine position
- Echocardiography and stress testing in the presence of cardiac symptoms

**Premedication**
- Short-acting benzodiazepine may be used to decrease anxiety
- Avoid sedatives if tracheal obstruction is suspected

**Preparation**
- Insert large bore IV cannulae
- Have cross-matched blood available

#### Intraoperative management

**Induction**
- Asymptomatic patients: Preoxygenation followed by IV induction
- Respiratory obstruction: Awake intubation under local anesthesia or inhalation induction followed by intubation under deep anesthesia
- Place the patient in a 20° head-up position

**Maintenance**
- IV and/or volatile anesthetics + neuromuscular blocking agent + short-acting opioid
- Ventilation of both lungs through a single-lumen endotracheal tube is usually sufficient

**Monitoring**
- Invasive arterial blood pressure monitoring, preferably in right arm
- Neuromuscular monitoring in patients with myasthenia gravis and Eaton –Lambert syndrome
- Observe ventilation presssure gauge for acute increases in airway pressure

#### Postoperative management

- Rapid emergence
- Extubation after full neuromuscular recovery
- A short period of ventilation may be required
- Chest X-ray or lung US in recovery room to exclude pneumothorax
- Observe for dyspnea and stridor
- Multimodal analgesia:
  - Local infiltration of the wound
  - Superficial cervical plexus block
  - Intercostal nerve block
  - Paracetamol and NSAIDs

**Complication management**
- Major hemorrhage:
  - Compression and packing to stop bleeding
  - Surgical exploration
  - Secure large bore IV access in the lower limbs
- Lung damage:
  - Tube thoracostomy

## SUGGESTED READING

- Ahmed-Nusrath A, Swanevelder J. Anaesthesia for mediastinoscopy. Continuing Education in Anaesthesia Critical Care & Pain. 2007;7(1):6-9.
- McNally PA, Arthur ME. Mediastinoscopy. [Updated 2022 Sep 12]. In: StatPearls [Internet]. Treasure Island (FL): StatPearls Publishing; 2022 Jan-. Available from: https://www.ncbi.nlm.nih.gov/books/NBK534863/

# OBSTRUCTIVE SLEEP APNEA

## LEARNING OBJECTIVES

- Manage a patient with obstructive sleep apnea (OSA) in the perioperative period

## DEFINITION AND MECHANISM

- Obstructive sleep apnea (OSA) is a disorder in which a person frequently stops breathing during their sleep due to obstruction of the upper airway
- This obstruction is caused by an inadequate motor tone of the tongue and/or airway dilator muscles and is exaggerated by excessive adipose tissue
- OSA accompanied by excessive daytime sleepiness is termed OSA syndrome (OSAS)

## OBSTRUCTIVE SLEEP APNEA (OSA)

### ABOUT

- Most common sleep-related breathing disorder
- Characterized by recurrent episodes of complete (apnea) or partial (hypopnea) obstruction of the upper airway leading to reduced or absent breathing during sleep → hypoxemia and hypercapnia
- Cause? Repeated episodes of complete or partial closure of the pharynx, accompanied with hypoventilation and desaturation and ↑ $CO_2$ → terminated by EEG arousal

### PATHOPHYSIOLOGY

- Upper airway collapsibility and patency are dependent on continuous balance between collapsing and expanding forces influenced by sleep-wake arousal
  - **Wakefulness:** Upper airway stability and patency are achieved by ↑ genioglossus muscle tone → pulls the tongue forward
  - **Sleep:** Upper airway collapse in OSA may occur due to the loss of upper airway dilating muscle tone, impaired response to mechanoreceptors sensing intrapharyngeal pressures, ventilator overshoot, and ↑ arousal threshold
- **Upper airway of patients with OSA is predisposed to collapse:** Occurs in the presence of smaller upper airway cross-sectional areas and ↑ critical closure pressures
- **NREM sleep and anesthesia:** ↓ wakeful cortical influences, reflex gain, and ventilatory drive → predispose to upper airway collapse and hypoventilation → effects are more intense during GA as the ↓ in tonic and phasic muscle activity is profound and the protective arousal response is abolished

### CLINICAL DIAGNOSTIC CRITERIA

- Diagnosis requires an overnight polysomnography (PSG) or sleep study

**Definitions**

- **Apnea:** ↓ in rate of airflow from intranasal pressure of ≥ 90%
- **Hypopnea:** ↓ in rate of airflow from intranasal pressure of 50-90%
  - → for at least 10 sec accompanied by a 3-4% ↓ in oxygen saturation or an EEG arousal

**Obstructive hypopnea:** Thoracoabdominal motion is out-of-phase or airflow limitation on nasal pressure signal

- **Central hypopnea:** Thoracoabdominal motion is in-phase and no evidence of airflow limitation on nasal pressure signal
- **Mixed apnea:** Events that begin as central for at least 10 sec and end as obstructive, with a min. of 3 obstructive efforts

**Apnea-hypopnea index (AHI)**

- Average number of abnormal breathing events per hour of sleep
- Determines OSA severity
  - **5-15 events/h:** Mild
  - **15-30 events/h:** Moderate
  - **> 30 events/h:** Severe

**Clinical diagnosis**

- Requires an AHI of ≥ 15 OR an AHI ≥ 5 with symptoms (excessive daytime sleepiness, unintentional sleep during wakefulness, unrefreshing sleep, loud snoring, or observed obstruction during sleep)

## BACKGROUND

- OSA affects 5-10% of the general population but is twice as prevalent in the population undergoing surgery

# PREDISPOSING FACTORS

- Obesity
- Age 40-70
- Male gender
- Alcohol abuse
- Smoking
- Pregnancy
- Low physical activity
- Unemployment
- Neck circumference > 40 cm
- Tonsillar and adenoidal hypertrophy
- Craniofacial abnormalities (e.g., Pierre Robin, Down's syndrome)
- Neuromuscular disease

# MEDICAL CONSEQUENCES

OSA is associated with

### Neurocognitive

- Increased risk of cerebrovascular accidents with poorer outcomes
- Psychosocial problems
- Decreased cognitive function
- Depression

### Endocrine

- Impaired glucose tolerance
- Dyslipidemia
- Increased adrenocorticotropic hormone and cortisol concentrations
- Testicular and ovarian dysfunction

### Cardiovascular

- Hypertension
- Brady- and tachyarrhythmias
- Pulmonary hypertension
- Congestive heart failure
- Myocardial infarction

# TREATMENT

- Weight loss is the preferred treatment for obese patients with OSA
- Continuous positive airway pressure (CPAP) therapy may reduce the risk of cardiac and cerebrovascular events, this effect is most pronounced in non-obese patients
- Surgical uvulo-palato-pharyngoplasty and various supportive airway devices promoting mandibular advancement can be offered to selected patients but have lower efficacy than weight loss and CPAP

# ANESTHESIOLOGIC IMPLICATIONS

- Assess the patient preoperatively for conditions associated with OSA
- Continue CPAP treatment during hospital admission and in the recovery room
- Avoid the administration of sedative medication unless the patient is properly monitored
- OSA is associated with difficult intubation so plan accordingly
- Use locoregional techniques where possible

# Obstructive sleep apnea (OSA): PREOPERATIVE EVALUATION

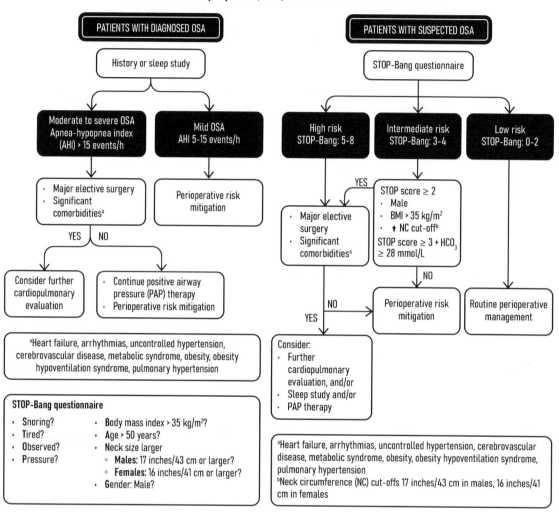

**PATIENTS WITH DIAGNOSED OSA**

History or sleep study

- **Moderate to severe OSA** Apnea-hypopnea index (AHI) > 15 events/h
- **Mild OSA** AHI 5-15 events/h

Moderate to severe OSA:
- Major elective surgery
- Significant comorbidities[a]

Mild OSA:
- Perioperative risk mitigation

YES → Consider further cardiopulmonary evaluation

NO → - Continue positive airway pressure (PAP) therapy
- Perioperative risk mitigation

[a]Heart failure, arrhythmias, uncontrolled hypertension, cerebrovascular disease, metabolic syndrome, obesity, obesity hypoventilation syndrome, pulmonary hypertension

**STOP-Bang questionnaire**
- Snoring?
- Tired?
- Observed?
- Pressure?
- Body mass index > 35 kg/m²?
- Age > 50 years?
- Neck size larger
  - **Males:** 17 inches/43 cm or larger?
  - **Females:** 16 inches/41 cm or larger?
- Gender: Male?

**PATIENTS WITH SUSPECTED OSA**

STOP-Bang questionnaire

- **High risk** STOP-Bang: 5-8
- **Intermediate risk** STOP-Bang: 3-4
- **Low risk** STOP-Bang: 0-2

High risk:
- Major elective surgery
- Significant comorbidities[a]

Intermediate risk → STOP score ≥ 2
- Male
- BMI > 35 kg/m²
- ↑ NC cut-off[b]
STOP score ≥ 3 + HCO₃ ≥ 28 mmol/L

YES →

NO → Perioperative risk mitigation

Low risk → Routine perioperative management

NO / YES → Consider:
- Further cardiopulmonary evaluation, and/or
- Sleep study and/or
- PAP therapy

[a]Heart failure, arrhythmias, uncontrolled hypertension, cerebrovascular disease, metabolic syndrome, obesity, obesity hypoventilation syndrome, pulmonary hypertension
[b]Neck circumference (NC) cut-offs 17 inches/43 cm in males, 16 inches/41 cm in females

# Obstructive sleep apnea (OSA): POSTOPERATIVE MANAGEMENT

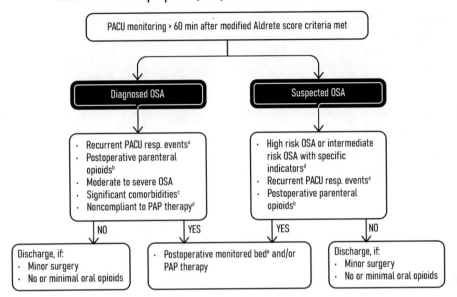

[a]Recurrent PACU respiratory event: Repeated occurrence of oxygen saturation < 90%, or bradypnea < 8 breaths/min, or apnea ≥ 10 sec, or pain-sedation mismatch (high pain and sedation scores concurrently)

[b]Postoperative parenteral opioid requirement more than usual standard of care such as multiple routes, long-acting preparations, or high dose infusions

[c]Uncontrolled systemic disease or additional problems with ventilation or gas exchange such as: hypoventilation syndromes, severe pulmonary hypertension, and resting hypoxemia in the absence of other cardiopulmonary disease

[d]Intermediate risk and specific risk indicators include: STOP score ≥ 2 + male or BMI > 35 kg/m$^2$ or ↑ NC cut-off (NC cut-offs: 17 inches/43 cm in males, 16 inches/41 cm in females) and STOP-Bang ≥ 3 + HCO$_3$ ≥ 28 mmol/L

[e]Monitored bed: Environment with continuous oximetry and the possibility of early medical intervention (e.g., ICU, step-down unit, or remote pulse oximetry with telemetry in surgical ward)

PAP, positive airway pressure; NC, Neck circumference

## SUGGESTED READING

- Martinez G, Faber P. Obstructive sleep apnoea. Continuing Education in Anaesthesia Critical Care & Pain. 2011;11(1):5-8.

# PNEUMONECTOMY

## LEARNING OBJECTIVES

- Describe the indications for and types of pneumonectomy
- Manage patients presenting for pneumonectomy

## DEFINITION AND MECHANISM

- Pneumonectomy involves the surgical removal of an entire lung
- Should only be considered if all other options, including sleeve lobectomy and non-anatomical resections, have been deemed inappropriate

## INDICATIONS

- Bronchial carcinoma
- Traumatic injury to the lung with uncontrolled hemorrhage
- Chronic infective disorders of the lung (e.g., tuberculosis)
- Fungal infections resulting in lung destruction

## TYPES OF PNEUMONECTOMY

- Standard pneumonectomy: Removal of the affected lung only
- Intrapericardial pneumonectomy: Longitudinal opening of the pericardium behind the phrenic nerve, indicated for locally advanced bronchogenic carcinoma
- Extrapleural pneumonectomy: Radical type of resection sometimes used for selected cases of mesothelioma
- It involves excision of the affected lung, ipsilateral pleura, hemidiaphragm, and hemipericardium, followed by patch reconstruction
- Completion pneumonectomy: Excision of the residual lung tissue following a previous lung resection surgery
- Carinal pneumonectomy: Excision of the lung and carina in patients with tumors of the distal trachea or carina

## MANAGEMENT
## PNEUMONECTOMY: PREOPERATIVE ASSESSMENT

Lung cancer staging
- Staging: Eighth edition of the tumour, node, metastasis classification
- CT & PET-CT to assess lymph node status
- If PET-CT-positive mediastinal lymph nodes are detected: Further mediastinal sampling via endobronchial ultrasound or mediastinoscopy

Functional assessment of cardiopulmonary interaction
- Shuttle walk test: Refer patients unable to walk more than 400 m for formal cardiopulmonary exercise testing
- Cardiopulmonary exercise testing: peak oxygen consumption < 10mL/kg/min is usually a contraindication for pneumonectomy

Suitability for surgery
- Operative mortality
  - Focus on exercise capacity and physiological reserve
- Perioperative myocardial events
  - Transthoracic echocardiography
  - Pulmonary hypertension is a relative contraindication
  - Optimize medical treatment for patients with active cardiac condition
  - Assess patients without active cardiac conditions using the Revised Cardiac Risk Index, refer those scoring $\geq 3$ for exercise stress testing and a cardiologist's opinion
- Postoperative dyspnea
  - Estimate the predicted postoperative forced expiratory volume in 1s (ppoFEV1)
  - Calculate diffusing capacity for carbon monoxide
  - Recommended limit of ppo values for both parameters: 30%
  - Make patients scoring < 30% aware of increased risk of postoperative dyspnea and needing long-term oxygen therapy and refer for formal exercise testing

# PNEUMONECTOMY: INTRAOPERATIVE MANAGEMENT

**Surgical approach**
- Preoperative rigid bronchoscopy after induction of anesthesia to confirm sufficient length of tumor-free bronchus to proceed
- Consider sleeve lobectomy as a surgical option for all cancers involving the bronchus
- Consider vascular sleeve resection for tumors localized near the pulmonary artery
- Most common approach: posterolateral thoracotomy at the fifth intercostal space
- Alternatively, access may be achieved via a video-assisted thoracoscopic approach

**Anesthetic technique**
- Confirm availability of a level 2 bed for postoperative care
- Cross-match two units of red blood cells
- Postoperative analgesia: mid-thoracic epidural or paravertebral catheter
- Vasopressors may be required to maintain arterial pressure without excessive volumes of IV fluids
- Volatile or IV anesthetic agents
- IV anesthesia for rigid bronchoscopy

**Monitoring**
- Invasive arterial pressure monitoring
- Central venous catheterization
- Temperature probe
- Urinary catheter

**Positioning**
- Left or right decubitus position with a table break
- Careful protection of eyes, pressure points and neck position
- Venous thromboembolism prophylaxis: Graduated compression stockings
- Maintain normothermia

**Lung isolation**
- Collapse operative lung using double-lumen tube or bronchial blocker
- Fiberoptic bronchoscopy to confirm appropriate positioning
- Initiate one lung ventilation before thoracotomy
- Lung-protective strategies. Pressure or volume control
- Targets:
  - Tidal volume: 5-6 mL/kg ideal body weight
  - Peak airway pressure: < 35 cmH$_2$O
  - Plateau airway pressure: < 35 cmH$_2$O
  - Aim for normal PaCO$_2$
  - PEEP 5 cmH$_2$O
  - Oxygen saturation: 94-98%

**Hemodynamic management**
- Restrict volume of IV fluid
- Avoid hypovolemia and acute kidney injury
- Exclude hemorrhage in the event of hypotension
- Treat hypotension with vasopressors
- In the event of significant cardiovascular collapse or excessive rise in central venous pressure following pulmonary artery clamping, evaluate if continuation of surgery is appropriate

# PNEUMONECTOMY: POSTOPERATIVE MANAGEMENT

**Postoperative care**
- Extubate when patient is awake
- Adequate analgesia (thoracic epidural or paravertebral catheter) to allow effective coughing and clearing of secretions
- Provide organ support if required
- Titrate vasopressors to maintain adequate mean arterial pressure
- Close monitoring to allow for early recognition and treatment of immediate postoperative complications (e.g., hemorrhage, post-pneumonectomy pulmonary edema, retained secretions, airway plugging within the contralateral lung, cardiac arrhythmias)
- Thoracic surgical ward on day 2
- Discharge within 7-10 days
- Remove chest drain on the first postoperative day

**Postoperative complications**
- Cardiac arrhythmias
  - Up to 40% of patients develop atrial fibrillation
  - Other arrhythmias: Atrial flutter, supraventricular tachycardia
  - Management: Correction of underlying acid/base and electrolyte abnormalities and appropriate pharmacological therapy
- Post-pneumonectomy pulmonary edema
  - Occurs in 2-5% of patients
  - Associated mortality > 50%
  - More likely after right pneumonectomy
  - Management: Chest closure without chest drain, attachment of chest drain to underwater seal, repeated unclamping of chest drain, use of a balanced chest drainage system
- Bronchopleural fistula
  - Incidence ranges from 4.5 to 20%
  - Associated mortality 18-67%
  - More likely after right pneumonectomy
  - Other risk factors: Prolonged postoperative ventilation, residual tumor in stump, large diameter stumps
  - Management: Draining pleural space, antibiotics, surgical repair
- Cardiac herniation
  - Rare complication, associated mortality > 50%
  - Immediate surgery to return the heart to its correct position and prevent recurrence

# SUGGESTED READING

- Beshara M, Bora V. Pneumonectomy. [Updated 2022 Sep 18]. In: StatPearls [Internet]. Treasure Island (FL): StatPearls Publishing; 2022 Jan-. Available from: https://www.ncbi.nlm.nih.gov/books/NBK555969/
- Hackett S, Jones R, Kapila R. Anaesthesia for pneumonectomy. BJA Educ. 2019;19(9):297-304.
- Lederman D, Easwar J, Feldman J, Shapiro V. Anesthetic considerations for lung resection: preoperative assessment, intraoperative challenges and postoperative analgesia. Ann Transl Med. 2019;7(15):356.

# 267

# PNEUMONIA

## LEARNING OBJECTIVES

- Signs and symptoms of pneumonia
- Management of pneumonia

## DEFINITION AND MECHANISM

- Pneumonia is an infection that inflames the alveoli in one or both lungs
- The alveoli may fill with fluid or pus causing cough with phlegm or pus, fever, and difficulty breathing
- Caused by bacteria (Streptococcus pneumoniae), bacteria-like organisms (Mycoplasma pneumoniae), viruses, or fungi
- Can also be caused by aspiration of food, fluids, vomit, or saliva
- Can be mild to life-threatening
- The disease may be classified by where it was acquired, such as community- or hospital-acquired or healthcare-associated pneumonia

## SIGNS AND SYMPTOMS

### General symptoms

- Chest pain when breathing or coughing
- Confusion/changes in mental awareness
- Cough, which may produce phlegm
- Fatigue
- Fever and sweating
- Hypothermia
- Loss of appetite
- Nausea, vomiting, or diarrhea
- Shortness of breath

### Symptoms of bacterial pneumonia

- High fever (up to 40.5 C)
- Cough with yellow, green, or bloody mucus
- Tiredness (fatigue)
- Rapid breathing
- Shortness of breath
- Rapid heart rate
- Sweating or chills
- Chest pain and/or abdominal pain, especially with coughing or deep breathing
- Loss of appetite
- Bluish skin, lips, or nails (cyanosis)
- Confusion or altered mental state

### Symptoms of viral pneumonia

- Symptoms similar to bacterial pneumonia
- Dry cough
- Headache
- Muscle pain
- Extreme tiredness or weakness

### Symptoms of pneumonia in babies and children

Babies and newborns may not show any symptoms of pneumonia or their symptoms may be different from adults, including:
- Fever, chills, general discomfort, sweating/flushed skin
- Cough
- Difficulty breathing or rapid breathing (tachypnea)
- Loss of appetite
- Vomiting
- Lack of energy
- Restlessness or fussiness

Signs in babies and young children include:
- Grunting sound with breathing or noisy breathing
- A decreased amount of pee or diapers that are less wet
- Pale skin
- Limpness
- Crying more than usual
- Difficulty feeding

# CLASSIFICATION

- Pneumonia is most commonly classified by where or how it was acquired:
  - Community-acquired pneumonia
  - Aspiration pneumonia
  - Community-acquired pneumonia
  - Hospital-acquired pneumonia
  - Ventilator-associated pneumonia
- It may also be classified by the area of the lung affected:
  - Lobar pneumonia
  - Bronchial pneumonia
  - Acute interstitial pneumonia

# RISK FACTORS

- Children < 2 years of age
- Adults > 65 years of age
- Hospitalization – ICU – long-term care facility
- Chronic disease: asthma, COPD, or heart disease
- Smoking
- Pregnancy
- Weakened or suppressed immune system: HIV/AIDS
- Neurological conditions making swallowing difficult: dementia, Parkinson's disease, or stroke

# DIAGNOSIS

- Medical history
- Physical exam
- Blood tests
- Chest X-ray
- Pulse oximetry
- Sputum test
- CT scan
- Arterial blood gas test
- Pleural fluid culture
- Bronchoscopy

# COMPLICATIONS

- Bacteremia or sepsis
- Difficulty breathing, requiring a ventilator
- Pleural effusion
- Lung abscess

# PREVENTION

- Vaccination: pneumococcal vaccine, flu, COVID-19
- Practice good hygiene
- Do not smoke

# MANAGEMENT

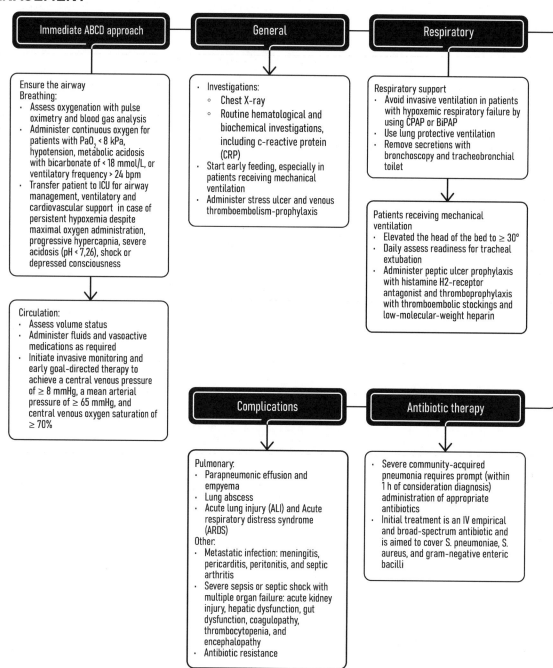

**Immediate ABCD approach**

Ensure the airway
Breathing:
· Assess oxygenation with pulse oximetry and blood gas analysis
· Administer continuous oxygen for patients with $PaO_2$ < 8 kPa, hypotension, metabolic acidosis with bicarbonate of < 18 mmol/L, or ventilatory frequency > 24 bpm
· Transfer patient to ICU for airway management, ventilatory and cardiovascular support in case of persistent hypoxemia despite maximal oxygen administration, progressive hypercapnia, severe acidosis (pH < 7,26), shock or depressed consciousness

Circulation:
· Assess volume status
· Administer fluids and vasoactive medications as required
· Initiate invasive monitoring and early goal-directed therapy to achieve a central venous pressure of ≥ 8 mmHg, a mean arterial pressure of ≥ 65 mmHg, and central venous oxygen saturation of ≥ 70%

**General**

· Investigations:
  ○ Chest X-ray
  ○ Routine hematological and biochemical investigations, including c-reactive protein (CRP)
· Start early feeding, especially in patients receiving mechanical ventilation
· Administer stress ulcer and venous thromboembolism-prophylaxis

**Respiratory**

Respiratory support
· Avoid invasive ventilation in patients with hypoxemic respiratory failure by using CPAP or BiPAP
· Use lung protective ventilation
· Remove secretions with bronchoscopy and tracheobronchial toilet

Patients receiving mechanical ventilation
· Elevated the head of the bed to ≥ 30°
· Daily assess readiness for tracheal extubation
· Administer peptic ulcer prophylaxis with histamine H2-receptor antagonist and thromboprophylaxis with thromboembolic stockings and low-molecular-weight heparin

**Complications**

Pulmonary:
· Parapneumonic effusion and empyema
· Lung abscess
· Acute lung injury (ALI) and Acute respiratory distress syndrome (ARDS)
Other:
· Metastatic infection: meningitis, pericarditis, peritonitis, and septic arthritis
· Severe sepsis or septic shock with multiple organ failure: acute kidney injury, hepatic dysfunction, gut dysfunction, coagulopathy, thrombocytopenia, and encephalopathy
· Antibiotic resistance

**Antibiotic therapy**

· Severe community-acquired pneumonia requires prompt (within 1 h of consideration diagnosis) administration of appropriate antibiotics
· Initial treatment is an IV empirical and broad-spectrum antibiotic and is aimed to cover S. pneumoniae, S. aureus, and gram-negative enteric bacilli

Be aware that:
- Anesthesia can contribute to postoperative pneumonia by causing gastric contents like stomach acid to enter the lungs, resulting in pulmonary complications and increased risk of infection
- Pulmonary infections and pneumonia are the most common cause of pulmonary ARDS

# SUGGESTED READING

- Morgan, A., Glossop, A., 2016. Severe community-acquired pneumonia. BJA Education 16, 167–172.
- Sadashivaiah, JB., Carr, B., 2009. Severe community-acquired pneumonia. Continuing Eduction in Anaesthesia Critical Care & Pain. 9;3:87-91.

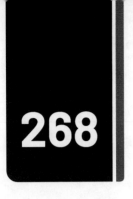

# POST-LUNG TRANSPLANT PATIENT

## LEARNING OBJECTIVES

- Pre- and perioperative management of a post-lung transplant patient

**268**

---

## DEFINITION AND MECHANISM

- A post-lung transplant patient may have one or both lungs replaced by a donor's lung, sometimes along with a donor's heart
- A lung transplant is a surgical procedure to replace a diseased or failing lung with a healthy lung from a deceased donor

- It usually takes at least 3-6 months to fully recover from transplant surgery
- Consider an increased risk of infection or rejection of the transplanted lungs

## INDICATIONS FOR A LUNG TRANSPLANTATION

- Chronic obstructive pulmonary disease (COPD), including emphysema
- Pulmonary fibrosis
- Cystic fibrosis
- Pulmonary hypertension
- Alpha-1-antitrypsin deficiency

## SYMPTOMS OF REJECTION

- Shortness of breath
- Fever
- Coughing
- Chest congestion

## MANAGEMENT

### Preoperative assessment

- Investigate:
  - The function of the transplanted lung
  - The possibility of rejection or infection of the transplanted lung
  - The effect of immunosuppressive therapy on other organs and the effect of organ dysfunction on the transplanted lung
  - Disease in the native lung
  - Indications for the surgical procedure and its effect on the lung
- Evaluate:
  - Need for supplemental oxygen
  - Pulmonary function tests
  - Arterial blood gas
  - Chest X-ray
  - CT
  - ECG
  - Echocardiogram
  - Complete blood count

  - Creatinine
  - Blood Urea Nitrogen (BUN)
  - Glucose
  - Electrolytes
  - Renal function tests
  - Liver function tests
  - Coagulation tests
  - Urinalysis
  - Exclude infections
- Take into account possible side effects of immunosuppressive therapy:
  - Hypertension
  - Renal failure
  - Hepatic dysfunction
  - Pancreatitis
  - Glucose intolerance or diabetes
  - Electrolyte abnormalities
  - Bone marrow depression

## PERIOPERATIVE MANAGEMENT

### General

- If possible, continue immunosuppressants until the day of surgery
- Be cautious with anxiolytics as they may lead to hypercarbia
- Administer:
  - Immunosuppressants IV if oral agents are precluded
  - Prophylactic antibiotics to avoid infection
- Perform standard monitoring

- Avoid:
  - Femoral lines → increased risk of infection
  - Nasal intubation → increased risk of infection
  - Invasive monitoring if not required → risk of infection or pneumothorax
- Place a central line in the antecubital fossa or internal jugular vein → a lower risk of pneumothorax than in the subclavian approach

## Anesthesia

- Local, regional, or general anesthesia are all considered safe to use, however, do not perform a block above T10
- Propofol is the anesthetic of choice
- Etomidate is preferred when there is a risk of hemodynamic instability
- Volatile anesthetics are also well tolerated
- Use short-acting relaxants (mivacurium) or intermediate-acting agents independent of kidney and liver function (cisatracurium, atracurium)
- Consider that vecuronium, rocuronium, and pancuronium can have prolonged effects with hepatic or renal insufficiency
- Note that immunosuppressive agents may interact with neuromuscular blocking agents
- Avoid:
  - Succinylcholine because of the possibility of hyperkalemia
  - Long-acting agents such as pancuronium or doxacurium

## Airway management

- Aim for early extubation to minimize the risk of infection
- The Trendelenberg position may further compromise pulmonary function and increase the work of breathing
- Place the endotracheal cuff just beyond the vocal cords to avoid trauma to the trachea or bronchial anastomosis
- Consider using a fiberoptic laryngoscope
- Positive pressure ventilation is complicated in single lung transplant recipients
- Consider differences in lung compliance between the native and transplanted lungs and consequently, two ventilator machines may be required with different ventilator settings
- Avoid:
  - Benzodiazepines
  - Nitrous oxide
  - Positive end-expiratory pressures
- Consider cardiac denervation in patients who have undergone double lung transplantation with tracheal anastomosis
  - These patients are sensitive to hypovolemia
  - Intraoperative bradycardia does not respond to atropine and direct agents such as epinephrine should be used

## Fluid balance

- Monitor central venous pressure, pulmonary artery pressure, and urine output
- Maintain a careful fluid balance
- Consider that altered lymphatic drainage in the transplanted lung may cause interstitial fluid accumulation
  - Treat these patients with diuretics and limited crystalloid infusion

# POSTOPERATIVE CARE

- Transfer the patient to the ICU
- Monitor oxygen saturation
- Administer adequate analgesia:
  - Parenteral paracetamol is an effective analgesic agent
  - Be cautious with the use of opioids as they can mediate CNS and respiratory depression
  - Transdermal buprenorphine and methadone appear to be safe to use even in patients with renal dysfunction
  - Avoid NSAIDs because of the risk of adverse reactions
- Seek and treat infection or rejection
- Continue immunosuppressive therapy

## SUGGESTED READING

- Brusich, K.T., Acan, I., 2018. Anesthetic Considerations in Transplant Recipients for Nontransplant Surgery. doi:10.5772/intechopen.74329
- Haddow, G.R., 1997. Anaesthesia for patients after lung transplantation. Canadian Journal of Anesthesia/Journal canadien d'anesthésie 44, 182–197.
- Seo M, Kim WJ, Choi IC. Anesthesia for non-pulmonary surgical intervention following lung transplantation: two cases report. Korean J Anesthesiol. 2014;66(4):322-326.

# PULMONARY EMBOLISM

## LEARNING OBJECTIVES

- Defining, diagnosing, and treating pulmonary embolism

---

## DEFINITION AND MECHANISM

- A pulmonary embolism (PE) is a blood clot that blocks blood flow to an artery in the lung
- Most often the blood clot originates in a deep leg vein and moves through the venous circulation to the heart
- Severe PE is an immediately life-threatening situation
- Low cardiac output and a ventilation/perfusion mismatch contribute to hypoxemia
- Right ventricular failure due to acute pressure overload is considered the primary cause of death in severe PE

## RISK FACTORS

- Predisposing factors for venous thromboembolism (VTE) are:

| Strong (OR > 10) | Moderate (OR 2–9) | Weak risk factors (OR < 2) |
|---|---|---|
| Fracture of the lower limb<br>Hospitalization for heart failure or atrial fibrillation/flutter ≤ 3 months<br>Hip or knee replacement<br>Major trauma<br>Myocardial infarction ≤ 3 months<br>Previous VTE<br>Spinal cord injury | Arthroscopic knee surgery<br>Autoimmune diseases<br>Blood transfusion<br>CVCs<br>IVs<br>Chemotherapy<br>Congestive heart failure<br>Respiratory failure<br>Erythropoiesis-stimulating agents<br>IVF<br>Oral contraceptive therapy<br>Postpartum period<br>Infection<br>IBD<br>Cancer<br>Paralytic stroke<br>Superficial vein thrombosis<br>Thrombophilia | Bed rest > 3 days<br>Diabetes mellitus<br>Arterial hypertension<br>Immobility due to sitting (e.g., prolonged car or air travel)<br>Increasing age<br>Laparoscopic surgery<br>Obesity<br>Pregnancy<br>Varicose veins |

OR, odds ratio; IBD, inflammatory bowel disease

## SYMPTOMS

| Symptoms | |
|---|---|
| Respiratory | Dyspnea<br>Hemoptysis<br>Hypoxemia<br>Hypocapnia<br>Chest pain |
| Cerebral | Syncope |
| Cardiac | Hemodynamic instability<br>ECG might show sinus tachycardia, S1Q3T3 pattern, incomplete or complete right bundle branch block (usually in more severe cases), or atrial arrhythmias |

Pulmonary embolism

# DIAGNOSIS

- Diagnostic scores like the pulmonary embolism rule-out Criteria (PERC) can help to determine whether further investigations for PE are warranted
- D-dimers have a high negative predictive value, meaning that a normal D-dimer level renders acute PE or deep vein thrombosis (DVT) unlikely
- The positive predictive value of elevated D-dimer levels is low, meaning it isn't useful as a test to confirm PE
- Use age-adjusted D-dimers (age x 10 µg/L) for patients aged > 50 years
- Computed tomographic pulmonary angiography (CTPA) is the gold standard for diagnosing PE

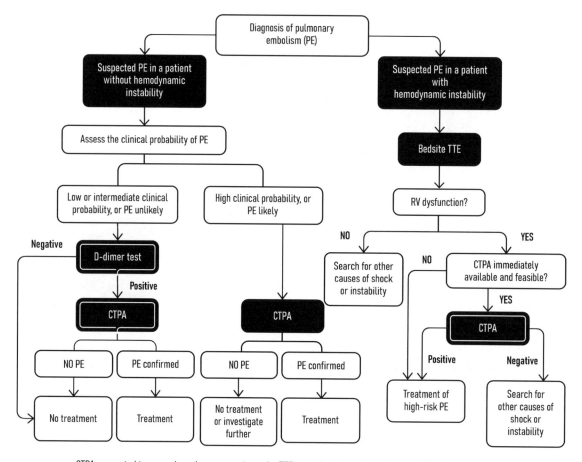

CTPA, computed tomography pulmonary angiography; TTE, transthoracic echocardiogram; RV, right ventricular

# MANAGEMENT

- The pulmonary embolism severity Index (PESI) reliably identifies patients with a low risk for 30-day mortality
- Administer supplemental oxygen to patients with PE and $SaO_2$ < 90%
- Initiate mechanical ventilation if necessary and start with non-invasive techniques if possible
- Treat right heart failure in hemodynamically unstable patients with PE
  - Fluids
  - Vasopressors
  - Mechanical circulatory support
- Anticoagulate patients with a high or intermediate clinical probability of PE while awaiting diagnostic test
- Low-molecular-weight heparin (LMWH) and fondaparinux are preferred over unfractionated heparin (UFH) for initial anticoagulation in PE
- Administer UFH in patients with overt hemodynamic instability and patients with renal impairment (≤ G4)
- When using vitamin K antagonists:
  - Continue anticoagulation with UFH, LMWH, or fondaparinux in parallel with the oral anticoagulant for ≥ 5 days
  - Until the international normalised ratio (INR) has been 2.0–3.0 for 2 consecutive days
- Start thrombolysis in patients with high-risk PE
- Perform a thrombectomy if thrombolysis is contraindicated or has failed, especially in high-risk patients with massive PE

Pulmonary embolism

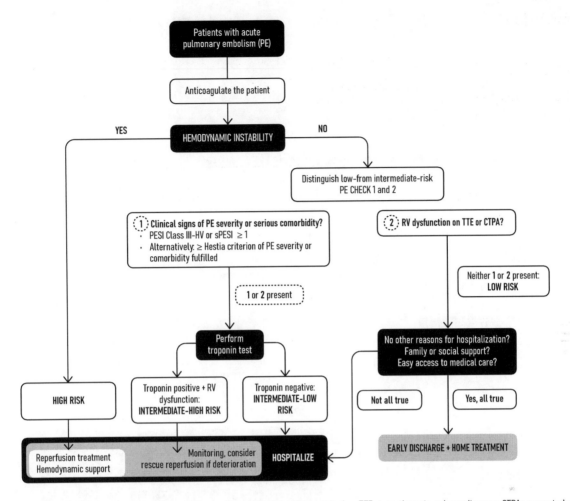

PESI, pulmonary embolism severity index; sPESI, simplified PESI; RV, right ventricular; TTE, transthoracic echocardiogram; CTPA; computed tomography pulmonary angiography

## SUGGESTED READING

- Konstantinides SV, Meyer G, Becattini C, et al. 2019 ESC Guidelines for the diagnosis and management of acute pulmonary embolism developed in collaboration with the European Respiratory Society (ERS). Eur Heart J. 2020;41(4):543-603.

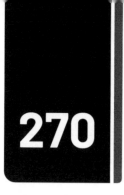

# RESTRICTIVE LUNG DISEASE

## 270

### LEARNING OBJECTIVES

- Description of restrictive lung disease
- Management of restrictive lung disease

- Diseases that restrict lung expansion, resulting in a decreased lung volume and total lung capacity, an increased work of breathing, and inadequate ventilation and/or oxygenation
- Often due to a decrease in the elasticity of the lungs themselves or caused by a problem related to the expansion of the chest wall during inhalation
- The normal lung tissue can be gradually replaced with scar tissue that is interspersed with pockets of air
- Characterized by a decrease in the forced vital capacity (FVC) and forced

## DEFINITION AND MECHANISM

expiratory volume in one second (FEV1), however, the decline in FVC is more than that of FEV1, resulting in a higher than 80% FEV1/FVC ratio
- May be caused by the destruction of distal lung parenchyma due to infiltrates from inflammation, toxins (intrinsic conditions) as well as extra parenchymal conditions (extrinsic causes)
- Examples of restrictive lung diseases are asbestosis, sarcoidosis, and pulmonary fibrosis

## SIGNS AND SYMPTOMS

- Progressive exertional dyspnea
- Cough
- Shortness of breath

- Wheezing
- Chest pain
- Respiratory failure

## CAUSES

| Intrinsic causes | Extrinsic causes |
|---|---|
| Pneumoconiosis: for example asbestosis | Nonmuscular diseases: kyphosis, pectus carinatum, pectus excavatum |
| Radiation fibrosis | Diseases restricting lower thoracic/abdominal volume, e.g., obesity, |
| Medication: amiodarone, bleomycin and methotrexate | diaphragmatic hernia, or the presence of ascites |
| As a consequence of rheumatoid arthritis | Pleural thickening |
| Hypersensitivity pneumonitis | |
| Acute Respiratory Distress Syndrome | |
| Infant respiratory distress syndrome | |
| Tuberculosis | |
| Idiopathic pulmonary fibrosis | |
| Idiopathic interstitial pneumonia | |
| Sarcoidosis | |
| Eosinophilic pneumonia | |
| Lymphangioleiomyomatosis | |
| Pulmonary Langerhans' cell histiocytosis | |
| Pulmonary alveolar proteinosis | |

## COMPLICATIONS

- Hypoxemia
- Muscle wasting and weight loss
- Chronic respiratory failure
- Obstructive sleep apnea
- Pulmonary hypertension
- Cor-pulmunale

## DIAGNOSIS

- Pulmonary function tests
- Chest X-ray
- CT
- Bronchoscopy
- Pulse oximetry
- Arterial blood gas

# TREATMENT

- Maximize pulmonary function with oxygen therapy, bronchodilators, inhaled beta-adrenergic agonists and diuretics
- Management varies depending on the etiology of the restriction:
  - Manage comorbid conditions
  - Idiopathic pulmonary fibrosis: immunosuppression or anti-fibrotic agents such as pirfenidone and nintedanib
  - Autoimmune conditions that lead to interstitial lung disease: immunosuppressants agents including steroids, mycophenolate mofetil, and cyclophosphamide
  - Obesity: diet and physical exercise to lose weight
- Acute exacerbations are treated with steroids

# MANAGEMENT

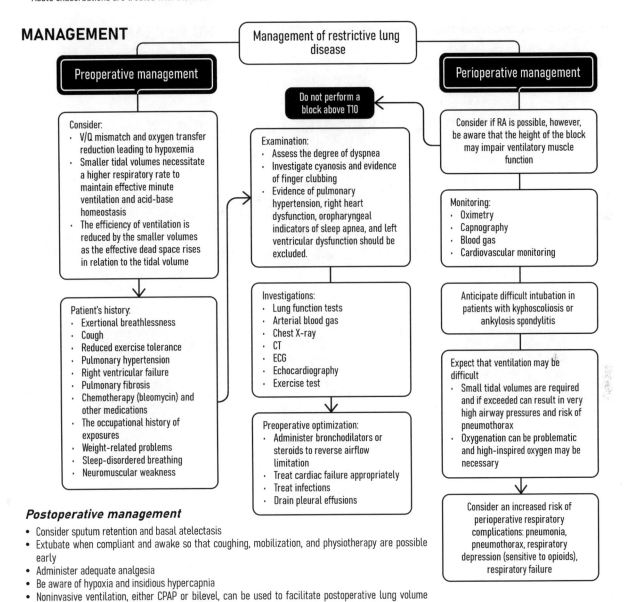

**Management of restrictive lung disease**

**Preoperative management**

Consider:
- V/Q mismatch and oxygen transfer reduction leading to hypoxemia
- Smaller tidal volumes necessitate a higher respiratory rate to maintain effective minute ventilation and acid-base homeostasis
- The efficiency of ventilation is reduced by the smaller volumes as the effective dead space rises in relation to the tidal volume

Patient's history:
- Exertional breathlessness
- Cough
- Reduced exercise tolerance
- Pulmonary hypertension
- Right ventricular failure
- Pulmonary fibrosis
- Chemotherapy (bleomycin) and other medications
- The occupational history of exposures
- Weight-related problems
- Sleep-disordered breathing
- Neuromuscular weakness

Examination:
- Assess the degree of dyspnea
- Investigate cyanosis and evidence of finger clubbing
- Evidence of pulmonary hypertension, right heart dysfunction, oropharyngeal indicators of sleep apnea, and left ventricular dysfunction should be excluded.

Investigations:
- Lung function tests
- Arterial blood gas
- Chest X-ray
- CT
- ECG
- Echocardiography
- Exercise test

Preoperative optimization:
- Administer bronchodilators or steroids to reverse airflow limitation
- Treat cardiac failure appropriately
- Treat infections
- Drain pleural effusions

**Do not perform a block above T10**

**Perioperative management**

Consider if RA is possible, however, be aware that the height of the block may impair ventilatory muscle function

Monitoring:
- Oximetry
- Capnography
- Blood gas
- Cardiovascular monitoring

Anticipate difficult intubation in patients with kyphoscoliosis or ankylosis spondylitis

Expect that ventilation may be difficult
- Small tidal volumes are required and if exceeded can result in very high airway pressures and risk of pneumothorax
- Oxygenation can be problematic and high-inspired oxygen may be necessary

Consider an increased risk of perioperative respiratory complications: pneumonia, pneumothorax, respiratory depression (sensitive to opioids), respiratory failure

## Postoperative management

- Consider sputum retention and basal atelectasis
- Extubate when compliant and awake so that coughing, mobilization, and physiotherapy are possible early
- Administer adequate analgesia
- Be aware of hypoxia and insidious hypercapnia
- Noninvasive ventilation, either CPAP or bilevel, can be used to facilitate postoperative lung volume recruitment and relieve the work of breathing as necessary

## SUGGESTED READING

- Mangera Z, Panesar G, Makker H. Practical approach to management of respiratory complications in neurological disorders. Int J Gen Med. 2012;5:255-263.
- Pollard BJ, Kitchen, G. Handbook of Clinical Anaesthesia. Fourth Edition. CRC Press. 2018. 978-1-4987-6289-2.
- Vyas, Varsha & Gehdoo, Raghbirsingh & Hazari, Shruti & Hirpara, Parthkumar & Kaur, Mankeerat & Vashwani, Jayshree. (2021). Anesthesia Management in a Case of Restrictive Lung Disease. Journal of Research & Innovation in Anesthesia. 6. 49-50. 10.5005/jp-journals-10049-0104.

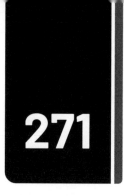

# SMOKING

## LEARNING OBJECTIVES

- Describe the perioperative complications associated with smoking
- Manage smoking patients scheduled for anesthesia

---

## DEFINITION AND MECHANISM

- Cigarette smoking is one of the primary causes of preventable illness and premature death
- Quitting smoking before surgery leads to a reduced incidence of postoperative complications
- The longer the period of cessation before surgery, the greater the benefit

## PERIOPERATIVE COMPLICATIONS ASSOCIATED WITH SMOKING

- There is a clear dose-response relationship between the amount smoked and perioperative morbidity
- Possible complications:

## MANAGEMENT

- Education regarding the benefits of preoperative smoking cessation when possible
- Ideally, smoking is stopped 8 weeks before surgery
- Stop smoking 24h before surgery to negate the effects of nicotine and carboxyhemoglobin (COHb)
- Effects of smoking cessation:
  - Symptoms of cough and wheeze decrease within weeks
  - Mucociliary clearance starts to improve after a week while lung infllmation takes much longer to subside
  - Goblet cell hyperplasia regresses and alveolar macrophages decrease
  - Decrease in all-cause mortality in patients with coronary artery disease by approximately 33%
  - Risk of coronary heart disease and cerebrovascular disease approaches the risk of never-smokers within 10-15 years

- Guidance
  - Patients who smoke are more likely to quit if they are offered a combination of interventions
  - Ask and record smoking history (pack-years)
  - Advise that the most effective way to quit is with a combination of medication and specialist support
- Pharmacological aid
  - Nicotine replacement therapy (patches, lozenges, chewing gum, or nasal sprays.)
  - Oral bupropion
  - Oral varenicline

| Perioperative complications associated with smoking | |
|---|---|
| Intraoperative | Reintubation after planned extubation<br>Laryngospasm<br>Bronchospasm<br>Aspiration<br>Hypoventilation and hypoxemia<br>Pulmonary edema |
| Postoperative | Increased mortality<br>Pneumonia<br>Unplanned intubation<br>Mechanical ventilation<br>Cardiac arrest<br>Myocardial infarction<br>Stroke<br>Superficial wound infection<br>Deep wound infection<br>Organ space infection<br>Septic shock |

---

## SUGGESTED READING

- Carrick MA, Robson JM, Thomas C. Smoking and anaesthesia. BJA Educ. 2019;19(1):1-6.

Smoking

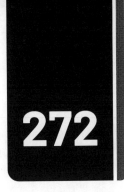

# THYMECTOMY

## LEARNING OBJECTIVES

- Describe the indications and techniques for thymectomy
- Manage patients presenting for thymectomy

## DEFINITION AND MECHANISM

- Thymectomy is the resection of the thymus gland
- The thymus can enlarge (myasthenia gravis and thymoma) and harbor malignant cells (thymic carcinoma or neuroendocrine tumors)

## INDICATIONS

- Most common: Myasthenia gravis (70%) and thymoma (10%)
- Less common: Malignant tumors (thymic carcinoma, neuroendocrine tumors), benign tumors (thymic cysts), ectopic parathyroid glands

## TECHNIQUES

- Median Sternotomy
- Video-Assisted Thoracoscopic Surgery
- Robotic surgery
- Video- and robot-assisted approaches are superior to traditional open approaches

## MANAGEMENT

### Preoperative assessment

- Optimize and stabilize condition in collaboration with neurologist
- Assess for bulbar symptoms (dysphagia, dysarthria and dysphonia, dyspnea, history of myasthenic crises)
- Consult a neurologist to optimize perioperative therapy
- Consider associated autoimmune diseases and their effects
- Full blood count, electrolytes, renal and hepatic function tests for patients taking non-steroidal immunosuppressive agents
- Thyroid function tests
- ECG
- Assess respiratory function especially in patients with muscoloskeletal weakness

### Review current and planned drug therapy

- Continue anticholinesterases and glucocorticoids
- Continue regular anticholinergics (e.g., propantheline), but note if further doses of anticholinergic drugs are planned
- Perioperative interruptions of non-steroidal immunosuppressive agents have no significant effect
- Regular glucocorticoid therapy may induce or exacerbate diabetes mellitus, cause hypothalamic-pituitary-adrenal axis suppression and adrenal insufficiency, which requires perioperative coverage with steroids

### Intraoperative management

- Sedation with short-acting agents, including premedication, can be given in carefully titrated doses with close observation
- Local and/or regional anesthesia may be used:
  - Use amide local anesthetics
  - Take caution when considering neuraxial and brachial plexus blocks in patients with significant respiratory or bulbar weakness
- Avoid hypokalemia

### General anesthesia

- Short-acting agents promote early recovery and minimize respiratory depression
- Avoid neuromuscular blocking agents
- When neuromuscular blocking is necessary, use rocuronium and sugammmadex
- Total IV anesthesia with propofol and remifentanil is adequate
- Inhalational induction can also be used
- Volatile anesthesia can reduce the use of neuromuscular blocking agents
- Mechanical positive-pressure ventilation
- Invasive arterial pressure monitoring
- Maintain normothermia
- Multimodal analgesia
- Be aware that an enlarged thymus can compress the trachea

### Postoperative management

- Closely monitor for signs of bulbar or respiratory muscle weakness and be aware of the augmented risk of aspiration

### Myasthenic crisis

- Severe respiratory or bulbar muscle weakness
- A vital capacity < 20-25 mL/kg is a common definition
- Requires intubation or delays extubation
- Urgent neurological input
- Treatment with high-dose steroids and IV immunoglobin or plasma exchange may be necessary

### Cholinergic crisis

- Resembles organophosphate poisoning with variable symptoms of excess cholinergic activity (paradoxical weakness, bradycardia, hypotension, bronchospasm, increased secretions, sweating, vomiting, diarrhea)
- Treatment with atropine up to 2 mg or glycopyrrolate in titrated IV doses
- Avoid further anticholinesterases
- Delayed extubation and critical care admission

## SUGGESTED READING

- Bennett B, Rentea RM. Thymectomy. [Updated 2022 Jul 25]. In: StatPearls [Internet]. Treasure Island (FL): StatPearls Publishing; 2022 Jan-. Available from: https://www.ncbi.nlm.nih.gov/books/NBK564302/
- Daum P, Smelt J, Ibrahim IR. Perioperative management of myasthenia gravis. BJA Education. 2021;21(11):414-9.

# TRANSFUSION-RELATED ACUTE LUNG INJURY (TRALI)

**273**

## LEARNING OBJECTIVES

- Describe the risk factors and pathophysiology of TRALI
- Diagnose and manage TRALI
- Prevent TRALI

## DEFINITION AND MECHANISM

- Transfusion-related acute lung injury (TRALI) is a transfusion reaction characterized by an acute, noncardiogenic pulmonary edema associated with hypoxia
- The leading cause of death from transfusion
- Caused by damage to pulmonary vasculature due to the immune response to antibodies or proinflammatory factors from the transfusion product that bind to antigens of the recipient
- Symptoms include acute dyspnea, fever, hypotension, and tachycardia

## RISK FACTORS

- Mechanical ventilation
- Sepsis
- Massive transfusion
- Coronary artery bypass graft
- End-stage liver disease
- Positive fluid balance
- Critically ill patient
- Blood products with high plasma contents

## PATHOPHYSIOLOGY

- Two-hit hypothesis:
  - First hit: Priming of neutrophils due to shock, sepsis, organ damage, previous surgery, stress, trauma
  - Second hit: Antibodies or proinflammatory factors in the transfusion product activate neutrophils, resulting in capillary leakage and subsequent pulmonary edema
- Threshold hypothesis:
  - No first hit, a threshold must be overcome to induce TRALI
  - Threshold depends on the susceptibility of the patient and the quantity of antibodies/proinflammatory factors in the transfusion product

## DIAGNOSIS

- Diagnostic criteria:
  - Symptoms develop during or within 6 hours of transfusion without any risk factors for developing acute lung injuries (sepsis from pneumonia, aspiration, shock)
- Clinical findings:
  - Exudative bilateral infiltrates on chest radiograph
  - No evidence of pulmonary vascular overload
  - Hypoxemia: $SpO_2$ < 90% on room air, ratio of partial oxygen pressure to fractional inspired oxygen concentration < 300 mmHg
  - Possible TRALI: Other risk factors for acute lung injury
  - Delayed TRALI: 6 – 72 hours after transfusion

## DIFFERENTIAL DIAGNOSIS

- Septic transfusion reaction: Signs of sepsis
- Anaphylactic transfusion reaction: Laryngeal and bronchial edema
- Transfusion-related circulatory overload: Increased pulmonary artery occlusion pressure (> 18 mmHg)

# TREATMENT

- There is no treatment, management is supportive
- Stop transfusion
- Additional oxygen
- Restrictive tidal volume ventilation
- Diuretics may be considered

## TRANSFUSION-RELATED ACUTE LUNG INJURY (TRALI) PREVENTION

**RESTRICTIVE TRANSFUSION POLICY**
- Restrictive transfusion policy for red blood cells and plasma
- Electronic decision support
- For non-emergency transfusions, delay the transfusion until the acute inflammation has subsided

**PATIENT-TAILORED TRANSFUSION POLICY**
- TRALI development is more dependent on patient-related factor than tansfusion product factors
- Patient-tailored approach aimed to reduce risk factors
- Monitor fluid balance
- Avoid shock before transfusion
- Avoid prior fluid overload
- Restrict airway pressures before transfusion in ventilated patients
- Ventilate with low tidal volumes

**SPECIFIC TRANSFUSION PRODUCTS FOR HIGH-RISK PATIENTS**
- Fresh blood products
- Washing of cell-containing transfusion products may be beneficial

**REPORTING OF TRALI**
- Report suspected TRALI reactions to the blood bank for identification and exclusion of involved donors to prevent future reactions

**BLOOD SERVICE PREVENTATIVE MEASURES**
- Exclusion of high-risk donors: Multiparous donors, donors exposed to blood transfusion
- Human leukocyte antigens (HLA) and HLA antibody screening
- Pooling of plasma
- Use of solvent-detergent plasma

# SUGGESTED READING

- Cho MS, Modi P, Sharma S. Transfusion-related Acute Lung Injury. [Updated 2022 Jul 25]. In: StatPearls [Internet]. Treasure Island (FL): StatPearls Publishing; 2022 Jan-. Available from: https://www.ncbi.nlm.nih.gov/books/NBK507846/
- Vlaar AP, Juffermans NP. Transfusion-related acute lung injury: a clinical review. Lancet. 2013;382(9896):984-994.

# SKIN & MUSCULOSKELETAL DISORDERS

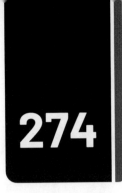

# 274

# ACHONDROPLASIA

## LEARNING OBJECTIVES

- Describe achondroplasia
- Understand the anatomical features associated with achondroplasia
- Anesthetic management of a patient with achondroplasia

## DEFINITION AND MECHANISM

- Achondroplasia is a bone growth disorder resulting in disproportionate dwarfism
- Genetic disorder of skeletal dysplasia → spontaneous fibroblast growth factor receptor 3 gene (FGFR3) mutation
- Inhibition of cartilage formation, resulting in premature ossification in the epiphyseal growth plates with concurrent restriction of growth → patients fail to achieve a height of 148 cm by adulthood

## SIGNS AND SYMPTOMS

### Facial deformities

- Macrocephaly with prominent forehead frontal bossing
- Macroglossia
- Short maxilla
- Large mandible
- Midfacial hypoplasia with flattened nasal bridge
- Small mouth

### Extremity deformities

- Long-bone shortening of proximal upper and lower extremities
- Short fingers and toes with "trident hands" (short hands with stubby fingers and a separation between the middle and ring fingers)

### Airway deformities

- Narrowed nasal passages from mucopolysaccharide deposition
- Tracheal narrowing
- Sternal prominence
- Rib hypoplasia
- Pharyngeal and maxillary hypoplasia
- Thickening of pharyngeal and laryngeal structures and this may hinder direct laryngoscopy and can cause obstruction of the upper aiway
- Tonsillar hyperplasia

### Spinal deformities

- Possibility of foramen magnum stenosis (avoid hyperextension of the neck)
- Short neck
- Cervical spine instability (odontoid hypoplasia)
- Possible atlantoaxial instability
- Spinal kyphosis or lordosis
- Thoracolumbar kyphosis
- Pelvic narrowing
- Spinal stenosis → can result in cauda equina syndrome, nerve root compression, thoracolumbar spinal cord compression, or high cervical cord compression secondary to stenosis of the foramen magnum (rarely)

### Other

- Varus or valgus deformities
- Hypotonia
- Hypersalivation

Achondroplasia

## COMPLICATIONS

- Obstructive sleep apnea
- Obesity
- Spinal stenosis
- Ear infections
- Hyperlordosis
- Back pain
- Hydrocephalus
- Severe scoliosis and rib cage deformities may result in restrictive lung diseases, pulmonary hypertension, cor pulmonale, and cardiovascular disease

## MANAGEMENT

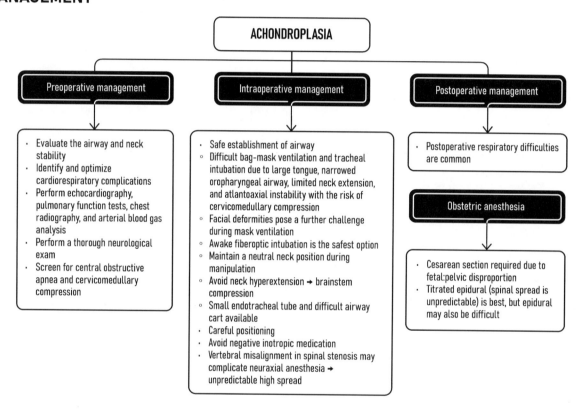

## KEEP IN MIND

- Anesthetic challenges in patients with achondroplasia include potentially difficult airways, often complicated by sleep apnea due to obesity, altered respiratory mechanics, and difficult neuraxial access with the unpredictable spread of local anesthetics

**SUGGESTED READING**

- Kim JH, Woodruff BC, Girshin M. Anesthetic Considerations in Patients With Achondroplasia. Cureus. 2021;13(6):e15832. Published 2021 Jun 22.
- Spiegel JE, Hellman M. Achondroplasia: Implications and Management Strategies in Anesthesia. December 23, 2015. Accessed January 24, 2023. https://anesthesiaexperts.com/uncategorized/achondroplasia-implications-management-strategies-anesthesia/.

Achondroplasia

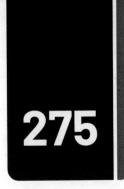

# ANKYLOSING SPONDYLITIS

## LEARNING OBJECTIVES

- Describe ankylosing spondylitis
- Recognize the symptoms and signs of ankylosing spondylitis
- Anesthetic management of a patient with ankylosing spondylitis

## DEFINITION AND MECHANISM

- Ankylosing spondylitis (AS), autoimmune seronegative spondyloarthropathy, is a painful chronic inflammatory arthritis characterized by exacerbations (flares) and quiescent periods
- AS primarily affects the spine and sacroiliac joints, eventually causing fusion and rigidity of the spine → bamboo spine
- Joint mobility in the affected areas worsens over time
- The areas most commonly affected are
  - Sacroiliac joints
  - Vertebrae in the lower back
  - Places where tendons and ligaments attach to bones, mainly in the spine
  - Cartilage between the breastbone and the ribs (sternum)
  - Hip and shoulder joints
- Linked to HLA-B27 gene

## SIGNS AND SYMPTOMS

Symptoms might worsen (flares), improve, or stop at irregular intervals
- Chronic dull pain in the lower back or gluteal region combined with stiffness of the lower back, especially in the morning and after periods of inactivity
- Hip pain
- Joint pain
- Neck pain
- Fatigue
- Difficulty breathing
- Loss of appetite and unexplained weight loss
- Abdominal pain and diarrhea
- Skin rash
- Vision problems

## COMPLICATIONS

- Spinal compression fractures
- Atlanto-axial subluxation possible (21% of AS patients)
- Eye inflammation (iritis or uveitis) and sensitivity to light (photophobia)
- Fused vertebrae (ankylosis)
- Kyphosis (forward curvature of the spine)
- Osteoporosis
- Cardiovascular abnormalities: Aortic insufficiency/aortitis, arrhythmias, angina, cardiomyopathy
- Respiratory abnormalities: Chest pain that affects breathing, restrictive disease, upper lobe fibrosis
- Jaw inflammation
- Cauda equina syndrome (rare)
- Patients with AS may also have psoriasis and/or inflammatory bowel disease

# EXTRA-ARTICULAR MANIFESTATIONS

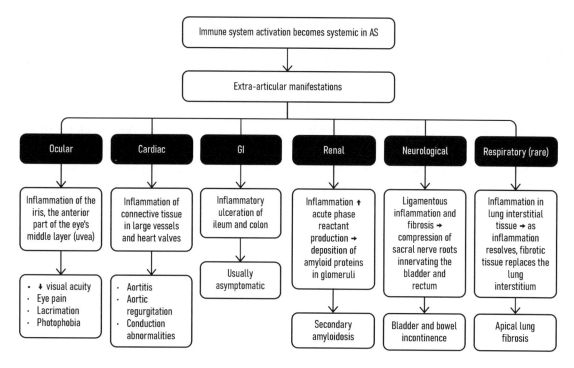

AS, ankylosing spondylitis; GI, gastrointestinal.

# TREATMENT

**Medications:** Relieve pain and reduce inflammation
- **Non-steroidal anti-inflammatory drugs (NSAIDs):** Ibuprofen and naproxen
- **Corticosteroids:** IV methylprednisolone
- **Disease-modifying anti-rheumatic drugs (DMARDs):** Sulfasalazine
- **TNF-α inhibitors:** Infliximab, adalimumab, and etanercept
- **Exercise:** To reduce pain and stiffness
- **Physical therapy:** Improve comfort and spinal flexibility
- **Surgery (rare):** Repair significantly damaged joints or correct severe bends in the spine

Ankylosing spondylitis

# MANAGEMENT

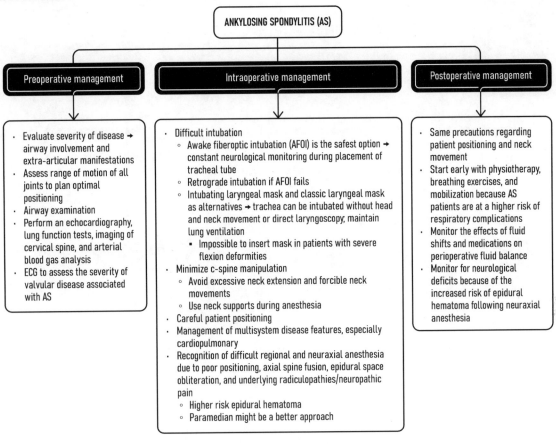

ANKYLOSING SPONDYLITIS (AS)

**Preoperative management**

- Evaluate severity of disease → airway involvement and extra-articular manifestations
- Assess range of motion of all joints to plan optimal positioning
- Airway examination
- Perform an echocardiography, lung function tests, imaging of cervical spine, and arterial blood gas analysis
- ECG to assess the severity of valvular disease associated with AS

**Intraoperative management**

- Difficult intubation
  - Awake fiberoptic intubation (AFOI) is the safest option → constant neurological monitoring during placement of tracheal tube
  - Retrograde intubation if AFOI fails
  - Intubating laryngeal mask and classic laryngeal mask as alternatives → trachea can be intubated without head and neck movement or direct laryngoscopy, maintain lung ventilation
    - Impossible to insert mask in patients with severe flexion deformities
- Minimize c-spine manipulation
  - Avoid excessive neck extension and forcible neck movements
  - Use neck supports during anesthesia
- Careful patient positioning
- Management of multisystem disease features, especially cardiopulmonary
- Recognition of difficult regional and neuraxial anesthesia due to poor positioning, axial spine fusion, epidural space obliteration, and underlying radiculopathies/neuropathic pain
  - Higher risk epidural hematoma
  - Paramedian might be a better approach

**Postoperative management**

- Same precautions regarding patient positioning and neck movement
- Start early with physiotherapy, breathing exercises, and mobilization because AS patients are at a higher risk of respiratory complications
- Monitor the effects of fluid shifts and medications on perioperative fluid balance
- Monitor for neurological deficits because of the increased risk of epidural hematoma following neuraxial anesthesia

## *Obstetrical anesthesia*

- Complicated due to difficult airway and difficult neuraxial techniques → have multiple plans in place
- Consider paramedian approach and ultrasound guidance for neuraxial anesthesia

## KEEP IN MIND

- AS is a challenge for the anesthesiologist because the rigid, immobile, fragile spine makes intubation, general anesthesia, and neuraxial anesthesia difficult
- Awake fiberoptic intubation is the safest method of securing the airway in AS patients, but supraglottic airway devices such as laryngeal masks can also be used
- The use of alternative approaches, such as the paramedian approach or the use of ultrasound guidance, may improve success with neuraxial anesthesia in AS patients

## SUGGESTED READING

- Pahwa D, Chhabra A, Arora MK. Anaesthetic management of patients with ankylosing spondylitis. Trends in Anaesthesia and Critical Care. 2013;3(1):19-24.
- Woodward LJ, Kam PC. Ankylosing spondylitis: recent developments and anaesthetic implications. Anaesthesia. 2009;64(5):540-548.

# 276

# EHLERS-DANLOS SYNDROME

## LEARNING OBJECTIVES

- Describe Ehlers-Danlos syndrome
- Recognize the symptoms and signs of Ehlers-Danlos syndrome
- Anesthetic management of a patient with Ehlers-Danlos syndrome

## DEFINITION AND MECHANISM

- Ehlers-Danlos syndrome (EDS) comprises a group of clinically and genetically heterogeneous heritable connective tissue disorders, characterized by joint hypermobility and instability, skin texture anomalies, and vascular and internal organ fragility
- Clinical manifestations range from extremely mild phenotypes to life-threatening complications depending on the specific subtype

- The current Villefranche nosology recognizes six major subtypes, comprising classic, hypermobile, vascular, kyphoscoliotic, arthrochalasia, and dermatosparaxis, most of which are linked to mutations in one of the genes encoding for fibrillar collagen proteins or enzymes involved in post-translational modification of these proteins

AD, autosomal dominant; AR, autosomal recessive.

| Common subtype | Major criteria | Minor criteria | Inheritance |
|---|---|---|---|
| Classic | Skin hyperextensibility<br>Widened atrophic scars<br>Joint hypermobility | Smooth, velvety skin<br>Molluscoid pseudotumors<br>Subcutaneous spheroids<br>Complications of joint hypermobility<br>Muscle hypotonia, motor delay<br>Easy bruising<br>Manifestations of tissue extensibility and fragility<br>Surgical complications<br>Positive family history | AD |
| Hypermobility | Hyperextensible and/or smooth, velvety skin<br>Generalized joint hypermobility | Recurring joint dislocations<br>Chronic joint/limb pain<br>Positive family history | AD (?) |
| Vascular | Thin, translucent skin<br>Arterial/intestinal/uterine fragility or rupture<br>Extensive bruising<br>Characteristic facial appearance | Acrogeria<br>Hypermobility of small joints<br>Tendon and muscle rupture<br>Talipes equinovarus<br>Early-onset varicose veins<br>Arteriovenous, carotid-cavernous sinus fistula<br>Pneumothorax/pneumohemothorax<br>Gingival recessions<br>Positive family history, sudden death in a close relative | AD |
| Kyphoscoliotic | Generalized joint hypermobility<br>Congenital hypotonia<br>Congenital and progressive scoliosis<br>Scleral fragility and rupture of the ocular globe | Tissue fragility, including atrophic scars<br>Easy bruising<br>Arterial rupture<br>Marfanoid habitus<br>Microcornea<br>Osteopenia, -porosis<br>Positive family history | AR |
| Arthrochalasia | Generalized joint hypermobility with recurrent subluxations<br>Congenital bilateral hip dislocation | Skin hyperextensibility<br>Tissue fragility, including atrophic scars<br>Easy bruising<br>Hypotonia<br>Kyphoscoliosis<br>Osteopenia, -porosis | AD |
| Dermatosparaxis | Severe skin fragility<br>Sagging, redundant skin | Soft, doughy skin texture<br>Easy bruising<br>Premature rupture of fetal membranes<br>Large hernias (umbilical, inguinal) | AR |

## SIGNS AND SYMPTOMS

- Loose joints
- Joint pain
- Stretchy, velvety skin
- Fragile skin
- Abnormal scar formation

## COMPLICATIONS

- Aortic dissection
- Joint dislocations
- Scoliosis
- Chronic pain
- Early osteoarthritis

## MANAGEMENT

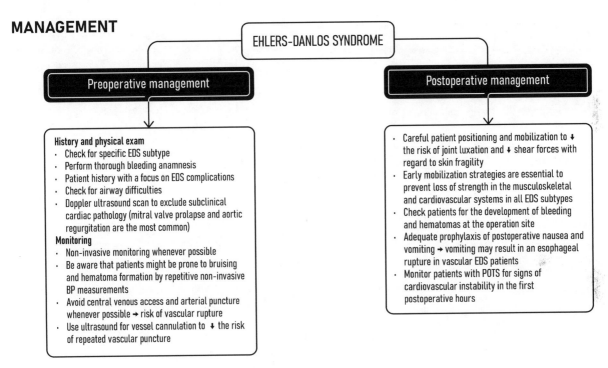

EDS, Ehlers-Danlos syndrome; BP, blood pressure; POTS, postural orthostatic tachycardia syndrome.

```
                        ┌─────────────────────────┐
                        │  EHLERS-DANLOS SYNDROME  │
                        └─────────────────────────┘
                                     │
                                     ▼
        ████████████████████████████████████████████████████████████
        ██              Intraoperative management                ██
        ████████████████████████████████████████████████████████████
```

**Positioning**
- Use padding to ↓ shear forces and external tissue pressure
- Protect the eye → direct force to the eyeball + the risk of retinal detachment and globe rupture
- Patient mobilization, positioning, and padding with great caution

**Crossmatching and bleeding prophylaxis**
- Crossmatch blood products (for patients at risk of bleeding) and prepare autotransfusion devices
- Use desmopressin in patients with positive bleeding history
- Strategies for bleeding therapy in vascular EDS subtypes
- Consider aggressive hemostatic therapy in acute bleeding

**Airway management and ventilator strategies**
- Mask ventilation, intubation, and laryngeal mask insertion are all possible
- Careful mask ventilation to avoid temporomandibular joint luxation
- Avoid BURP and hypertensive response during intubation → vessel rupture
- Repeated intubation attempts may cause bleeding
- Use smaller endotracheal tubes to ↓ mucosal damage
- Keep low airway pressures due to ↑ risk of pneumothorax

**Pharmacology**
- General anesthesia can be performed as balanced anesthesia with volatile aesthetics, nitrous oxide, or as TIVA
- Depolarizing (e.g., succinylcholine) and non-depolarizing neuromuscular blockers are safe
- Advised to monitor neuromuscular block as EDS patients present with muscular weakness
- Avoid succinylcholine in immobilized patients

**Circulatory issues**
- POTS is sometimes a feature in EDS, mainly in the hypermobile variant
- Preoperative infusion of crystalloid and early use of vasopressors may be helpful

**Use of tourniquets**
- Avoid tourniquets → high risk of hematoma, compartment syndromes, and untreatable diffuse bleeding

EDS, Ehlers-Danlos syndrome; BURP, backward, upward, rightward pressure; POTS, postural orthostatic tachycardia syndrome; TIVA, total intravenous anesthesia.

### *Obstetrical anesthesia*

- Difficult management, requires multidisciplinary effort
- High risk of preterm labor, uterine rupture, and hemorrhage
- Neuraxial anesthesia is relatively contraindicated, may need general anesthesia
- If vascular subtype → recommendations are termination of pregnancy or cesarean section before 32 weeks

## KEEP IN MIND

- Avoid ambulatory surgery in EDS patients
- Be aware of typical EDS-related emergency-like situations such as difficult airway status, bleeding risks, and organ rupture in specific subtypes
- Vascular ELS is a risk factor for vascular, skin, ocular and respiratory complications

═══════════════════════════════════ **SUGGESTED READING** ═══════════════════════════════════

- Malfait F, Francomano C, Byers P, et al. The 2017 international classification of the Ehlers-Danlos syndromes. Am J Med Genet C Semin Med Genet. 2017;175(1):8-26.
- Wiesmann T, Castori M, Malfait F, Wulf H. Recommendations for anesthesia and perioperative management in patients with Ehlers-Danlos syndrome(s). Orphanet J Rare Dis. 2014;9(109).

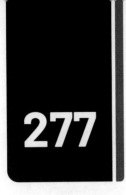

# MARFAN SYNDROME

**277**

## LEARNING OBJECTIVES

- Describe Marfan syndrome
- Recognize signs and symptoms of Marfan syndrome
- Anesthetic management of a patient with Marfan syndrome

## DEFINITION AND MECHANISM

- Marfan syndrome (MFS) is an autosomal dominant condition of connective tissue, mainly involving the cardiovascular, musculoskeletal, and ocular systems
- MFS is caused by a mutation in the FBN1 gene on chromosome 15 that encodes the protein fibrillin
- The connective tissue abnormalities lead to connective tissue weakness with hyperextensible joints, eyes (dislocation of the lens), increased risk of valvular/aortic dissection, and spontaneous pneumothorax

## SIGNS AND SYMPTOMS

- **Ocular:** Lens dislocation, myopia, retinal detachment, glaucoma
- **Cardiovascular:** Aortic root dilatation with aortic regurgitation, aneurysm formation, aortic dissection, mitral valve prolapse with mitral regurgitation
- **Musculoskeletal:** Long bone overgrowth, scoliosis, kyphosis, kyphoscoliosis, joint hypermobility, pectus carinatum/excavatum, high-arched palate
- **Respiratory:** Spontaneous pneumothorax
- **Skin:** Striae
- **Central nervous system:** Dural ectasia

## COMPLICATIONS

- Patients with MFS and left ventricular dilatation are at risk of ventricular arrhythmias
- Aortic root diameter > 4 cm carries a risk of aortic dissection

## TREATMENT

- Medications
  - β-blockers
  - Calcium channel blockers or angiotensin-converting enzyme (ACE) inhibitors if β-blockers are contraindicated/not tolerated
- Surgery to repair the aorta or replace a heart valve

# MANAGEMENT

```
┌─────────────────────────┐
│     MARFAN SYNDROME     │
└─────────────────────────┘
```

| Preoperative management | Intraoperative management | Postoperative management |

**Preoperative management**
- Assess cardiopulmonary status
  - Presence of mitral valvular disease, aortic valvular disease, angina, and heart failure
  - Echocardiography to determine aortic root size
  - Chest radiograph
  - Arterial blood gas analysis and lung function test only in the presence of significant kyphoscoliosis
- Preoperative control of blood pressure to minimize shear forces and wall stress in the aorta → ↓ risk of aortic rupture or dissection

**Intraoperative management**
- Possible difficult airway
  - High-arched palate and retrognathia
  - Potential cervical spine ligamentous instability → avoid neck hyperextension
  - Temporomandibular joint may sublux or dislocate during tracheal intubation
- Smooth laryngoscopy to prevent hypertension and subsequent ↑ risk of aortic dissection
- Proper patient positioning, handling, and limb support to avoid joint trauma and dislocation, and eye trauma
- Antibiotic prophylaxis because of the ↑ risk of subacute bacterial endocarditis
- Intraoperative cardiovascular monitoring
- Maintain blood pressure and avoid maneuvers leading to tachycardia and hypertension to ↓ the risk of aortic dissection or rupture
- Maintain intravascular status to ↓ chances of aortic and/or mitral valve prolapse
- Keep ventilatory pressure low to prevent barotrauma and pneumothorax
- Continue β-blockers perioperatively to ↓ myocardial contractility and control aortic wall tension
- Avoid cardiodepressive drugs in patients with significant cardiovascular disease
- Avoid long-acting neuromuscular blockers
- Regional anesthesia not contraindicated; presence of dural ectasia may lead to inadequate spinal anesthesia

**Postoperative management**
- Adequate postoperative pain management to avoid hypertension and tachycardia

## Obstetric anesthesia

- **If no symptoms and aorta diameter < 4 cm:** No special considerations and vaginal delivery ok
- **If aortic root dilation and aortic regurgitation:** Multidisciplinary management with cardiology/cardiac surgery/obstetrics
- Some recommend cesarean section if aorta diameter > 4.5 cm and labor if aorta diameter > 4 and < 4.5 cm
- Problems
  - Airway might be even more difficult
  - Neuraxial anesthesia for vaginal delivery and cesarean section
  - Aortic dilatation with risk of dissection or rupture
  - Perform monthly echocardiography during pregnancy
  - Reduce shear forces on aorta
  - Consider very early epidural placement
  - Need for invasive monitoring
  - Drug therapy to prevent hypertension and tachycardia (e.g., labetalol)
- Dural ectasia
  - Higher risk for failed epidural, dural puncture, and postdural puncture headache
  - Consider CT/MRI

# KEEP IN MIND

- Prevent a sudden increase in myocardial contractility, producing an increase in aortic wall tension, which could lead to aortic dissection
- Preexisting cardiovascular disease and the potential for acute cardiovascular and respiratory complications in patients with MFS require careful preoperative assessment and the use of a skillful anesthetic technique to avoid fatal complications
- Blood pressure control is the central component of perioperative management

# SUGGESTED READING

- Allyn J, Guglielminotti J, Omnes S, Guezouli L, Egan M, Jondeau G, Longrois D, Montravers P. Marfan's Syndrome During Pregnancy: Anesthetic Management of Delivery in 16 Consecutive Patients. Anesthesia & Analgesia. 2013;116(2): 392-398.
- Araújo MR, Marques C, Freitas S, Santa-Bárbara R, Alves J, Xavier C. Marfan Syndrome: new diagnostic criteria, same anesthesia care? Case report and review. Braz J Anesthesiol. 2016;66(4):408-413.
- Castellano JM, Silvay G, Castillo JG. Marfan Syndrome: Clinical, Surgical, and Anesthetic Considerations. Seminars in Cardiothoracic and Vascular Anesthesia. 2014;18(3):260-271.
- Marfan Syndrome. In: Bissonnette B, Luginbuehl I, Marciniak B, Dalens BJ. eds. Syndromes: Rapid Recognition and Perioperative Implications. Mgraw Hill; 2006. Accessed January 26, 2023.

# 278

# OSTEOGENESIS IMPERFECTA

## LEARNING OBJECTIVES

- Describe osteogenesis imperfecta
- Recognize signs and symptoms of osteogenesis imperfecta
- Anesthetic management of a patient with osteogenesis imperfecta

## DEFINITION AND MECHANISM

- Osteogenesis imperfecta (OI), or brittle bone disease, is a group of genetic disorders present at birth, characterized by fragile bones that break easily
- The underlying mechanism is usually a connective tissue disorder caused by a lack of or poorly formed type I collagen
- In more than 90% of the cases, OI occurs due to mutations in the COL1A1 and COL1A2 genes
- Inherited in an autosomal dominant manner or de novo mutations
- There are at least 8 different types of the disease. and types vary greatly, both within and between types.
- Types are based on the type of inheritance, and signs and symptoms, including findings on X-rays and other imaging tests

| Types | OI syndromic names | Clinical features | Radiographic or histological features |
|---|---|---|---|
| Type I | Nondeforming OI with blue sclera | Blue sclera<br>Normal stature<br>Fractures<br>Hearing loss<br>Presence of DI rare | Fractures |
| Type II | Perinatally lethal OI | Perinatal lethal<br>Blue-gray sclera<br>Small for gestational age<br>Respiratory distress<br>Limb deformities<br>"Frog leg" positioning<br>Soft calvarium | Multiple fractures "crumpled appearance"<br>Beaded ribs<br>Short thoracic cage<br>Osteopenia<br>Long bone deformities<br>Limited calvarial mineralization |
| Type III | Progressively deforming OI | Severe phenotype<br>Short stature<br>Multiple fractures<br>Progressive deformities<br>Usually non-ambulatory<br>May have DI<br>Adolescent onset hearing loss | Osteopenia<br>Multiple fractures<br>Long bone deformity<br>Thin ribs |
| Type IV | Common variable OI with normal sclera | Milder than OI III<br>Typically ambulatory DI is common<br>Adult onset hearing loss<br>Normal-gray sclera | Intermediate appearance between OI II and III |
| Type V | Osteogenesis Imperfecta Type V | Hyperplastic callus formation, calcification of the interosseous membrane, radial head dislocations | Interosseous membrane calcification, dense hyperplastic calluses |
| Type VI | Osteogenesis Imperfecta Type VI | Moderate to severe phenotype, often without blue sclera, fish scale bone pattern under microscope | Fish scale bone pattern, severe osteopenia |
| Type VII | Osteogenesis Imperfecta Type VII | Coxa vara, severe scoliosis, primarily in a Quebec population with founder mutation | Severe osteopenia, coxa vara deformity |
| Type VIII | Osteogenesis Imperfecta Type VIII | Extremely low bone mineral density, severe bone deformities, high fracture rate | Severe osteoporosis, minimal trabecular bone |

OI, osteogenesis imperfecta; DI, dentinogenesis imperfecta.

## SIGNS AND SYMPTOMS

Signs and symptoms vary from mild to severe
- Bones that break easily, brittle bones
- Bone deformity and pain
- Easy bruising
- Blue sclera
- Joint hypermobility
- Loose joints

- Muscle weakness
- Curved spine, kyphoscoliosis
- Short height
- Hearing loss
- Dentinogenesis imperfecta (weak, brittle, or discolored teeth)
- Difficulty breathing
- Triangle-shaped face

## COMPLICATIONS

- Respiratory infections (e.g., pneumonia)
- Pulmonary valve insufficiency secondary to distortion of the thoracic cage
- Cardiovascular problems (e.g., valvular disease, aorta dissection)
- Kidney stones
- Vision loss

## TREATMENT

Treatment focuses on managing symptoms and increasing bone strength to prevent deformities and fractures
- Maintain a healthy lifestyle via exercise, eat a balanced diet sufficient in vitamin D and calcium, and avoid smoking
- Biphosphonate medicines
- Acute care of fractures
- Orthopedic treatment (e.g., bracing and splinting)
- Rodding surgery
- Physical and occupational therapy
- Assistive devices (e.g., leg braces and wheelchairs)
- Oral and dental care

## ANESTHETIC CONCERNS

| Types | Anesthetic concerns | |
|---|---|---|
| Type I | Bone fractures during extremity manipulation (e.g., positioning, peripheral IV placements with tourniquet)<br>Dental damage during oropharyngeal instrumentation<br>Difficulty of hearing<br>Hyperthermia or malignant hyperthermia<br>Platelet dysfunction<br>Capillary fragility | |
| Type II | Most prenatally diagnosed pregnancies are terminated; patients rarely survive to adulthood | |
| Type III | Bone fractures during extremity manipulation<br>Posterior fossa compression syndromes due to basilar impression from cervical manipulation<br>Pulmonary insufficiency or hypertension<br>Cardiopulmonary failure<br>Hyperthermia or malignant hyperthermia<br>Platelet dysfunction<br>Capillary fragility<br>Postoperative pain control | |
| Type IV | Bone fracture or dislocation<br>Dental damage<br>Posterior fossa compression syndromes<br>Pulmonary insufficiency or hypertension | Cardiopulmonary failure<br>Hyperthermia or malignant hyperthermia<br>Platelet dysfunction<br>Postoperative pain control |
| Type V | Hypertrophic callus formation<br>Increased bleeding tendency due to vascular abnormalities<br>Bone fractures during minor procedures<br>Joint hypermobility and dislocations<br>Dentinogenesis imperfecta causing dental complications | |
| Type VI | Increased risk of vertebral compression fractures<br>Bone fragility with minimal trauma<br>Risk of hypercalcemia | Respiratory complications from rib fractures<br>Dentinogenesis imperfecta causing dental complications |
| Type VII | Coxa vara (malformed hip joint)<br>Severe scoliosis impacting respiratory function | High risk of long bone fractures during positioning<br>Increased bleeding tendency |
| Type VIII | Severe growth deficiency impacting pediatric anesthesia equipment sizing<br>Extremely fragile long bones<br>High risk of respiratory failure from minimal rib cage deformities<br>Dentinogenesis imperfecta with severe dental implications<br>Severe scoliosis requiring careful monitoring of respiratory status | |

Osteogenesis imperfecta

# MANAGEMENT

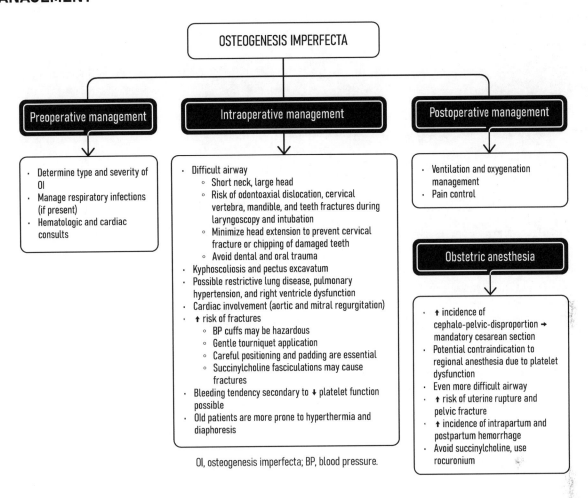

**OSTEOGENESIS IMPERFECTA**

**Preoperative management**

- Determine type and severity of OI
- Manage respiratory infections (if present)
- Hematologic and cardiac consults

**Intraoperative management**

- Difficult airway
  - Short neck, large head
  - Risk of odontoaxial dislocation, cervical vertebra, mandible, and teeth fractures during laryngoscopy and intubation
  - Minimize head extension to prevent cervical fracture or chipping of damaged teeth
  - Avoid dental and oral trauma
- Kyphoscoliosis and pectus excavatum
- Possible restrictive lung disease, pulmonary hypertension, and right ventricle dysfunction
- Cardiac involvement (aortic and mitral regurgitation)
- ↑ risk of fractures
  - BP cuffs may be hazardous
  - Gentle tourniquet application
  - Careful positioning and padding are essential
  - Succinylcholine fasciculations may cause fractures
- Bleeding tendency secondary to ↓ platelet function possible
- Old patients are more prone to hyperthermia and diaphoresis

OI, osteogenesis imperfecta; BP, blood pressure.

**Postoperative management**

- Ventilation and oxygenation management
- Pain control

**Obstetric anesthesia**

- ↑ incidence of cephalo-pelvic-disproportion → mandatory cesarean section
- Potential contraindication to regional anesthesia due to platelet dysfunction
- Even more difficult airway
- ↑ risk of uterine rupture and pelvic fracture
- ↑ incidence of intrapartum and postpartum hemorrhage
- Avoid succinylcholine, use rocuronium

## SUGGESTED READING

- Gupta D, Purohit A. Anesthetic management in a patient with osteogenesis imperfecta for rush nail removal in femur. Anesth Essays Res. 2016;10(3):677-679.
- Frost EAM. Osteogenesis imperfecta and anesthetic implications. October 21, 2019. Accessed January 27, 2023. https://anesthesiaexperts.com/uncategorized/16596/#:~:text=In%20 OI%2C%20the%20need%20for,or%20chipping%20of%20damaged%20teeth.
- Wang H, Huang X, Wu A, Li Q. Management of anesthesia in a patient with osteogenesis imperfecta and multiple fractures: a case report and review of the literature. Journal of International Medical Research. 2021;49(6).

# 279

# PSORIASIS

## LEARNING OBJECTIVES

- Define and classify the different types of psoriasis
- Describe psoriasis triggers
- Anesthetic management of a patient with psoriasis

## DEFINITION AND MECHANISM

- Psoriasis is a chronic skin disorder characterized by an accelerated epidermal turnover and epidermal hyperplasia
- Autoimmune disease resulting from an increased rate of epidermal protein synthesis, rapid epidermal cell growth, shortened epidermal cell cycle, and increase in the proliferative cell population
- Lesions consist of sharply demarcated, loosely adherent, thickened, noncoherent, silver skin scales with increased vascularity → they most commonly appear on the extensor surfaces (i.e., elbows and knees), lumbosacral area, and scalp
- Injury to the skin can trigger psoriatic skin changes at that spot (Koebner phenomenon)

## CLASSIFICATION

- Plaque psoriasis or psoriasis vulgaris
  - Most common type (85-90%)
  - Causes dry, itchy, raised skin patches (plaques) covered with scales
  - Most commonly found on the elbows, knees, scalp, and back
- Nail psoriasis
  - Affecting fingernails and toenails
  - Causes pitting, abnormal nail growth, and discoloration
  - Nails might loosen and separate from the nail bed (onycholysis)
- Guttate psoriasis
  - Primarily affects young adults and children
  - Triggered by a bacterial infection (e.g., strep throat)
  - Marked by small, drop-shaped, scaling spots on the trunk, arms, or legs

- Inverse psoriasis
  - Mainly affects the skin folds of the armpits, groin, buttocks, and breasts
  - Causes smooth patches of inflamed skin that worsen with friction and sweating
  - Fungal infections may trigger this type of psoriasis
- Pustular psoriasis
  - Causes clearly defined pus-filled blisters
  - Occur in widespread patches or on small areas of the palms or soles
- Erythrodermic psoriasis (erythroderma)
  - Least common type
  - Widespread inflammation and exfoliation of the skin over most of the body surface (> 90% of the body surface area)
  - Accompanied by severe dryness, itching, swelling, and pain
  - Can develop from any type of psoriasis

## SIGNS AND SYMPTOMS

- Patchy rash ranging from spots of dandruff-like scaling to major eruptions across the entire body
- Rashes that vary in color (purple with gray scale to pink-red with silver scale)
- Small scaling spots
- Dry, cracked skin that may bleed
- Itching, burning, or soreness
- Cyclic rashes that flare for a few weeks or months and then subside
- Psoriatic lesions become colonized by bacteria (especially Staphylococcus aureus, Streptococcus pyogenes)
- Severe psoriasis may be associated with hyperuricemia, anemia, negative nitrogen balance, iron loss, and hypoalbuminemia

## COMPLICATIONS

- Psoriatic arthritis, which resembles seronegative rheumatoid arthritis
- Temporary skin color changes (postinflammatory hypo- or hyperpigmentation) where plaques have healed
- Eye conditions (e.g., conjunctivitis, blepharitis, and uveitis)
- Obesity
- Diabetes type 2
- Hypertension
- Cardiovascular disease

- Other autoimmune diseases (e.g., ulcerative colitis, Crohn's disease, celiac disease, multiple sclerosis, systemic lupus erythematosus, autoimmune thyroid disease, Sjögren's syndrome, vitiligo, or alopecia areata)
- Increased risk of developing non-melanoma skin cancer
- Mental health conditions (e.g., low self-esteem and depression)

# RISK FACTORS

- Genetic (HLA-Cw6)
- Family history
- Smoking

## *Psoriasis triggers*
- Infections (e.g., strep throat or skin infections)
- Weather (cold and dry)
- Injury to the skin (e.g., cut or scrape, bug bite, or severe sunburn)
- Stress
- Smoking and exposure to secondhand smoke
- Obesity
- Heavy alcohol consumption
- Certain medications (e.g., lithium, beta-blockers, calcium channel blockers, antimalarial drugs, NSAIDs)
- Rapid withdrawal of oral or injected corticosteroids

# TREATMENT

- Topical therapy
  - Corticosteroids (i.e., hydrocortisone)
  - Vitamin D3 analogs (i.e., calcipotriene and calcitriol) to slow skin cell growth
  - Retinoids/vitamin A derivatives (i.e., tazarotene)
  - Calcineurin inhibitors (i.e., tacrolimus and pimecrolimus) to calm the rash and reduce the scaly buildup
  - Salicylic acid to reduce the scaling of scalp psoriasis
  - Coal tar to reduce scaling, itching, and inflammation
  - Anthralin to slow skin cell growth
- Phototherapy
  - Sunlight
  - UVB broadband and narrowband
  - UVB
  - PUVA
- Oral or injected (systemic) medications
  - Corticosteroids
  - Retinoids/vitamin A derivatives
  - Biologics (i.e., apremilast, etanercept, infliximab, adalimumab, etc.) to suppress the immune system
  - Methotrexate to decrease the production of skin cells and suppress inflammation
  - Cyclosporine to suppress the immune system

# MANAGEMENT

```
┌──────────────────────────────────────────┐
│   PSORIASIS: PREOPERATIVE MANAGEMENT       │
└──────────────────────────────────────────┘
```

**History and examination**

- Assess the disease and the extent, duration, distribution, and severity of lesions
- Assess nutritional state
- Exclude hypovolemia (due to increased transepidermal water loss or pyrexia) in erythroderma
- Check core temperature in erythroderma and pustular psoriasis
- Note drug therapy and dose, especially immunosuppressants and steroids
- Airway assessment (especially if psoriasis is complicated by arthropathy): Possible limited joint mobility → requiring awake fiberoptic intubation

**Investigations**

- Full blood count
  - Anemia (chronic illness or deficiencies of iron, vitamin B12, or folate)
  - Leukopenia and thrombocytopenia (immunosuppressant therapy)
- Urea and electrolytes
  - Abnormalities in renal function and electrolyte balance may exist in erythroderma
  - Immunosuppressants and methotrexate can impair renal function
  - Measure calcium levels if hypoalbuminemia exists
- Liver function tests: Immunosuppressants and methotrexate can impair liver function
- ECG and chest X-ray: Proceed to echocardiography if there is evidence of heart failure
- Crossmatch blood in erythroderma: Risk of blood loss

## PSORIASIS: INTRAOPERATIVE MANAGEMENT

### Premedication

- Start perioperative steroid supplementation
- Do not inject intramuscular premedication into areas of psoriasis

### General anesthesia

**Induction of anesthesia**
- Avoid nitrous oxide (potentiates cytotoxic effects of methotrexate)
- Avoid using psoriatic sites for IV access (risk of infection due to skin colonization)
- Suture IV cannula in place (adhesive tape may denude skin, cause bleeding, or new lesions)
- Hyperdynamic circulation in erythroderma may alter the onset of IV and inhalational anesthetic agents
- Hypervolemia, hypovolemia, congestive heart failure, hypoalbuminemia, and reduced renal blood flow may affect the kinetics of drug distribution and excretion

**Maintenance of anesthesia**
- Increased skin blood flow and high cardiac output in erythroderma may lead to excessive bleeding during surgery
- Use warming blankets with care in erythroderma → risk of hyperthermia (patients have difficulty in regulating body temperature, increased metabolic rate, not able to sweat)

### Regional anesthesia

- Avoid using psoriatic sites for regional techniques
- Use swabs soaked in an aqueous solution of antiseptic for skin cleaning, avoid skin scrubbing
- Secure extradural catheters using bandages (adhesive tape may cause skin loss)
- Consider the risk of postoperative pruritus with neuraxial opioids (highest with morphine, lowest with fentanyl)

### Monitoring

- Attach ECG electrodes and pulse oximeter to unaffected skin areas
- Consider central venous pressure or cardiac output monitoring in erythroderma (fluid replacement)
- Monitor core temperature in erythroderma
- Blood pressure cuffs can cause the Koebner phenomenon → padding to reduce this risk

## SUGGESTED READING

- Baluch A, Kak A, Saleh O, Lonadier L, Kaye AD. Psoriasis and anesthetic considerations. Middle East J Anaesthesiol. 2010;20(5):621-629.
- Pollard BJ, Kitchen G. Handbook of Clinical Anaesthesia. 4th ed. Taylor & Francis group; 2018. Chapter 9 Connective tissue, Lomas JP.

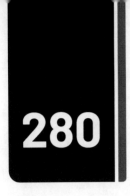

# RHABDOMYOLYSIS

## LEARNING OBJECTIVES

- Definition, signs, and symptoms of rhabdomyolysis
- Causes of rhabdomyolysis
- Treament and anesthetic management of rhabdomyolysis

## DEFINITION AND MECHANISM

- Rhabdomyolysis occurs when damaged skeletal muscle breaks down rapidly and releases its content in the bloodstream
- Characterized by skeletal muscle disintegration and the release of myoglobin and other intercellular proteins and electrolytes into the circulation
- Hyperkalemia, hyperuricemia, and hyperphosphatemia can all develop rapidly
- This can lead to heart or kidney failure and can even be fatal
- Rhabdomyolysis ranges from an asymptomatic illness with elevation in the creatine kinase (CK) level to a life-threatening condition associated with extreme elevations in CK, electrolyte imbalances, acute kidney injury, and disseminated intravascular coagulation
- Most often caused by direct traumatic injury, however, can also result from a wide array of other causes

## SIGNS AND SYMPTOMS

- Muscle pains or cramps
- Weakness
- Swelling of affected muscles
- Nausea and vomiting
- Confusion
- Coma
- Tea-colored urine due to the presence of myoglobin
- Abdominal pain
- Fever
- Tachycardia
- Arrhythmias
- Hypotension and shock
- Acute kidney injury

## ACUTE KIDNEY INJURY AND RHABDOMYOLYSIS

- Myoglobin interacts with the Tamm-Horsfall protein in the renal tubules to form brown granular casts which lead to tubular obstruction
- This process is favored when the urine is acidic
- The heme group of myoglobin could lead to lipid peroxidation
- Myoglobin also scavenges nitrous oxide leading to renal vasoconstriction
- Renal blood flow is furter reduced by hypovolemia, activation of the renin-angiotensin-aldosterone system (RAAS), and other vascular mediators

## COMPLICATIONS

- Hyperkalemia
- Hypocalcemia
- Acute kidney injury
- Disseminated intravascular coagulation
- Compartment syndrome

## CAUSES

- Strenuous exercise
- Delirium tremens
- Tetanus
- Prolonged seizures
- Crush injuries
- Arterial thrombosis or embolism
- Clamping of an artery during surgery
- Hyperthermia
- Hypothermia

- Drugs and toxins
  □ Statins and fibrates
  □ Antipsychotic medications may cause the neuroleptic malignant syndrome
  □ Succinylcholine or the inhalational anesthetics (e.g., sevoflurane, isoflurane, halothane, desflurane, enflurane, ether) may trigger malignant hyperthermia, also associated with rhabdomyolysis
  □ Medications that cause serotonin syndrome, such as selective serotonin reuptake inhibitors (SSRIs)
  □ Medications that interfere with potassium levels, such as diuretics
  □ Heavy metals
  □ Venom from insects or snakes

□ Drugs: alcohol, amphetamine, cocaine, heroin, ketamine, and MDMA
- Infection
- Electrical injury
- Immobilization
- Metabolism:
  □ Hyperglycemic hyperosmolar state
  □ Hyper- and hyponatremia
□ Hypokalemia
□ Hypocalcemia
□ Hypophosphatemia
□ Ketoacidosis
□ Hypothyroidism

## RISK FACTORS

| Endogenous risks | Exogenous risks |
|---|---|
| Advanced age (> 80 years)<br>Small body frame and frailty<br>Multisystem disease<br>- Renal dysfunction<br>- Hepatic dysfunction<br>Thyroid disorders, especially hypothyroidism<br>Hypertriglyceridemia<br>Metabolic muscle disease<br>- Carnitine palmitoyltransferase II deficiency<br>- McArdle disease<br>Myoadenylate deaminase deficiency | Alcohol consumption<br>Heavy exercise<br>Surgery with severe metabolic demands<br>Agents affecting the cytochrome P450 system, especially<br>- Fibrates<br>- Nicotinic acid<br>- Cyclosporine<br>- Azole antifungals<br>- Macrolide antibiotics<br>- HIV protease inhibitors<br>- Nefazodone<br>- Verapamil<br>- Amiodarone<br>- Warfarin<br>- Consumption of > 1 quart daily of grapefruit juice |

## DIAGNOSIS

- Blood test: creatine kinase (CK) > 5000 U/L
  □ Note that myoglobin levels peak before increases in CK
  □ However, myoglobin is metabolized rapidly at sites outside of the kidney
  □ This makes CK a more reliable marker of rhabdomyolysis
- A metabolic acidosis with a high anion gap is commonly reported in rhabdomyolysis with associated acute kidney injury

| Investigations | Possible findings |
|---|---|
| Serum and urine myoglobin | Present |
| Urinary dipstick + pH | Positive for blood |
| Urea and creatinine | Raised |
| Potassium | Raised |
| Calcium | Low |
| Phosphate, uric acid | Raised |
| Coagulation studies | Prologend in severe cases |
| Blood gas | Lactic acidosis |
| Calculation of anion gap | Raised |
| ECG | Raised |

Rhabdomyolysis

## MANAGEMENT

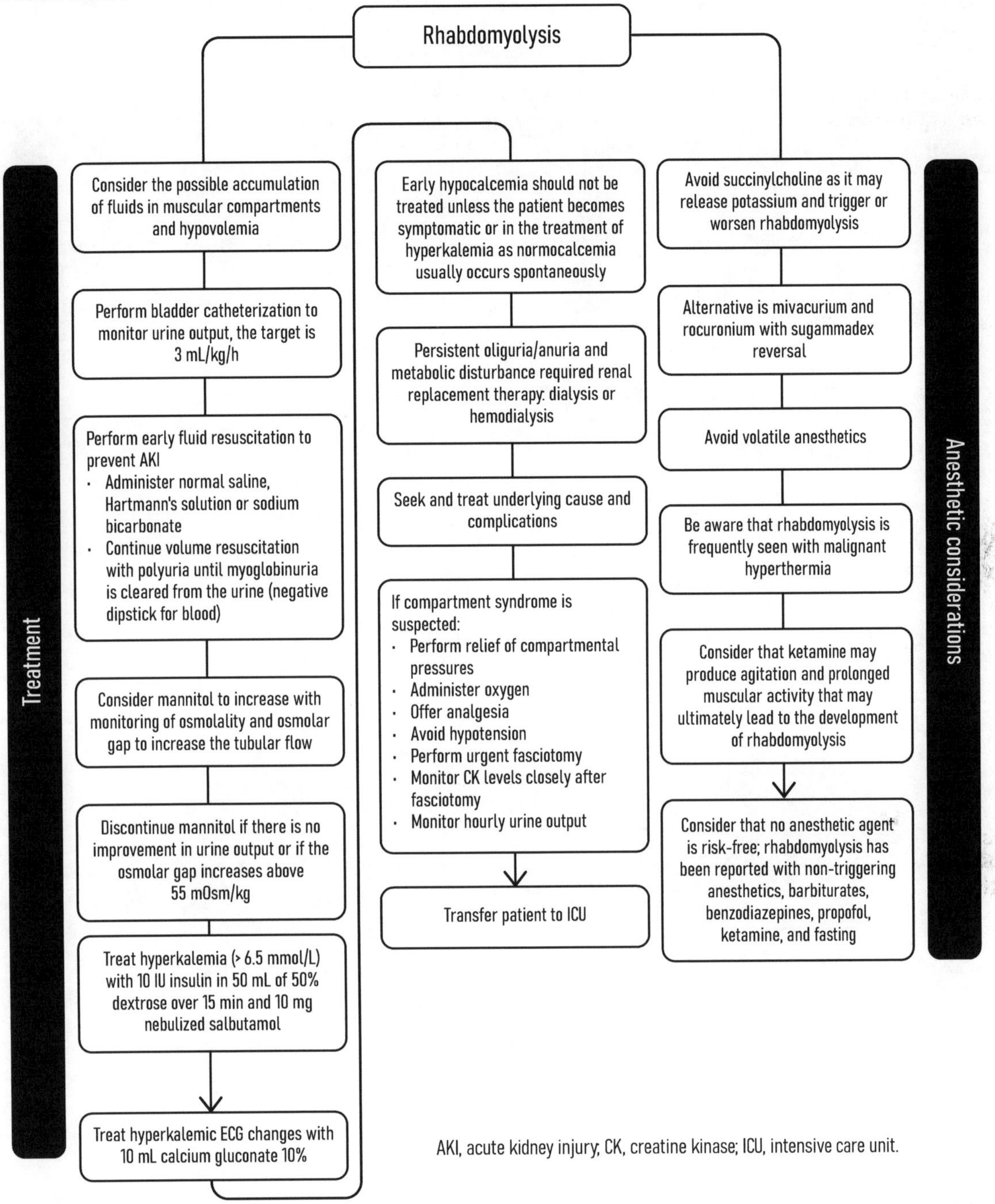
Rhabdomyolysis
Treatment
Consider the possible accumulation of fluids in muscular compartments and hypovolemia
Perform bladder catheterization to monitor urine output, the target is 3 mL/kg/h
Perform early fluid resuscitation to prevent AKI
· Administer normal saline, Hartmann's solution or sodium bicarbonate
· Continue volume resuscitation with polyuria until myoglobinuria is cleared from the urine (negative dipstick for blood)
Consider mannitol to increase with monitoring of osmolality and osmolar gap to increase the tubular flow
Discontinue mannitol if there is no improvement in urine output or if the osmolar gap increases above 55 mOsm/kg
Treat hyperkalemia (> 6.5 mmol/L) with 10 IU insulin in 50 mL of 50% dextrose over 15 min and 10 mg nebulized salbutamol
Treat hyperkalemic ECG changes with 10 mL calcium gluconate 10%
Early hypocalcemia should not be treated unless the patient becomes symptomatic or in the treatment of hyperkalemia as normocalcemia usually occurs spontaneously
Persistent oliguria/anuria and metabolic disturbance required renal replacement therapy: dialysis or hemodialysis
Seek and treat underlying cause and complications
If compartment syndrome is suspected:
· Perform relief of compartmental pressures
· Administer oxygen
· Offer analgesia
· Avoid hypotension
· Perform urgent fasciotomy
· Monitor CK levels closely after fasciotomy
· Monitor hourly urine output
Transfer patient to ICU
Anesthetic considerations
Avoid succinylcholine as it may release potassium and trigger or worsen rhabdomyolysis
Alternative is mivacurium and rocuronium with sugammadex reversal
Avoid volatile anesthetics
Be aware that rhabdomyolysis is frequently seen with malignant hyperthermia
Consider that ketamine may produce agitation and prolonged muscular activity that may ultimately lead to the development of rhabdomyolysis
Consider that no anesthetic agent is risk-free; rhabdomyolysis has been reported with non-triggering anesthetics, barbiturates, benzodiazepines, propofol, ketamine, and fasting

AKI, acute kidney injury; CK, creatine kinase; ICU, intensive care unit.

## SUGGESTED READING


- Floridis, J., Barbour, R., 2022. Postoperative weakness and anesthetic-associated rhabdomyolysis in a pediatric patient: a case report and review of the literature. Journal of Medical Case Reports 16.
- Hunter JD, Greggg K, Damani S. 2006. Rhabdomyolysis. Continuing Education in Anaesthesia Critical Care. 6;4:141-143.
- Pollard BJ, Kitchen, G. Handbook of Clinical Anaesthesia. Fourth Edition. CRC Press. 2018. 978-1-4987-6289-2.
- Torres PA, Helmstetter JA, Kaye AM, Kaye AD. Rhabdomyolysis: pathogenesis, diagnosis, and treatment. Ochsner J. 2015;15(1):58-69.
- Williams J, Thrope C. 2014. Rhabdomyolysis. Continuing Education in Anaesthesia Critical Care & Pain. 14;4:163-166.

# RHEUMATOID ARTHRITIS

## LEARNING OBJECTIVES

- Describe rheumatoid arthritis
- Recognize the symptoms and signs of rheumatoid arthritis
- Anesthetic management of a patient with rheumatoid arthritis

## DEFINITION AND MECHANISM

- Rheumatoid arthritis (RA) is a chronic autoimmune inflammatory disorder that mainly affects the synovial joints → symmetrical erosive polyarthropathy
- Early RA affects the smaller joints first (hands and feet)
- As RA progresses, symptoms spread to the wrists, knees, ankles, elbows, hips, and shoulders as well as the cervical spine
- Periods of increased disease activity (flares) alternate with periods of relative remission
- RA also affects other organs in more than 15-25% of the cases → systemic

## SIGNS AND SYMPTOMS

- Tender, warm, swollen joints
- Joint stiffness that is usually worse in the mornings and after inactivity
- Fatigue, fever, loss of appetite
- The painful swelling can eventually result in bone erosion and joint deformity

## RISK FACTORS

- Female gender
- Family history
- Increasing age
- Smoking
- Overweight

## COMPLICATIONS

- Osteoporosis
- Rheumatoid nodules
- Dry eyes and mouth (Sjogren's syndrome)
- Infections
- Abnormal body composition
- Carpal tunnel syndrome
- Cardiovascular disease
- Lung disease
- Lymphoma

## EXTRA-ARTICULAR MANIFESTATIONS

- **Neurological:** Central neuropathy, peripheral neuropathy (carpal tunnel syndrome), autonomic neuropathy
- **Ocular:** Kerato-conjuctivitis
- **Cardiovascular:** Pericarditis, pericardial effusion, cardiac tamponade, valvular heart disease (usually regurgitation), conduction abnormalities, granulomatous disease, endocarditis or myocarditis, coronary artery disease
- **Respiratory:** Reduced chest wall compliance (costochondral disease), pleural effusion, restrictive lung disease, pulmonary nodule

- **Hematological:** Anemia [chronic disease, iron deficiency (bleeding) and bone marrow suppression from medication], thrombocytopenia, Felty's syndrome, lymphoma
- **Hepatic:** Hepatic fibrosis, hepatomegaly with splenomegaly, hypoalbuminemia
- **Renal:** Glomerulonephritis, tubulointerstitial nephritis, amyloidosis
- **Skin:** Fragile skin, pyoderma gangrenosum, Sicca syndrome, scleritis, scleromalacia perforans
- **Musculoskeletal:** Osteoporosis

## TREATMENT

- **Medications:** Relieve pain, reduce inflammation, slow down the progression of RA
  - **Non-steroidal anti-inflammatory drugs (NSAIDs):** Ibuprofen and naproxen
  - **Corticosteroids:** Prednisone
  - **Conventional disease-modifying anti-rheumatic drugs (DMARDs):** Methotrexate, leflunomide, hydroxychloroquine, and sulfasalazine
  - **Biological DMARDs:** Abatacept, adalimumab, anakinra, certolizumab, etanercept, golimumab, infliximab, rituximab, sarilumab, and tocilizumab
  - **Targeted synthetic DMARDs:** Baricitinib, tofacitinib, and upadacitinib
- **Physical therapy:** To reduce pain and stiffness

- **Surgery:** Repair damaged joints to restore function and reduce pain
  - Synovectomy
  - Tendon repair
  - Joint fusion
  - Total joint replacement

# MANAGEMENT

RHEUMATOID ARTHRITIS

**Preoperative management**

- Evaluate RA disease severity and duration, systemic involvement, and medication status
- Physical examination
  - Airway
  - Anatomical landmarks for regional anesthesia
  - Range of motion in the position-related joint for the surgery
- Rule out systemic disease and manage any existing abnormalities, especially cardiopulmonary
- Document preexisting neurological symptoms
- Continue or stop medication (see table)
  - Corticosteroid coverage
  - Thromboprophylaxis

**Intraoperative management**

- Potential for difficult airway and unstable c-spine due to temporomandibular joint involvement, cricoarytenoid arthritis, atlantoaxial instability, sub-axial subluxation, and/or bony and ligamentous destruction of the lower cervical vertebrae (C3-C7) causing instability and/or spinal stenosis
- Establish a safe airway with preservation of c-spine integrity
  - Careful positioning
  - Minimize c-spine manipulation
  - Avoid excessive neck extension and forcible neck movements
- The use of laryngeal mask airway can exacerbate laryngeal rheumatoid arthritis, which may be undiagnosed prior to surgery. This possibility must be included in the differential diagnosis in the setting of acute upper airway obstruction particularly following extubation
- Aseptic technique and appropriate antibiotic prophylaxis
- Monitor for systemic disorder
  - Carefully monitor cardiovascular and respiratory systems
  - Increased risk of blood transfusion
  - Change of pharmacokinetics and pharmacodynamics

**Postoperative management**

- Closely monitor airway and breathing status and prepare for emergency airway management
- Perform standard breathing exercises to prevent respiratory problems
- Control postoperative pain to allow for early recovery and mobilization
- Infection control

**Obstetric anesthesia**

- Vaginal delivery is preferred over Cesarean section (only for obstetrical indications)
- Regional anesthesia if platelets are within normal limits
- Document preexisting injuries
- Cautious airway management in case of GA

*Recommendations on how to deal with RA medications during elective surgical procedures*

| Medication | Administration during surgical procedure |
|---|---|
| Corticosteroids | See next table |
| Conventional DMARDs | Continue |
| Biological DMARDs | Withhold before surgery and schedule surgery at the end of the dosing cycle |
| Targeted synthetic DMARDs | Withhold at least 3 to 7 days prior to surgery depending on the drug |

*Recommended steroid doses during surgery*

| Type of surgery | Endogeneous cortisol secretion rate | Examples | Recommended steroid dosing |
|---|---|---|---|
| Superficial | 8-10 mg/day (baseline) | Dental surgery, biopsy EGD, colonoscopy | Usual daily dose |
| Minor | 50 mg/day | Inguinal hernia, uterine curettage, hand surgery | Usual daily dose plus hydrocortisone 50 mg IV before incision + hydrocortisone 25 mg IV every 8 hrs for 1 day + usual daily dose |
| Moderate | 75-150 mg/day | Low extremity revascularization, total joint replacement, cholecystectomy, colon cancer, abdominal hysterectomy | Usual daily dose plus hydrocortisone 50 mg IV before incision + hydrocortisone 25 mg IV every 8 hrs for 1 day + usual daily dose |
| Major | 75-150 mg/day | Esophagectomy, total proctocolectomy, major cardiac/vascular surgery, hepaticojejenostomy, delivery, trauma | Usual daily dose plus hydrocortisone 100 mg IV before incision + continuous IV infusion of hydrocortisone 200 mg for > 1 day or hydrocortisone 50 mg IV every 8 hours/day + taper dose by half/day until usual daily dose reached and continuous IV fluids with 5% dextrose and 0.2-0.45% sodium chloride, based on degree of hypoglycemia |

## KEEP IN MIND

- Carefully perform a preoperative evaluation to prevent complications and minimize injury
- Anesthetic management strategies should consider RA-related systemic problems
- Individualize postoperative management

## SUGGESTED READING

- Chilkoti GT, Singh A, Mohta M, Saxena AK. Perioperative "stress dose" of corticosteroid: Pharmacological and clinical perspective. J Anaesthesiol Clin Pharmacol. 2019;35(2):147-152.
- Kim HR, Kim SH. Perioperative and anesthetic management of patients with rheumatoid arthritis. Korean J Intern Med. 2022;37(4):732-739.
- Krause ML, Matteson EL. Perioperative management of the patient with rheumatoid arthritis. World J Orthop. 2014;5(3):283-291.
- Samanta R, Shoukrey K, Griffiths R. Rheumatoid arthritis and anaesthesia. Anaesthesia. 2011;66(12):1146-1159.

Rheumatoid arthritis

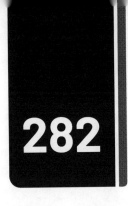

# SCLERODERMA

## LEARNING OBJECTIVES

- Describe scleroderma
- Recognize the symptoms and signs of scleroderma
- Anesthetic management of a patient with scleroderma

## DEFINITION AND MECHANISM

- Scleroderma or systemic sclerosis (SSc) is a systemic, immune-mediated disease characterized by abnormal cutaneous and organ-based fibrosis, resulting in hardening and tightening of the skin, and progressive end-organ dysfunction
- SSc is characterized by increased synthesis of collagen (leading to sclerosis), damage to small blood vessels, activation of T lymphocytes, and production of altered connective tissue

## SIGNS, SYMPTOMS, AND COMPLICATIONS

- **Cardiovascular:** Raynaud's phenomenon, healed pitting ulcers on the fingertips, skin and mucosal telangiectasis, palpitations, irregular heart rate, fainting due to conduction abnormalities, hypertension, and congestive heart failure (CHD)
- **Pulmonary:** Progressive worsening of dyspnea, chest pain (due to pulmonary hypertension), and dry, persistent cough due to interstitial lung disease (ILD)
- **Digestive:** Gastroesophageal reflux disease (GERD), bloating, indigestion, loss of appetite, diarrhea alternating with constipation, sicca syndrome and its complications, loosening of teeth, and hoarseness (due to acid reflux)
- **Musculoskeletal:** Joint and muscle aches, loss of joint range of motion, carpal tunnel syndrome, calcinosis, and weight loss
- **Genitourinary:** Erectile dysfunction, kidney failure
- **Other:** Facial pain due to trigeminal neuralgia, hand paresthesias, headache, stroke, and fatigue
- **Cancer:** Increased risk of developing malignancy in SSc patients with breast, lung and hematologic subtypes most prevalent

## RISK FACTORS

- Family history
- Certain genetic factors
- Gender: Occurs more in women than in men
- Exposure to silica, viruses, medications, and drugs

## TREATMENT

There is no treatment that can cure or stop the overproduction of collagen, which is characteristic of SSc. Treatment mainly focuses on controlling symptoms and preventing complications.

- **Raynaud's phenomenon:** Vasodilators (e.g., calcium channel blockers, α-blockers, serotonin receptor antagonists, angiotensin II receptor inhibitors, statins, local nitrates, or iloprost)
- **Digital ulcers:** Phosphodiesterase-5-inhibitors or iloprost
- **Prevention of new digital ulcers:** Bosentan
- **Malnutrition:** Tetracycline antibiotics
- **Interstitial lung disease:** Cyclophosphamide, azathioprine with or without corticosteroids
- **Pulmonary arterial hypertension:** Endothelin receptor antagonists, phosphodiesterase-5-inhibitors, and prostanoids
- **Gastroesophageal reflux disease:** Antacids or prokinetics
- **Kidney crises:** Angiotensin-converting enzyme inhibitors and angiotensin II receptor antagonists

Scleroderma

# MANAGEMENT

*Preoperative risk identification and stratification*

- Airway
  - Microstomia
  - Limited cervical extension
- Neurological
  - Peripheral neuropathies (paresthesias, numbness)
  - Autonomic dysfunction risk factors (orthostatic hypotension)
- Pulmonary hypertension risk factors (dyspnea, increased PASP, RVSP)
  - Progressive cardiomyopathy (TTE)
  - Conduction abnormalities (ECG)
- ILD risk factors
  - DLCO < 50%
  - CRP $\geq$ 5 or ESR $\geq$ 20
  - Decreased 6-minute walk test
- Sleep-disordered breathing risk (apnea, daytime somnolence)
  - STOP-Bang questionnaire
  - Sleep study findings
- Esophageal dilation: GERD symptoms
- Malnutrition
  - Pseudo-obstruction
  - Presence of sarcopenia
- Venous thromboembolic disease risk factors
  - SSc diagnosis < 12 months
  - Atrial fibrillation
  - CHD
- Anemia: Preoperative complete blood count

*Intraoperative risk mitigation*

- Difficult airway preparedness
- Aspiration chemoprophylaxis
- Appropriate padding and positioning
- Availability of ultrasound for difficult intravenous access
- Cardiac monitoring: Arterial line, possible TEE, PA catheter
- Lung protective ventilation strategy
- Minimize adverse drug interactions
- Ensure adequate prophylactic anticoagulation

*Postoperative complication surveillance*

- Sleep-disordered breathing: Continuous postoperative pulse oximetry
- Increased myocardial infarction: Continuous postoperative telemetry
- ILD deterioration: Presence of increased oxygen requirements > 24 hours after surgery; consider early workup for postoperative pneumonia or exacerbation of ILD
- Venous thromboembolic disease: Surveillance in surgery, trauma, and those administered glucocorticoids
- SSc renal crisis: Refractory HTN, encephalopathy, CHF

PASP, pulmonary arterial systolic pressure; RVSP, right ventricular systolic pressure; TTE, transthoracic echocardiogram; DLCO, diffusing capacity of the lungs for carbon monoxide; CRP, C-reactive protein; ESR, erythrocyte sedimentation rate; GERD, gastroesophageal reflux disease; CHD, congenital heart disease; HTN, hypertension; CHF, congestive heart failure.

# KEEP IN MIND

- Patients with SSc often have well-compensated mechanisms for their underlying disease, which may be unmasked with anesthetic interventions
- Anticipate a difficult airway and the potential risk of aspiration
- SSc patients are at risk for postoperative myocardial infarction, and prolonged mechanical ventilation may result in substantial morbidity, specifically in patients with interstitial lung disease

## ■ SUGGESTED READING ■

- Bernal-Bello D, de Tena JG, Guillén-Del Castillo A, et al. Novel risk factors related to cancer in scleroderma. Autoimmun Rev. 2017;16(5):461-468.
- Carr ZJ, Klick J, McDowell BJ, Charchaflieh JG, Karamchandani K. An Update on Systemic Sclerosis and its Perioperative Management. Curr Anesthesiol Rep. 2020;10:512-521.
- Denton CP, Khanna D. Systemic sclerosis. Lancet. 2017;390(10103):1685-1699.
- Efrimescu CI, Donnelly S, Buggy DJ. Systemic sclerosis. Part II: perioperative considerations. BJA Educ. 2023;23(3):101-109.

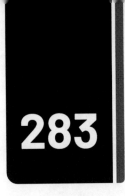

# SJOGREN'S SYNDROME

## LEARNING OBJECTIVES

- Describe Sjogren's syndrome
- Recognize the symptoms and signs of Sjogren's syndrome
- Anesthetic management of a patient with Sjogren's syndrome

## DEFINITION AND MECHANISM

- Sjogren's syndrome is a frequent autoimmune disease (autosomal recessive disorder) characterized by dysfunction and destruction of exocrine glands (e.g., lacrimal and salivary glands), associated with lymphocytic infiltrates and immunological hyperreactivity
- The hallmark symptoms of Sjogren's syndrome are dry eyes and a dry mouth
- The condition often accompanies other immune system disorders (e.g., rheumatoid arthritis, systemic lupus erythematosus, and multiple sclerosis)
- An incidence of 0.3-2.7% in the general population (primary syndrome), however, mostly affects women (female:male ratio is 9:1)

## SIGNS AND SYMPTOMS

- Dry eyes (keratoconjunctivitis sicca)
- Dry mouth (xerostomia)
- Joint pain, swelling, and stiffness
- Swollen salivary glands
- Skin rashes or dry skin (xeroderma)
- Vaginal dryness
- Chronic dry cough
- Prolonged fatigue
- Thyroid problems

## CAUSES

- **Genetic factors:** Mutations in HLA-DR and HLA-DQ genes
- **Environmental factors:** Viruses (e.g., Epstein-Barr virus, hepatitis C, and human T-cell leukemia virus type 1), hormones (e.g., estrogen, prolactin), etc.

## COMPLICATIONS

- Dental cavities
- Yeast infections
- Vision problems: Light sensitivity, blurred vision, and corneal damage
- Lymphoma
- Inflammation can cause pneumonia, bronchitis, or other problems in the lungs; lead to problems with kidney function; and cause hepatitis or cirrhosis of the liver
- Peripheral neuropathy (numbness, tingling, and burning of the hands and feet)

## RISK FACTORS

- Age > 40 years
- Female gender
- Rheumatic disease (i.e., rheumatoid arthritis or lupus)

# PATHOPHYSIOLOGY

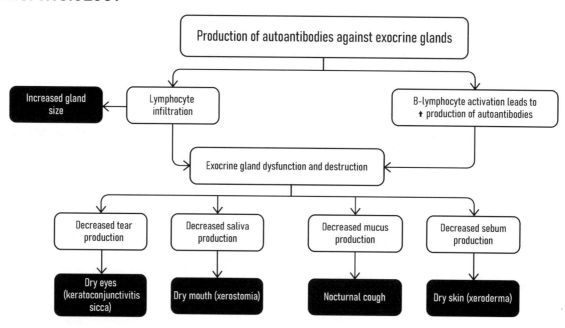

# TREATMENT

- Medications
  - Decrease eye inflammation (artificial tears): Cyclosporine or lifitegrast
  - Increase production of saliva (and sometimes tears): Pilocarpine and cevimeline
  - Address specific complications: NSAIDs or other arthritis medications, antifungal medications for yeast infections
- Surgery to seal the nasolacrimal ducts that drain tears from the eyes

# MANAGEMENT

### Preoperative management

- Complete medical history: Evolution and symptomatology of the disease
- Thorough physical examination
- Continue chronic therapy until the morning of surgery

### Intraoperative management

- Goal: Humidify the mucous membranes rigorously during the anesthetic procedure
- Lubricate the eyes to prevent corneal damage
- Avoid respiratory dryness by using humidified oxygen
- Suction efficiently to prevent mucous plugs
- Avoid parasympatholytic and anticholinergic drugs due to their decrease in gland secretions
- The administration of anesthetic agents, hypnotics and local anesthetics must be done slowly and in presence of blood pressure monitoring because of the possibility of autonomic nervous system dysfunction

### Postoperative management

- No increased risk for postoperative complications

## SUGGESTED READING

- Brito-Zerón, P., Baldini, C., Bootsma, H. et al. Sjögren syndrome. Nat Rev Dis Primers 2, 16047 (2016).
- Negrini, S., Emmi, G., Greco, M. et al. Sjögren's syndrome: a systemic autoimmune disease. Clin Exp Med 22, 9–25 (2022).
- Sjögren Syndrome. In: Bissonnette B, Luginbuehl I, Marciniak B, Dalens BJ. eds. Syndromes: Rapid Recognition and Perioperative Implications. Mgraw Hill; 2006. Accessed February 20, 2023. https://accessanesthesiology.mhmedical.com/content.aspx?bookid=852&sectionid=49518220

Sjogren's syndrome

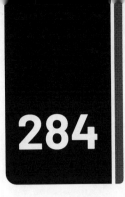

# STEVENS-JOHNSON SYNDROME

## LEARNING OBJECTIVES

- Describe Stevens-Johnson syndrome
- Understand the course of Stevens-Johnson syndrome
- Anesthetic management of a patient with Stevens-Johnson syndrome

## DEFINITION AND MECHANISM

- Stevens-Johnson syndrome (SJS) is a rare and acute exfoliating disease of the skin and mucous membranes with systemic manifestations of variable severity
- SJS is a delayed-type hypersensitivity reaction in which SJS-inducing drugs or their metabolites stimulate cytotoxic T cells (i.e., CD8+ T cells) or T helper cells (i.e., CD4+ T cells) to initiate autoimmune responses
- The initial lesions of SJS are diffuse erythematous macules with purpuric, necrotic centers, and overlying blisters that may progress to skin shedding, resulting in widespread superficial ulcers and loss of the epidermal barrier ➜ fluid and protein loss ➜ fluid and electrolyte imbalance with hypoproteinemia

## SIGNS AND SYMPTOMS

One to three days before a rash develops, early signs of SJS include
- Fever
- A sore mouth and throat
- Fatigue
- Burning, red eyes

As the condition develops, other signs and symptoms include
- Unexplained widespread skin pain
- A red or purple rash that spreads
- Blisters on the skin and mucous membranes of the mouth, nose, eyes, and genitals
- Shedding of skin within days after blisters form

## CAUSES

- Infections (e.g., pneumonia and HIV)
- Drug-induced
  - Anti-gout medications (e.g., allopurinol)
  - Medications to treat seizures and mental illness (e.g., anticonvulsants and antipsychotics)
  - Antibacterial sulfonamides (e.g., sulfasalazine)
  - Antiretroviral therapy, e.g., nevirapine
  - Analgesics (e.g., acetaminophen, ibuprofen, and naproxen sodium)
- Malignancy-related
- Idiopathic

## RISK FACTORS

- HIV infection
- Weakened immune system: Organ transplant patients, HIV/AIDS, and autoimmune disease (e.g., systemic lupus erythematosus)
- Cancer: Particularly blood cancer
- History of SJS
- Family history of SJS
- Genetic factors

## COMPLICATIONS

- Dehydration
- Sepsis
- Eye problems (e.g., eye inflammation, dry eyes, and light sensitivity)
- Pneumonia
- Acute respiratory failure
- Permanent skin damage
- Multiple organ failure

# TREATMENT

- Treatment requires hospitalization, in an ICU or burn unit
- Stop nonessential medications → stop taking SJS-inducing drugs
- Fluid replacement and nutrition
- Wound care
- Eye care
- Temperature management

- Medications
  - Pain medications to reduce discomfort
  - Medication to reduce inflammation of the eyes and mucous membranes (e.g., topical steroids)
  - Antibiotics to control infection, when needed
  - Other oral or IV medications (e.g., corticosteroids, intravenous immunoglobulin therapy)

# MANAGEMENT

- Maintain skin and mucous membrane integrity
  - Minimize handling and transfer of patients to prevent further epithelial damage or rupture of bullae
- Safe airway management
  - Mucous membranes of the respiratory tract and pleura may be involved
  - Ulcers in the nose, oropharynx, trachea, and bronchi increase the risk of hematemesis
  - Avoid manipulation and trauma to the oral, tracheal, and laryngeal mucosa (lesions are often present)
  - Avoid desquamation of the skin on the face during mask pre-oxygenation
- Difficulties getting venous access, application of monitors and anesthesia face masks, airways, laryngoscopy, and intubation
  - Establish access over areas of normal epidermis
  - Use invasive BP monitoring
  - Use one smaller than the standard size for laryngeal mask airways and because of the risk of airway swelling
- Adhere to strict aseptic precautions at all stages (immune-compromised state and susceptibility to respiratory infection due to disruption of skin barrier and mucous membranes)
- Induction with etomidate or ketamine could provide better hemodynamic stability when compared to propofol or thiopental
- Avoid succinylcholine due to risk of hyperkalemia and use non-depolarizing muscle relaxants instead
- Fluid and electrolyte replacement
- Avoid hypothermia
  - OR temperature 28°C
  - Warm IV fluids
  - Water mattresses/forced air-warmers
- Adequate postoperative analgesia

# KEEP IN MIND

- Proper preoperative evaluation, identification of the precipitating agents in order to avoid them, a continuation of preoperative medications, and other immunosuppressants or steroids is essential
- Extreme care should be taken while transferring patients with fresh lesions
- Patients with involvement of the respiratory tract and pleura require special attention, including the application of a face mask, laryngoscopy, intubation, and suction with extra lubrication when general anesthesia is chosen
- Anesthetic drugs can be safely used in SJS patients
- Note that fluid requirements are much higher win case of major skin lesions due to insensible perspiration

# SUGGESTED READING

- Ramsali MV, Puduchira KG, Maganti SP, Vankaylapatti SD, Pasupuleti S, Kulkarni D. Anesthetic management and outcomes of patients with Steven-Johnson Syndrome-A retrospective review study. J Anaesthesiol Clin Pharmacol. 2021;37(1):119-123.
- Kwass WK, Chow J. Anesthetic Management in Stevens-Johnson syndrome: Case Report. Integr Anesthesiol. 2019;2(1):001-004.

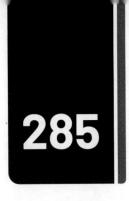

# 285

# SYSTEMIC LUPUS ERYTHEMATOSUS

## LEARNING OBJECTIVES

- Describe systemic lupus erythematosus
- Understand the potential complications associated with systemic lupus erythematosus
- Anesthetic management of a patient with systemic lupus erythematosus

## DEFINITION AND MECHANISM

- Systemic lupus erythematosus (SLE) is a chronic autoimmune connective tissue disorder with a heterogeneous presentation and systemic involvement in which tissues and multiple organs are damaged by pathogenic autoantibodies and immune complexes
- There are often periods of illness (flares) and periods of remission during which there are few symptoms

## SIGNS AND SYMPTOMS

- Fatigue
- Fever
- Joint pain, stiffness, and swelling
- Butterfly-shaped rash on the face that covers the cheeks and bridge of the nose or rashes elsewhere on the body
- Skin lesions that appear or worsen with sun exposure
- Fingers and toes that turn white or blue when exposed to cold or during stressful periods and Raynaud's phenomenon
- Shortness of breath
- Chest pain
- Dry eyes
- Photosensitivity
- Headaches, confusion, and memory loss
- Hair loss
- Mouth ulcers
- Swollen lymph nodes

## RISK FACTORS

- Gender: Female > male
- Age: 15-45 years
- Race: More common in African, Asian and Hispanic patients

## CAUSES

SLE is probably caused by a genetic susceptibility coupled with an environmental trigger, resulting in a defect in the immune system
- **Genetics:** Mutations in HLA-DR2/HLA-DR3 genes, complement genes, cytokine genes, etc.
- **Environmental:** UV-light (UV-A, UV-B), viruses (e.g., EBV, CMV, retroviruses), drugs (e.g., minocycline, hydralazine, procainamide), hormones (e.g., estrogen, prolactin), heavy metals

## COMPLICATIONS

- **Dermatologic:** Malar rash, chronic discoid lesions
- **Brain and central nervous system:** Headaches, dizziness, behavior changes, vision problems, strokes or seizures
- **Cardiovascular:** Symptomatic pericarditis, pericardial tamponade, myocarditis, Libman-Sacks endocarditis, valvular dysfunction, Raynaud's phenomenon
- **Pulmonary:** Pleuritis, pneumonitis, diffuse alveolar hemorrhage, pulmonary arterial hypertension
- **Renal:** Lupus nephritis, end-stage renal disease
- **Hematology:** Anemia of chronic disease, autoimmune hemolytic anemia, autoimmune thrombocytopenia
- **Gastrointestinal:** Oral ulcers, Sjogren's syndrome, dysphagia, acute abdominal pain, abnormal liver function tests, autoimmune hepatitis
- **Musculoskeletal:** Arthritis, osteoporosis, fractures, asymptomatic atlantoaxial subluxation
- **Infection:** SLE and treatment can weaken the immune system
- **Pregnancy complications:** Increased risk of miscarriage, high blood pressure during pregnancy, and preterm birth

Systemic lupus erythematosus

# PATHOPHYSIOLOGY

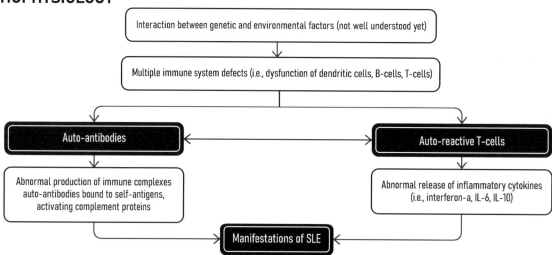

# TREATMENT

| Drug | Indication | Anesthetic implications |
|------|-----------|------------------------|
| Aspirin/NSAIDs (ibuprofen, naproxen sodium) | Antiphospholipid syndrome<br>SLE arthritis | Peptic ulceration<br>Platelet inhibition<br>Renal impairment<br>Fluid retention/electrolyte disturbance<br>Hepatic dysfunction<br>Bronchospasm |
| Antimalarial drugs (hydroxychloroquine) | Cutaneous SLE<br>Pleuritis/pericarditis<br>Arthritis<br>Reduced renal flares | Retinotoxicity<br>Neuromyotoxicity<br>Cardiotoxicity |
| Corticosteroids (prednisone, methylprednisone, topical preparation) | Cutaneous SLE<br>Nephritis<br>Pleuritis/pericarditis<br>Diffuse alveolar hemorrhage<br>Neuropsychiatric SLE<br>Mesenteric vasculitis<br>SLE pancreatitis | Hyperglycemia<br>Hypercholesterolemia<br>Hypertension<br>Osteoporosis |
| **Immunosuppressants** | | |
| Cyclophosphamide | Nephritis<br>Neuropsychiatric SLE | Myelosuppression<br>Pseudocholinesterase inhibition<br>Cardiotoxicity<br>Leucopenia<br>Hemorrhagic cystitis |
| Azathioprine | Arthritis | Myelosuppression<br>Hepatotoxicity |
| Methotrexate | Arthritis<br>Cutaneous SLE | Myelosuppression<br>Hepatic fibrosis/cirrhosis<br>Pulmonary infiltrates/fibrosis |
| Mycophenolate mofetil | Nephritis<br>Hemolytic anemia, thrombocytopenia | GI upset<br>Pancytopenia |

Systemic lupus erythematosus

# MANAGEMENT

## *Preoperative management*

- **History:** Review disease activity index, accrued organ damage, and drug history
- **Examination:** Thorough examination of cardiovascular, respiratory, and neurological systems, including testing for atlantoaxial subluxation symptoms and signs or with an X-ray
- **Full blood count:** Test for anemia, thrombocytopenia, and leucopenia; consider further testing for hemolysis if anemia is present
- **Serum electrolytes, creatinine, urea:** Any abnormality requires further investigation for lupus nephritis
- **Liver function tests:** Abnormalities should prompt review for autoimmune or drug hepatotoxicity
- **Coagulation studies:** Elevated aPTT requires investigation for the presence of lupus anticoagulant
- **Anti-dsDNA, complement levels:** May reflect lupus activity after comparison with previous baseline measurements
- **Urinalysis:** Proteinuria, red cells, white cells, and cellular casts may indicate clinically silent disease and prompt further investigation
- **ECG:** Silent ischemia, myocarditis, pericarditis, and conduction abnormalities may be identified
- **Chest radiograph:** Pleural effusion, interstitial pneumonitis, pericardial effusion, or subglottic stenosis may be seen

## *Intraoperative management*

- **5-lead ECG:** Accelerated coronary artery disease, conduction abnormalities
- **Intra-arterial blood pressure monitoring:** Case-dependent, consider in the presence of myocarditis, conduction abnormalities, valvular abnormalities, or autonomic dysfunction
- **Laryngeal mask airway if appropriate:** Minimize airway manipulation due to the risk of inflammation and post-extubation airway edema
- **Difficult airway precautions with immediate access to smaller-size endotracheal tubes:** Vocal cord paralysis, subglottic stenosis, or laryngeal edema may make intubation difficult
- **Standard antibiotic prophylaxis:** Innate susceptibility to infection and immunosuppressive therapy predispose to infection risk therefore maintain strict asepsis and temperature control
- **Caution with muscle relaxants:** Azathioprine and cyclophosphamide may interact with muscle relaxants (azathioprine lowers the effectivity of rocuronium and cisatracurium while azathioprine and cyclophosphamide increase the potency of succinylcholine)
- **Renal protective strategies:** Maintain urine output, avoid hypoperfusion and hypotensive states, and use nephrotoxic drugs cautiously due to the possibility of subclinical lupus nephritis
- **Careful patient positioning:** Predisposition to peripheral neuropathies and osteoporosis
- **Antithrombotic prophylaxis:** Institute mechanical and pharmacological measures early, especially in the presence of antiphospholipid antibodies
- **Eye protection and artificial tears/lubrication:** Sjogren's syndrome may predispose to corneal abrasions despite adequate eye taping
- **Temperature monitoring:** Hypothermic state may induce vasospasm and may also increase the risk of infections, in patients with Raynaud's phenomenon
- **Pain management:** Consider side effects of systemic analgesics; regional techniques may be helpful if neuropathies, myelitis, and coagulopathies are excluded
- **Corticosteroid cover:** Adrenal suppression may have resulted from long-term corticosteroid therapy with the need for a "stress dose" perioperatively

## *Postoperative management*

- **Pain management:** Minimize systemic side effects

# KEEP IN MIND

- The anesthetic plan must be individualized based on the preoperative evaluation, degree of involvement of various systems, current medications, and laboratory results, but also on the magnitude of the expected surgery

## SUGGESTED READING

- Ameer MA, Chaudhry H, Mushtaq J, et al. An Overview of Systemic Lupus Erythematosus (SLE) Pathogenesis, Classification, and Management. Cureus. 2022;14(10):e30330.
- Erez BM. Systemic Lupus Erythematosus: A Review for Anesthesiologists. Anesthesia & Analgesia. 2010;111(3):665-676.
- Kaul, A., Gordon, C., Crow, M. et al. Systemic lupus erythematosus. Nat Rev Dis Primers 2, 16039 (2016).

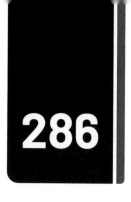

# GRANULOMATOSIS WITH POLYANGIITIS

**286**

## LEARNING OBJECTIVES

- Describe Granulomatosis with polyangiitis
- Recognize the symptoms and signs of Granulomatosis with polyangiitis
- Anesthetic management of a patient with Granulomatosis with polyangiitis

## DEFINITION AND MECHANISM

- Granulomatosis with polyangiitis (GPA) is a chronic, immunologic, systemic disease, characterized by a triad of necrotizing granulomas in the upper and lower respiratory tract, small- and medium-sized vessel vasculitis, and glomerulonephritis
- Involvement of the upper respiratory tract (i.e., nose and sinuses) is seen in nearly all GPA patients
- Early diagnosis and treatment might lead to a full recovery
- Without treatment, the condition can be fatal

## SIGNS AND SYMPTOMS

Signs and symptoms develop suddenly or over several months
- Pus-like drainage with crusts from the nose, stuffiness, sinus infections, and nosebleeds
- Coughing, sometimes with bloody phlegm
- Shortness of breath or wheezing
- Fever
- Fatigue
- Joint pain

- Numbness in the limbs, fingers, or toes
- Weight loss
- Hematuria
- Skin sores, bruising, or rashes
- Eye redness, burning or pain, and vision problems
- Ear inflammation and hearing problems

## COMPLICATIONS

- Hearing loss
- Skin scarring
- Chronic kidney disease
- A loss of height in the bridge of the nose (saddling) caused by weakened cartilage
- Deep vein thrombosis

## TREATMENT

Combination of corticosteroids and cytotoxic agents to induce and maintain remission

| Severe disease | Induce remission with immunosuppressants (e.g., rituximab or cyclophosphamide) in combination with high-dose corticosteroids (e.g., prednisone)<br>Plasmapheresis if kidneys are involved<br>Steroid dose is tapered slowly after remission → focus shifts to maintain remission state and prevent subsequent GPA flares → less toxic immunosuppressants (e.g., rituximab, methotrexate, azathioprine, leflunomide, or mycophenolate) |
|---|---|
| Limited disease | Combination of methotrexate and corticosteroids<br>Steroid dose is reduced after remission and methotrexate is continued as maintenance therapy |

# MANAGEMENT

```
                    ┌─────────────────────────────────────────┐
                    │   GRANULOMATOSIS WITH POLYANGIITIS        │
                    └─────────────────────────────────────────┘
```

| Preoperative management | Intraoperative management | Postoperative management |

**Preoperative management**

- Indirect laryngoscopy to rule out involvement of the larynx and upper airway and potential subglottis stenosis
- Complete examination of the lungs and kidneys to evaluate their involvement: Chest X-ray, chest CECT, and renal function profile
- Corticosteroid coverage → administer IV hydrocortisone → prolonged steroid therapy in GPA patients is associated with an immunocompromised state, increased risk of infection, easy bruisability, gastrointestinal bleeding and ulceration, decreased bone density, and hyperglycemia

**Intraoperative management**

- Anticipate a difficult airway due to laryngeal stenosis, subglottic stenosis, tracheal stenosis, and friable bleeding tissue and have a difficult airway cart available
- Careful airway management (i.e., laryngoscopy and intubation), avoid repeated attempts → can lead to bleeding from the granulomas or migration of the ulcerated tissue down into the trachea or larynx, causing airway compromise
- Anticipate a difficult ventilation due to pulmonary infiltrates and nodules, cavities, hemorrhage, and rarely bronchial stenosis
- Maintain a stable hemodynamic status, avoid variations in heart rate and blood pressure → can lead to myocardial ischemia or infarct
- Minimize the number of arterial and venous punctures due to vasculitis of peripheral veins and arteries → use ultrasound guidance
- Altered excretion of drugs, fluid, and electrolytes due to progressive kidney failure (75% of patients)
  - Loading doses of inducing agents remain the same
  - Maintenance doses of highly protein-bound agents will be lowered with 30-50%
  - Anesthetic agents depending on renal excretion: Vecuronium, pancuronium, atropine, glycopyrrolate, and neostigmine
  - Drugs producing active or toxic metabolites depending on renal excretion: Midazolam, diazepam, and morphine
- Use succinylcholine sparingly → cyclophosphamide inhibits pseudocholinesterase
- Determine adequate coagulation status and document neurologic deficits prior to regional anesthesia

**Postoperative management**

- More prone to develop airway edema after tracheal extubation, which may lead lead to airway obstruction
- IV dexamethasone to decrease postoperative airway and oral edema (be careful if hydrocorticoids as a stress dose are administered)

## SUGGESTED READING

- Frost EAM. Wegener's Granulomatosis, PHACE Syndrome: Rarities With Anesthetic Implications. December 20, 2018. Accessed January 26, 2023. https://anesthesiaexperts.com/uncategorized/wegeners-granulomatosis-phace-syndrome-rarities-anesthetic-implications/.
- Sharma J, Lal J, Gehlaut P, Amanpreet, Dhawan G, Yadav A. Wegener's Granulomatosis and Anaesthetic Implications: A Case Report. Int J Med Res Prof. 2018; 4(1): 479-81.

# ANESTHETIC TECHNIQUES

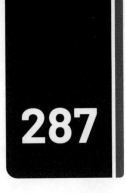

# BLIND NASAL INTUBATION

## LEARNING OBJECTIVES

- Describe the indications and contraindications for blind nasal intubation
- Describe the technique for blind nasal intubation
- Describe the possible repositioning actions and complications of blind nasal intubation

## DEFINITION AND MECHANISM

- Blind nasal intubation was originally used in spontaneously breathing patients anesthetized with an inhalational agent, but has been modified for intubating awake patients, with or without sedation
- Useful technique for patients with a difficult airway
- Has been largely replaced by fiber-optic intubation, but remains a relevant and easy alternative when a fiber-optic scope is not available or fiber-optic intubation has failed
- Indicated when there are structural abnormalities in the mouth or limited mouth opening

## INDICATIONS & CONTRAINDICATIONS

- Indications
  - Known difficult intubation or previous nasal intubation
  - Anticipated difficult intubation
  - Known or suspected difficult mask ventilation
  - Unstable C-spine

- Contraindications
  - Absolute
    - Patient refusal or inability to cooperate
  - Relative
    - Lack of trained personnel
    - Risk of impending airway obstruction
    - Coagulopathy or bleeding in airway
    - Allergy to local anesthetic
    - Base of skull fracture (as this poses an additional risk)

## TECHNIQUE

- Awake patients must be able to cooperate and respond to commands
- Adequate airway anesthesia is essential (4% lidocaine spray, nebulized lidocaine)
- Sedation and a topical vasoconstrictor will facilitate improved tolerance and reduce bleeding

**Preparation**
- Have all the necessary equipment and emergency medications available
- Gain IV access
- Have a trained assistant familiar with blind nasal intubation available
- Ensure that the patient is spontaneously breathing at all times

**Positioning**
Position the patient with the neck flexed and head extended at the atlantoaxial joint (sniffing position) (without neck manipulation in case of concern about C-spine stability)

Identify a suitable nostril (assess size, patency and history of epistaxis or polyps)

**Insertion procedure**
- Insert a well-lubricated 6-7 mm internal diameter nasotracheal tube, which has been softened in warm water
- Have the bevel face the septum to reduce trauma to the inferior turbinate

Direct the tube posteriorly along the floor of the nasal cavity, gentle pressure and twisting may be needed

While keeping the other nostril and mouth closed, gently advance the nasotracheal tube into the hypopharynx toward the glottis, taking care to stay in the midline

Listen for breath sounds as a guide to the position of the tube tip: As the tube approaches the glottis, breath sounds get louder and misting of the tube may occur

Once at the laryngeal inlet, ask the patient to take a deep inspiration to abduct the vocal cords and intubate the trachea in one smooth motion (transient coughing and a degree of laryngospasm suggests correct tube placement where gag reflex is still intact, and should quickly cease)

**Confirm tube position**
Confirm correct placement in the trachea (breath sounds through the tube, movement of the reservoir bag when connected to the breathing system, inability to phonate and capnography)

Inflate cuff and secure tube

Induce anesthesia in awake patients

- Clinical findings for tube repositioning to facilitate successful intubation:

| Position | Clinical findings | Action |
|---|---|---|
| Trachea | Breath sounds through tube maintained as it is advanced, coughing through tube | Confirm ETCO$_2$, bilateral air entry |
| Anterior | Breath sounds heard through tube but unable to advance further, bulge felt anteriorly at level of hyoid, coughing mostly through tube | Withdraw tube 2 cm, reduce neck extension or externally manipulate larynx before readvancing |
| Left/right piriform fossa | No breath sounds, unable to advance tube, no coughing, a bulge may be seen or palpated superior-lateral to larynx | Withdraw tube until breath sounds return, rotate tube to midline or turn head towards bulge and readvance |
| Esophagus | Tube advances smoothly with loss of breath sounds, no cough, larynx elevated | Withdraw tube until breath sounds return and try the following maneuvers before readvancing:<br>· Head extension<br>· Cricoid pressure<br>· Inflate cuff with 5-10 mL of air to direct the tip anteriorly. Advance until resistance met, ensure breath sounds retained (at laryngeal inlet), slowly deflate cuff while maintaining some advancing pressure on tube to enter trachea |

## COMPLICATIONS

- General complications:
  - Oversedation
  - Respiratory depression
  - Airway obstruction
  - Apnea
  - Trauma
  - Bleeding
  - Laryngospasm
  - Vomiting
  - Local anesthetic allergy
  - Toxicity
  - Risk of aspiration due to loss of laryngeal reflexes
- Specific complications related to nasal route
  - Epistaxis
  - Turbinate or polyp fracture
  - Retropharyngeal laceration
  - Retropharyngeal abscess and mediastinitis
  - Intracranial placement in basal skull fracture and pneumocephalus
- Specific complications related to blind technique:
  - Airway trauma from multiple intubation attempts
  - Obstruction caused by the epiglottis being pushed into the glottic opening
  - Esophageal intubation

## SUGGESTED READING

- Pollard BJ, Kitchen, G. Handbook of Clinical Anaesthesia. Fourth Edition. CRC Press. 2018. 978-1-4987-6289-2.

Blind nasal intubation

# CLOSED CIRCLE ANESTHESIA

## LEARNING OBJECTIVES

- Describe the purpose and composition of closed circle anesthesia
- Describe the technique and safety precautions of closed circle anesthesia
- Describe the advantages and disadvantages of closed circle anesthesia

## DEFINITION AND MECHANISM

- The current inhalational anesthetic agents with low blood solubility sparked renewed interest in closed circle anesthesia, due to their cost and environmental concerns
- The circle system's components are arranged in a circular manner
- The system allows rebreathing of anesthetic agents while avoiding rebreathing of $CO_2$
- This allows the use of low or minimal fresh gas flow

## SYSTEM COMPOSITION

- The circle system consists of:
  - Fresh gas flow (FGF)
  - Inspiratory and expiratory unidirectional valves
  - Inspiratory and expiratory tubing
  - Y-piece connector
  - Adjustable pressure limiting (APL) valve
  - Reservoir bag
  - $CO_2$ absorber
- The most efficient arrangement:
  - FGF enters the system before the inspiratory unidirectional valve
  - The APL valve and reservoir are situated between the expiratory valve and the $CO_2$ absorber
  - The $CO_2$ absorber is situated before the FGF entry point

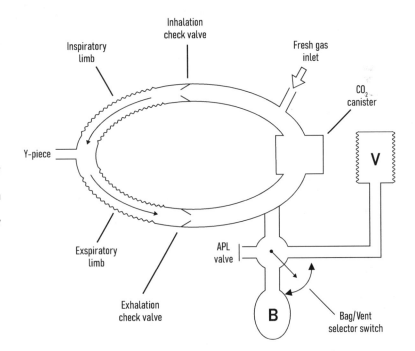

## DEFINITIONS

- Closed circle anesthesia:
  - FGF is just sufficient to replace the volume of gas and vapor absorbed by the patient (Basal oxygen requirements, volatile agent uptake, and nitrous oxide uptake if used)
  - No gas leaves through the APL valve
  - Exhaled gases are rebreathed after $CO_2$ absorption
- Low flow anesthesia
  - FGF < alveolar ventilation (usually < 1.5 L/min)
  - Excess gases are eliminated via the APL valve
- Ultra-low flow anesthesia
  - FGF < 0.5 L/min
  - Excess gases are eliminated via the APL valve

# TECHNIQUE

## ANESTHETIC AGENT ADMINISTRATION

- Vaporizers are usually outside of the circle
- Vaporizer in circuit (VIC): Low resistance to gas flow to minimize the work of breathing required for spontaneous breathing, allows vaporization of agent into recirculated gas already containing anesthetic agent

## PRINCIPLES OF LOW FLOW ANESTHESIA

- High fresh gas flow (FGF) is needed initially to denitrogenate the circle and functional residual capacity (FRC) (up to 15 min in closed circle anesthesia, 5 min in low flow anesthesia)
- Time constant for circle = Volume of circle system/FGF
- Side-stream/vapor monitors remove 150-200 mL/min from the system for analysis, these are returned to the system for ultra-low flow or closed circle anesthesia
- A ventilator with rising bellows is necessary which will collapse if there is a leak in the system
- FGF is intermittently increased to facilitate removal of accumulated undesired gases
- At the end of anesthesia, anesthetic agents are switched off and oxygen flow is increased to rapidly elminate the anesthetic agents

## VOLATILE REQUIREMENTS

- Components needed to calculate the dose of an anesthetic agent: Minimum alveolar concentration (MAC), amount of vapor needed to achieve MAC, amount of vapor required for uptake into the circulation, amount required for uptake into the tissues
- The ED95 dose of a volatile agent is achieved at concentrations of $\geq 1.3$ MAC
- Ventilation-priming dose = target concentration x (system volume + lung volume)/100 = mL in liquid phase of anesthetic vapor

## DENITROGENATION

- With a high initial FGF (10 L/min), > 95% of nitrogen is eliminated from the FRC and circle in ~5 min
- Nitrogen builds up slowly due to release by tissues

## $CO_2$ ABSORPTION

- Achieved with soda lime (94% calcium hydroxide, 2-5% sodium hydroxide, 0.2% silica, indicator dye and a zeolite) or baralyme (80% barium hydroxide and 20% barium octahydrate)
- Absorber granules are consumed more rapidly the lower the FGF used
- Avoid drying out the absorber to prevent carbon monoxide formation when using enflurane, isoflurane, or desflurane
- When Sevoflurane is used with carbon dioxide ($CO_2$) absorbents, particularly those containing strong bases like sodium hydroxide or potassium hydroxide, Compound A is formed (with potential toxic effects)

## CONTROL OF MOISTURE

- Condensation due to prolonged use can cause sticking of the one-way valves due to surface tension, potentially turning the entire volume of the system into dead space
- Can be avoided by using a hydrophobic filter at the end of the expiratory limb before the $CO_2$ absorber or by changing the breathing tubing between cases

## MONITORING

- Inspired and end tidal oxygen, $CO_2$, $N_2O$, and anesthetic agent
- Tidal volume
- Standard monitoring

# SAFETY

- Monitor inspired oxygen, end-tidal carbon dioxide, and inhalational agent
- Prevent unidirectional valves from sticking due to water vapor condensation
- Resistance to breathing is increased during spontaneous ventilation due to the unidirectional valves
- Prevent compound A formation (due to potential toxic effects): Newer designs of soda lime claim less or no production of compound A, baralyme is worse than soda lime, and Amsorb© is the safest
- Methane, acetone, ethanol, and hydrogen can accumulate but generally do not become clinically significant
- Uneven filling of the canister with soda lime leads to channeling of gases and reduced efficiency
- There is an increased risk for leaks and disconnection due to the many connections

# ADVANTAGES & DISADVANTAGES

| Advantages | Disadvantages |
|---|---|
| Economy of gases and inhalational agents | Need for expensive/advanced anesthesia stations |
| Humidification of the inspired gases + retention of heat | Accumulation of unwanted gases (less of a problem with modern systems) |
| Reduced atmospheric pollution | |

## SUGGESTED READING

- Herbert L, Magee P. Circle systems and low-flow anaesthesia. BJA Education. 2017;17(9):301-5.
- Pollard BJ, Kitchen, G. Handbook of Clinical Anaesthesia. Fourth Edition. CRC Press. 2018. 978-1-4987-6289-2.

Closed circle anesthesia

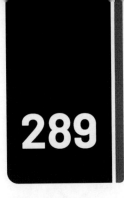

# FIBEROPTIC INTUBATION

## LEARNING OBJECTIVES

- Describe the principles, indications, and contraindications of fiberoptic intubation
- Perform fiberoptic intubation
- Describe the possible complications of fiberoptic intubation

## DEFINITION AND MECHANISM

- Fiberoptic intubation can be performed in awake (with or without sedation) or anesthetized patients
- Awake fiberoptic intubation is the gold standard for anticipated difficult airways
- Based on the optical characteristics of very thin flexible glass fibers that are capable of transmitting light over their length
- Insulation of these fibers by a glass layer with a different optical density facilitates transmission by the internal reflection of light
- In combination with a light source and lenses on both ends of the fiberoptic bronchoscope, images can be transmitted from the tip of the scope to the eyepiece

## INDICATIONS & CONTRAINDICATIONS

- Indications
  - Known difficult intubation or previous awake fiberoptic intubation
  - Anticipated difficult intubation
  - Known or suspected difficult mask ventilation
  - Unstable C-spine
  - Abnormal anatomy (congenital airway deformities, head and neck cancers)
  - Face/neck/upper airway trauma

- Contraindications
  - Absolute
    - Patient refusal or inability to cooperate
  - Relative
    - Lack of trained personnel
    - Risk of impending airway obstruction
    - Coagulopathy or bleeding in the airway
    - Allergy to local anesthetic
    - Base of skull fracture (for nasal route)

Fiberoptic intubation

# TECHNIQUE

*Fiberoptic intubation: preparation, sedation and anesthesia*

| **Preparation** | **Sedation** | **Local anesthesia** |
|---|---|---|

**Preparation**

- Ensure that all necessary equipment and emergency medications are available
- Two anesthesiologists (one to perform intubation, one to provide sedation) and a trained assistant familiar with fiberoptic intubation are required
- Gain IV access
- Monitoring throughout the procedure: ECG, pulse oximetry, noninvasive blood pressure, capnography, sedation level
- Administer glycopyrronium (400 μg IM or 200 μg IV), atropine, or hyoscine to reduce airway secretions

**Sedation**

- Conscious sedation improves patient comfort and cooperation, but is not essential
- If the airway is acutely compromized, avoid sedation as it may lead to complete obstruction

**Methods**

- Remifentanil: Target-controlled infusion at an effect site concentration of 1-5 ng/mL, as a sole agent or in conjunction with propofol or midazolam
- Propofol: Infusion or intermittent boluses, as a sole agent or in combination with fentanyl, remifentanil or midazolam (when used with a second agent by target-controlled infusion, an effect site concentration of 0.5-1 μg/mL is sufficient)
- Midazolam: 0.5-1 mg boluses to maximum of 0.05 mg/kg, usually in combination with an opioid
- Dexmedetomidine: Loading dose of 0.7-1 μg/kg over 10-20 minutes, maintenance infusion of 0.3-0.7 μg/kg/h

**Local anesthesia**

- Identify the preferred nasal passage based on patency and history of epistaxis
- Administer supplemental oxygen at 4 L/min via nasal sponge in the opposite nostril (alternatively, nasal cannulae can be used for oral fiberoptic intubation)
- Administer local anesthetic in a stepwise manner, do not exceed a topical lidocaine dose of 7 mg/kg

**Nose**

- Co-phenylcaine (0.5% phenylephrine + 5% lidocaine) given via mucosal atomiser to each nostril
- Co-phenylcaine, xylocaine (2% lidocaine + adrenaline) or 4% lidocaine soaked cotton buds/ribbon gauze inserted into nasal cavity and left for 3 minutes
- 2 mL of 4% lidocaine via nebulizer

**Oropharynx**

- 10 sprays of 10% lidocaine to tongue and posterior pharynx

**Larynx**

- 4% lidocaine sprayed above the vocal cords during endoscopy
- Cricothyroid injection of 2 mL 2% lidocaine via 20G cannula or 22G needle

**Trachea**

- 4% lidocaine sprayed below vocal cords during endoscopy

Fiberoptic intubation

## Fiberoptic intubation: Technique

Place the patient in a semi-recumbent position

Check the orientation of the fiberscope and perform white balance

Load the scope with a lubricated 6 mm internal diameter endotracheal tube and fix with tape to the handle of the endoscope in a way to allow rapid release

If using "spray as you go" technique: Pass epidural catheter down suction port

Insert the fiberscope through the nostril or mouth (for oral intubation, use a Berman airway or Breathesafe as a bite block to maintain the scope in the midline)

- Once in the oropharynx, identify the epiglottis and slowly advance toward the glottis opening
- Visualization may be improved by asking the patient to stick out their tongue
- In anesthetized patients, have the assistant pull the tongue with a swab or provide jaw thrust

- Keep the black air cavity in the center of the screen
- When the whole screen is pink, the tip of the scope is against mucosa: Withdraw slightly until relevant anatomy can be identified before advancing further

Spray local anesthetic onto the laryngeal inlet, warn the patient that this will cause them to cough

Enter the subglottic space to identify the trachea and spray an additional dose of local anesthetic

Advance the scope until the tip is just proximal to the carina

- Release the endotracheal tube and railroad this gently over the fiberscope
- In case of resistance, do not use force but rotate the tube counter clockwise as it is advanced

Confirm that the tip of the endotracheal tube is in the trachea on removal of the fiberscope

Connect to breathing system and check for correct placement with capnography

Proceed with induction of anesthesia

Plan for difficult extubation if necessary

## COMPLICATIONS

- Oversedation
- Respiratory depression
- Airway obstruction
- Apnea
- Trauma
- Bleeding

- Laryngospasm
- Vomiting
- Local anesthetic allergy
- Toxicity
- Risk of aspiration due to loss of laryngeal reflexes

■ SUGGESTED READING ■

- Collins SR, Blank RS. Fiberoptic intubation: an overview and update. Respir Care. 2014;59(6):865-880.
- Pollard BJ, Kitchen, G. Handbook of Clinical Anaesthesia. Fourth Edition. CRC Press. 2018. 978-1-4987-6289-2.

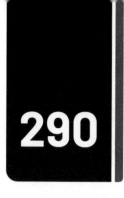

# ONE-LUNG ANESTHESIA

## LEARNING OBJECTIVES

- Describe the indications & contraindications of one-lung anesthesia
- Perform one-lung anesthesia
- Manage hypoxia during one-lung anesthesia

## DEFINITION AND MECHANISM

- One-lung anesthesia defines the process of complete functional separation of the lungs
- Involves ventilating one lung and collapsing the other
- Facilitates certain types of surgery, but can cause significant physiological disturbance

## INDICATIONS

- Protective isolation
  - Prevent contamination or spillage of infectious material (pus or secretions) from the contralateral lung
  - Prevent contamination of the good lung from massive hemorrhage in the contralateral lung
- Control the distribution of ventilation between the two lungs in the presence of:
  - Bronchopleural fistula
  - Giant unilateral cyst/bulla
  - Surgical opening of major airway
  - Tracheobronchial tree disruption
- Unilateral bronchopulmonary lavage (e.g., for alveolar proteinosis)
- Video-assisted thoracoscopic surgery
- Facilitate surgical exposure (e.g., pneumonectomy, lobectomy, thoracoscopy, esophageal surgery, thoracic aneurysm, thoracic spinal surgery)

## CONTRAINDICATIONS

- Patient dependent on bilateral ventilation
- Intraluminal airway masses
- Hemodynamic instability
- Severe hypoxia
- Severe chronic obstructive pulmonary disease (COPD)
- Severe pulmonary hypertension
- Known or suspected difficult intubation

## LUNG SEPARATION

- Double lumen tube: Allows rapid transition between one-lung ventilation and two-lung ventilation, also allows rapid deflation of lung and suctioning, most commonly used technique
- Bronchial blockers: Do not facilitate ventilation or suction distal to the blocker, can be useful if placement of a double lumen tube expected to be difficult
- Uncut tracheal tube: Can be advanced into the relevant main bronchus, generally only used in emergency situations
- Papworth BiVent tube: New double lumen tube designed to facilitate rapid and reliable lung isolation using a bronchus blocker without endoscopic guidance

# TECHNIQUE (DOUBLE LUMEN TUBE)

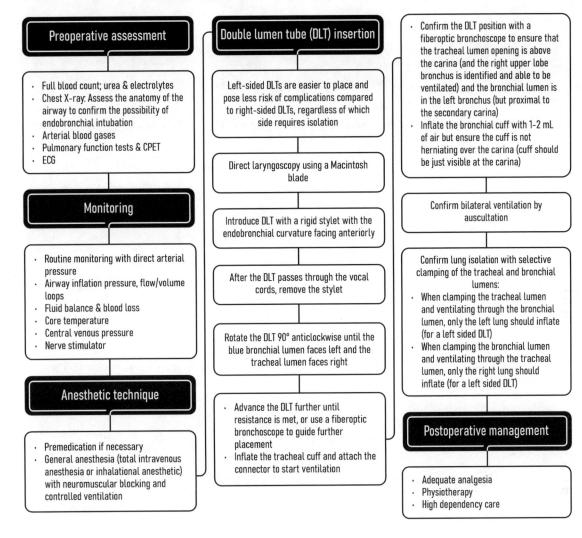

**Preoperative assessment**

- Full blood count; urea & electrolytes
- Chest X-ray: Assess the anatomy of the airway to confirm the possibility of endobronchial intubation
- Arterial blood gases
- Pulmonary function tests & CPET
- ECG

**Monitoring**

- Routine monitoring with direct arterial pressure
- Airway inflation pressure, flow/volume loops
- Fluid balance & blood loss
- Core temperature
- Central venous pressure
- Nerve stimulator

**Anesthetic technique**

- Premedication if necessary
- General anesthesia (total intravenous anesthesia or inhalational anesthetic) with neuromuscular blocking and controlled ventilation

**Double lumen tube (DLT) insertion**

Left-sided DLTs are easier to place and pose less risk of complications compared to right-sided DLTs, regardless of which side requires isolation

Direct laryngoscopy using a Macintosh blade

Introduce DLT with a rigid stylet with the endobronchial curvature facing anteriorly

After the DLT passes through the vocal cords, remove the stylet

Rotate the DLT 90° anticlockwise until the blue bronchial lumen faces left and the tracheal lumen faces right

- Advance the DLT further until resistance is met, or use a fiberoptic bronchoscope to guide further placement
- Inflate the tracheal cuff and attach the connector to start ventilation

- Confirm the DLT position with a fiberoptic bronchoscope to ensure that the tracheal lumen opening is above the carina (and the right upper lobe bronchus is identified and able to be ventilated) and the bronchial lumen is in the left bronchus (but proximal to the secondary carina)
- Inflate the bronchial cuff with 1-2 mL of air but ensure the cuff is not herniating over the carina (cuff should be just visible at the carina)

Confirm bilateral ventilation by auscultation

Confirm lung isolation with selective clamping of the tracheal and bronchial lumens:
- When clamping the tracheal lumen and ventilating through the bronchial lumen, only the left lung should inflate (for a left sided DLT)
- When clamping the bronchial lumen and ventilating through the tracheal lumen, only the right lung should inflate (for a left sided DLT)

**Postoperative management**

- Adequate analgesia
- Physiotherapy
- High dependency care

## COMPLICATIONS

- Hypoxemia is one of the most important complications encountered during one-lung anesthesia
- Management of hypoxemia:
  - Increase inspired oxygen to 100%
  - Check the position of the tube with a fiberoptic bronchoscope
  - Ensure adequate blood pressure and cardiac output
  - Positive end-expiratory pressure 5-10 $cmH_2O$ to the dependent lung to decrease atelectasis and increase functional residual capacity
  - Continuous positive airway pressure 5-10 $cmH_2O$ with 100% oxygen to the non-ventilated lung (if this can be tolerated by the surgeon)
  - If hypoxemia is severe and does not resolve with the aforementioned steps: Abandon one-lung ventilation and intermittently ventilate the collapsed lung after warning the surgeon
  - Early clamping of the appropriate pulmonary artery to stop the shunt (if possible / appropriate)

## SUGGESTED READING

- Ashok V, Francis J. A practical approach to adult one-lung ventilation. BJA Educ. 2018;18(3):69-74.
- Mehrotra M, Jain A. Single Lung Ventilation. [Updated 2022 Jul 25]. In: StatPearls [Internet]. Treasure Island (FL): StatPearls Publishing; 2022 Jan-. Available from: https://www.ncbi.nlm.nih.gov/books/NBK538314/
- Pollard BJ, Kitchen, G. Handbook of Clinical Anaesthesia. Fourth Edition. CRC Press. 2018. 978-1-4987-6289-2.

# 291

# PREOPERATIVE FASTING

## LEARNING OBJECTIVES

- Minimum preoperative fasting times
- Recommendations regarding preoperative fasting

## DEFINITION AND MECHANISM

- Preoperative fasting is defined as abstaining from eating or drinking for some time by surgical patient before having an operation
- Preoperative fasting allows sufficient time for gastric emptying of ingested food and liquid
- This minimizes the risk of pulmonary aspiration during anesthesia as aspiration of as little as 30-40 mL can be a significant cause of morbidity and mortality
- Pulmonary aspiration of gastric contents is a rare but potentially life-threatening complication
- Aspiration is uncommon in healthy ASA I or II patients, 1.1/10,000 adults, and 1.3/10,000 children, but may lead to pneumonitis, pneumonia, bronchospasm, and acute respiratory distress syndrome

### MINIMUM FASTING TIMES

| Age | Solids | Clear liquids |
|---|---|---|
| < 6 months | 4h (formula or breast milk) | 2h |
| 6-36 months | 6h | 2h |
| > 36 months (including adults) | 6h | 2h |

## FACTORS AFFECTING GASTRIC EMPTYING

| | Factor increasing emptying | Factor decreasing emptying |
|---|---|---|
| Physiological factors | Large gastric volume<br>Liquid gastric contents<br>Solids < 2 mm<br>Parasympathetic stimulation<br>Secretion of motilin and gastrin<br>Sitting position (for non-caloric liquids) | Large duodenal volume<br>High-calorie chyme<br>Acidic chyme<br>Hypo-/hyper-osmolar chyme<br>Fatty and amino acid-rich chyme<br>Hot and cold chyme<br>Sympathetic stimulation<br>Secretion of cholecystokinin, secretin, somatostatin, vasoactive intestinal peptide, and gastric inhibitory peptide |
| Pharmacological factors | Anticholinergics<br>Metoclopramide<br>Domperidone<br>Erythromycin | Antimuscarinics<br>Opioids |
| Patient factors | Hyperthyroidism | Pain<br>Anxiety and stress<br>Trauma<br>Pregnancy<br>Alcohol ingestion<br>Hypothyroidism<br>Diabetes<br>Pyloric stenosis<br>Intestinal obstruction<br>Vagotomy |

# RECOMMENDATIONS

- Clear liquids such as water, black coffee, black tea, and juice without pulp are safe to drink until 2h before general anesthesia
- Healthy adults are allowed to drink carbohydrate-containing clear liquids until 2h before elective procedures requiring general anesthesia, regional anesthesia, or procedural sedation
  - In this way, the patient is hydrated and in a more normal metabolic state
- Protein-containing clear liquids should not be recommended over other clear liquids before elective procedures requiring general anesthesia, regional anesthesia, or procedural sedation
- Elective procedures requiring general anesthesia, regional anesthesia, or procedural sedation should not be delayed in healthy adults chewing gum
- Avoid prolonged fasting in children by allowing children at low risk of aspiration to drink clear liquids as close to 2h before procedures when possible
  - Consider even a 1-h fast for clear liquids in healthy children as there is no increased risk for pulmonary aspiration (an acceptable rate of drinking clear fluids in healthy children is a maximum of 3 ml/kg/hr)

## SUGGESTED READING

- Coté CJ. Preoperative preparation and premedication. Br J Anaesth. 1999;83(1):16-28.
- Fawcett, W.J., Thomas, M., 2019. Pre-operative fasting in adults and children: clinical practice and guidelines. Anaesthesia 74, 83-88.
- Girish P. Joshi, Basem B. Abdelmalak, Wade A. Weigel, Monica W. Harbell, Catherine I. Kuo, Sulpicio G. Soriano, Paul A. Stricker, Tommie Tipton, Mark D. Grant, Anne M. Marbella, Madhulika Agarkar, Jaime F. Blanck, Karen B. Domino; 2023 American Society of Anesthesiologists Practice Guidelines for Preoperative Fasting: Carbohydrate-containing Clear Liquids with or without Protein, Chewing Gum, and Pediatric Fasting Duration—A Modular Update of the 2017 American Society of Anesthesiologists Practice Guidelines for Preoperative Fasting. Anesthesiology 2023; 138:132-151
- Mesbah, A., Thomas, M., 2017. Preoperative fasting in children. BJA Education 17, 346-350.
- Pollard BJ, Kitchen, G. Handbook of Clinical Anaesthesia. Fourth Edition. CRC Press. 2018. 978-1-4987-6289-2.
- Wilson, G.R., Dorrington, K.L., 2017. Starvation before surgery: is our practice based on evidence?. BJA Education 17, 275-282.

# 292

# PROLONGED ANESTHESIA

## LEARNING OBJECTIVES

- Describe the possible consequences of prolonged anesthesia
- Manage patients scheduled for prolonged anesthesia

## DEFINITION AND MECHANISM

- Prolonged anesthesia is associated with an increased risk of postoperative complications
- Careful preparation, management, and attention to detail can reduce these risks

## NEGATIVE EFFECTS OF PROLONGED ANESTHESIA

- Accumulation of anesthetic agents leads to delayed emergence, depending on the pharmacokinetics of the agent used (e.g., isuflurane > desflurane, fentanyl > remifentanil) and retention of anesthetic agents can lead to undesired effects postoperatively (sedation, PONV)
- Potential toxicity of anesthetic agents
  - Degradation of inhalational agents by $CO_2$ absorber may lead to accumulation of toxins (e.g., sevoflurane to compound A)
  - Inorganic fluoride production from the hepatic metabolism of sevoflurane and enflurane may be nephrotoxic in patients with chronic renal impairment
  - Prolonged exposure to nitrous oxide may result in acute vitamin B12 deficiency with megaloblastic anemia and neurological complications (e.g., neuropathies and subacute combined degeneration of the spinal cord)
- Impairment of gas exchange and respiratory mechanics (hypoxemia and hypercarbia secondary to slowly developing dependent atelectasis)
- The effects of anesthetic agents on renal function can lead to water and salt retention
- Disturbances in intermediary carbohydrate metabolism promote the development of metabolic acidosis
- Retention of anesthetic agents in the body can lead to undesired effects postoperatively
- Metabolic effects
  - Disturbances in intermediary carbohydrate metabolism promote the development of metabolic acidosis
  - Decreased carbohydrate metabolism results in intraoperative hyperglycemia
- Problems with accurate fluid and electrolyte management
- Inadvertent perioperative hypothermia can lead to:
  - Increased wound infection
  - Surgical bleeding
  - Impaired immune function
  - Increased incidence of myocardial ischemia and infarction
  - Malignant arrhythmias
  - Postoperative shivering
- Prolonged immobility can lead to:
  - Increased risk of deep vein thrombosis
  - Nerve damage and pressure sores
  - Bilateral compartment syndrome
  - Rhabdomyolysis
  - Corneal damage if the eyes are left open
- Postoperative delirium
- Immunosuppression and increased susceptibility to infections
- Increased risk of human error due to fatigue

# MANAGEMENT

## PROLONGED ANESTHESIA

| Preparation | Intraoperative management | Postoperative management |
|---|---|---|

### Preparation

Discuss the risks of prolonged procedures with the operating room team prior to the procedure and plan appropriately

**Patient positioning**
- Pad pressure areas
- Ensure neutral joint placement and support of the lower back
- Avoid traction on at-risk nerves (e.g., brachial plexus)
- Ensure documentation of every event

**Protection of the operating room team**
Recommended maximum accepted concentration over 8 hours: 100 ppm $N_2O$, 50 ppm enflurane/desflurane, 10 ppm halothane

Use a low-flow circle system to reduce gas and vapor consumption

Maintain body temperature

### Intraoperative management

**Monitoring**
- Standard monitoring with invasive blood pressure
- Core and skin temperature
- Blood loss
- Bispectral index analysis
- Tracheal tube cuff pressure
- Peripheral nerve stimulator
- Blood gases, electrolytes, glucose, coagulation
- Pressure-volume loop and lung compliance
- Inspiratory and expired concentration of oxygen, nitrous oxide, anesthetic vapor and $CO_2$
- Fluid balance (central venous pressure, hourly urine output)
- Cardiac output

**Anesthetic technique**
- The technique is chosen based on the procedure, anticipated blood loss, and chronic health status of the patient
- Regional anesthesia may be used, but light general anesthesia or sedation is often necessary for patient comfort
- Consider using oxygen/air technique
- Consider total intravenous anesthesia/target-controlled anesthesia
- Use a high-volume low-pressure cuff with regular tracheal tube suctioning
- Pay careful attention to body positioning with frequent repositioning of the head
- Passive movement of joints periodically may reduce the incidence of postoperative arthralgia
- Cover exposed body surfaces
- Use eye protection (lubrication, tapes, padding, eye shields)
- Deep vein thrombosis prophylaxis
- Be aware of the increased risk of errors due to fatigue

### Postoperative management
- Intensive care/high dependency unit for continued ventilation until warm and stable, slow emergence
- Regular physiotherapy
- Maintain deep vein thrombosis prophylaxis
- Adequate fluid management

## SUGGESTED READING

- Cheng H, Clymer JW, Po-Han Chen B, et al. Prolonged operative duration is associated with complications: a systematic review and meta-analysis. J Surg Res. 2018;229:134-144.
- Pollard BJ, Kitchen, G. Handbook of Clinical Anaesthesia. Fourth Edition. CRC Press. 2018. 978-1-4987-6289-2.

# TOTAL INTRAVENOUS ANESTHESIA (TIVA)

## LEARNING OBJECTIVES

- Describe the indications for total intravenous anesthesia
- Describe the techniques and models used for total intravenous anesthesia
- Describe the advantages, disadvantages, and safety measures for total intravenous anesthesia

## DEFINITION AND MECHANISM

- Total intravenous anesthesia (TIVA) is a technique where intravenous agents are used to induce and maintain general anesthesia, avoiding the use of inhalational anesthetics
- Continuous intravenous infusion is commonly done by a target-controlled infusion (TCI) pump, but can also be achieved using intermittent boluses or manual infusion techniques
- TCI allows precise and individualized administration of intravenous anesthetics
- Both hypnosis and analgesia can be achieved using an intravenous technique
- Goals for TIVA: Smooth induction, reliable and titratable maintenance, and rapid emergence
- Careful preparation, management, and attention to detail reduce risks

## INDICATIONS

- Malignant hyperthermia susceptibility
- Long QT syndrome
- History of severe PONV
- Surgery requiring neurophysiological monitoring
- Anesthesia in non-theatre environments
- Transfer of anesthetized patients between different locations
- Sedation in intensive care
- Tubeless ENT procedures and rigid bronchoscopy
- Thoracic surgery
- Intracranial surgery
- Procedures requiring sedation (e.g., endoscopy, cardioversion)

## ANESTHETIC AGENTS

- Propofol is the hypnotic agent of choice for TIVA
- Analgesia can be achieved using short-acting opioids (alfentanil, remifentanil)

## TARGET-CONTROLLED INFUSION (TCI)

- Sophisticated TCI syringe drivers incorporate real-time pharmacokinetic models that deliver the appropriate dose to achieve and maintain the requested target concentration
- The microprocessor within the syringe driver continuously calculates the appropriate infusion rates
- A bolus/elimination/transfer principle is used to maintain an appropriate plasma level of anesthetic agents
- Induction is achieved by a rapid propofol infusion, giving a bolus calculated to achieve the required plasma concentration
- This is followed by a progressively decreasing infusion rate calculated to match the transfer between compartments and elimination of the drug, maintaining the required plasma level
- Once the compartments reach a steady-state concentration, the infusion rate slows to match elimination only
- To increase the target plasma level, the syringe driver delivers an additional bolus to achieve the desired concentration and then maintains a higher infusion rate
- To decrease the target plasma level, the syringe driver stops infusing until the microprocessor calculates that the new target has been achieved, and the new level is maintained
- Modern TCI pumps also have software that allows titrating to effect-site concentration (the concentration in the brain)
- Depth of anesthesia monitoring (e.g., bispectral index) is required, as there is considerable variation in the uptake and effect of anesthetic agents in individual patients

# PROPOFOL TCI MODELS

- Propofol TCI allows easy control and rapid change of the target propofol concentration
- Unpremedicated adult patients < 55 years: Target propofol concentration 4-8 µg/mL for induction (usually takes 60-120 seconds)
- When co-administering an analgesic, maintenance at 3-6 µg/mL
- Lower target concentrations are used in the elderly population due to the risk of side-effects
- Propofol TCI is not routinely used in children
- Propofol TCI models:
  - Marsh
    - Calculations based on the assumption that the central compartment volume is proportional to the patient's weight, ignoring age
    - Assumes that the central compartment volume is 19.4 L for an 85 kg patient
    - Designed primarily to target plasma concentrations
    - Only used for patients > 16 years of age
  - Schnider
    - Requires age, height, and body weight
    - Calculates a sex-specific lean body mass and determines the dosages accordingly
    - Assumes that the fixed central compartment volume is 4.27 L for an 85 kg patient (4-fold difference with the Marsh model)
    - Allows for effect site concentration to be targeted
    - More commonly used in the elderly population
  - Paedfusor
    - Variant of the Marsh model for patients 1-16 years of age
    - Uses weight to calculate target plasma concentration and features a nonlinear scaling of central compartment volume as age exceeds 12 years
  - Kataria
    - Can be used for patients 3-16 years of age with a minimum weight of 15 kg
    - Uses weight to calculate target plasma concentration

# OTHER TCI MODELS

- Minto: For remifentanil
- Bergmann: For fentanyl
- Maitre: For alfentanil
- Gepts: For sufentanil

- Eleveld: For propofol & remifentanil
- Domino: For ketamine
- Dick & Hannivoort: For dexmedetomidine
- Greenblatt: For midazolam

# ANALGESIA

- Since propofol has no analgesic properties, TIVA is commonly achieved by combining propofol infusion with a regional block or supplemental opioids
- Supplemental short-acting opioids:
  - Remifentanil
    - Elimination half-time: 3-10 min
    - Does not accumulate in hepatic or renal failure
    - Context insensitive: the time required for the drug concentration to fall by 50% is always the same (~3 min), regardless of age, weight, sex, or hepatic or renal function
    - Opioid of choice for TIVA for many anesthesiologists
    - Can be given using the Minto model (allows easy titration based on patient age, gender, weight and height)
    - Target plasma concentration: 3-8 ng/mL for induction, up to 15 ng/mL in stimulating procedures
    - Ensure adequate analgesia after remifentanil has worn off
  - Alfentanil
    - Short onset time (90 s)
    - Given using Maitre model (calculations based on age, gender and weight)
  - Sufentanil
    - Much more potent than remifentanil
    - Longer duration of action
    - Tends to accumulate during prolonged infusion
    - Two TCI models: Gepts (fixed compartment volume) and Bovill (assumes that the central compartment volume is proportional to body weight)

Total intravenous anesthesia (TIVA)

## ADVANTAGES & DISADVANTAGES

| Advantages | Disadvantages |
| --- | --- |
| More predictable onset and stability of maintenance | Pharmacokinetic and pharmacodynamic variability of response to the injected agent(s) |
| Elimination of volatile anesthetics along with their possible liver and kidney toxicity, potential rise in intracranial pressure, their effect on the uterus, and their detrimental environmental effects | Lack of ability to accurately assess actual blood levels |
| No need for accurately calibrated vaporizers | Variations in the hemodynamic state of the patient |
| Fast recovery with fewer complications, decreased time to discharge | Requirement for dedicated IV access, and risk of disconnection |
| Propofol is a powerful antiemetic | Risk of accidental awareness |
| Avoidance of nitrous oxide with its effect on air emboli, pneumothoraces, and bone marrow suppression | |

## SAFETY

- Ensure the cannula is visible and accessible at all times and checked regularly to prevent disconnection or tissuing
- Check the pump setup regularly to prevent tubing disconnection, ensure clamps are open/closed accordingly, pump alarms are rectified and no backtracking of drug occurs
- Ensure the drug concentration matches the programmed concentration
- Ensure the correct syringe is placed in the correct syringe driver
- Use anti-reflux and anti-syphon valves with clamps in multilumen tubing for safe delivery
- Use a processed EEG monitor when a neuromuscular blocker is used

## SUGGESTED READING

- Al-Rifai Z, Mulvey D. (2016). Principles of total intravenous anaesthesia: Basic pharmacokinetics and model descriptions. BJA Educ 16(3): 92–7.
- Nimmo AF, Absalom AR, Bagshaw O, Biswas A, Cook TM, Costello A, et al. Guidelines for the safe practice of total intravenous anaesthesia (TIVA). Anaesthesia. 2019;74(2):211-24.
- Pollard BJ, Kitchen, G. Handbook of Clinical Anaesthesia. Fourth Edition. CRC Press. 2018. 978-1-4987-6289-2.

Total intravenous anesthesia (TIVA)

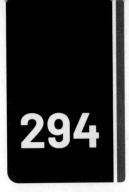

# 294

# VIDEOLARYNGOSCOPY

## LEARNING OBJECTIVES

- Background of videolaryngoscopy
- Advantages and disadvantages of videolaryngoscopy

## DEFINITION AND MECHANISM

- Videolaryngoscopy utilizes video camera technology to visualize airway structures and facilitate endotracheal intubation
- Videolaryngoscopy is an alternative to direct laryngoscopy for airway intubation in adults and children as it improves airway safety and is associated with fewer failed attempts and complications
- Different types of videolaryngoscope blades - hyperangulated vs non-hyperangulated/Macintosh blades - are available, each of which has advantages and disadvantages, and choice of optimal blade is dependant on the clinical scenario
- Is also a new diagnostic and therapeutic tool in head and neck surgery
- Has the great advantage of reducing difficult views of the laryngeal opening (glottis)
- Despite a good view of the cords with videolaryngoscopy, difficulty may still be encountered in advancing a tube through the glottis into the trachea
- Use the mnemonic aid "CCLL" to prepare for videolaryngoscopy:
  - Choose the right tube
  - Check the endotracheal tube cuff
  - Lubricate the stylet and the endotracheal tube
  - Load the stylet (bend it according to the curvature of the videolaryngoscopy blade)
- Consider the possibility of airway trauma during videolaryngoscopy as the operator's attention is diverted from the direct view of the proximal airway to the indirect view of the glottis on the monitor
- Therefore, introduce the tip of the tube and stylet into the oropharynx under direct vision and then advance as guided by the indirect view on the monitor

## INDICATIONS AND CONTRAINDICATIONS

- Indications
  - Difficult airway
  - Limited neck mobility or cervical spine injuries
  - Obesity
  - Pediatric patients
  - Rescue device when traditional methods have failed
  - Pathological airway changes (tumor, swelling or other anatomical variations that obscure the airway)
- Contraindications
  - Lack of equipment or expertise
  - Severe oropharyngeal bleeding

## COMPLICATIONS

- Palatal perforation
- Palatopharyngeal arch tear
- Injury to tonsilar pillars
- Oropharyngeal soft tissue trauma
  - Palatal perforation
  - Palatopharyngeal arch tear
  - Injury to tonsilar pillars
- Dental trauma during tube insertion
- Vomiting and aspiration during tube insertion
- Incorrect tube placement (eg, esophageal intubation)
- Hypoxia during the intubation attempt

## CLINICAL USE

- Orotracheal intubation
- Nasotracheal intubation
- Intubation in the presence of cervical spine pathology
- Awake intubation
- Conduit for flexible fiberoptic bronchoscope
- To assist with insertion of e.g. TEE probe, gastric tube etc
- Diagnosis and recording of upper airway pathology

# ADVANTAGES AND DISADVANTAGES OF VIDEOLARYNGOSCOPY

| Advantages | Disadvantages |
|---|---|
| Easier to learn and maintain the skill (by observing the video screen) Effective tool for those who infrequently intubate as well as students learning to intubate | Succes rate is not 100% |
| Less workforce is needed to view the glottis Improved glottic visualization | Unknown efficacy in routine airway management and the efficacy of different videolaryngoscopes differs |
| A higher first-pass success rate of tracheal intubation in patients with difficult airways versus direct laryngoscopy and thus a lower incidence of multiple attempts | A higher incidence of oropharyngeal injury |
| Superior view of the glottic opening versus direct laryngoscopy | Prolonged intubation time due to difficult tracheal tube delivery into the glottic opening or difficulty advancing the tracheal tube through the glottis into the trachea |
| A lower incidence of inadvertent esophageal intubation versus direct laryngoscopy | The camera view can frequently be blurred by fogging, secretions, blood, or emesis in the oropharynx |
| Easier to confirm pathological changes (laryngeal edema) after repeated attempts at tracheal intubation | Two-dimensional view with loss of depth perception |
| It is not necessary to align airway axes (oral-pharyngeal-laryngeal) to achieve line of sight | More expensive and not universally available |
| Less cervical manipulation | Potential weakening in development/maintenance of direct laryngoscopy skill set |
| Possible awake assessment/intubation | Potential for false sense of security and lack of preparation for a difficult airway |

# OROTRACHEAL RAPID SEQUENCE INTUBATION TECHNIQUE

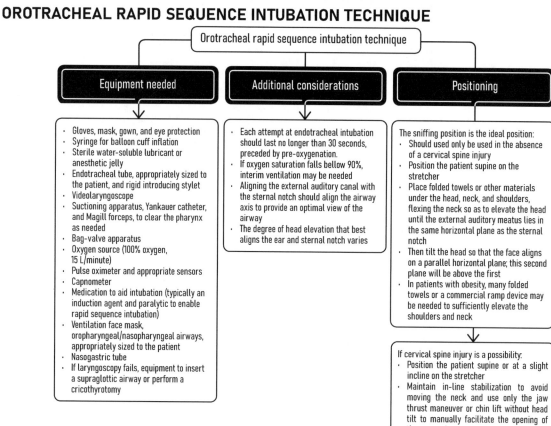

Orotracheal rapid sequence intubation technique

**Equipment needed**

- Gloves, mask, gown, and eye protection
- Syringe for balloon cuff inflation
- Sterile water-soluble lubricant or anesthetic jelly
- Endotracheal tube, appropriately sized to the patient, and rigid introducing stylet
- Videolaryngoscope
- Suctioning apparatus, Yankauer catheter, and Magill forceps, to clear the pharynx as needed
- Bag-valve apparatus
- Oxygen source (100% oxygen, 15 L/minute)
- Pulse oximeter and appropriate sensors
- Capnometer
- Medication to aid intubation (typically an induction agent and paralytic to enable rapid sequence intubation)
- Ventilation face mask, oropharyngeal/nasopharyngeal airways, appropriately sized to the patient
- Nasogastric tube
- If laryngoscopy fails, equipment to insert a supraglottic airway or perform a cricothyrotomy

**Additional considerations**

- Each attempt at endotracheal intubation should last no longer than 30 seconds, preceded by pre-oxygenation.
- If oxygen saturation falls bellow 90%, interim ventilation may be needed
- Aligning the external auditory canal with the sternal notch should align the airway axis to provide an optimal view of the airway
- The degree of head elevation that best aligns the ear and sternal notch varies

**Positioning**

The sniffing position is the ideal position:
- Should used only be used in the absence of a cervical spine injury
- Position the patient supine on the stretcher
- Place folded towels or other materials under the head, neck, and shoulders, flexing the neck so as to elevate the head until the external auditory meatus lies in the same horizontal plane as the sternal notch
- Then tilt the head so that the face aligns on a parallel horizontal plane; this second plane will be above the first
- In patients with obesity, many folded towels or a commercial ramp device may be needed to sufficiently elevate the shoulders and neck

If cervical spine injury is a possibility:
- Position the patient supine or at a slight incline on the stretcher
- Maintain in-line stabilization to avoid moving the neck and use only the jaw thrust maneuver or chin lift without head tilt to manually facilitate the opening of the upper airway

## Orotracheal rapid sequence intubation technique

| Before tube insertion | Tube insertion in the mouth and passing behind the tongue | Advancing the tube through the vocal cords |
|---|---|---|
| • Establish IV access<br>• Ventilate and pre-oxygenate the patient with 100% oxygen<br>• Inflate the balloon cuff of an appropriately sized endotracheal tube to verify it does not leak<br>• Perform rapid sequence intubation<br>• Perform cricoid pressure<br>• Clear the oropharynx, if necessary, of obstructing secretions, vomitus, or foreign material<br>• Continue oxygenation | • Insert the videolaryngoscope blade into the patient's mouth, following the curve of the tongue<br>• Once the tip of the videolaryngoscope blade is behind the patient's tongue, look at the video laryngoscope monitor and manipulate the blade so the glottic opening is in the middle of the upper half of the video screen<br>• Optimize the view with bimanual laryngoscopy by manipulating the larynx with the operator's right hand while operating the video laryngoscope with the left hand.<br>• Applying backward, upward, and rightward pressure on the thyroid cartilage will usually optimize the view<br>• Insert the endotracheal tube in the right side of the mouth and pass it behind the tongue, carefully avoiding damaging the balloon on the teeth | • At this point, watch the monitor to guide the tip of the tube through the vocal cords<br>• Because some stylets used with certain videolaryngoscopes are rigid, this maneuver may require having an assistant pull the stylet out 1 to 2 cm while the tube is gently advanced<br>• Then advance the tube an additional 3 to 4 cm<br>• Inflate the cuff and fully remove the stylet<br>• Ventilate the patient (8 to 10 breaths/minute, each about 6 to 8 mL/kg or 500 mL and lasting about 1 second)<br>• If unable to intubate, the use of adjuncts such as the bougie may be helpful<br>• If adjunct use does not result in a successful airway, quickly pursue an alternate airway: rescue bag-valve-mask ventilation, laryngeal mask airway, King laryngeal tube, esophageal-tracheal double lumen tube or cricothyrotomy |

## SUGGESTED READING

• Asai T, Jagannathan N. Videolaryngoscopy Is Extremely Valuable, But Should It Be the Standard for Tracheal Intubation?. Anesth Analg. 2023;136(4):679-682.
• Chemsian R, Bhananker S, Ramaiah R. Videolaryngoscopy. Int J Crit Illn Inj Sci. 2014;4(1):35-41.
• Goranović, T., 2021. Videolaryngoscopy, the Current Role in Airway Management. https://doi.org/10.5772/intechopen.93490
• Hansel, J., Rogers, A.M., Lewis, S.R., Cook, T.M., Smith, A.F., 2022. Videolaryngoscopy versus direct laryngoscopy for adults undergoing tracheal intubation: a Cochrane systematic review and meta-analysis update. British Journal of Anaesthesia 129, 612-623.
• Pollard BJ, Kitchen, G. Handbook of Clinical Anaesthesia. Fourth Edition. CRC Press. 2018. 978-1-4987-6289-2.
• Prekker ME, Driver BE, Trent SA, et al. Video versus Direct Laryngoscopy for Tracheal Intubation of Critically Ill Adults [published online ahead of print, 2023 Jun 16]. N Engl J Med. 2023;10.1056/NEJMoa2301601.

# TOXICITIES

# BETA-BLOCKER OVERDOSE

## LEARNING OBJECTIVES

- Diagnose and treat beta-blocker overdose

**295**

---

## DEFINITION AND MECHANISM

- Beta-blockers are a type of medicine used to treat high blood pressure and heart rhythm disturbances
- Also used in the treatment of thyroid disease, migraine, and glaucoma
- Isolated beta-blocker overdose is usually benign
- Two beta-blockers require special consideration because of cardiac instability:
  - Propanolol → causes sodium channel blockade → QRS widening → treat with $NaHCO_3$
  - Sotalol → causes potassium efflux blockade → long QT → monitor for Torsades
- Beta-blockers competitively block beta-1 and beta-2 receptors
- Results in a decreased production of intracellular cyclic adenosine monophosphate (cAMP) with a resultant blunting of multiple metabolic and cardiovascular effects of circulating catecholamines
  - This leads to a reduced heart rate and blood pressure
  - An overdose causes the heart to enter a shock state
- Comorbid disease (CAD, CHF, atrial fibrillation, dysrhythmias, hypertrophic obstructive cardiomyopathy)

## SIGNS AND SYMPTOMS

- Proportional to the type and amount ingested

| Signs and symptoms | |
|---|---|
| Respiratory system | Bronchospasm |
| Visual system | Blurred vision<br>Double vision |
| Cardiovascular system | Hypotension<br>Bradycardia<br>AV block<br>Heart failure |
| Metabolic system | Hypoglycemia<br>Hyperkalemia |
| Nervous system | Weakness<br>Nervousness<br>Excessive sweating<br>Drowsiness<br>Confusion<br>Seizures<br>Fever<br>Stupor<br>Coma |

# MANGEMENT

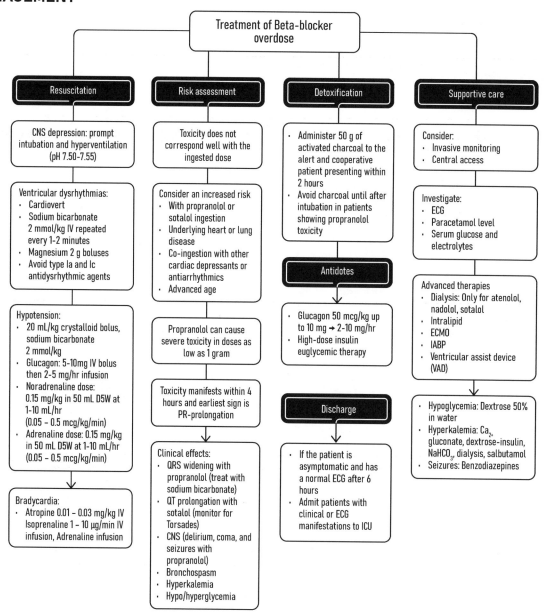

**Treatment of Beta-blocker overdose**

## Resuscitation

CNS depression: prompt intubation and hyperventilation (pH 7.50-7.55)

Ventricular dysrhythmias:
- Cardiovert
- Sodium bicarbonate 2 mmol/kg IV repeated every 1-2 minutes
- Magnesium 2 g boluses
- Avoid type Ia and Ic antidysrhythmic agents

Hypotension:
- 20 mL/kg crystalloid bolus, sodium bicarbonate 2 mmol/kg
- Glucagon: 5-10mg IV bolus then 2-5 mg/hr infusion
- Noradrenaline dose: 0.15 mg/kg in 50 mL D5W at 1-10 mL/hr (0.05 – 0.5 mcg/kg/min)
- Adrenaline dose: 0.15 mg/kg in 50 mL D5W at 1-10 mL/hr (0.05 – 0.5 mcg/kg/min)

Bradycardia:
- Atropine 0.01 – 0.03 mg/kg IV Isoprenaline 1 – 10 µg/min IV infusion, Adrenaline infusion

## Risk assessment

Toxicity does not correspond well with the ingested dose

Consider an increased risk
- With propranolol or sotalol ingestion
- Underlying heart or lung disease
- Co-ingestion with other cardiac depressants or antiarrhythmics
- Advanced age

Propranolol can cause severe toxicity in doses as low as 1 gram

Toxicity manifests within 4 hours and earliest sign is PR-prolongation

Clinical effects:
- QRS widening with propranolol (treat with sodium bicarbonate)
- QT prolongation with sotalol (monitor for Torsades)
- CNS (delirium, coma, and seizures with propranolol)
- Bronchospasm
- Hyperkalemia
- Hypo/hyperglycemia

## Detoxification

- Administer 50 g of activated charcoal to the alert and cooperative patient presenting within 2 hours
- Avoid charcoal until after intubation in patients showing propranolol toxicity

### Antidotes

- Glucagon 50 mcg/kg up to 10 mg → 2-10 mg/hr
- High-dose insulin euglycemic therapy

### Discharge

- If the patient is asymptomatic and has a normal ECG after 6 hours
- Admit patients with clinical or ECG manifestations to ICU

## Supportive care

Consider:
- Invasive monitoring
- Central access

Investigate:
- ECG
- Paracetamol level
- Serum glucose and electrolytes

Advanced therapies
- Dialysis: Only for atenolol, nadolol, sotalol
- Intralipid
- ECMO
- IABP
- Ventricular assist device (VAD)

- Hypoglycemia: Dextrose 50% in water
- Hyperkalemia: Ca$_{2+}$, gluconate, dextrose-insulin, NaHCO$_3$, dialysis, salbutamol
- Seizures: Benzodiazepines

CNS, central nervous system; D5W, 5% dextrose in water; ECMO, extracorporeal membrane oxygenation; IABP, intra-aortic balloon pump; VAD, ventricular assist device; METs, metabolic equivalents of task

## SUGGESTED READING

- Shepherd G. Treatment of poisoning caused by beta-adrenergic and calcium-channel blockers. Am J Health Syst Pharm. 2006;63(19):1828-1835.

Beta-blocker overdose

# 296

# CALCIUM CHANNEL BLOCKER TOXICITY

## LEARNING OBJECTIVES

- Diagnose and treat calcium blocker toxicity

## DEFINITION AND MECHANISM

- Calcium channel blockers (CCBs) are used to treat hypertension, supraventricular tachycardia, vasospasm, and migraine headaches
- Ingestion of excessive CCB agents is one of the most potentially lethal prescription medication overdoses
- Overdoses of immediate-release CCBs are characterized by rapid progression to hypotension, bradydysrhythmia, and cardiac arrest
- Overdoses of extended-release formulations result in delayed onset of dysrhythmias, shock, sudden cardiac collapse, and bowel ischemia
- Symptoms occur within six hours after ingestion, although some forms of medication do not start until after 24 hours
- Calcium channel blockers target the L-type voltage-gated calcium channels, wich are responsible for the depolarization of the sinoatrial node and impulse propagation through the atrioventricular node
- Three main classes of CCBs:
  - Phenylalkylamines (verapamil)
  - Benzothiazepines (diltiazem)
  - Dihydropyridines (nifedipine, amlodipine, felodipine, isradipine, nicardipine, nimodipine)

## SIGNS AND SYMPTOMS

- Dizziness
- Fatigue
- Nausea and vomiting
- Lightheadedness
- Altered mental status
- Coma
- Dyspnea
- Hypotension
- Bradycardia
- Hyperglycemia
- Metabolic acidosis
- Hypokalemia
- Hypocalcemia
- Pulmonary edema
- Renal failure

## DIAGNOSIS

- Hyperglycemia
- Blood gas: hyperlactatemia, metabolic acidosis, impaired oxygen delivery
- ECG:
  - Bradycardia
  - QT prolongation
  - Bundle branch block
  - First-degree atrioventricular block
  - Junctional rhythms
  - Reflex tachycardia (dihydropyridines)
- Echocardiography
- Chest X-ray: pulmonary edema

## COMPLICATIONS

| Complications from toxicity |
| --- |
| Refractory cardiogenic and distributive shock |
| Acute respiratory distress syndrome |
| Severe hypoperfusion and resultant end-organ injury like ischemic bowel, myocardial infarction, acute tubular necrosis, limb necrosis |
| Pulseless electrical activity with cardiac arrest (PEA) |

| Complications from treatment |
| --- |
| Multiorgan failure from calciphylaxis with overaggressive calcium infusion |
| Hypokalemia and hypoglycemia |
| Acute respiratory distress syndrome, hypertriglyceridemia, pancreatitis, and fat overload syndrome with lipid emulsion therapy |
| Nausea, vomiting, ileus, and hypokalemia with glucagon |
| Arterial and venous thrombosis and limb ischemia with interventions like ECMO |

# MANAGEMENT

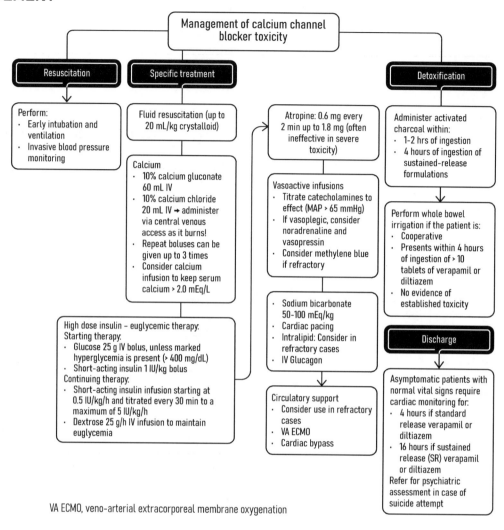

**Management of calcium channel blocker toxicity**

**Resuscitation**

Perform:
- Early intubation and ventilation
- Invasive blood pressure monitoring

**Specific treatment**

Fluid resuscitation (up to 20 mL/kg crystalloid)

Calcium
- 10% calcium gluconate 60 mL IV
- 10% calcium chloride 20 mL IV → administer via central venous access as it burns!
- Repeat boluses can be given up to 3 times
- Consider calcium infusion to keep serum calcium > 2.0 mEq/L

High dose insulin – euglycemic therapy.
Starting therapy:
- Glucose 25 g IV bolus, unless marked hyperglycemia is present (> 400 mg/dL)
- Short-acting insulin 1 IU/kg bolus
Continuing therapy:
- Short-acting insulin infusion starting at 0.5 IU/kg/h and titrated every 30 min to a maximum of 5 IU/kg/h
- Dextrose 25 g/h IV infusion to maintain euglycemia

Atropine: 0.6 mg every 2 min up to 1.8 mg (often ineffective in severe toxicity)

Vasoactive infusions
- Titrate catecholamines to effect (MAP > 65 mmHg)
- If vasoplegic, consider noradrenaline and vasopressin
- Consider methylene blue if refractory

- Sodium bicarbonate 50-100 mEq/kg
- Cardiac pacing
- Intralipid: Consider in refractory cases
- IV Glucagon

Circulatory support
- Consider use in refractory cases
- VA ECMO
- Cardiac bypass

**Detoxification**

Administer activated charcoal within:
- 1-2 hrs of ingestion
- 4 hours of ingestion of sustained-release formulations

Perform whole bowel irrigation if the patient is:
- Cooperative
- Presents within 4 hours of ingestion of > 10 tablets of verapamil or diltiazem
- No evidence of established toxicity

**Discharge**

Asymptomatic patients with normal vital signs require cardiac monitoring for:
- 4 hours if standard release verapamil or diltiazem
- 16 hours if sustained release (SR) verapamil or diltiazem
Refer for psychiatric assessment in case of suicide attempt

VA ECMO, veno-arterial extracorporeal membrane oxygenation

## SUGGESTED READING

- Alshaya, O.A., Alhamed, A., Althewaibi, S., Fetyani, L., Alshehri, S., Alnashmi, F., Alharbi, S., Alrashed, M., Alqifari, S.F., Alshaya, A.I., 2022. Calcium Channel Blocker Toxicity: A Practical Approach. Journal of Multidisciplinary Healthcare Volume 15, 1851–1862.
- Jackson, R., Bellamy, M., 2015. Antihypertensive drugs. BJA Education 15, 280–285.
- Kerns W 2nd. Management of beta-adrenergic blocker and calcium channel antagonist toxicity. Emerg Med Clin North Am. 2007;25(2):309-viii.
- St-Onge M, Dubé PA, Gosselin S, et al. Treatment for calcium channel blocker poisoning: a systematic review. Clin Toxicol (Phila). 2014;52(9):926–944.

# CARBON MONOXIDE POISONING

## LEARNING OBJECTIVES

• Diagnose and treat carbon monoxide (CO) poisoning

## DEFINITION AND MECHANISM

• Carbon monoxide is a colorless, odorless, tasteless gas produced by burning gasoline, wood, propane, charcoal, or other fuel
• Volatile anesthetics can produce CO when used with $CO_2$ absorbents
• CO intoxication causes tissue hypoxia in three ways:
  ◦ CO binds with hemoglobin with about 250 times the affinity of oxygen, thereby, preventing oxygen binding
  ◦ CO leads to a shift in the oxygen dissociation curve to the left, thereby, impending delivery
  ◦ CO competitively inhibits the binding of oxygen with cytochrome oxidase, a key mitochondrial enzyme, significantly impairing cellular utilization of oxygen
• Mortality is 1-3%

| Acute poisoning | |
| --- | --- |
| Central nervous system | Headache |
| | Dizziness |
| | Confusion |
| | Altered mental status |
| | Incoordination |
| | Ataxia |
| | Seizures |
| | Coma |
| Cardiovascular system | Dysrhythmias |
| | Ischemia |
| | Hypertension |
| | Hypotension |

| Acute poisoning | |
| --- | --- |
| Gastrointestinal tract | Abdominal pain |
| | Nausea |
| | Vomitting |
| | Diarrhea |
| Respiratory system | Dyspnea |
| | Tachypnea |
| | Chest pain |
| | Palpitations |
| Other | Non-cardiogenic pulmonary edema |
| | Lactic acidosis |
| | Rhabdomyolysis |
| | Hyperglycemia |
| | Disseminated intravascular coagulation (DIC) |
| | Bullae |
| | Alopecia |
| | Sweat gland necrosis |

## COMPLICATIONS

• Chronic fatigue
• Permanent brain damage
• Damage to the heart, possibly leading to life-threatening cardiac complications
• Fetal death or miscarriage
• Death

| Chronic exposure | |
| --- | --- |
| May have similar effects to acute poisoning, but often with a gradual, insidious onset, and symptoms may fluctuate with varying levels of exposure to CO over time | Headache |
| | Personality changes |
| | Poor concentration |
| | Dementia |
| | Psychosis |
| | Parkinson's disease |
| | Ataxia |
| | Peripheral neuropathy |
| | Hearing loss |

Carbon monoxide poisoning

# DIAGNOSIS

- Co-oximetry
- Standard $SpO_2$ does not identify CO poisoning
- HbCO level of more than 3% among nonsmokers and more than 10% among smokers
- ECG indication of ischemia
- Clinically significant acidosis

# MANAGEMENT

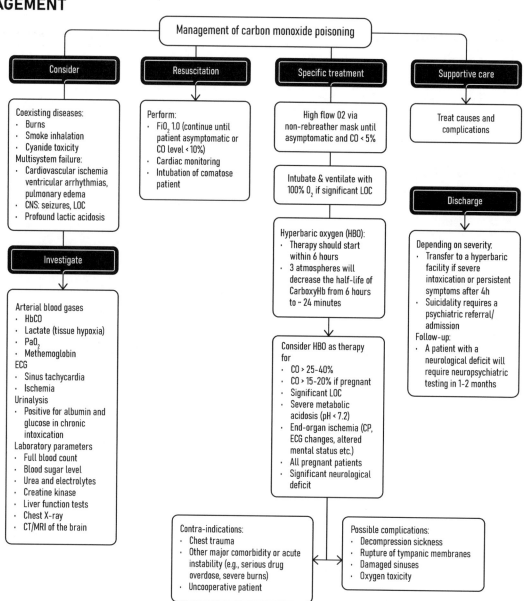

**Management of carbon monoxide poisoning**

**Consider**

Coexisting diseases:
- Burns
- Smoke inhalation
- Cyanide toxicity

Multisystem failure:
- Cardiovascular ischemia ventricular arrhythmias, pulmonary edema
- CNS: seizures, LOC
- Profound lactic acidosis

**Investigate**

Arterial blood gases
- HbCO
- Lactate (tissue hypoxia)
- $PaO_2$
- Methemoglobin

ECG
- Sinus tachycardia
- Ischemia

Urinalysis
- Positive for albumin and glucose in chronic intoxication

Laboratory parameters
- Full blood count
- Blood sugar level
- Urea and electrolytes
- Creatine kinase
- Liver function tests
- Chest X-ray
- CT/MRI of the brain

**Resuscitation**

Perform:
- $FiO_2$ 1.0 (continue until patient asymptomatic or CO level < 10%)
- Cardiac monitoring
- Intubation of comatose patient

**Specific treatment**

High flow O2 via non-rebreather mask until asymptomatic and CO < 5%

Intubate & ventilate with 100% $O_2$ if significant LOC

Hyperbaric oxygen (HBO):
- Therapy should start within 6 hours
- 3 atmospheres will decrease the half-life of CarboxyHb from 6 hours to ~ 24 minutes

Consider HBO as therapy for
- CO > 25-40%
- CO > 15-20% if pregnant
- Significant LOC
- Severe metabolic acidosis (pH < 7.2)
- End-organ ischemia (CP, ECG changes, altered mental status etc.)
- All pregnant patients
- Significant neurological deficit

Contra-indications:
- Chest trauma
- Other major comorbidity or acute instability (e.g., serious drug overdose, severe burns)
- Uncooperative patient

Possible complications:
- Decompression sickness
- Rupture of tympanic membranes
- Damaged sinuses
- Oxygen toxicity

**Supportive care**

Treat causes and complications

**Discharge**

Depending on severity:
- Transfer to a hyperbaric facility if severe intoxication or persistent symptoms after 4h
- Suicidality requires a psychiatric referral/ admission

Follow-up:
- A patient with a neurological deficit will require neuropsychiatric testing in 1-2 months

$FiO_2$, fraction of inspired oxygen; LOC, loss of consciousness; $PaO_2$, partial pressure of oxygen in arterial blood; HBO, hyperbaric oxygen

## SUGGESTED READING

- Chenoweth JA, Albertson TE, Greer MR. Carbon Monoxide Poisoning. Crit Care Clin. 2021;37(3):657-672.
- Gill, P., Martin, R.V., 2015. Smoke inhalation injury. BJA Education 15, 143-148.
- Horncastle, E., Lumb, A.B., 2019. Hyperoxia in anaesthesia and intensive care. BJA Education 19, 176-182.

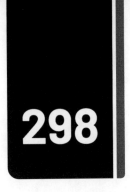

# COCAINE INTOXICATION

## LEARNING OBJECTIVES

- Diagnose and treat cocaine toxicity

**DEFINITION AND MECHANISM**

- Cocaine intoxication refers to the subjective, desired and adverse effects of cocaine on the mind and behavior of users
- Cocaine has an indirect sympathomimetic effect
- It is often mixed with adulterants which can cause health problems on their own
- The drug was the first local anesthetic discovered
- Cocaine is available in two forms – the hydrochloride (white powder) and free-base ('crack' cocaine) form, the latter is made by combining the hydrochloride form and an alkali
- Intranasal or intravenous administration results in rapid euphoria and a sensation of power and tirelessness
- In higher doses, agitation, insomnia, hallucinations, and seizures may occur
- These effects are mediated by an increase in catecholamines acting at central receptors, but peripheral effects of sympathetic stimulation (e.g., raised heart rate and blood pressure) are also prominent
- The most serious threat posed by a cocaine overdose is the potential for cardiovascular complications
- Levamisole is an anthelmintic agent found in up to 70% of cocaine samples and can cause agranulocytosis and vasculitis

| Signs and symptoms | |
|---|---|
| Cardiovascular | Tachycardia and hypertension<br>Arrhythmia and cardiac conduction abnormalities<br>Acute coronary syndromes: Vasospastic and /or coronary thrombotic<br>QT prolongation<br>Aortic dissection |
| Neurological | Euphoria<br>Anxiety, dysphoria, agitation, and aggression<br>Paranoid psychosis<br>Hyperthermia, rigidity and myoclonic movements<br>Seizures<br>Depression, sometimes with tentamen suicide |
| Respiratory | Pulmonary edema<br>Pneumothorax<br>Pneumomediastinum |
| Peripheral sympathomimetic | Hyperthermia<br>Muscle fasciculations<br>Mydriasis, sweating and tremor |
| Other | Hyperthermia induced rhabdomyolysis, renal failure, and cerebral edema<br>Subarachnoid/intracerebral hemorrhage<br>Ischemic colitis<br>Ileus (body packers)<br>Epistaxis |

# MANAGEMENT

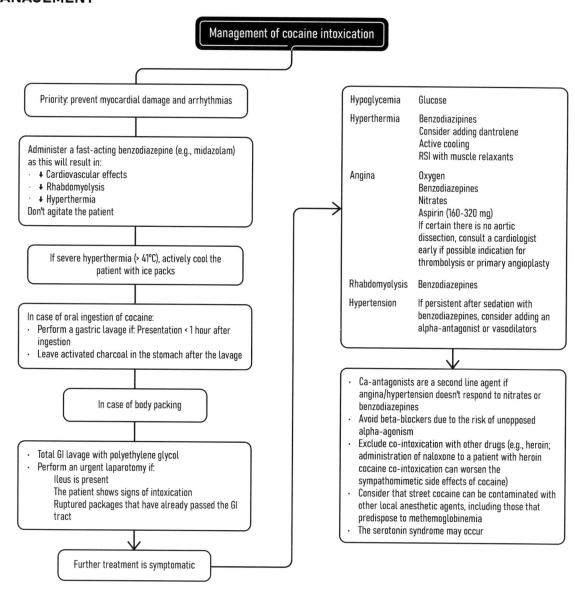

**Management of cocaine intoxication**

Priority: prevent myocardial damage and arrhythmias

Administer a fast-acting benzodiazepine (e.g., midazolam) as this will result in:
- ↓ Cardiovascular effects
- ↓ Rhabdomyolysis
- ↓ Hyperthermia

Don't agitate the patient

If severe hyperthermia (> 41°C), actively cool the patient with ice packs

In case of oral ingestion of cocaine:
- Perform a gastric lavage if: Presentation < 1 hour after ingestion
- Leave activated charcoal in the stomach after the lavage

In case of body packing

- Total GI lavage with polyethylene glycol
- Perform an urgent laparotomy if:
  Ileus is present
  The patient shows signs of intoxication
  Ruptured packages that have already passed the GI tract

Further treatment is symptomatic

| | |
|---|---|
| Hypoglycemia | Glucose |
| Hyperthermia | Benzodiazipines<br>Consider adding dantrolene<br>Active cooling<br>RSI with muscle relaxants |
| Angina | Oxygen<br>Benzodiazepines<br>Nitrates<br>Aspirin (160-320 mg)<br>If certain there is no aortic dissection, consult a cardiologist early if possible indication for thrombolysis or primary angioplasty |
| Rhabdomyolysis | Benzodiazepines |
| Hypertension | If persistent after sedation with benzodiazepines, consider adding an alpha-antagonist or vasodilators |

- Ca-antagonists are a second line agent if angina/hypertension doesn't respond to nitrates or benzodiazepines
- Avoid beta-blockers due to the risk of unopposed alpha-agonism
- Exclude co-intoxication with other drugs (e.g., heroin; administration of naloxone to a patient with heroin cocaine co-intoxication can worsen the sympathomimetic side effects of cocaine)
- Consider that street cocaine can be contaminated with other local anesthetic agents, including those that predispose to methemoglobinemia
- The serotonin syndrome may occur

RSI, rapid sequence induction

## SUGGESTED READING

- Kramers C. et al. Toxicologische behandel informatie: Cocaïne, 2020, accessed 25/01/2023, https://toxicologie.org/cocaine
- Nicholson Roberts, T., Thompson, J.P., 2013. Illegal substances in anaesthetic and intensive care practices. Continuing Education in Anaesthesia Critical Care & Pain 13, 42–46.
- Jenkins BJ. 2002. Drug abusers and anaesthesia, BJA CEPD Reviews. 2;1:15-19.

Cocaine intoxication

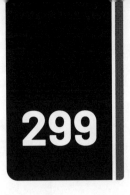

# CYANIDE POISONING

## LEARNING OBJECTIVES

- Diagnose and treat cyanide poisoning

## DEFINITION AND MECHANISM

- Cyanide can be a colorless gas, such as hydrogen cyanide (HCN) or cyanogen chloride (CNCl), or a crystal form such as sodium cyanide (NaCN) or potassium cyanide (KCN)
- Hydrogen cyanide is described as having a "bitter almond" odor, which is discernible by approximately 40-60% of the population
- Cyanide poisoning may result from structural fires, smoke inhalation, industrial exposures, medical exposures such as sodium nitroprusside, and certain foods (lima beans and almonds)
- Cyanide inhibits oxidative phosphorylation by binding to the enzyme cytochrome C oxidase and blocks the mitochondrial transport chain
- The result is cellular hypoxia and the depletion of ATP leading to metabolic acidosis
- Signs and symptoms begin at blood cyanide concentrations of approximately 40 mol/L
- The average lethal dose of hydrogen cyanide taken by mouth is between 60 and 90 mg (adult)

## SIGNS AND SYMPTOMS

Acute inhalation or ingestion
- Rapid loss of consciousness and seizures with inhalation
- Onset of symptoms over ~30 minutes with ingestion (depending on the dose)

| Signs and symptoms | |
|---|---|
| Early symptoms | Headache<br>Dizziness<br>Confusion<br>Mydriasis<br>Nausea and vomiting<br>Weakness<br>Tachypnea<br>Tachycardia |
| Late symptoms | Apnea<br>Hypotension<br>Arrhythmia<br>Myocardial ischemia<br>Seizures<br>Loss of consciousness<br>Bradycardia |
| Severe exposure | Progressive features will result from end-organ damage secondary to anaerobic respiration and histotoxic hypoxia<br>Hypotension<br>Bradycardia<br>Reduced Glasgow Coma Scale<br>Respiratory depression<br>Cardiovascular collapse<br>Hyperlactatemia<br>The patient may appear 'pink' due to high SvO$_2$ following oxygen administration<br>The smell of bitter almonds may be present |

## COMPLICATIONS

- Parkinson
- Other forms of neurological sequelae
- Headache
- Abnormal taste
- Vomiting
- Chest pain
- Anxiety

## DIAGNOSIS

- Methemoglobin level
- Carboxyhemoglobin level (in case of smoke inhalation due to fire)
- Lactate > 7 mmol/L
- Elevated anion gap acidosis
- Reduced arteriovenous oxygen gradient

# MANAGEMENT

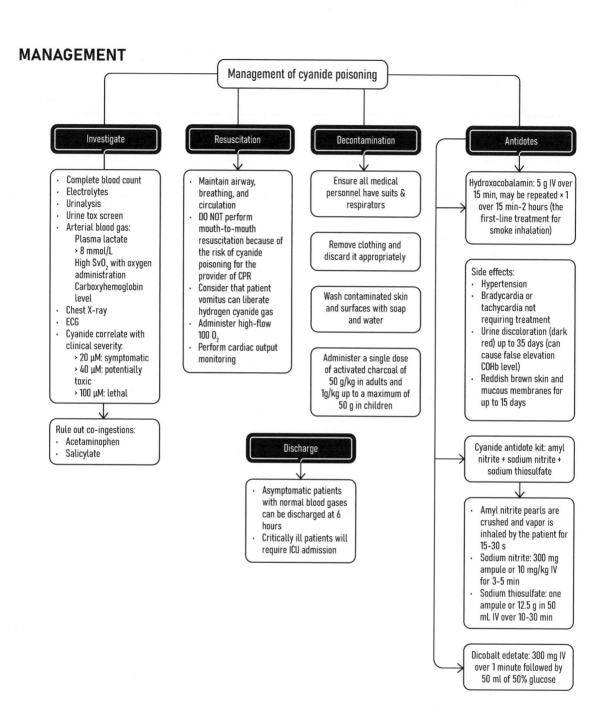

**Management of cyanide poisoning**

## Investigate

- Complete blood count
- Electrolytes
- Urinalysis
- Urine tox screen
- Arterial blood gas:
  - Plasma lactate > 8 mmol/L
  - High $SvO_2$ with oxygen administration
  - Carboxyhemoglobin level
- Chest X-ray
- ECG
- Cyanide correlate with clinical severity:
  - > 20 μM: symptomatic
  - > 40 μM: potentially toxic
  - > 100 μM: lethal

Rule out co-ingestions:
- Acetaminophen
- Salicylate

## Resuscitation

- Maintain airway, breathing, and circulation
- DO NOT perform mouth-to-mouth resuscitation because of the risk of cyanide poisoning for the provider of CPR
- Consider that patient vomitus can liberate hydrogen cyanide gas
- Administer high-flow 100 $O_2$
- Perform cardiac output monitoring

## Discharge

- Asymptomatic patients with normal blood gases can be discharged at 6 hours
- Critically ill patients will require ICU admission

## Decontamination

Ensure all medical personnel have suits & respirators

Remove clothing and discard it appropriately

Wash contaminated skin and surfaces with soap and water

Administer a single dose of activated charcoal of 50 g/kg in adults and 1g/kg up to a maximum of 50 g in children

## Antidotes

Hydroxocobalamin: 5 g IV over 15 min, may be repeated × 1 over 15 min–2 hours (the first-line treatment for smoke inhalation)

Side effects:
- Hypertension
- Bradycardia or tachycardia not requiring treatment
- Urine discoloration (dark red) up to 35 days (can cause false elevation COHb level)
- Reddish brown skin and mucous membranes for up to 15 days

Cyanide antidote kit: amyl nitrite + sodium nitrite + sodium thiosulfate

- Amyl nitrite pearls are crushed and vapor is inhaled by the patient for 15–30 s
- Sodium nitrite: 300 mg ampule or 10 mg/kg IV for 3–5 min
- Sodium thiosulfate: one ampule or 12.5 g in 50 mL IV over 10–30 min

Dicobalt edetate: 300 mg IV over 1 minute followed by 50 ml of 50% glucose

---

## SUGGESTED READING

- Gill, P., Martin, R.V., 2015. Smoke inhalation injury. BJA Education 15, 143–148.
- Huzar TF, George T, Cross JM. Carbon monoxide and cyanide toxicity: etiology, pathophysiology, and treatment in inhalation injury. Expert Rev Respir Med. 2013;7(2):159-170.

Cyanide poisoning

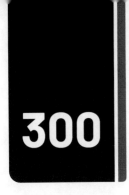

# DIGOXIN TOXICITY

## LEARNING OBJECTIVES

- Diagnose and treat digoxin toxicity

## DEFINITION AND MECHANISM

- Digoxin is a cardiac glycoside indicated for the treatment of chronic heart failure and persistent atrial fibrillation as it has ionotropic and AV nodal blocking effects
- Digoxin toxicity can present acutely after an overdose or chronically
- Toxicity can also occur from exposure to a number of plants and animals that contain cardioactive corticosteroids, including dogbane, foxglove, lily of the valley, oleander, red quill, and the Bufo species toad
- In therapeutic doses (0.5-0.9 ng/mL), digoxin increases cardiac contractility and controls the heart rate
- Because of the narrow therapeutic index, chronic toxicity is more likely in the elderly and those with renal impairment
- Toxic level > 2 ng/mL and fatal dose is > 10 mg/kg in adults and 0.1 mg/kg in children
- Digoxin inhibits the sodium-potassium ATPase, leading to an increase in intracellular sodium. As a result, less calcium is expelled through the sodium-calcium cation exchanger, causing intracellular calcium levels to rise
- Higher intracellular calcium increases inotropy which can be of symptomatic benefit in CHF

## SIGNS AND SYMPTOMS

| Acute ingestion | |
|---|---|
| Gastrointestinal tract | Anorexia <br> Nausea <br> Vomiting <br> Diarrhea <br> Abdominal pain |
| Metabolic system | Hyperkalemia |
| Cardiovascular system | Enhanced automaticity: Atrial tachycardia (e.g. flutter, atrial fibrillation (AF)) with AV block, ventricular fibrillation, ventricular tachycardia, ventricular ectopic beats <br> Bradyarrhythmias: Conduction delays/blocks, slow or regularised AF <br> Hypotension <br> Shock |
| Central nervous system | Lethargy <br> Confusion |
| **Chronic ingestion** | |
| | Fatigue <br> Malaise <br> Visual disturbances: Blurred vision, color disturbances, haloes, and scotomas |

## RISK FACTORS

- Low potassium
- Low magnesium
- High calcium

## DIAGNOSIS

- ECG
  - Premature ventricular contractions (PVCs)
  - Sinus bradycardia
  - Trigeminal rhythms
  - Ventricular bigeminy
  - Bidirectional ventricular tachycardia
- Laboratory tests
  - Hyperkalemia is characteristic of digoxin toxicity
  - Digoxin levels

## MANAGEMENT

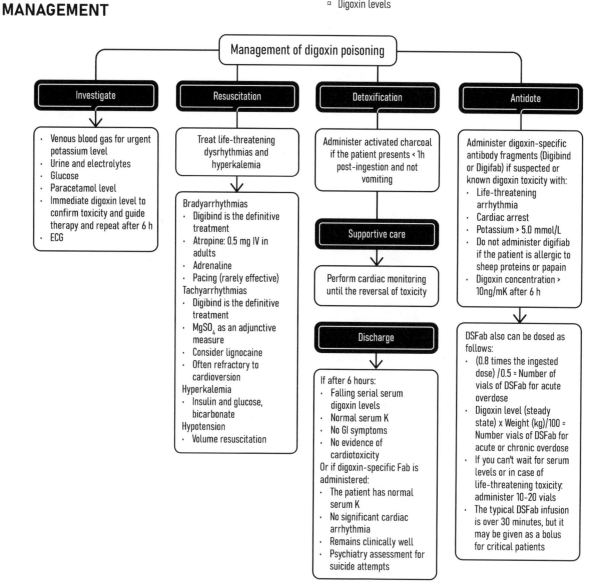

## SUGGESTED READING

- Kotzé, A., Howell, S.J., 2008. Heart failure: pathophysiology, risk assessment, community management and anaesthesia. Continuing Education in Anaesthesia Critical Care & Pain 8, 161–166.
- Levine M, O'Connor A. Digitalis (cardiac glycoside) poisoning. UpToDate. 2016.
- Pincus M. Management of digoxin toxicity. Aust Prescr. 2016;39(1):18-20.

Digoxin toxicity

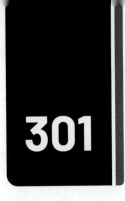

# HEROIN OR OPIOID TOXICITY

**301**

## LEARNING OBJECTIVES

- Signs and symptoms of heroin or opioid toxicity
- Treatment and perioperative management of heroin or opioid toxicity

## DEFINITION AND MECHANISM

- Heroin, also known as diacetylmorphine, is a potent opioid mainly used as an illegal recreational drug for its euphoric effects
- Very addictive and known for causing significant withdrawal symptoms and can be sniffed, smoked, or injected
- When administered intravenously, heroin has two to three times the effect of a similar dose of morphine
- Heroin has an average half-life of three minutes in blood after intravenous administration, requiring drug users to use it several times per day to maintain the effect
- Tolerance usually develops over time
- Heroin levels peak after five minutes of intranasal or intravenous uptake, but its potency after intranasal usage is about half of intravenous usage
- The three most clinically relevant opioid receptors are the μ-, κ-, and δ-receptors:
  - Stimulation of central μ-receptors causes respiratory depression, analgesia (supraspinal and peripheral), and euphoria
  - κ- and δ-receptors also have potent analgesic effects, and stimulation of κ-receptors leads to dissociation, hallucinations, and dysphoria
  - δ-receptors are thought to influence mood

## SIGNS AND SYMPTOMS

| Signs and symptoms | |
|---|---|
| Respiratory system | Respiratory depression<br>- No breathing<br>- Shallow breathing<br>- Slow and difficult breathing |
| Nervous system | Dry mouth<br>Extremely small pupils (pinpoint pupils)<br>Delirium<br>Disorientation<br>Drowsiness<br>Seizures<br>Muscle spasms<br>Coma |
| Cardiovascular system | Hypotension<br>Weak pulse |
| Skin | Bluish-colored nails and lips |
| Gastrointestinal system | Constipation<br>Spasms of the stomach and intestines |

## DIAGNOSIS

- Blood and urine test
- Chest X-ray
- CT scan
- ECG

## OPIATE WITHDRAWAL SYMPTOMS

- Symptoms are not life-threatening
  - Alertness
  - Muscle pain
  - Dilated pupils
  - Piloerection
  - Sweating
  - Vomiting and diarrhea
  - Pain
  - Aspiration
  - Insomnia
  - Yawning
- Medications to treat opiate withdrawal symptoms
  - Methadone (long-acting opioid)
  - Buprenorphine (partial mu agonist and K antagonist)
  - Clonidine and lofexidine (alpha-2 adrenergic agents)

## COMPLICATIONS

- Intravascular infections and infectious disease transmission (HIV, hepatitis B, and C) due to shared needles
- The needle can break off → Embedded foreign body
- Skin infections: Cellulitis and abscess
- Compartment syndrome
- Intravascular infections can grow on the heart valves → Valve replacement
- Septic emboli → Empyema
- Hypoxic end-organ damage secondary to hypoventilation
- Acute lung injury
- Narcotic bowel syndrome
- Withdrawal symptoms

# MANAGEMENT

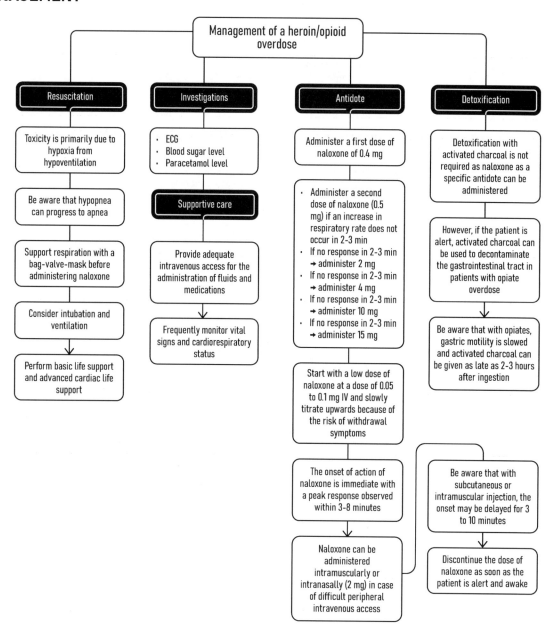

## Management of a heroin/opioid overdose

### Resuscitation

- Toxicity is primarily due to hypoxia from hypoventilation
- Be aware that hypopnea can progress to apnea
- Support respiration with a bag-valve-mask before administering naloxone
- Consider intubation and ventilation
- Perform basic life support and advanced cardiac life support

### Investigations

- ECG
- Blood sugar level
- Paracetamol level

### Supportive care

- Provide adequate intravenous access for the administration of fluids and medications
- Frequently monitor vital signs and cardiorespiratory status

### Antidote

- Administer a first dose of naloxone of 0.4 mg
- Administer a second dose of naloxone (0.5 mg) if an increase in respiratory rate does not occur in 2-3 min
- If no response in 2-3 min → administer 2 mg
- If no response in 2-3 min → administer 4 mg
- If no response in 2-3 min → administer 10 mg
- If no response in 2-3 min → administer 15 mg
- Start with a low dose of naloxone at a dose of 0.05 to 0.1 mg IV and slowly titrate upwards because of the risk of withdrawal symptoms
- The onset of action of naloxone is immediate with a peak response observed within 3-8 minutes
- Naloxone can be administered intramuscularly or intranasally (2 mg) in case of difficult peripheral intravenous access

### Detoxification

- Detoxification with activated charcoal is not required as naloxone as a specific antidote can be administered
- However, if the patient is alert, activated charcoal can be used to decontaminate the gastrointestinal tract in patients with opiate overdose
- Be aware that with opiates, gastric motility is slowed and activated charcoal can be given as late as 2-3 hours after ingestion
- Be aware that with subcutaneous or intramuscular injection, the onset may be delayed for 3 to 10 minutes
- Discontinue the dose of naloxone as soon as the patient is alert and awake

# PERIOPERATIVE MANAGEMENT

▫ Refer to opioid tolerance or methadon-using patients

## SUGGESTED READING

- Boyer EW. Management of opioid analgesic overdose. N Engl J Med. 2012;367(2):146-155.
- Nicholson Roberts, T., Thompson, J.P., 2013. Illegal substances in anaesthetic and intensive care practices. Continuing Education in Anaesthesia Critical Care & Pain 13, 42–46.
- Simpson, G., Jackson, M., 2017. Perioperative management of opioid-tolerant patients. BJA Education 17, 124–128.
- Volkow ND, Jones EB, Einstein EB, Wargo EM. Prevention and Treatment of Opioid Misuse and Addiction: A Review. JAMA Psychiatry. 2019;76(2):208-216.
- World Health Organization. 2021. Opioid overdose. https://www.who.int/news-room/fact-sheets/detail/opioid-overdose

Heroin or opioid toxicity

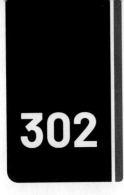

# LITHIUM TOXICITY

## LEARNING OBJECTIVES

- Diagnose and treat lithium toxicity

---

## DEFINITION AND MECHANISM

- Lithium is a very powerful, antimanic medication with a narrow therapeutic index
- Excessive intake or impaired excretion can result in lithium accumulation
- Decreased excretion may occur as a result of dehydration such as from vomiting or diarrhea, a low sodium diet, or from kidney problems
- Co-ingestants can increase the risk of lithium toxicity
  - NSAIDs
  - Indomethacin
  - Selective COX-2 inhibitors
  - Acetaminophen
  - Metronidazole
  - Calcium channel blockers
  - ACE inhibitors
  - Diuretics

- Acute toxicity: Lithium overdose in a patient who does not regularly take lithium
- Acute-on-chronic toxicity: Acute overdose in a patient who takes lithium daily, a sudden decline in renal function in a patient taking lithium can also lead to acute-on-chronic toxicity
- Chronic toxicity: Typically a patient on chronic lithium therapy who, due to toxic drug effects, physical disability, or concurrent illness, becomes hypovolemic, leading to reduced renal excretion of lithium
- Alternatively, toxicity can develop solely from the effects of mediations that reduce kidney function

## SIGNS AND SYMPTOMS

- Mild symptoms occur at a level of 1.5-2.5 mEq/L
  - Nausea and fatigue
- Moderate symptoms occur at a level of 2.5-3.5 mEq/L
  - Confusion, increased heart rate, and low muscle tone
- Severe symptoms occur at a level > 3.5 mEq/L
  - Coma, hypotension, and increased body temperature

## COMPLICATIONS

- Cerebellar dysfunction
- Extrapyramidal symptoms
- Brainstem dysfunction
- Memory deficits
- Cognitive deficits
- Sub-cortical dementia

## DIAGNOSIS

- Lithium levels > 1.2 mEq/L
- ECG
- Fingerstick glucose
- Renal function
- Serum acetaminophen and salicylate concentrations

| Signs and symptoms | |
| --- | --- |
| Neurological effects | Tremor<br>Hyperreflexia<br>Nystagmus<br>Ataxia<br>Confusion<br>Delirium |
| Renal effects | Renal toxicity<br>Impaired urinary concentrating ability<br>Nephrogenic diabetes insipidus<br>Sodium-losing nephritis<br>Nephrotic syndrome |
| Cardiovascular effects | T wave flattening<br>Sinus node dysfunction<br>QT prolongation<br>Intraventricular conduction defects<br>U waves |
| Gastrointestinal effects | Nausea<br>Vomiting<br>Diarrhea<br>Abdominal pain |
| Endocrine effects | Hypothyroidism |

# MANAGEMENT

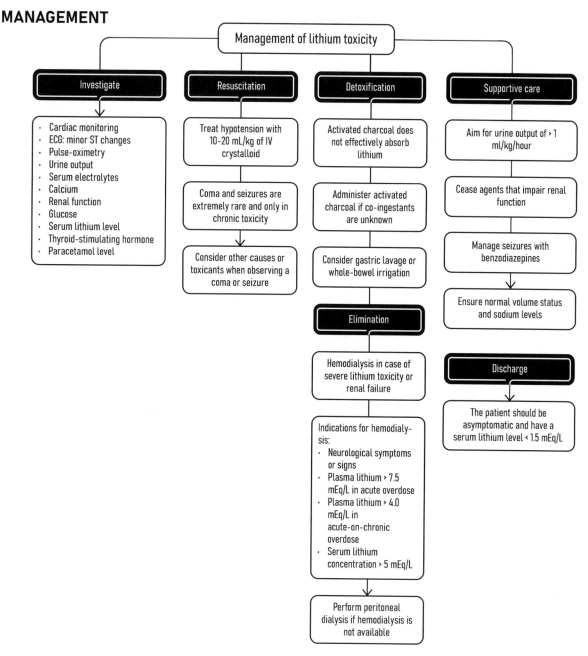

## ANESTHETIC IMPLICATIONS

- Lithium prolongs both depolarizing and non-depolarizing neuromuscular blocks
- Perform neuromuscular monitoring in patients on lithium undergoing general anesthesia with the use of neuromuscular blocking agents
- Consider conduction defects and ST changes on ECG in patients on lithium undergoing GA
- Access to free water may be impaired during the perioperative period and lead to volume depletion and hypernatremia, consider increased attention to fluid and electrolyte monitorin

## SUGGESTED READING

- Gitlin, M., 2016. Lithium side effects and toxicity: prevalence and management strategies. International Journal of Bipolar Disorders 4.
- Flood S, Bodenham A. 2010. Lithium: mimicry, mania, and muscle relaxants. Continuing Education in Anaesthesia Critical Care & Pain. 10;3:77-80.

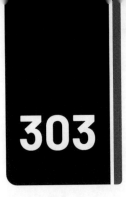

# MAOI TOXICITY

## LEARNING OBJECTIVES

- Diagnose and treat MAOI toxicity

---

## DEFINITION AND MECHANISM

- Monoamine oxidase inhibitors (MAOIs) are a class of antidepressants
- MAOIs prevent the breakdown of monoamine neurotransmitters serotonin and norepinephrine, and thereby increasing their availability
- MAOIs interact severely with commonly used anesthetic agents
- MAOI toxicity can be difficult to distinguish from much more common clinical entities
- Without MAO to break down epinephrine, norepinephrine, dopamine, serotonin, and tyramine, the storage, and release of these monoamines are increased
- This can lead to tachycardia, hyperthermia, myoclonus, hypertension, and agitation
- Plasma concentrations peak within two to three hours
- Three ways in which MAOI toxicity can occur:
  - Medication-food interaction with tyramine-containing foods such as aged cheeses, beer, wine, ginseng, avocado
    - When MAO in the gut and liver is inhibited, dietary tyramine can indirectly cause an increase in adrenergic activity
  - Overdose as MAOIs have a low therapeutic index
  - Drug-drug interaction when a MAOI is combined with other agents that increases the synthesis, release, and effect of monoamines or decreases the metabolism or reuptake of these
    - E.g., dextromethorphan, linezolid, methylene blue, selective serotonin reuptake inhibitors, serotoninergic agents, and tramadol

## SIGNS AND SYMPTOMS

- MAOI toxicity can present with diaphoresis whereas an anticholinergic syndrome presents with dry skin
- MAOI toxicity is much more likely to present with generalized or ocular clonus than neuroleptic malignant syndrome

## DIAGNOSIS

- History and physical examination
- Frequent temperature measurements
- Electrolytes and lactic acid
- Salicylate, acetaminophen, and alcohol levels should be obtained

| Signs and symptoms | |
|---|---|
| Mild signs | Agitation<br>Diaphoresis<br>Tachycardia<br>Mild temperature elevation |
| Moderate signs | Altered mental status<br>Tachypnea<br>Vomiting<br>Dysrhythmias<br>Hypertension |
| Severe signs | Severe hyperthermia<br>Seizures<br>Central nervous system (CNS) depression<br>Coma<br>Cardiorespiratory depression<br>Muscle rigidity<br>Myoclonus |

# MANAGEMENT

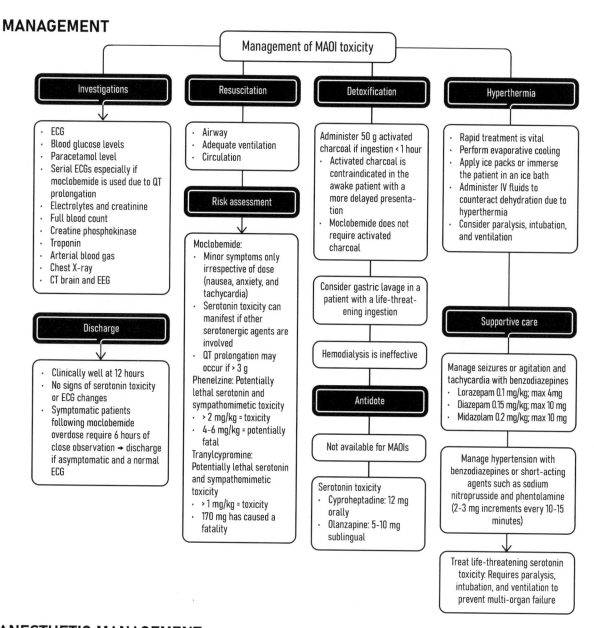

**Management of MAOI toxicity**

**Investigations**

- ECG
- Blood glucose levels
- Paracetamol level
- Serial ECGs especially if moclobemide is used due to QT prolongation
- Electrolytes and creatinine
- Full blood count
- Creatine phosphokinase
- Troponin
- Arterial blood gas
- Chest X-ray
- CT brain and EEG

**Discharge**

- Clinically well at 12 hours
- No signs of serotonin toxicity or ECG changes
- Symptomatic patients following moclobemide overdose require 6 hours of close observation → discharge if asymptomatic and a normal ECG

**Resuscitation**

- Airway
- Adequate ventilation
- Circulation

**Risk assessment**

Moclobemide:
- Minor symptoms only irrespective of dose (nausea, anxiety, and tachycardia)
- Serotonin toxicity can manifest if other serotonergic agents are involved
- QT prolongation may occur if > 3 g

Phenelzine: Potentially lethal serotonin and sympathomimetic toxicity
- > 2 mg/kg = toxicity
- 4-6 mg/kg = potentially fatal

Tranylcypromine: Potentially lethal serotonin and sympathomimetic toxicity
- > 1 mg/kg = toxicity
- 170 mg has caused a fatality

**Detoxification**

Administer 50 g activated charcoal if ingestion < 1 hour
- Activated charcoal is contraindicated in the awake patient with a more delayed presentation
- Moclobemide does not require activated charcoal

Consider gastric lavage in a patient with a life-threatening ingestion

Hemodialysis is ineffective

**Antidote**

Not available for MAOIs

Serotonin toxicity
- Cyproheptadine: 12 mg orally
- Olanzapine: 5-10 mg sublingual

**Hyperthermia**

- Rapid treatment is vital
- Perform evaporative cooling
- Apply ice packs or immerse the patient in an ice bath
- Administer IV fluids to counteract dehydration due to hyperthermia
- Consider paralysis, intubation, and ventilation

**Supportive care**

Manage seizures or agitation and tachycardia with benzodiazepines
- Lorazepam 0.1 mg/kg; max 4mg
- Diazepam 0.15 mg/kg; max 10 mg
- Midazolam 0.2 mg/kg; max 10 mg

Manage hypertension with benzodiazepines or short-acting agents such as sodium nitroprusside and phentolamine (2-3 mg increments every 10-15 minutes)

Treat life-threatening serotonin toxicity. Requires paralysis, intubation, and ventilation to prevent multi-organ failure

# ANESTHETIC MANAGEMENT

- Consider the risk of serotonin syndrome if combined with other serotonergic agents
- Avoid phenelzine as it prolonges neuromuscular blockade with succinylcholine
- Consider a risk of hypertensive crisis:
  - Avoid indirect sympathomimetics, caution with direct agents
  - Avoid cocaine
  - Avoid Ketamine

# SUGGESTED READING

- Bartakke, A., Corredor, C., Van Rensburg, A., 2020. Serotonin syndrome in the perioperative period. BJA Education 20, 10–17.
- Gillman, P.K., 2005. Monoamine oxidase inhibitors, opioid analgesics and serotonin toxicity. British Journal of Anaesthesia 95, 434–441.
- Harbell MW, Dumitrascu C, Bettini L, Yu S, Thiele CM, Koyyalamudi V. Anesthetic Considerations for Patients on Psychotropic Drug Therapies. Neurol Int. 2021 Nov 29;13(4):640-658.
- Peck T, Wong A, Norman E. 2010. Anaesthetic implications of psychoactive drugs. Continuing Education in Anaesthesia Critical Care & Pain.10;(6); 177-181.

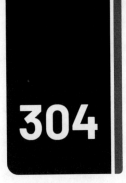

# MDMA (EXCTASY) TOXICITY

## LEARNING OBJECTIVES

- Diagnose and treat MDMA toxicity

---

## DEFINITION AND MECHANISM

- MDMA (3,4-methylenedioxymethamphetamine) ecstasy is a synthetic compound with structural and pharmacologic similarities to both amphetamines and mescaline
- Typical effects include feelings of euphoria, wakefulness, intimacy, excitement, and a loss of inhibitions
- It is mistakenly believed that it is a safe drug with little toxicity and a long duration of action
- The effects of MDMA typically last 3 to 6 hours
- The effects are believed to result from changes in serotonin, dopamine, and norepinephrine levels
- The drug is commonly ingested orally in tablet form, however, the powder itself can be snorted
- Absorbed via the GI tract with an onset of effect between 20 minutes and 1 hour after consumption
- MDMA is profoundly serotonergic and can precipitate serotonin syndrome

## SIDE EFFECTS ASSOCIATED WITH MDMA

| Minor side effects | Life-threatening side effects |
| --- | --- |
| Trismus | Hyperpyrexia > 41.5 °C |
| Tachycardia | Rhabdomyolysis |
| Bruxism | Serotonin syndrome |
| Anxiety | Acute liver failure |
| Prolonged hangover | Hyponatremia and cerebral edema |

# SIGNS AND SYMPTOMS

| System | Minor or moderate overdose | Severe overdose |
|---|---|---|
| Cardiovascular | | Disseminated Intravascular Coagulation (DIC)<br>Intracranial hemorrhage<br>Severe hypotension or hypertension<br>Hypotensive bleeding |
| Central nervous system | Hyperreflexia<br>Agitation<br>Mental confusion<br>Paranoia<br>Stimulant psychosis | Cognitive and memory impairment potentially to the point of retrograde or anterograde amnesia<br>Coma<br>Convulsions<br>Hallucinations<br>Loss of consciousness<br>Serotonin syndrome |
| Musculoskeletal | | Muscle rigidity<br>Rhabdomyolysis |
| Respiratory | | Acute respiratory distress syndrome |
| Urinary | | Acute kidney injury (AKI) |
| Other | | Cerebral edema<br>Hepatitis<br>Hyperpyrexia<br>Hyponatremia |

# COMPLICATIONS

- Neurological
  - Delirium
  - Seizures
- Cardiovascular
  - Cardiac dysrhythmias
  - Myocardial infarction
  - Aortic dissection
  - Intracranial hemorrhages
- GI
  - Hepatotoxicity
  - Liver failure

- Renal
  - Rhabdomyolysis
  - Acute renal failure
- Endocrine
  - SIADH resulting in life-threatening hyponatremia
- Minor complications
  - Increased muscle activity (such as bruxism, restless legs, and jaw clenching)
  - Hyperactivity
  - Insomnia
  - Difficulty concentrating
  - Feelings of restlessness

# RISK FACTORS

- Ingestion of several doses at once or in a short period
- Mixing MDMA with alcohol or other drugs

- Vigorous physical activity
- Use of MDMA in a hot environment

# DIAGNOSIS

- Blood glucose levels
- Electrolyte abnormalities
- Urine, potassium, BUN, creatinine, creatine phosphokinase levels, and myoglobin levels for the evaluation of rhabdomyolysis and renal injury

- Liver function tests for hepatotoxicity
- Aspirin, alcohol, acetaminophen levels, and urine drug screening
- ECG
- Head CT, lumbar puncture

MDMA (exctasy) toxicity

# MANAGEMENT

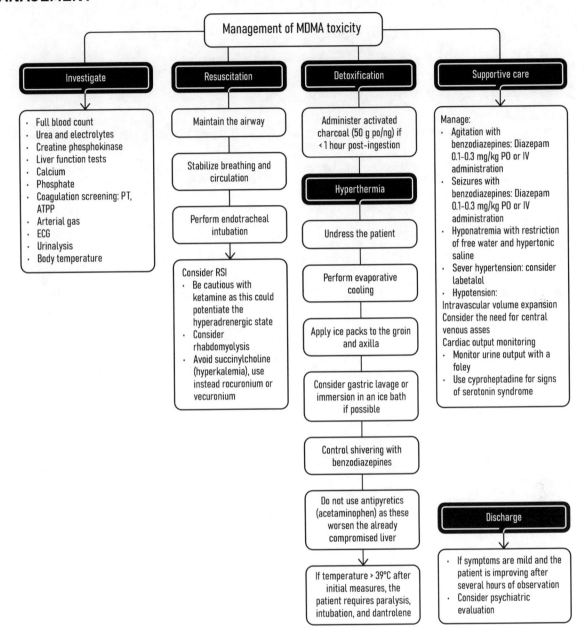

```
                    Management of MDMA toxicity
```

**Investigate**
- Full blood count
- Urea and electrolytes
- Creatine phosphokinase
- Liver function tests
- Calcium
- Phosphate
- Coagulation screening: PT, ATPP
- Arterial gas
- ECG
- Urinalysis
- Body temperature

**Resuscitation**

Maintain the airway

Stabilize breathing and circulation

Perform endotracheal intubation

Consider RSI
- Be cautious with ketamine as this could potentiate the hyperadrenergic state
- Consider rhabdomyolysis
- Avoid succinylcholine (hyperkalemia), use instead rocuronium or vecuronium

**Detoxification**

Administer activated charcoal (50 g po/ng) if < 1 hour post-ingestion

**Hyperthermia**

Undress the patient

Perform evaporative cooling

Apply ice packs to the groin and axilla

Consider gastric lavage or immersion in an ice bath if possible

Control shivering with benzodiazepines

Do not use antipyretics (acetaminophen) as these worsen the already compromised liver

If temperature > 39°C after initial measures, the patient requires paralysis, intubation, and dantrolene

**Supportive care**

Manage:
- Agitation with benzodiazepines: Diazepam 0.1-0.3 mg/kg PO or IV administration
- Seizures with benzodiazepines: Diazepam 0.1-0.3 mg/kg PO or IV administration
- Hyponatremia with restriction of free water and hypertonic saline
- Sever hypertension: consider labetalol
- Hypotension:
Intravascular volume expansion
Consider the need for central venous asses
Cardiac output monitoring
- Monitor urine output with a foley
- Use cyproheptadine for signs of serotonin syndrome

**Discharge**
- If symptoms are mild and the patient is improving after several hours of observation
- Consider psychiatric evaluation

RSI, rapid sequence induction; PT, prothrombin time; APTT, activated partial thromboplastin time

## SUGGESTED READING

- Davies N, English W, Grundlingh J. MDMA toxicity: management of acute and life-threatening presentations. Br J Nurs. 2018;27(11):616-622.
- Hall, A.P., Henry, J.A., 2006. Acute toxic effects of 'Ecstasy' (MDMA) and related compounds: overview of pathophysiology and clinical management. British Journal of Anaesthesia 96, 678-685.
- Nicholson Roberts, T., Thompson, J.P., 2013. Illegal substances in anaesthetic and intensive care practices. Continuing Education in Anaesthesia Critical Care & Pain 13, 42-46.

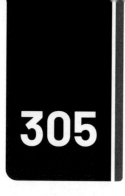

# METHAMPHETAMINE TOXICITY

## 305

## LEARNING OBJECTIVES

- Diagnose and treat methamphetamine toxicity or overdose

## DEFINITION AND MECHANISM

- Methamphetamine is a highly addictive psychostimulant drug that is a derivative of amphetamine and may be snorted, ingested, injected, or smoked
- Methamphetamine hydrochloride is FDA-approved for the long-term treatment of ADHD and the short-term treatment of exogenous obesity
- Methamphetamine promotes the release of the monoamine neurotransmitters dopamine, serotonin, and norepinephrine within central and peripheral nerve endings
- It also blocks the reuptake of dopamine similar to cocaine
- As a result, the drug produces euphoria and stimulant effects similar to cocaine
- Oral administration: peak concentrations are observed within 2-4 hours
- Snorting, smoking, and injection: peak concentrations occur within minutes

## SIGNS AND SYMPTOMS

- Euphoria
- Tachycardia
- Hypertension
- Sweating
- Restlessness
- Dry mouth
- Elevated body temperature
- Agitation
- Chest pain
- Coma or unresponsiveness (in extreme cases)

- Heart attack
- Irregular or stopped heartbeat
- Difficulty breathing
- Kidney damage and possibly kidney failure
- Paranoia
- Seizures
- Severe stomach pain
- Stroke
- Mydriasis

## COMPLICATIONS

- Intracranial hemorrhage
- Seizures
- Ischemic stroke
- Coma
- Heart failure
- Arrhythmias
- Delusional behavior

- Extreme paranoia
- Major mood swings
- Insomnia (severe inability to sleep)
- Missing and rotted teeth (called "meth mouth")
- Repeated infections
- Severe weight loss
- Abscesses or boils

# MANAGEMENT

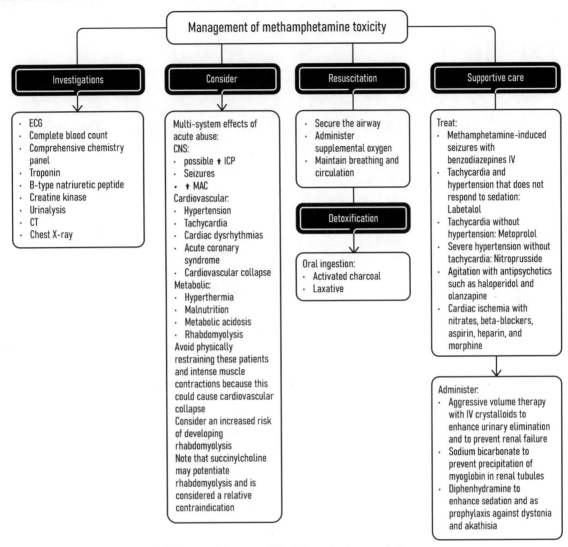

**Management of methamphetamine toxicity**

**Investigations**
- ECG
- Complete blood count
- Comprehensive chemistry panel
- Troponin
- B-type natriuretic peptide
- Creatine kinase
- Urinalysis
- CT
- Chest X-ray

**Consider**

Multi-system effects of acute abuse:
CNS:
- possible ↑ ICP
- Seizures
- ↑ MAC

Cardiovascular:
- Hypertension
- Tachycardia
- Cardiac dysrhythmias
- Acute coronary syndrome
- Cardiovascular collapse

Metabolic:
- Hyperthermia
- Malnutrition
- Metabolic acidosis
- Rhabdomyolysis

Avoid physically restraining these patients and intense muscle contractions because this could cause cardiovascular collapse

Consider an increased risk of developing rhabdomyolysis

Note that succinylcholine may potentiate rhabdomyolysis and is considered a relative contraindication

**Resuscitation**
- Secure the airway
- Administer supplemental oxygen
- Maintain breathing and circulation

**Detoxification**

Oral ingestion:
- Activated charcoal
- Laxative

**Supportive care**

Treat:
- Methamphetamine-induced seizures with benzodiazepines IV
- Tachycardia and hypertension that does not respond to sedation: Labetalol
- Tachycardia without hypertension: Metoprolol
- Severe hypertension without tachycardia: Nitroprusside
- Agitation with antipsychotics such as haloperidol and olanzapine
- Cardiac ischemia with nitrates, beta-blockers, aspirin, heparin, and morphine

Administer:
- Aggressive volume therapy with IV crystalloids to enhance urinary elimination and to prevent renal failure
- Sodium bicarbonate to prevent precipitation of myoglobin in renal tubules
- Diphenhydramine to enhance sedation and as prophylaxis against dystonia and akathisia

ICP, intracranial pressure; MAC, minimum alveolar concentration

---

**SUGGESTED READING**

- Dignam, G., Bigham, C., 2017. Novel psychoactive substances: a practical approach to dealing with toxicity from legal highs. BJA Education 17, 172-177.
- Richards JR, Laurin EG. Methamphetamine Toxicity. In: StatPearls. Treasure Island (FL): StatPearls Publishing; October 10, 2022

# METHANOL AND ETHYLENE GLYCOL POISONING

**306**

## LEARNING OBJECTIVES

- Diagnose and treat intoxication with the toxic alcohols methanol and ethylene glycol (EG)

- EG is a common component of antifreeze and deicing solutions
- Methanol is present as a solvent in many household products, such as antifreeze, cleaning solutions, dyes, and paint removers
- Onset of symptoms of methanol poisoning can range from 40 minutes to 72 hours, depending on the dose and co-ingestion of ethanol

## PATHOPHYSIOLOGY

- Toxicity of methanol and EG is related to the production of toxic metabolites by the hepatic enzyme alcohol dehydrogenase (ADH)

## METABOLISM OF ETHYLENE GLYCOL AND METHANOL

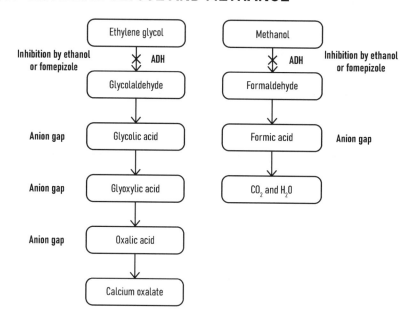

- Oxalic acid
  - The main toxic metabolite of EG
  - Binds to calcium, forming insoluble calcium oxalate crystals, this can cause hypocalcemia and crystal deposition in several organs causing organ dysfunction
- Formic acid
  - The main toxic metabolite of methanol
  - Directly toxic to the retina which can cause visual disturbances and even blindness
  - Inhibits the mitochondrial cytochrome oxidase, which deranges ATP synthesis

# SIGNS AND SYMPTOMS

|  | Ethylene glycol | Methanol |
|---|---|---|
| Early | Confusion<br>Stupor<br>Nausea<br>Vomiting | Mild euphoria<br>Drunkenness<br>Headache<br>Lethargy<br>Confusion |
| Progression | Metabolic acidosis<br>Küssmaul breathing<br>Hypocalcemia<br>Hyperreflexia | Vision abnormalities<br>Extrapyramidal symptoms (in severe intoxication)<br>Seizures<br>Metabolic acidosis<br>Küssmaul breathing |
| Late | Coma<br>Acute renal failure (earlier in severe intoxication)<br>Cardiovascular shock<br>Multi organ failure<br>Death | Blindness<br>Coma<br>Cardiovascular shock<br>Respiratory failure<br>Sudden respiratory arrest<br>Death |

# MANAGEMENT

- Decreased consciousness
  - Requires endotracheal intubation if the airway is at risk
  - Administer a pre-intubation bolus of 1-2 mmol/kg sodium bicarbonate to avoid exacerbating acidosis, which will worsen symptoms
- Supportive care
  - IV fluids
  - Vasopressors as needed
  - Correct acidemia (pH < 7.3) by administering sodium bicarbonate
  - Supplement calcium in EG intoxication
- Decontamination
  - Activated charcoal and gastric lavage are not recommended for the treatment of toxic alcohol intoxication
- Seizures
  - Treat with a benzodiazepine
- Antidotal therapy.

# ETHYLENE GLYCOL (EG) AND METHANOL POISONING: ANTIDOTAL TREATMENT

**Antidotal treatment**
- Ethanol and fomepizole are used to block the ADH-mediated metabolism of EG and methanol
- Fomepizole:
  - (+) No need to monitor blood levels, higher affinity for ADH, minimal adverse effects
  - (−) Expensive, limited availability
- Ethanol:
  - (+) Inexpensive, high availability, more clinical experience
  - (−) Significant side effects, lower affinity for ADH, treatment needs to be monitored in intensive care
- Start antidotal treatment if:
  - Plasma concentration ≥ 200 mg/L (3.2 mol/L for EG and 6.2 mmol/L for methanol)
  - or
  - Recent history of ingesting toxic amounts of EG/methanol and osmolal gap > 10 mOsm/L
  - or
  - Suspected EG/methanol ingestion and at least 3 (for EG poisoning) or 2 (for methanol poisoning) of the following criteria:
    - Arterial pH < 7.3
    - Serum bicarbonate < 20 mmol/L
    - Osmolal gap > 10 mOsm/L
    - Oxalate crystalluria (for EG exposure)
- Treat until blood methanol or EG < 200 mg/L and normal arterial pH and the patient is asymptomatic

| | Fomepizole | Ethanol |
|---|---|---|
| No hemodialysis | Loading dose 15 mg/kg<br><br>Maintenance dose<br>10 mg/kg at t = 12, 24 and 36 h<br><br>After 48 hours, increase the dose to 15 mg/kg every 12 hours | Loading dose<br>0.6–1.0 g/kg IV in glucose 5% or 2.5 mL/kg 40% ethanol solution orally<br><br>Maintenance dose<br>Continuous infusion: Maintenance dose (g/h) = (target ethanol concentration x Vmax* x body weight in kg / (Km** + target ethanol concentration***)<br>(*) Vmax in adults = 0.125 g/kg/h (occasional alcohol intake); 0.175 g/kg/h (alcohol abusers)<br>(**) Km = 0.138 g/L<br>(***) Target ethanol concentration = 1000–1500 mg/L |
| If hemodialysis | Loading dose: 15 mg/kg<br>Administer maintenance dose* 6 hours after the initial loading dose<br>and every 4 hours thereafter<br>or<br>Start continuous infusion at 1–1.5 mg/kg/h after the initial loading dose<br><br>(*) All doses are given IV over 30 min | Loading dose<br>0.6–1.0 g/kg IV in glucose 5% or 2.5 mL/kg 40% ethanol solution orally<br>Maintenance dose (continuous infusion)<br>An additional dose of 1.9 mL ethanol 10% solution in glucose/kg/h should be administered IV (in addition to the calculated maintenance dose) |

- Hemodialysis
Start hemodialysis if any of the following conditions are met:
- Clinical Signs and Symptoms:
  - Coma
  - Convulsions
  - Renal failure
  - Metabolic acidosis with pH < 7.15
  - Persisting acidosis despite treatment
  - Serum anion gap > 24 mmol/L
- Plasma concentration ≥ 500 mg/L if not yet antidotal treatment, ≥ 600 mg/L if ethanol, ≥ 700 mg/L if fomepizole
  - Plasma concentration ≥ 500 mg/L if no antidotal treatment has been initiated
  - Plasma concentration ≥ 600 mg/L if ethanol is being used as the antidote
  - Plasma concentration ≥ 700 mg/L if fomepizole is being used as the antidote

**SUGGESTED READING**

- Grouls R. et al. Toxicologie behandel informatie: Methanol, 2022, accessed 25/01/2023 https://toxicologie.org/methanol
- Rietjens SJ at al. Ethylene glycol or methanol intoxication: which antidote should be used, fomepizole or ethanol? Neth J Med. 2014 Feb;72(2):73-9. PMID: 24659589

Methanol and ethylene glycol poisoning

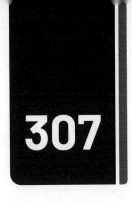

# OPIOID TOLERANCE OR METHADONE-USING PATIENTS

## 307

### LEARNING OBJECTIVES

- Definition of opioid tolerance
- Adverse effects of methadone and buprenorphine
- The pre-, peri- and postoperative management of opioid-tolerant or methadone-using patients

## DEFINITION AND MECHANISM

- Opioid tolerance is characterized by neuroadaptations that result in reduced drug effects, and is:
  - Characterized by reduced responsiveness to an opioid agonist such as morphine
  - Usually manifested by the need to use increasing doses to achieve the desired effect
  - A common occurrence in individuals taking high doses of opioids for extended periods
- Addiction to opioids is common among recreational opioid users (heroin), but relatively rare in chronic pain patients
- The six most common clinically used opioids are morphine, oxycodone, hydromorphone, fentanyl, buprenorphine, and methadone
- Successful approaches to pharmacotherapy of opioid addiction continue to rely largely on the substitution of short-acting agonists such as heroin with oral administration of long-acting high-efficacy agonists such as methadone or the partial agonist buprenorphine
- **Methadone**
  - Is a synthetic opioid agonist used as an analgesic for chronic pain (often in rotation with other opioids) and also for opioid dependence
  - Is a μ-agonist as well as an NMDA-antagonist and monoamine reuptake inhibitor
  - Relieves cravings and removes withdrawal symptoms
  - Detoxification using methadone can be accomplished in less than a month
- **Buprenorphine**
  - Is an opioid used to treat opioid use disorder, acute pain, and chronic pain
  - Is a partial agonist at μ-receptors and an antagonist at κ- and δ-receptors
  - It is used in addiction medicine to suppress opioid withdrawal and craving for 24–48 hours

## ADVERSE EFFECTS

| Methadone | Buprenorphine |
|---|---|
| Sedation | Nausea and vomiting |
| Constipation | Drowsiness |
| Flushing | Dizziness |
| Perspiration | Headache |
| Heat intolerance | Memory loss |
| Dizziness | Cognitive and neural inhibition |
| Weakness | Perspiration |
| Chronic fatigue | Itching |
| Insomnia | Dry mouth |
| Constricted pupils | Constricted pupils |
| Dry mouth | Hypotension |
| Nausea and vomiting | Urinary retention |
| Hypotension | Respiratory depression |
| Headache | |
| Tachycardia | |
| Abnormal heart rhythms | |
| Trouble breathing, slow or shallow breathing | |
| Weight gain | |
| Memory loss | |
| Itching | |
| Difficulty urinating | |
| Swelling of the hands, arms, feet, and legs | |
| Mood changes, euphoria, disorientation | |
| Blurred vision | |
| Skin rash | |
| Central sleep apnea | |

# MANAGEMENT

## PREOPERATIVE MANAGEMENT

- Obtain a detailed medical history
- Perform a physical exam
- Obtain pain and medication history

## PERIOPERATIVE MANAGEMENT

### Perioperative management

**Assessment and monitoring**
- Assess the overall effectiveness of the pain management
- Consider other important factors such as the presence of opioid-related side-effects, signs of opioid withdrawal, patient expectations, patient satisfaction, mood, and levels of physical function

**Acute pain management plan**
- Identify complex patients early
- Adhere to a clear multi-disciplinary pain management plan
- Consider opioid-sparing techniques

**Opioid-sparing techniques**
- Use paracetamol, NSAIDs or COX-2s
- Use local, regional, or neuraxial anesthesia where possible
- Administer ketamine in a low dose as a continuous IV or as a subcataeous infusion for 1–3 days in the acute pain management of opioid-tolerant patients
- Consider the use of:
  - Gabapentinoids (e.g., gabapentin/pregabalin)
  - IV lidocaine infusions

**Prevention of withdrawal**
- Maintain the usual 24-hour opioid dose and continue the patient's baseline opioid into the postoperative period
- Convert the dose of oral morphine to IV morphine
- Manage acute post-surgical pain with the addition of an appropriate dose of immediate-release opioids
- Continue the use of a buprenorphine path (up to 70 µg/h) as this is unlikely to interfere with the use of full opioid agonists
- The patient may need parenteral replacement if unable to take oral opioids

**Additional opioids**
- Note that opioid-tolerant patients may require a greater amount of immediate-release oral opioids than expected
- Consider IV patient-controlled analgesia and base the size of the bolus dose on the patient's usual 24-hour opioid requirement

**Opioid rotation**
- Switch from one opioid to another to improve pain relief and to reduce side-effects
- Reduce the calculated equianalgesic dose by 30–50% because of the possibility of incomplete crosstolerance

**Converting back from IV to oral opioid**
- Identify the IV opioid consumption in the previous 24 hours and convert this to an equivalent oral dose
- Administer 50% of this oral equivalent dose in a sustained-release form and prescribe 1/6th of the equivalent dose as an immediate-release preparation every four hours

**Opioid tolerance or opioid-induced hyperalgesia**
- Increase the opioid dose or consider an opioid rotation in opioid-tolerant patients
- Reduce the opioid dose in opioid-induced hyperalgesia patients

Opioid tolerance or methadone-using patients

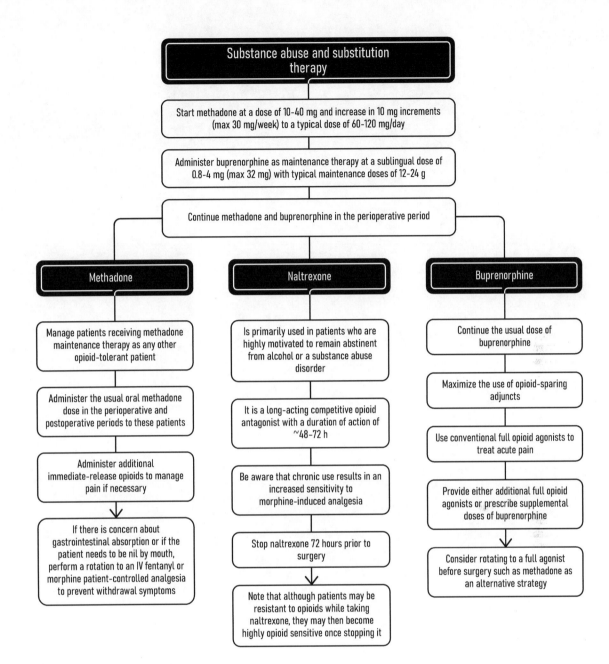

**Substance abuse and substitution therapy**

Start methadone at a dose of 10-40 mg and increase in 10 mg increments (max 30 mg/week) to a typical dose of 60-120 mg/day

Administer buprenorphine as maintenance therapy at a sublingual dose of 0.8-4 mg (max 32 mg) with typical maintenance doses of 12-24 g

Continue methadone and buprenorphine in the perioperative period

**Methadone**

Manage patients receiving methadone maintenance therapy as any other opioid-tolerant patient

Administer the usual oral methadone dose in the perioperative and postoperative periods to these patients

Administer additional immediate-release opioids to manage pain if necessary

If there is concern about gastrointestinal absorption or if the patient needs to be nil by mouth, perform a rotation to an IV fentanyl or morphine patient-controlled analgesia to prevent withdrawal symptoms

**Naltrexone**

Is primarily used in patients who are highly motivated to remain abstinent from alcohol or a substance abuse disorder

It is a long-acting competitive opioid antagonist with a duration of action of ~48-72 h

Be aware that chronic use results in an increased sensitivity to morphine-induced analgesia

Stop naltrexone 72 hours prior to surgery

Note that although patients may be resistant to opioids while taking naltrexone, they may then become highly opioid sensitive once stopping it

**Buprenorphine**

Continue the usual dose of buprenorphine

Maximize the use of opioid-sparing adjuncts

Use conventional full opioid agonists to treat acute pain

Provide either additional full opioid agonists or prescribe supplemental doses of buprenorphine

Consider rotating to a full agonist before surgery such as methadone as an alternative strategy

## POSTOPERATIVE MANAGEMENT

- **Methadone**
  - Continue preoperative dose
  - Continue the multimodal pain management
- **Buprenorphine**
  - Continue preoperative dose
  - If not on the maximal dose, increase the dose to 24-32 mg/day, divide the daily dose to every 6-8 hours
  - Continue the multimodal pain management
  - Consider converting buprenorphine to methadone to prevent acute withdrawal

## SUGGESTED READING

- Morgan MM, Christie MJ. Analysis of opioid efficacy, tolerance, addiction and dependence from cell culture to human. Br J Pharmacol. 2011;164(4):1322-1334.
- Rajan, J., Scott-Warren, J., 2016. The clinical use of methadone in cancer and chronic pain medicine. BJA Education 16, 102-106.
- Simpson, G., Jackson, M., 2017. Perioperative management of opioid-tolerant patients. BJA Education 17, 124-128.
- Sritapan Y, Clifford S, Bautista A. Perioperative Management of Patients on Buprenorphine and Methadone: A Narrative Review. Balkan Med J. 2020;37(5):247-252.
- Srivastava, D., Hill, S., Carty, S., Rockett, M., Bastable, R., Knaggs, R., Lambert, D., Levy, N., Hughes, J., Wilkinson, P., 2021. Surgery and opioids: evidence-based expert consensus guidelines on the perioperative use of opioids in the United Kingdom. British Journal of Anaesthesia 126, 1208-1216.

Opioid tolerance or methadone-using patients

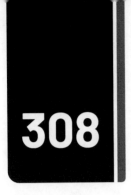

# ORGANOPHOSPHATES TOXICITY

## LEARNING OBJECTIVES

- Diagnose and treat organophosphates toxicity

## DEFINITION AND MECHANISM

- Organophosphates toxicity often results from contact with organophosphate insecticides
- The majority of organophosphate toxicity occurs in farmers and people who work in agriculture
- The onset of symptoms is often within minutes and can persist for weeks
- Organophosphate pesticide exposure may occur through inhalation, ingestion, or dermal contact
- Organophosphate insecticides inhibit carboxyl ester hydrolases and acetylcholinesterase (AChE), an essential enzyme in the breakdown of acetylcholine
- Resulting in the accumulation of acetylcholine and overstimulation of the nicotinic and muscarinic receptors
- Organophosphates stimulate both the sympathetic and parasympathetic nervous system

## SIGNS AND SYMPTOMS

- Mnemonics to remember the symptoms and the responsible receptor:

| For nicotinic signs of acetylcholinesterase inhibitor toxicity, think of the days of the week: | The more common mnemonic that captures the muscarinic effects of organophosphate poisoning is DUMBELS: | Additional symptoms |
|---|---|---|
| Monday = Mydriasis<br>Tuesday = Tachycardia<br>Wednesday = Weakness<br>Thursday = Hypertension<br>Friday = Fasciculations | D = Defecation/diaphoresis<br>U = Urination<br>M = Miosis<br>B = Bronchospasm/bronchorrhea<br>E = Emesis<br>L = Lacrimation<br>S = Salivation | Increased saliva and tear production<br>Diarrhea<br>Vomiting<br>Small pupils<br>Sweating<br>Muscle tremors<br>Anxiety<br>Confusion<br>Drowsiness<br>Emotional lability<br>Seizures<br>Hallucinations<br>Headaches |

## COMPLICATIONS

- Neck flexions
- Weakness
- Decreased deep tendon reflexes
- Cranial nerve abnormalities
- Proximal muscle weakness
- Respiratory insufficiency
- Neuropathy
- Neuropsychiatric deficits:

- Confusion
- Memory impairment
- Lethargy
- Psychosis
- Irritability
- Parkinson like symptoms

# DIAGNOSIS

- Based on clinical suspicion
- Some organophosphates have a distinct garlic or petroleum odor
- Measurement of AChe in red blood cells
- Complete blood count
- Serum glucose levels

- Troponin levels
- Liver and renal function tests
- Arterial blood gas
- ECG

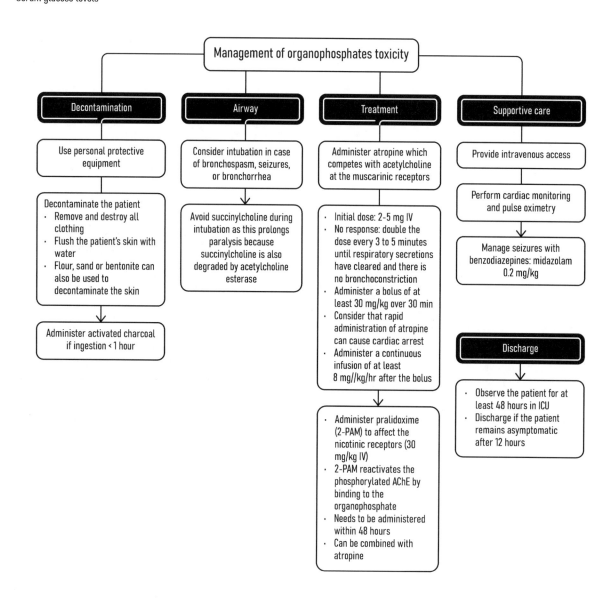

**SUGGESTED READING**

- Geoghegan, J., Tong, J.L., 2006. Chemical warfare agents. Continuing Education in Anaesthesia Critical Care & Pain 6, 230–234.
- Ward C, Sair M. 2010. Oral poisoning: an update. Continuing Education in Anaesthesia Critical Care & Pain. 10;1: 6-11.

Organophosphates toxicity

# PARACETAMOL OVERDOSE

**309**

## LEARNING OBJECTIVES

- Assess paracetamol (acetaminophen) overdose and recognise treatment indications

---

### DEFINITION AND MECHANISM

- Paracetamol is a mild analgesic and antipyretic medication and is safe if used in therapeutic doses
- Most medication overdoses, either accidentally or intentionally, are due to paracetamol overdose
- The most common cause of acute liver failure in the western world
- A dose of $\geq$ 150 mg/kg can cause liver damage and this threshold might be lower in people with chronic alcohol abuse or anorexia
- The preferred treatment is an n-acetylcysteine infusion

| Toxicity | |
|---|---|
| Hepatic effects | Acute liver failure<br>Hepatoxicity may also occur with doses within the therapeutic range secondary to deficiencies in glutathione, because of inadequate nutrition, P450 enzyme induction by chronic alcohol excess, or concomitant use of other medications |
| Renal effects | Thought to have only minor effects on renal function<br>Rare effects observed after an acute overdose or chronic abuse include:<br>· Acute kidney injury (AKI)<br>· Acute tubular necrosis<br>· Interstitial nephritis |
| Gastro-inestinal effects | Paracetamol can be associated with:<br>Nausea and vomiting<br>Dyspepsia<br>Abdominal pain<br>Bloating<br>Acute pancreatitis (rarely) |
| Hemodynamic effects | Hypotension (rare)<br>Increased skin blood flow |
| Respiratory effects | Difficulty breathing<br>Bronchospasm<br>Paracetamol may causally be linked with the development of asthma |
| Hematological/oncological effects | Very rare:<br>Thrombocytopenia<br>Leucopenia<br>Neutropenia<br>Methemoglobinemia |
| Dermatological effects | Extremely rare:<br>Erythema<br>Flushing<br>Peripheral edema and pruritus<br>Bullous erythema<br>Purpura fulminans<br>Toxic epidermal necrolysis (TEN)<br>Stevens-Johnson syndrome<br>Acute generalized exanthematous pustulosis |

# MANAGEMENT

- The SNAP-12 protocol is one of the preferred regimens over the Classe 21-hour regimen for intravenous N-acetylcysteine (NAC) infusion as this has some advantages:
  - Simple to use
  - Fewer adverse drug reactions
  - A shortened length of hospital stay for most patients
- Clinical judgment is important:
  - Ensure that there is no doubt about the time of ingestion or the type of drug or the total ingested dose
  - Some patients have chronically raised ALT/INR
  - If ALT is abnormal despite a normal paracetamol concentration, consider treating for an overdose
  - If uncertain, treat and review

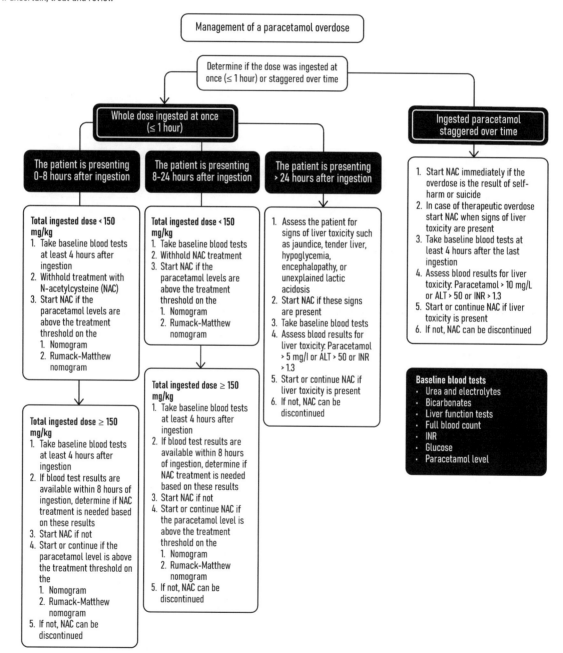

Paracetamol overdose

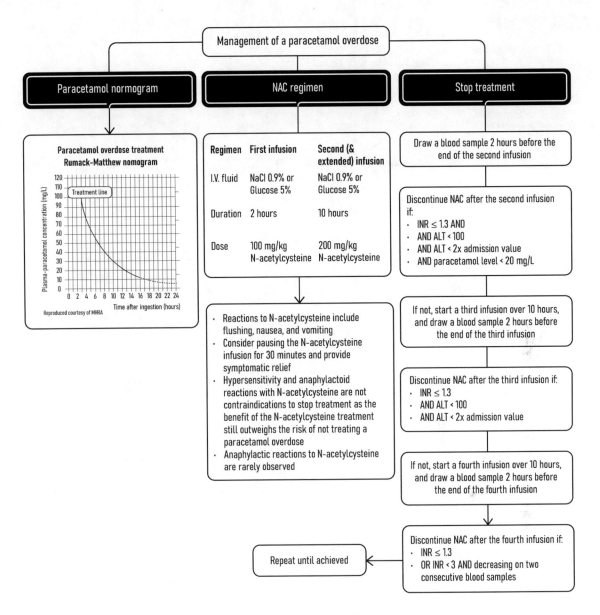

**Management of a paracetamol overdose**

**Paracetamol normogram** | **NAC regimen** | **Stop treatment**

**Paracetamol overdose treatment**
**Rumack-Matthew nomogram**

Plasma-paracetamol concentration (mg/L)

Treatment line

Time after ingestion (hours)

Reproduced courtesy of MHRA

| Regimen | First infusion | Second (& extended) infusion |
|---|---|---|
| I.V. fluid | NaCl 0.9% or Glucose 5% | NaCl 0.9% or Glucose 5% |
| Duration | 2 hours | 10 hours |
| Dose | 100 mg/kg N-acetylcysteine | 200 mg/kg N-acetylcysteine |

- Reactions to N-acetylcysteine include flushing, nausea, and vomiting
- Consider pausing the N-acetylcysteine infusion for 30 minutes and provide symptomatic relief
- Hypersensitivity and anaphylactoid reactions with N-acetylcysteine are not contraindications to stop treatment as the benefit of the N-acetylcysteine treatment still outweighs the risk of not treating a paracetamol overdose
- Anaphylactic reactions to N-acetylcysteine are rarely observed

Draw a blood sample 2 hours before the end of the second infusion

Discontinue NAC after the second infusion if:
- INR ≤ 1.3 AND
- AND ALT < 100
- AND ALT < 2x admission value
- AND paracetamol level < 20 mg/L

If not, start a third infusion over 10 hours, and draw a blood sample 2 hours before the end of the third infusion

Discontinue NAC after the third infusion if:
- INR ≤ 1.3
- AND ALT < 100
- AND ALT < 2x admission value

If not, start a fourth infusion over 10 hours, and draw a blood sample 2 hours before the end of the fourth infusion

Repeat until achieved

Discontinue NAC after the fourth infusion if:
- INR ≤ 1.3
- OR INR < 3 AND decreasing on two consecutive blood samples

NAC, N-acetylcysteine; ALT, alanine aminotransferase; INR, international normalized ratio

**SUGGESTED READING**

- NHS Greater Glasgow and Clyde Area Drug and Therapeutics Committee. (2022). Paracetamol Overdose Protocol and Shortened N-acetylcysteine (NAC) Administration Chart. Adult paracetamol overdose protocol and shortened N-acetylcysteine (NAC) administration chart (904). https://rightdecisions.scot.nhs.uk/ggc-clinical-guideline-platform/emergency-department/substance-related/adult-paracetamol-overdose-protocol-and-shortened-n-acetylcysteine-nac-administration-chart-904/
- Pettie JM, Caparrotta TM, Hunter RW, et al. Safety and Efficacy of the SNAP 12-hour Acetylcysteine Regimen for the Treatment of Paracetamol Overdose. Clinical medicine. 2019;11:11-17.
- Sharma CV, Mehta V. 2014. Paracetamol: mechanisms and updates, Continuing Education in Anaesthesia Critical Care & Pain, 14;4:153-158.

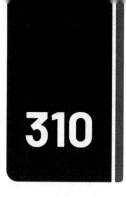

# SALICYLATE TOXICITY

## LEARNING OBJECTIVES

- Diagnose and manage salicylate toxicity of salicylate toxicity

## DEFINITION AND MECHANISM

- Salicylate toxicity is the result of ingestion of, or (rarely) topical exposure to, chemicals metabolized to salicylate
- Poisoning may occur due to acute or chronic salicylate exposure:
  - Uncouples oxidative phosphorylation
  - Interferes with the Krebs cycle
  - Leads to accumulation of lactic acid & ketoacids
- Characterized by acid-base disturbances, electrolyte abnormalities, and effects on the central nervous system
- Unintentional salicylate toxicity is more common than intentional intoxication
- The most common source of salicylate poisoning is aspirin itself (acetylsalicylic acid) which is rapidly hydrolyzed to salicylate in the gastrointestinal tract, liver, and bloodstream
  - Acute toxicity may occur after ingestion of a single dose of aspirin or the equivalent of > 150 mg/kg or > 6.5 g
  - Chronic poisoning tends to occur as a result of repeated exposure to high-dose aspirin or equivalent (150 mg/kg/day), particularly in the setting of renal insufficiency
  - Beware that many over-the-counter medications contain salicylates, such as Pepto-Bismol, etheric oils, vapors, or analgesic ointments
- Herbs and spices such as ginger or mint also contain salicylates which can add to the drug burden
- Initially, symptoms such as tachypnea, lung crackles, and fever often mimic a viral infection
- The classic triad of mild toxicity:
  - Nausea
  - Vomiting
  - Tinnitus

## PATHOPHYSIOLOGY

### Therapeutic levels of salicylates

- Irreversibly block COX-1 and modify COX-2 leading to a decrease in inflammation and platelet aggregation

### Toxic levels of salicylates

- Stimulate the respiratory center causing hyperpnea
- Shift in metabolism to glycolysis for energy production → ↑ oxygen consumption and heat production → lactic acidosis

## SIGNS AND SYMPTOMS

| Signs and symptoms | |
|---|---|
| Nervous system | Tinnitus<br>Listlessness<br>Vertigo and ataxia<br>Hallucinations<br>Muscle rigidity<br>Seizures<br>Cerebral edema<br>Coma |
| Gastro-intestinal | Nausea<br>Vomiting |

| Signs and symptoms | |
|---|---|
| Respiratory | Hyperpnea<br>Noncardiogenic pulmonary edema |
| Cardiac | Cardiovascular collapse |
| Metabolic | Fever<br>Respiratory alkalosis<br>Increased anion-gap metabolic acidosis (late sign)<br>Hypernatremia due to fluid deficit<br>Hypokalemia |

# DIAGNOSIS

- Arterial blood gas
- Serum electrolyte panel
- Serum salicylate level
- BUN and creatinine
- ECG
- Head CT scan
- EEG

# MANAGEMENT

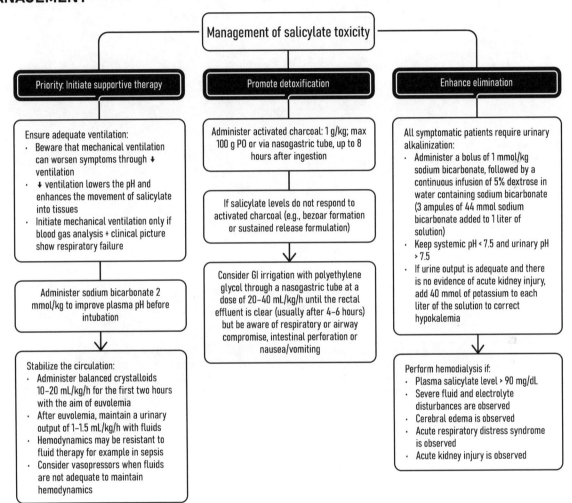

**Management of salicylate toxicity**

**Priority: Initiate supportive therapy**

Ensure adequate ventilation:
- Beware that mechanical ventilation can worsen symptoms through ↓ ventilation
- ↓ ventilation lowers the pH and enhances the movement of salicylate into tissues
- Initiate mechanical ventilation only if blood gas analysis + clinical picture show respiratory failure

Administer sodium bicarbonate 2 mmol/kg to improve plasma pH before intubation

Stabilize the circulation:
- Administer balanced crystalloids 10–20 mL/kg/h for the first two hours with the aim of euvolemia
- After euvolemia, maintain a urinary output of 1–1.5 mL/kg/h with fluids
- Hemodynamics may be resistant to fluid therapy for example in sepsis
- Consider vasopressors when fluids are not adequate to maintain hemodynamics

**Promote detoxification**

Administer activated charcoal: 1 g/kg; max 100 g PO or via nasogastric tube, up to 8 hours after ingestion

If salicylate levels do not respond to activated charcoal (e.g., bezoar formation or sustained release formulation)

Consider GI irrigation with polyethylene glycol through a nasogastric tube at a dose of 20–40 mL/kg/h until the rectal effluent is clear (usually after 4–6 hours) but be aware of respiratory or airway compromise, intestinal perforation or nausea/vomiting

**Enhance elimination**

All symptomatic patients require urinary alkalinization:
- Administer a bolus of 1 mmol/kg sodium bicarbonate, followed by a continuous infusion of 5% dextrose in water containing sodium bicarbonate (3 ampules of 44 mmol sodium bicarbonate added to 1 liter of solution)
- Keep systemic pH < 7.5 and urinary pH > 7.5
- If urine output is adequate and there is no evidence of acute kidney injury, add 40 mmol of potassium to each liter of the solution to correct hypokalemia

Perform hemodialysis if:
- Plasma salicylate level > 90 mg/dL
- Severe fluid and electrolyte disturbances are observed
- Cerebral edema is observed
- Acute respiratory distress syndrome is observed
- Acute kidney injury is observed

**SUGGESTED READING**

- Palmer BF, Clegg DJ. Salicylate Toxicity. N Engl J Med. 2020;382(26):2544-2555.

# TCA TOXICITY

## LEARNING OBJECTIVES

- Diagnose and treat TCA toxicity

---

## DEFINITION AND MECHANISM

- Tricyclic antidepressants (TCAs) are used to treat depression, chronic pain, and some forms of acute pain
- The mode of action is by prevention of presynaptic re-uptake of norepinephrine and serotonin
  - Also anti-muscarinic, antihistaminergic, and anti-α1-adrenergic effects
- TCA toxicity is caused by excessive intake (can be intentional or accidental) of:
  - Amitriptyline
  - Imipramine
  - Nortriptyline
  - Doxepin
  - Dothiepin
  - Clomipramine
- TCAs have a narrow therapeutic index which carries a high risk of toxicity
- Most poisonings present from acute ingestion; however chronic poisoning can also present acutely
- A dose > 10 mg/kg can be potentially life-threatening
- Severe toxicity usually manifests within 2 and no later than 6 hours after ingestion
- Exclude co-ingestion of other toxic agents (e.g., paracetamol)
- Excess sodium bicarbonate can be lethal due to severe hypernatremia, hypokalemia, and alkalemia, don't give more than 6 mmol/kg
- The goals and limitations of sodium bicarbonate treatment are:
  - pH 7.50-7.55
  - Sodium 155 mmol/L
  - QRS < 140 ms

## SIGNS AND SYMPTOMS

| Signs and symptoms | |
| --- | --- |
| Anticholinergic effects | Fever<br>Inability to sweat<br>Dry mouth<br>Mydriasis<br>Blurred vision<br>Constipation<br>Urinary retention |
| Cardiovascular effects | Sinus tachycardia<br>Hypotension<br>ABG: Mixed acidosis with both respiratory depression and ↑ lactate<br>ECG: QRS and PR/QT prolongation<br>Large terminal R wave in aVR, Predisposing to broad complex tachyarrhythmia (VT) |
| Central nervous system | Altered mental status<br>Agitation<br>Seizures<br>Coma |

# TREATMENT

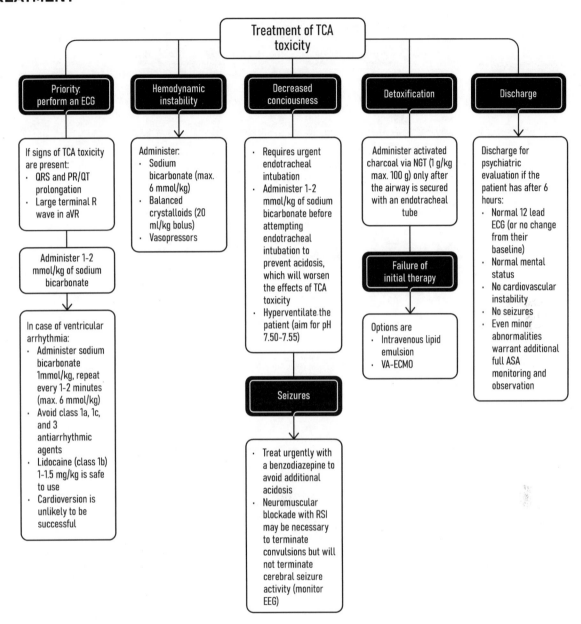

**Treatment of TCA toxicity**

**Priority: perform an ECG**

If signs of TCA toxicity are present:
- QRS and PR/QT prolongation
- Large terminal R wave in aVR

Administer 1-2 mmol/kg of sodium bicarbonate

In case of ventricular arrhythmia:
- Administer sodium bicarbonate 1mmol/kg, repeat every 1-2 minutes (max. 6 mmol/kg)
- Avoid class 1a, 1c, and 3 antiarrhythmic agents
- Lidocaine (class 1b) 1-1.5 mg/kg is safe to use
- Cardioversion is unlikely to be successful

**Hemodynamic instability**

Administer:
- Sodium bicarbonate (max. 6 mmol/kg)
- Balanced crystalloids (20 ml/kg bolus)
- Vasopressors

**Decreased conciousness**

- Requires urgent endotracheal intubation
- Administer 1-2 mmol/kg of sodium bicarbonate before attempting endotracheal intubation to prevent acidosis, which will worsen the effects of TCA toxicity
- Hyperventilate the patient (aim for pH 7.50-7.55)

**Seizures**

- Treat urgently with a benzodiazepine to avoid additional acidosis
- Neuromuscular blockade with RSI may be necessary to terminate convulsions but will not terminate cerebral seizure activity (monitor EEG)

**Detoxification**

Administer activated charcoal via NGT (1 g/kg max. 100 g) only after the airway is secured with an endotracheal tube

**Failure of initial therapy**

Options are
- Intravenous lipid emulsion
- VA-ECMO

**Discharge**

Discharge for psychiatric evaluation if the patient has after 6 hours:
- Normal 12 lead ECG (or no change from their baseline)
- Normal mental status
- No cardiovascular instability
- No seizures
- Even minor abnormalities warrant additional full ASA monitoring and observation

TCA, tricyclic antidepressant; aVR, augmented vector right, a lead in ECG; ASA, American society of anesthesiologists; VA-ECMO, veno-arterial extracorporeal membrane oxygenation; RSI, rapid sequence induction and intubation

# MANAGEMENT

```
┌────────────────────────────────────────────────────────┐
│           Anesthetic management of TCA toxicity          │
└────────────────────────────────────────────────────────┘
```

Consider
- Co-ingestants
- Life-threatening multi-system effects:
- CNS: sedation, coma, seizures CVS: tachycardia, hypotension, myocardial dysfunction, lethal arrhythmias

Be aware of the potentiation of the effect of indirectly acting sympathomimetics (e.g., ephedrine and metaraminol) by TCAs

- Avoid indirecty acting sympathomimetics
- Use directly acting sympathomimetics with caution to prevent hypertensive crises

Avoid abrupt withdrawal of TCAs because of the risk of cholinergic symptoms

Contraindicated therapies
- Class IA (e.g., procainamide) & class IC agents (e.g., flecainide) due to their inhibition of rapid sodium channels (similar to TCA effect)
- Class III agents (e.g., amiodarone) due to QTc prolonging effect
- Phenytoin
- Flumazenil as this can induce seizures

## SUGGESTED READING

- Kerr GW, Mguffie AC, Wilkie S. Tricyclic antidepressant overdose: a review. Emerg Med J. 2001;18(4):236-241. doi:10.1136/emj.18.4.236
- Lott C, Truhlář A, Alfonzo A, et al. European Resuscitation Council Guidelines 2021: Cardiac arrest in special circumstances [published correction appears in Resuscitation. 2021 Oct;167:91-92]. Resuscitation. 2021;161:152-219.
- Peck, T., Wong, A., Norman, E., 2010. Anaesthetic implications of psychoactive drugs. Continuing Education in Anaesthesia Critical Care & Pain 10, 177-181.

TCA toxicity

# VASCULAR
# DISORDERS

# ABDOMINAL AORTIC ANEURYSM (AAA) REPAIR

## 312

### LEARNING OBJECTIVES

- Etiology and complications of abdominal aortic aneurysm (AAA)
- Anesthetic management of AAA through an open incision or through EndoVascular Aneurysma Repair (EVAR)

## DEFINITION AND MECHANISM

- Abdominal aortic aneurysm (AAA) repair is a procedure used to treat an aneurysm of the abdominal aorta
- An aneurysm is a bulging, weak spot in the aorta that may be at risk for rupturing
  - Small AAA: 3-4.4 cm across
  - Medium AAA: 4.5-5.4 cm across
  - Large AAA: $\geq$ 5.5 cm more across
- The incidence of AAA increases with age
- Repair of an abdominal aortic aneurysm may be performed surgically through an open incision or in a minimally-invasive procedure called endovascular aneurysm repair (EVAR)
- In the EVAR procedure, a stent graft is inserted into the aneurysm through the arteries in the groin accessed by small incisions in the groin

## ETIOLOGY

| Etiology | |
|---|---|
| Atherosclerosis | |
| Cystic medial necrosis | |
| Connective tissue disorders | Marfan's syndrome<br>Ehlers Danlos syndrome type IV<br>Turner's syndrome<br>Polycystic kidney disease |
| Arteritis | Giant cell arteritis<br>Takayasu's disease<br>Relapsing polychondritis |
| Infections | Acute: Syphilis, salmonella, staphylococcus, brucellosis<br>Chronic: Tuberculosis, fungal (mycotic) |
| Posttraumatic | |
| Inflammatory | |

## RISK FACTORS

- Age > 60 years
- Male
- Family history
- Hyperlipidemia
- Hypertension
- Chronic obstructive pulmonary disease
- Smoking
- Diabetes
- Caucasian race
- Sedentary life style
- Coronary artery disease
- Peripheral vascular disease

## MANAGEMENT

### Preoperative management

Similar for open repair and EVAR
- Start patients on statins and antiplatelet medication
- Control arterial blood pressure
- Perform standard investigations: Full blood count, creatinine, GFR, electrolytes, ECG, chest X-ray, urinalysis
- Assess major cardiac risk factors:
  - Decompensated heart failure
  - Acute coronary syndrome
  - Arrhythmias
  - Valvular disease
  - Worsening ischemic heart disease
  - Recent myocardial infarction
- Consider:
  - Diuretics and ACE inhibitors
  - Potential for major hemorrhage, large fluid shifts & hypothermia

## *Perioperative management: open incision*

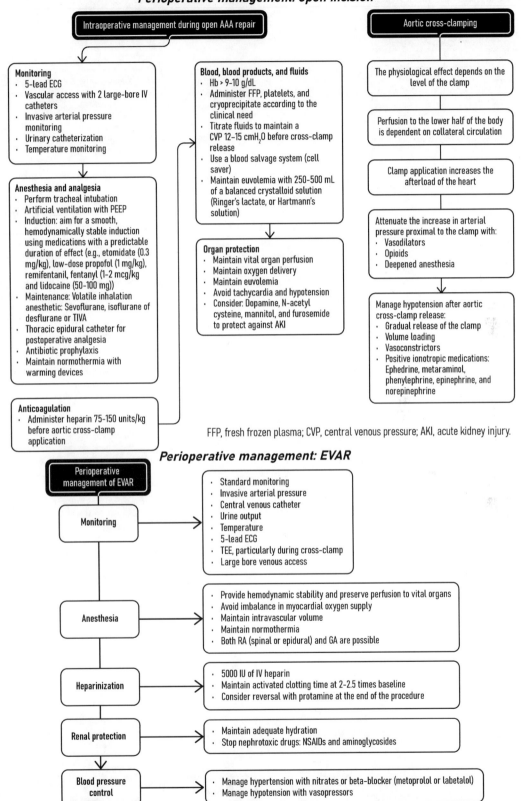

**Intraoperative management during open AAA repair**

**Monitoring**
- 5-lead ECG
- Vascular access with 2 large-bore IV catheters
- Invasive arterial pressure monitoring
- Urinary catheterization
- Temperature monitoring

**Anesthesia and analgesia**
- Perform tracheal intubation
- Artificial ventilation with PEEP
- Induction: aim for a smooth, hemodynamically stable induction using medications with a predictable duration of effect (e.g., etomidate (0.3 mg/kg), low-dose propofol (1 mg/kg), remifentanil, fentanyl (1-2 mcg/kg and lidocaine (50-100 mg))
- Maintenance: Volatile inhalation anesthetic: Sevoflurane, isoflurane of desflurane or TIVA
- Thoracic epidural catheter for postoperative analgesia
- Antibiotic prophylaxis
- Maintain normothermia with warming devices

**Anticoagulation**
- Administer heparin 75-150 units/kg before aortic cross-clamp application

**Blood, blood products, and fluids**
- Hb > 9-10 g/dL
- Administer FFP, platelets, and cryoprecipitate according to the clinical need
- Titrate fluids to maintain a CVP 12-15 cmH$_2$O before cross-clamp release
- Use a blood salvage system (cell saver)
- Maintain euvolemia with 250-500 mL of a balanced crystalloid solution (Ringer's lactate, or Hartmann's solution)

**Organ protection**
- Maintain vital organ perfusion
- Maintain oxygen delivery
- Maintain euvolemia
- Avoid tachycardia and hypotension
- Consider: Dopamine, N-acetyl cysteine, mannitol, and furosemide to protect against AKI

**Aortic cross-clamping**

The physiological effect depends on the level of the clamp

Perfusion to the lower half of the body is dependent on collateral circulation

Clamp application increases the afterload of the heart

Attenuate the increase in arterial pressure proximal to the clamp with:
- Vasodilators
- Opioids
- Deepened anesthesia

Manage hypotension after aortic cross-clamp release:
- Gradual release of the clamp
- Volume loading
- Vasoconstrictors
- Positive ionotropic medications: Ephedrine, metaraminol, phenylephrine, epinephrine, and norepinephrine

FFP, fresh frozen plasma; CVP, central venous pressure; AKI, acute kidney injury.

## *Perioperative management: EVAR*

**Perioperative management of EVAR**

**Monitoring**
- Standard monitoring
- Invasive arterial pressure
- Central venous catheter
- Urine output
- Temperature
- 5-lead ECG
- TEE, particularly during cross-clamp
- Large bore venous access

**Anesthesia**
- Provide hemodynamic stability and preserve perfusion to vital organs
- Avoid imbalance in myocardial oxygen supply
- Maintain intravascular volume
- Maintain normothermia
- Both RA (spinal or epidural) and GA are possible

**Heparinization**
- 5000 IU of IV heparin
- Maintain activated clotting time at 2-2.5 times baseline
- Consider reversal with protamine at the end of the procedure

**Renal protection**
- Maintain adequate hydration
- Stop nephrotoxic drugs: NSAIDs and aminoglycosides

**Blood pressure control**
- Manage hypertension with nitrates or beta-blocker (metoprolol or labetalol)
- Manage hypotension with vasopressors

Abdominal Aortic Aneurysm (AAA) Repair

## Perioperative management: ruptured AAA

**Anesthetic management for ruptured AAA**

Consider:
- Full stomach, limited time to optimize
- Emergency procedure requiring immediately an OR
- Need for extra help, second anesthesiologist
- Hemorrhagic shock with high mortality (85%)

Evaluation of the patient in the OR:
- History
- Comorbidities
- Details of resuscitation
- Results of laboratory tests and diagnostic imaging
- Hemodynamic status

Provide:
- Intravenous access to allow for adequate fluid resuscitation
- Type-specific (cross-matched) blood:
  10 units of packed red cells
  10 units of FFP and platelets

Place invasive arterial lines

Preoxygenate the patient

---

Administer fluid and blood to target systolic blood pressure between 50 and 100 mmHg

Perform RSI with etomidate and succinylcholine

Titrate fentanyl, midazolam and inhalation anesthetics very carefully

Administer vasopressors and fluids cautiously before clamping as aggressive resuscitation may unplug the hemostatic clot and cause bleeding

Obtain an arterial blood gas and determine:
- Acidosis
- Electrolyte abnormalities
- Hematocrit

Administer a 1:1 mixture of packed red blood cells (PRBCs) and fresh frozen plasma (FFP) if massive blood transfusion is required to prevent dilutional coagulopathy

---

Once the aneurysm is clamped, maintain hemodynamics and preserve cardiac function:
- Administer vasopressors if the patient is hypotensive with a normal cardiac function despite adequate fluid resuscitation
- Administer inotropic agents if the patient has a decreased cardiac function despite adequate fluid resuscitation
- Consider that intraoperative use of thoracic epidural analgesia will blunt the physiological effects of aortic cross clamping

Administer calcium if the patient has citrate toxicity due to massive transfusions

Guide further transfusion after the repair by the use of:
- Prothrombin time
- Activated partial thromboplastin time
- Platelet count
- Thrombin time

Early use of visco-elastic testing following the release of the aortic cross-clamp guides transfusion of fresh frozen plasma, thrombocytes, fibrinogen, and clotting factors

Consider activated factor VII if bleeding continues despite massive transfusion of blood products

Maintain normothermia to prevent coagulopathy and arrhythmias

Fluid management: 2-4 L crystalloid IV

Ruptured AAA:
- RSI with etomidate and succinylcholine or rocuronium (1.2 mg/kg)
- Guide transfusion by early visco-elastic testing
- FVII in critical situation: High incidence of prothrombotic complications

---

FFP, fresh frozen plasma; RSI, rapid sequence induction and intubation

Abdominal Aortic Aneurysm (AAA) Repair

*Postoperative management: open repair and EVAR*

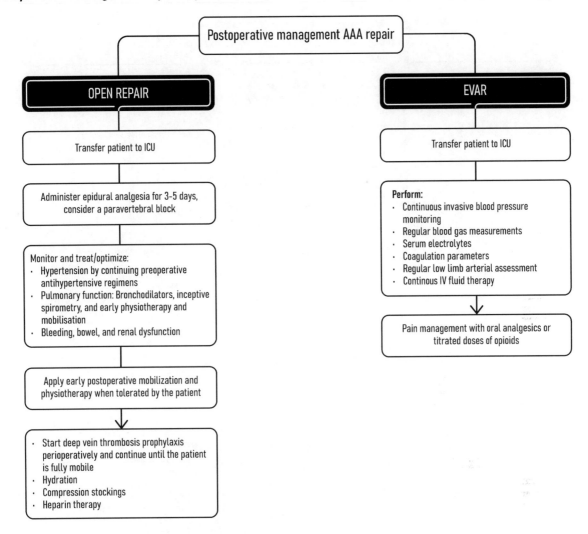

Postoperative management AAA repair

**OPEN REPAIR**

Transfer patient to ICU

Administer epidural analgesia for 3-5 days, consider a paravertebral block

Monitor and treat/optimize:
- Hypertension by continuing preoperative antihypertensive regimens
- Pulmonary function: Bronchodilators, inceptive spirometry, and early physiotherapy and mobilisation
- Bleeding, bowel, and renal dysfunction

Apply early postoperative mobilization and physiotherapy when tolerated by the patient

- Start deep vein thrombosis prophylaxis perioperatively and continue until the patient is fully mobile
- Hydration
- Compression stockings
- Heparin therapy

**EVAR**

Transfer patient to ICU

**Perform:**
- Continuous invasive blood pressure monitoring
- Regular blood gas measurements
- Serum electrolytes
- Coagulation parameters
- Regular low limb arterial assessment
- Continous IV fluid therapy

Pain management with oral analgesics or titrated doses of opioids

# POSTOPERATIVE COMPLICATIONS EVAR

| Surgical | Medical |
|---|---|
| Maldeployment of malposition of graft | Acute coronary syndromes |
| Arterial rupture/arterial dissection | Acute congestive cardiac failure |
| Delayed AAA rupture | |
| Stent-graft limb thrombosis leading to lower limb ischemia | Acute kidney injury (AKI)/CIN |
| Graft migration | Arrhythmia |
| Endoleak | Respiratory infection |
| Rupture of iliac artery | Venous thromboembolism |
| Ischemia of spinal cord, kidneys, liver, bowel, legs | Cerebrovascular accident |
| Graft infection | Postimplantation syndrome |
| Paralysis | |

CIN, contrast-induced nephropathy.

Abdominal Aortic Aneurysm (AAA) Repair

# POSTOPERATIVE COMPLICATIONS OPEN REPAIR

| Postoperative complications open repair | |
|---|---|
| Respiratory complications | Pneumonia<br>Atelectasis<br>Respiratory failure<br>Pulmonary thromboembolism |
| Cardiovascular complications | Myocardial ischemia<br>Myocardial infarction<br>Dysrhythmias |
| Cerebrovascular complications | Stroke<br>Intracerebral hemorrhage<br>Postoperative cognitive dysfunction<br>Delirium |
| Renal complications | AKI<br>CKD<br>Terminal renal disease/renal insufficiency OR need for acute dialysis due to volume overload or AKI<br>Acute tubular necrosis<br>Renal vascular injury<br>Ureteral injury |
| Gastrointestinal complications | Bowel ischemia<br>Abdominal compartment syndrome<br>Paralytic Ileus |
| Neurological complications | Spinal cord ischemia<br>Paraplegia |
| Surgical complications | Bleeding<br>Wound dehiscence<br>Incisional hernia<br>Venous thromboembolism<br>Wound infection<br>Leg ischemia<br>Graft infection<br>Graft thrombosis |

## ▰ SUGGESTED READING ▰

- Al-Hashimi M, Thompson J. Anaesthesia for elective open abdominal aortic aneurysm repair, Continuing Education in Anaesthesia Critical Care & Pain, Volume 13, Issue 6, December 2013, Pages 208–212.
- Gelzinis TA, Subramaniam K. Anesthesia for Open Abdominal Aortic Aneurysm Repair. Anesthesia and Perioperative Care for Aortic Surgery. 2010;301-327.
- Kothandan H, Haw Chieh GL, Khan SA, Karthekeyan RB, Sharad SS. Anesthetic considerations for endovascular abdominal aortic aneurysm repair. Ann Card Anaesth. 2016;19(1):132-141.
- Nataraj V, Mortimer AJ. Endovascular abdominal aortic aneurysm repair, Continuing Education in Anaesthesia Critical Care & Pain, Volume 4, Issue 3, June 2004, Pages 91–94.

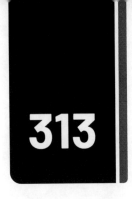

# CAROTID ENDARTERECTOMY

## LEARNING OBJECTIVES

- Recognise complications and manage anesthesia for carotid endarterectomy

## DEFINITION AND MECHANISM

- A surgical procedure to remove a build-up of fatty deposits (plaque), which cause narrowing of a carotid artery
- The carotid arteries are the main blood vessels that supply blood to the neck, face, and brain
- The carotid artery may become blocked or a clot is formed leading to a stroke or a transient ischemic attack (TIA)
- Carotid endarterectomy (CEA) significantly reduces the risk in patients at risk of a stroke or TIA

## COMPLICATIONS

- Ischemic or hemorrhagic stroke or TIA
- Prolonged postoperative observation on HDU
- Any change in peroperative neurological status requires immediate surgical consultation
- Myocardial infarction
- Cranial and/or laryngeal nerve injury (causing unilateral paralysis of vocal cord)
- Hematoma formation around incisional site causing gross swelling to the neck
- Seizures
- Thrombotic (re-)occulsion of the carotid artery
- Bleeding at the incision site in the neck
- Surgical site infection
- Hyperperfusion syndrome presenting with acute hypertension and reperfusion cephalgia, may lead to hemorrhagic stroke
- Arrhythmia
- Acute airway obstruction due to postoperative hematoma formation or airway edema

## CEA OPERATION

- After careful surgical exposure, the external, internal, and common carotid arteries are cross-clamped
- The carotid bifurcation is isolated from the circulation
- The artery is opened and the plaque will be removed
- An intravascular stent/bypass may be placed to perfuse the brain during surgery
- The artery may be then reconstructed using a patch to prevent narrowing of the vessel
- The vascular clamps are consecutively removed and cerebral blood flow reestablished
- The overlying tissue is closed layer by layer, a subcutaneous drain may be placed and the skin is closed with a continuous suture

# MANAGEMENT

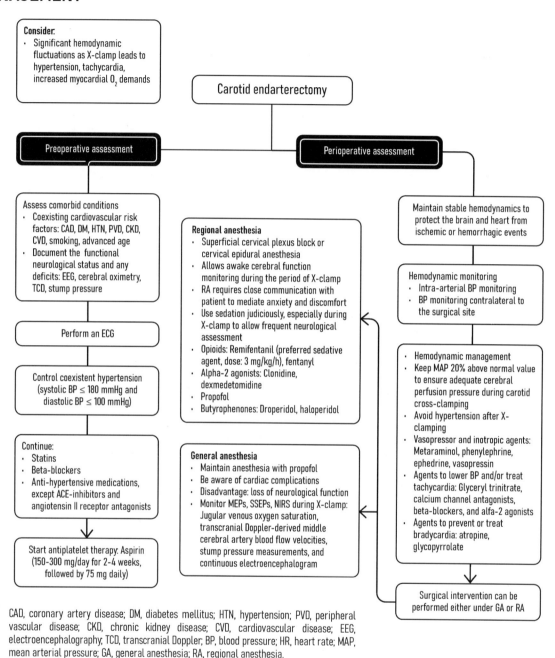

**Consider:**
- Significant hemodynamic fluctuations as X-clamp leads to hypertension, tachycardia, increased myocardial $O_2$ demands

**Carotid endarterectomy**

**Preoperative assessment**

**Perioperative assessment**

**Assess comorbid conditions**
- Coexisting cardiovascular risk factors: CAD, DM, HTN, PVD, CKD, CVD, smoking, advanced age
- Document the functional neurological status and any deficits: EEG, cerebral oximetry, TCD, stump pressure

**Perform an ECG**

**Control coexistent hypertension** (systolic BP ≤ 180 mmHg and diastolic BP ≤ 100 mmHg)

**Continue:**
- Statins
- Beta-blockers
- Anti-hypertensive medications, except ACE-inhibitors and angiotensin II receptor antagonists

**Start antiplatelet therapy:** Aspirin (150-300 mg/day for 2-4 weeks, followed by 75 mg daily)

**Regional anesthesia**
- Superficial cervical plexus block or cervical epidural anesthesia
- Allows awake cerebral function monitoring during the period of X-clamp
- RA requires close communication with patient to mediate anxiety and discomfort
- Use sedation judiciously, especially during X-clamp to allow frequent neurological assessment
- Opioids: Remifentanil (preferred sedative agent, dose: 3 mg/kg/h), fentanyl
- Alpha-2 agonists: Clonidine, dexmedetomidine
- Propofol
- Butyrophenones: Droperidol, haloperidol

**General anesthesia**
- Maintain anesthesia with propofol
- Be aware of cardiac complications
- Disadvantage: loss of neurological function
- Monitor MEPs, SSEPs, NIRS during X-clamp: Jugular venous oxygen saturation, transcranial Doppler-derived middle cerebral artery blood flow velocities, stump pressure measurements, and continuous electroencephalogram

**Maintain stable hemodynamics to protect the brain and heart from ischemic or hemorrhagic events**

**Hemodynamic monitoring**
- Intra-arterial BP monitoring
- BP monitoring contralateral to the surgical site

- Hemodynamic management
- Keep MAP 20% above normal value to ensure adequate cerebral perfusion pressure during carotid cross-clamping
- Avoid hypertension after X-clamping
- Vasopressor and inotropic agents: Metaraminol, phenylephrine, ephedrine, vasopressin
- Agents to lower BP and/or treat tachycardia: Glyceryl trinitrate, calcium channel antagonists, beta-blockers, and alfa-2 agonists
- Agents to prevent or treat bradycardia: atropine, glycopyrrolate

**Surgical intervention can be performed either under GA or RA**

CAD, coronary artery disease; DM, diabetes mellitus; HTN, hypertension; PVD, peripheral vascular disease; CKD, chronic kidney disease; CVD, cardiovascular disease; EEG, electroencephalography; TCD, transcranial Doppler; BP, blood pressure; HR, heart rate; MAP, mean arterial pressure; GA, general anesthesia; RA, regional anesthesia.

## SUGGESTED READING

- Howell SJ. Carotid endarterectomy, BJA: British Journal of Anaesthesia, Volume 99, Issue 1, July 2007, Pages 119-131.
- Zdrehuş C. Anaesthesia for carotid endarterectomy – general or loco-regional?. Rom J Anaesth Intensive Care. 2015;22(1):17-24.

Made in United States
Orlando, FL
19 June 2025

62254323R00455